KU-013-117

Clinical Endocrinology
and
Diabetes Mellitus
(A Comprehensive Text)

Derby Hospitals NHS Foundation
Trust

B16917

WITHDRAWN

Derby Hospitals NHS Foundation
Trust
Library and Knowledge Service

Volume Two

Clinical Endocrinology and
Diabetes Mellitus
(A Comprehensive Text)

Editor
Y Sachdev (Lt Gen) AVSM
MBBS (Pb), DCH (Osm) Gold Medalist
MD Gen Med (Pune), MD Paed (Osm) Gold Medalist
MAMS, FICP, FGSI, FAMS
Post-doctorate fellowship (Endocrinology), Universities
of NewCastle-upon-Tyne and South Wales, Cardiff

Senior Consultant (Endocrinology, Diabetology, Paediatrics and Medicine)
Pushpawati Singhania Research Institute
New Delhi, India

Founder Chairman, National Medical Education and Research Forum
India

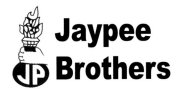

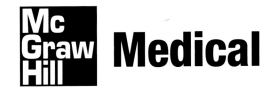

© 2009, Y Sachdev
First published in India in 2009 by

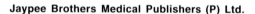

Jaypee Brothers Medical Publishers (P) Ltd.

Corporate Office
4838/24 Ansari Road, Daryaganj, **New Delhi** - 110002, India, +91-11-43574357

Registered Office
B-3 EMCA House, 23/23B Ansari Road, Daryaganj, **New Delhi** 110 002, India
Phones: +91-11-23272143, +91-11-23272703, +91-11-23282021,
+91-11-23245672, Rel: +91-11-32558559 Fax: +91-11-23276490, +91-11-23245683
e-mail: jaypee@jaypeebrothers.com, Website: www.jaypeebrothers.com

First published in USA by The McGraw-Hill Companies, 2 Penn Plaza, New York, NY 10121. Exclusively
worldwide distributor except South Asia (India, Nepal, Sri Lanka, Bhutan, Pakistan, Bangladesh, Malaysia).

All rights reserved. No part of this publication may be reproduced, stored in a retrieval system, or transmitted,
in any form or by any means, electronic, mechanical, photocopying, recording, or otherwise, without the prior
permission of the publisher or in accordance with the provisions of the Copyright, Designs and Patents Act
1988 or under the terms of any licence permitting limited copying issued by the Copyright Licensing Agency,
90 Tottenham Court Road, London W1P 0LP.

Vol 2 P/Ns 9780071634342 • 0071634347

Part of 2-Vols set:
ISBN-13: 978-0-07-163626-1
ISBN-10: 0-07-163626-9

The book is dedicated
to

- *My dear and ever-loving late parents for what I am today. It is they who taught me the importance of diligence, honesty, integrity, courtesy, humility and compassion.*

- *My teachers and innumerable patients for the knowledge and experience I gained.*

- *My dear friend and guide Late Professor R Hall CBE and other colleagues and associates at Universities of NewCastle-upon-Tyne and South Wales, Cardiff, for making me understand the finer points and intricacies of clinical and laboratory endocrinology. It was Reg Hall who taught me how to plan and execute various dynamic tests in a cost-effective manner for an endocrine patient to reach an early and definitive diagnosis.*

- *Last but certainly not the least, to my most affectionate and understanding wife for her constant support, encouragement and inspiration.*

Contributors

JK Agrawal
MD (Med), DM (Endo), FICP, FFIACM, FAMS
Senior Consultant Diabetologist and
Endocrinologist, Varanasi
Formerly, Professor and Head
Department of Endocrinology, IMS, BHU, Varanasi
President, Endocrine Society of India
Examiner, DM and DNB (Endo)

NK Agrawal
MD (Med), DM (Endo)
Assistant Professor
Department of Endocrinology and Metabolism
IMS, BHU, Varanasi

AC Anand (Brigadier) VSM
MD (Med), DM (Gastro), FICP, FACG
Professor and Head, Department of Gastroenterology
Army Hospital (Research and Referral), New Delhi
Formerly, Professor and Head, Department of
Medicine and Gastroenterology
Armed Forces Medical College (AFMC), Pune

Punita Arora (Surgeon Vice-Admiral) SM, VSM
MD (Obstetrics and Gynaecology)
Director General Medical Services (Navy)
Naval Head Quarter, New Delhi
Formerly Professor and Head, Department of Obstetrics
and Gynaecology, AFMC, Pune
and Army Hospital (Research and Referral), New Delhi

JS Bajaj
MD, FRCP (London), FRCP (Edin), FAMS, DM (hc Karolinska)
Hon DSc (BHU); DSc (hc MGR Med Univ)
DSc (hc GND Univ), DSc (hc Univ Health Science (Andhra)
Padma Bhushan Awardee (1982)
Hony. President (life time)
International Diabetic Federation
Emeritus Professor (life time)
National Academy Medical Sciences
Chief Consultant and Director
Diabetes, Endocrine and Metabolic Medicine
Batra Hospital and Medical Research Centre, New Delhi
Formerly, Member Planning Commission (Health)
Govt. of India, Professor and Head
Department of Medicine, AIIMS, New Delhi
President, Endocrine Society of India
President, Diabetic Association of India

Mandeep Bajaj
MD (Med), FACP, FACE
Associate Professor (Med) and
Director, Stark Diabetes Centre (Endo. Division)
Formerly Senior Consultant
Diabetes and Endocrinology
Indraprastha Apollo Hospital and Research Centre
New Delhi

KV Baliga (Colonel)
MD (Med), DM (Nephrology)
Professor and Head, Department of Nephrology and
Renal Transplantation
AH (R & R), New Delhi

Madhu Bhadauria (Colonel)
MS (Ophthal), FMRF (Sankara Nethralya)
Specialist in Anterior Chamber Microsurgery
Associate Professor, AFMC, Pune
Formerly, Associate Professor, AH (R & R)
New Delhi

Mir Iftikhar Bashir
MD (Med), DM (Endo)
Assistant Professor
Department of Endocrinology and Metabolism
Sher-e-Kashmir Institute of Medical Sciences, Srinagar

ML Chawla (Lt Gen) PVSM, VSM
MD (Med), DM (Cardiology), FICP
Director General Hospital Services (Armed Forces)
Ministry of Defence, Govt. of India
New Delhi
Formerly, Professor and Head
Department of Medicine and
Cardiology AH (R & R), New Delhi

AK Das
MD (Med), PhD, FICP, FAMS
Addl. Director General Medical Services (GOI)
Dean and Head, Department of Medicine
Jawahar Lal Institute of Postgraduate Medical Education
and Research (JIPMER), Pondicherry
Dean, Indian College of Physicians
Formerly, President, Association of Physicians of India
President, Diabetic Association of India
President, Endocrine Society of India

SR Gadela (Brigadier)
MD (Med), DM (Nephrology)
Director Professor and Head
Department of Med and Nephrology
Command Hospital (Central Command), Lucknow
Formerly, Professor and Head, Department of
Nephrology and Renal Transplantation, AH (R & R)
New Delhi

SP Gorthi (Colonel)
MD (Med), DM (Neurology)
Associate Professor, Department of Neurosciences
AH (R & R), New Delhi

VS Gurunadh (Lt. Col)
MD (Ophthalmol)
Specialist in Anterior Chamber Microsurgery
Associate Professor, Department of Ophthalmology
AFMC and Command Hospital
Pune

RG Holla (Colonel)
MD (Paediatrics), DM (Neonatology)
Associate Professor and Head
Department of Neonatology AH (R & R)
New Delhi

IK Indrajit (Surgeon Commander)
MD, DNB
Associate Professor and Head, MRI Wing
Department of Radiodiagnosis and Imaging
Army Hospital (R & R), New Delhi

SP Kalra (Lt. Gen) AVSM
MD (Medicine)
Director General Medical Services
'L' Block, Army Head Quarters, New Delhi.
Formerly, Professor and Head
Department of Medicine
AFMC, Pune

Umesh Kapil
MD DNB, FAMS
Additional Professor
Department of Human Nutrition
AIIMS, New Delhi

Dheeraj Kapoor
MD (Med), DM (Endo)
Consultant, Diabetologist and Endocrinologist
Max Heart and Vascular Hospital
New Delhi

Atul Kotwal (Colonel) SM
MD (PSM), FIPHA, Post-doctorate Fellowship (Epidemiology)
Advisor, Planning Commission, Govt. of India
New Delhi
Formely, Associate Professor and Joint Director
(Medical and Health), MS Organisation
Integrated HQ, Ministry of Defence (Army)
New Delhi

Jyoti Kotwal
MD (Pathology), Post-doctorate Fellowship (Haematology)
Associate Professor
AH (R & R), New Delhi

Narendra Kotwal (Lt.Col)
MD (Med), DNB (Med), DM (Endo)
Associate Professor
Department of Endocrinology and Metabolism
AH (R & R), New Delhi

Rajiv Kumar
MD (Med), DM (Endo)
Consultant Endocrinologist and Diabetologist
Max Hospital, Rohini
New Delhi

Surender Kumar
MD (Med), DM (Endo)
Chairman, Department of Endocrinology and
Metabolism
Sir Ganga Ram Hospital, New Delhi
Formerly, Professor and Head
Department of Endocrinology
AH (R & R)
New Delhi

BN Kapur (Colonel)
MD (Med), DM (Med Onco)
Professor, Department of Medical Oncology
AH (R & R)
New Delhi

Ajit Singh Kashyap (Colonel)
MD (Med), DM (Endo)
Professor and Head
Department of Endocrinology, Command Hospital (CC)
Lucknow

Nitin Chandra Mathur
MD (Paed), DCH
Consultant Paediatrician
Aditya Hospital, Hyderbad

Rajiv Chandra Mathur
DNB, MD (Paed), DCH, MNAMS
Consultant Paediatrician, Aditya Hospital
Hyderabad

YC Mathur
MD (Paed), DCH, FIAP, FAMS
Senior Consultant, Professor and Head
Department of Paediatrics
CRD Children Hospital, Hyderabad
Formerly, Additional Professor, Preventive and
Social Paediatrics
Nilofour Hospital, Osmania University, Hyderabad
IAP Advisor on Growth and Development
President, Indian Academy of Paediatrics

Chander Mohan (Brigadier) SM
MD, DNB, MNAMS
Director Professor
Department of Radiodiagnosis and Imaging
(R & R) Hospital
New Delhi

Velu Nair (Colonel) VSM
MD, MNAMS, FICP
Professor and Head, Department of Haematology and
Bone Marrow Transplantation, AH (R & R)
New Delhi

AA Pawar (Surgeon Captain)
MD (Psychiatry)
Professor and Head, Department of Psychiatry
INHS Ashvini
Colaba Mumbai

BNBM Prasad (Colonel) SM
MD (Med) DNB (Med), DTCD, DNB (Pulmonary Med)
MD (Pul. Med), FCCP, FNCCP
Professor and Head
Department of Pulmonary Medicine
AH (R & R), New Delhi
Formerly, Professor and Head, Department of Pulmonary
Medicine
Cardio Thoracic Centre (CTC) Military Hospital
Galibar Maidan
Pune

Ritu Priya
MBBS, PhD
Associate Professor
Centre of Social Medicine and Community Health
Jawaharlal Nehru Univeristy, New Delhi

Rajul Rastogi
MD (Radiodiagnosis)
Senior Resident, Department of Radiology and Imaging
University College of Medical Sciences and GTB Hospital
New Delhi

P Prusty (Colonel)
MD (Med), DM (Endo)
Professor and Head
Department of Endocrinology and Metabolism
AH (R & R), New Delhi
Formerly, Associate Professor
Department of Medicine, AFMC, Pune

Imrana Qadeer
MD (Paed), MD (PSM)
Centre of Social Medicine and Community Health
Jawaharlal Nehru University, New Delhi

Y Sachdev (Lt. Gen) AVSM
MD (Med), MD (Paed), Gold Medalist, DCH (Gold Medalist)
FICP, FGSI, FCCP (USA), FICA(N York), FRIPHH (London), FAMS
Senior Consultant (Endocrinology, Diabetology,
Paediatrics and Medicine), Pushpawati Singhania
Research Institute, New Delhi
Founder Chairman, Medical Education and
Research Forum
Visiting Professor, Various Universities and Medical
Institutions, India and Abroad
Postgraduate Teacher and Examiner, Universities of
Pune, Lucknow, BHU Varanasi, CMC Vellore
AIIMS New Delhi and PGIMER Chandigarh
Founder Fellow, Geriatric Society of India
Formerly, Chief Consultant (Med, Endo)
Armed Forces Medical Services
Professor and Head
Department of Medicine and Endocrinology
AFMC and CH (SC), Pune
President, Endocrine Society of India
President, Geriatric Society of India
Associate Professor, Department of Paediatrics
AFMC, Pune
Senior Consultant and National Coordinator
CTC Integrated Child Development Services
Advisor, ICMR and WHO

SK Sayal (Colonel)
MD (Dermatology), DVD, MNAMS
Professor, Department of Dermatology
Santosh Medical College, Ghaziabad (UP)
Formerly, Professor and Head
Department of Dermatology, AFMC, Pune

D Saldanha (Colonel)
BSc, MD (Psychiatry)
Professor and Head
Department of Psychiatry, AFMC, Pune

Ms Vani Sethi
MSc (Nutrition)
Research Associate, Department of Human Nutrition
AIIMS, New Delhi

RK Sharma (Colonel) VSM
MD (Obst & Gynae)
Special Training Infertility Management
Professor and Head, Assisted Reproduction Technologies
(ART) Centre, AH (R & R), New Delhi

HB Singh (Colonel)
MD (Med), DM (Med Onco)
Professor, Department Departmentof Medical Oncology
AH (R & R), New Delhi

SK Singh
MD (Med), DM (Endo)
Professor and Head
Department of Endocrinology and Metabolism
Institute of Medical Sciences (IMS)
Banaras Hindu University (BHU), Varanasi
Formerly, President Endocrine Society of India

Yashpal Singh (Lt Colonel) MD (Med), DM (Endo)
Command Hospital (EC), Kolkata

MN Sree Ram (Colonel)
MD (Radiodiagnosis), FICR, FIMSA
Professor and Head, Department of Radiodiagnosis and
Imaging, AFMC, Pune

GR Sridhar
MD (Med), DM (Endo)
Senior Consultant and Head, Endocrine and
Diabetes Centre, Vishakhapatnam
Formerly, Chief Editor Indian Journal of
Endocrinology and Metabolism
General Secretary, Endocrine Society of India

KM Suryanarayan (Air Commodore)
MD (Med), DM (Endo), FICP
Professor and Head
Department of Med. and Endocrinology
Command Hospital (Air Force), Bangalore
Examiner MD (Med), DM (Endo) and DNB for various
Universities
Formerly, Professor and Head, Department of
Endocrinology and Metabolism, AH (R & R), New Delhi

Sudhir Tripathi (Lt Colonel)
MD (Med), DM (Endo)
Senior Consultant Endocrinologist
Sir Ganga Ram Hospital, New Delhi
Formerly, Associate Professor
Department of Endocrinology and Metabolism,
AH (R & R)
New Delhi

Devender Paul Vats (Brigadier) SM VSM
MD (Ophth)
Specialised in Anterior Chamber Microsurgery
Director Professor and Head, Department of
Ophthalmology and Dean (Academics)
AH (R & R), New Delhi
Formerly, Professor and Head, Department of
Ophthalmology AFMC
Pune

AG Unnikrishnan
MD, DM (Endo), DNB, MNAMS
Assistant Professor
Department of Endocrinology and Diabetes
Amrita Institute of Medical Sciences
Cochin

S Venkataraman VSM
MD (Med), DM (Neurology)
Senior Consultant (Neurology)
Mata Chanan Devi Hospital
New Delhi
Formerly, President, Association of Physicians of India

Ms Shaveta Vedehra
MSc. (Foods and Nutrition)
Nutritionist and Dietician
Pushpawati Singhania Research Institute
New Delhi

Ajit Venniyoor (Surg Captain)
MD (Med), DM (Med Onco)
Professor and Head
Department of Medical Oncology
INHS Ashvini
Mumbai

AH Zargar
MD (Med), DM (Endo), FICP
Professor and Head
Department of Endocrinology and Metabolism
Sher-e-Kashmir Postgraduate Institute of Medicine
Srinagar
President, Endocrine Society of India

Foreword

It gives me great pleasure to write this Foreword for the book *Clinical Endocrinology and Diabetes Mellitus: A Comprehensive Text* edited by Lt Gen (Prof) Y Sachdev, AVSM. I know Yash Sachdev for over 40 years. He is a par excellence educator, a super teacher, masterful endocrinologist, a passionate researcher, a prolific writer and a well-known institute builder. As an editor, he has ensured to involve many of his illustrious associates to write various chapters on the topics of their choice.

Over the past 8 to 10 years, with the better understanding of molecular and cellular biology, the Science of Endocrinology has seen many new developments in its clinical, laboratory and management approach. I am glad, the book contains an authoritative, balanced and evidence-based account of various endocrine problems. The book makes an easy and pleasant reading with several coloured illustrations, photographs, algorithms, etc. The contributors have left no stone unturned to fashion the text to provide an expert and a comprehensive resource and an accurate information on various problems of endocrine glands and diabetes mellitus. I am certain the book will be of great benefit to all those involved in patients care. These appear to be the best of time for those interested in the study of endocrine glands and diabetes.

Lt Gen DN Gupta PVSM, AVSM
MD, FRCP (London), FRCP (Edin)
DTM & H (Edin), FIMSA , FAMS
Formerly Director General Armed Forces Medical Services
New Delhi

Preface

World Health Organisation (WHO) has estimated that by 2025 there will be approximately 300 million diabetics in the world. India will be housing over 60 million diabetics by that time. Presently, there are approximately 43 million individuals with diabetes in our country. Besides this phenomenal increase in diabetic population, one is horrified to see more and more of obese children and teenagers having T2DM. The incidence of ischaemic heart disease, hypertension and stroke in the young is also on the increase. The prevalence of goitre again has not shown any sign of abatement despite implimentation of the National Iodine Deficiency Diseases Control Programme (NIDDCP).

The medical professionals are fully conscious of this dismal scenario and a lot of research is going on all over the world including India to tackle the problems of T2DM, obesity, hypertension, osteoporosis, dyslipidaemia, male and female infertility and to find out an easy way to ensure population control and eradication of iodine and other deficiency diseases. Several new strategies and formulations are being worked out to improve the situation. The result of these research projects has confirmed that T2DM is potentially preventable with lifestyle modifications and in certain instances with medication. Similarly, other conditions like obesity, hyperlipidaemia, osteoporosis, nutritional deficiency diseases like goitre, cretinism, rickets, osteomalacia and some other metabolic bone diseases are also preventable.

Since early 1990s, new developments and new thinking have appeared about the endocrines and their dysfunctional states. As a result of these advances in endocrine disorders especially T2DM, the therapeutic decisions faced by health care providers have become extremely complex. An endocrinologist is expected to identify high risk individuals, motivate them for coming to the clinic, initiate intervention in the form of appropriate tests to reach an early and definite diagnosis, prevent/delay the onset of disease and organise optimal surveillance to prevent complications and side effects.

To ensure this, it is important; therefore, to have an authoritative reference book available to medical fraternity. Unfortunately, so far there has not been a comprehensive updated text available in the market. Hence, this endeavour to bring out a book which draws on the experiences of some of the most senior and reputed Professors, Consultants, Researchers and Professionals to write on different aspects of endocrinology.

It has been a great pleasure to edit the book *Clinical Endocrinology and Diabetes Mellitus: A Comprehensive Text*. A book of this magnitude bringing out the latest in each topic will not have been possible without the magnanimity and kindness of our star-studded and elite group of contributors, who agreed upon to write on the topics of their own choice. It was a great experience to be associated with some of the topmost medical scientists and experts in the country, belonging to defence and civil medical services and their younger colleagues. A great care has been taken to make the text an easy and pleasant reading.

The book is presented in two volumes and is divided into six parts. Each part is subdivided into sections and each section has several subsections. Each subsection begins with a brief account of relevant embryology, applied anatomy and physiology before dealing with the main topic. A sincere effort has been made by the contributors to deal with the subject in a comprehensive but concise manner avoiding repetitions. To help the readers understand better, the clinical problem and management approach, several tables, figures, algorithms, flow charts, diagrammatic sketches, pictures, etc. have been included, wherever possible.

This is probably the first comprehensive textbook on Endocrinology and Diabetes Mellitus which is authored by some of the senior-most Indian experts in the field. It is intended to provide a linking bridge between the practice of clinical medicine and science of Endocrinology. The text is aimed to provide a condensed and authoritative approach to the management of various types of endocrinopathies. The treatise is based on an updated scientific information obtained after screening the vast literature and expert clinical experience of some of the famed and better-known teachers and medical scientists.

The book is targeted at medical consultants, general physicians, paediatricians, endocrinologists, diabetologists, ophthalmologists, graduates, postgraduates and post-doctorate scholars. It should also be of immense value to the undergraduates, nursing officers, nutritionists, dieticians, medical educators, teachers, researchers and all those who look after endocrine and diabetic patients. I am sure they will find it a useful aid in their day-to-day medical practice. It is hoped the readers will enjoy reading it as much as we did in writing it.

It is well appreciated that advancement in medical sciences is taking place at an extremely fast pace. What is the latest in the morning might well be outdated in the evening. Therefore, in a problem with divergent views, the readers may like to confirm the information given in this book from yet another source, if they so desire. This advice is being given, despite the fact that each contributor and the editor have tried their very best to provide as complete and as accurate an information as was possible at the time of publication.

Lt Gen (Prof) Y Sachdev AVSM

Acknowledgements

I acknowledge with a great sense of pride and gratitude the tremendous contributions made by the illustrious teachers, senior endocrinologists for writing an excellent account of the various topics of their choice for this book. I am extremely happy to note that many of them involved their junior colleagues in this project. They have done a phenomenal job in bringing out the very best and the latest in the endocrine field. It was indeed very magnanimous of them to spare their precious time for this project.

I also thank my loving wife, Mumta Sachdev, for several free hand line drawings, numerous sketches and figures and to our dear friend Ms. Jarna Das Gupta who supervised all the complicated and complex computer work. Both these ladies have done a great job.

My profound gratitude to M/s Jaypee Brothers Medical Publishers (P) Ltd., New Delhi, especially their Group Chairman and CEO, Shri Jitendar P Vij, who provided a dynamic leadership to his staff. It was great to know Mr Vij, a thorough gentleman and a very good human being (a rare commodity indeed, these days). I am also thankful to Mr Tarun Duneja, the young and youthful GM (Publishing), Mr DC Gupta, Mr Sukhdev Prasad, Mr Deepak Goyal, Mr Manoj Pahuja, Ms Samina Khan, and many other engaged in various phases of publication of this book. Some of them have become my personal friends.

I also thank my elder brother, Laj Sachdev, my associates and friends at PSRI and AH (R & R), New Delhi, especially *Generals* Jai Prakash, Prem Chandra, Rajagopal, *Colonels* Prusty, Narendra Kotwal, Drs Sudeep Khanna, Ajanta Hazarika, Ms Neelanjana Singh, Ms Hema Rani, Mr Raja Tarafdar and Mr Ravi Kumar Lakra for their constructive criticism, suggestions, proofreading and encouraging support, which I needed quite frequently.

Contents

Derby Hospitals NHS Foundation
Trust
Library and Knowledge Service

VOLUME TWO

PART 3: PAEDIATRIC ENDOCRINOLOGY

SECTION 18: GROWTH AND DEVELOPMENT......603

SECTION 19: HYPO- AND HYPERTHYROIDISM IN CHILDREN......659

SECTION 20: CONGENITAL ADRENAL HYPERPLASIA (CAH)......673
RG Holla

PART 4: IMAGING AND RADIO-DIAGNOSIS IN ENDOCRINOLOGY

SECTION 21: IMAGING IN ENDOCRINOLOGY......685
MN Shree Ram

SECTION 30: SPECIAL TOPICS IN DIABETES MELLITUS......1045

APPENDICES

Part 3

PAEDIATRIC ENDOCRINOLOGY

SECTION

GROWTH AND DEVELOPMENT

18

18.1 Growth and Development in Early Childhood

YC Mathur, NC Mathur

INTRODUCTION

Growth and development is a continuous and dynamic process. Throughout the span of development, interactive aspects of physical, cognitive, social and emotional development play their role. It is imperative for any endocrinologist to evaluate the growth of the child and take note of any aberration.

The trauma of dysfunctional families and socio-economic status affects optimal development outcome. Genetic and environmental aspects play a major part in growth. Development occurs at a variable pace in each child.

NEWBORN

Newborns are endowed with rooting and sucking reflexes and remarkable sensory abilities. Hearing is well developed at birth and speech sounds are preferred. Infant becomes alert to a female voice with high-pitched tones more than to a low-pitched male voice. Within the first few weeks, they learn to recognize mother's voice. Smell is well developed at birth. By one week of age, they recognize the smell of mother's breast pads, the smell of milk and their mother. Infant has more taste buds than adults and they avoid bitter tastes.

At birth retina is well developed but lens is immobile. By two months of age, fixation and tracking is well developed. Infants prefer to gaze at a human face than geometric designs. They prefer curved lines and bright colour. Visual acuity is poor at birth but improves rapidly in first 6 months. Strabismus resolves by 3 months of age. Crying is the main modality by which infants express responses to stimuli like hunger, wet diaper, fear and fatigue. Crying gradually decreases by 3 months of age

as smiling or reaching out and self-soothing modalities like sucking the fingers or thumb start. The first year of child is an oral stage. Mother and child attachment process is known as bonding. By 8 months infant develops separation and stranger anxiety.

Growth in First Three Years

i. Newborn may lose 10% of body weight in first few days of life. Birth weight is regained by 10 days. Gain in weight is 30 gm/day for the first several months. After 6 months genetic factors influence ultimate height.

By one year of age infant is 3 times the birth-weight and 1½ times as long.

Gain in weight thereafter is 2 to 3 kg per year and height gain is 5 to 7.5 cm per year. At the second birthday child attains approximately 50% of adult height.

After two years the energy requirement progressively decreases from 90 to 60 kcal/kg/day during middle childhood.

At birth the head is 75% of its adult size and 25% of baby's length. Cerebellum develops last. It begins growth at 30 weeks of age and ends at one year. The spinal cord doubles its weight in the first year and is 8-fold by adulthood.

ii. Development progression of grasp through first year illustrates gradual improvement. Grasp starts developing at 3 to 4 months involving ulnar aspect and thumb is used by 5 months. Thumb opposes the finger for picking up a cube by 7 months. Next, pincer grasp for smaller objects develops around 9 months, sitting with support at about 6 months and without support at 8 months. Standing and walking begin at 12 months (with a range of 9 to 17 months).

iii. In the second year, they take a jump in independence and develop a sense of 'self.' They begin to understand right or wrong. They develop cognitive, emotional and physical abilities in relation to brain development.

Stage is set for toilet training by 18 months of age when bladder and bowel control starts developing.

iv. By 2 months, vocalization like cooing and reciprocal vocal play with mother begins. Babbling begins at 6 to 10 months and repetition of sounds such as 'da, da, da' starts. Babbling reaches a peak at one year. They start expressing their needs by pointing to objects. By 18 months, 20 to 50 words are expressed. Receptive language develops faster than expressive languages: from 18 to 24 months expressive and receptive vocabulary takes a leap. Major change in cognitive development is also seen. After two years, children begin to put verbs into phrases like "I go out."

v. Early language milestones scale (ELM) is a simple tool for assessing the child in growth clinics and it is scored like Denver II. Brain reaches 90% of adult weight by 5 to 7 years. At 6 years remodelling of cortex occurs. By 5½ years most children have mastered conservation of length and by 6½ years they are conservative of mass and weight, and by 8 years volume.

Weight

The newborn baby regains birth weight by 1½ to 2 weeks. Then gains 200 gm/week (wk) in the first 3 months, 150 gm/wk in the next 3 months and 100 gm/week in the next 6 months. Healthy term infants will gain approximately 20 to 30 grams per day in the first three months. Birth weight doubles by 5 months and trebles by one year (i.e. nearly 6 kg at 5 months and 9 kg at 1 year). The child gains about 2 kg per year of age from 1 to 6 years and about 3 kg per year of age beyond 7 years. The normal range of weight of a child 1 to 6 years of age is given by the formula:

Normal range of weight varies from $(age + 3) \times 2$ to $(age + 4) \times 2$

Weight of a child > 7 years is given by the formula:

Age in years $\times 3$

Height

Height of a child beyond one year of age = $(Age \times 6) + 77$ cm

At 2 years the child may be 87 cm tall, at 3 years 94 cm and at 4 years 100 cm. Beyond one year the child gains about 6 cm per year. Any gain below 4 cm per year is pathological at any age during childhood. Separate growth curves are available for specific ethnic groups. Turner's syndrome, Down's syndrome, etc.

Head Circumference

At birth it is about 34 cm for a full term baby. Increases by 2 cm/month for the first 2 months (0 to 2 months), then 1.5 cm/month for the next 2 months (3 to 4 months), 1 cm/month for the next 2 months (5 to 6 months) and 0.5 cm/month for the next 6 months (7 to 12 months).

Small head size is not always pathological. Isolated microcephaly or familial microcephaly may be a normal variation and may not be associated with developmental retardation. However, microcephaly associated with genetic or dysmorphic syndromes usually are associated with mental retardation. Large head early in infancy is another condition where dismal prognosis should not be given early. Most of the hydrocephalus get arrested in course of time and the child develops normally; familial macrocephaly is likely to be benign. Macrocephaly without hydrocephalus may be due to metabolic or anatomic abnormalities and the prognosis may not be good. Macrocephaly associated with progressive hydrocephalus also may be associated with developmental retardation.

Mid Arm Circumference

Normal mid arm circumference is constant at 13 to 16 cm in children of 1 to 6 years of age. It is measured at a point mid-way between the acromion and the olecranon of the left arm. Table 18.1.1 gives the normal growth parameters in children up to 3 years.

Dysmorphism

Dysmorphic features are usually given undue importance. Isolated dysmorphic features are inconsequential (e.g. isolated low set ear, slant of eye, single palmar crease etc.).

Bone Age

Approximate bone age can be determined by the X-ray demonstration of the appearance of centres of ossification. If one is not sure of the usual age of appearance, the best method is to compare the film with an age matched control. If charts are available one can also determine the bone age depending on the degree of

TABLE 18.1.1

Age	Head circumference	Weight	Height	Dentition
Fulf term baby at birth	34 cm	3-3.5 kg	50 cm	Neonatal teeth if present may fall off before the primary dentition or remain as the primary teeth
0-1 year	2 months—38 cm	1 month—3.5-4 kg	Birth—50 cm	**Deciduous teeth:**
	4 months—41 cm	3 months—5 kg	3 months—60 cm	Incisor I: 6-12 months
	6 months—43 cm	6 months—6.75 kg	6 months—65 cm	Incisor II: 8-14 months
	8 months—44 cm	9 months—8 kg	9 months—70 cm	Molars I: 16 months
	10 months—45 cm	1 year—9 kg	1 year—75 cm	Canines: 20 months
	1 year—46 cm			Molars II: 25 months
1-2 years	Gains—2 cm	Gains—2 kg	Gains—12 cm	Molar I: 6.5-10 years
				Incisors: 7-10 years
2-3 years	Gains—1 cm	Gains—2 kg	Gains—6 cm	Premolars: 10-12 years
				Canines: 10-12 years
				Molar II: 10-14 years
				Molar III: 17-22 years

Physical growth parameters

fusion of epiphysis with the shaft. Radiologist may be able to give further refined opinion depending on the form and shape of ossification centres rather than the mere presence of it. Table 18.1.2 enumerates the time of appearance of epiphyseal ossification centres of hand, wrist and extremities

Milestones of Development

The motor development proceeds from cephalic to caudal and proximal to distal end. That is, the head control develops far ahead of walking and arm movements earlier than precise pincer movements of fingers.

The language includes receptive (ability to understand) and expressive skills (speech, gestures, writing, etc.). Speech is just the vocal expression of language. Thus, language and speech are not synonymous. Speech delay need not be a language delay. There are many children who have speech delay but normal receptive language. For example, the child may not be able to say tiger, but when asked to show a tiger; he will be able to show it in a picture book.

More fine and adaptive developments may be considered synonymous. Adaptive skills are fine motor skills related to independence, like feeding, dressing, etc.

Social milestones are the ones that help in inter-personal relationships.

Developmental quotient (DQ) = (development age in any of the domains divided by chronological age) × 100. A DQ above 85 is normal. 70 to 85 is gray zone, may be normal or abnormal, and the final answer comes only as the child grows up. Such children may benefit from early intervention of the type practised by the child development centre (CDC), Thiruvananthapuram.

NORMAL DEVELOPMENT AND ITS ASSESSMENT

Points to remember are:
  i. Development proceeds from cephalic to caudal and head control comes first, upper limb next, and lower limbs next.
 ii. Development proceeds from proximal to distal and precision of arm movement comes first and precision of finger movement later.
iii. Development proceeds from non-specific reaction to stimulus to specific stimulus-directed reaction.
 iv. Deficits in one domain of development may affect acquisition and assessment of skills of other domains.
  v. Speech and language are not the same. One can have speech delay but normal receptive language.

TABLE 18.1.2

Age (yr/month)			Hand and wrist	Age (yr/month)		
Percentile (boys)			bones and	Percentile (girls)		
5	50‡	95	epiphyseal centres	5	50‡	95
Birth	0//2.5	0//4	Capitate	<term¶	0//2.25	0//4
Birth	0//3.5	Q//6	Hamate	<term¶	0//2.5	0//5
8//8	1//0	2//0	Distal radius	8//6	0//10	1//6
1//0	1//6	2//0	Prox, III carpal	0//9	0//11	1//3
1//0	1//6	2//0	Prox II, IV carpal	0//9	0//11	1//6
1//3	1//6	2//3	Metacarpal II	0//9	0//11	1//6
1//0	1//6	2//3	Distal I carpal	0//9	1//0	1//6
1//3	1//9	2//6	Metacarpal III	0//9	1//0	1//6
1//6	2//0	2//6	Metacarpal IV	1//9	1//10	1//9
1//6	2//0	2//6	Prox. V carpal	1//0	1//3	2//0
1//6	2//0	2//6	Middle III, IV carpal	1//0	1//3	2//0
1//6	2//3	3//0	Metacarpal V	1//0	1//6	2//0
1//6	2//3	3//0	Middle II carpal	1//0	1//6	2//0
1//0	2//3	4//6	Triquetrum	1//0	1//6	3//0
2//0	2//3	3//0	Metacarpal I	1//6	1//6	2//6
2//6	3//0	3//6	Proximal I carpal**	1//3	1//9	2//6
2//6	3//6	5//0	Middle V carpal**	1//6	2//0	3//3
1//6	4//0	5//6	Lunate**	2//6	3//0	4//0
3//6	5//3	6//6	Greater multang**	2//6	4//0	5//6
3//0	5//3	S//6	Lesser multang**	2//6	4//0	5//6
4//0	5//3	7//0	Navicular**	3//0	4//0	6//6
6//0	7//0	8//0	Distal ulna	5//0	5//6	7//0
10//0	11//0	13//0	Pisiform	7//6	8//0	10//6
			Extremities (excluding hand and wrist)			
<term¶	<term¶	2 wk	Distal femur	<term¶	<term¶	1 wk
<term¶	<term¶	2 wk	Prox. tibia	<term¶	<term¶	1 wk
<term¶	2 wk	6 wk	Tarsal cuboid	<term¶	1 wk	2 wk
Birth	3 wk	0//2	Head of humerus	Birth	2 wk	0//1
0//3	0//4	0//9	Distal tibia	0//2	0//3	0//8
0//4	0//5	0//10	Head of femur	0//3	0//4	0//8
0//5	0//7	1//6	Capit of humerus	0//3	0//5	1//0
0//7	1//0	2//0	Gr tuber, humerus	0//4	0//8	1//6
0//8	1//0	2//0	Distal fibula	0//8	0//9	1//6
2//6	3//6	4//6	Gr. troch. femur	2//0	2//6	4//0
3//0	4//0	5//6	Prox. fibula	2//0	2//6	4//6
3//6	5//0	7//6	Prox. radius	3//0	4//0	6//0
4//6	6//0	8//0	Med. epicond. humerus	3//0	3//6	6//0
7//6	10//0	12//0	Trochlea of humerus	6//0	8//0	10//0
8//0	10//6	12//0	Prox. ulna	6//6	8//0	9//6
10//0	12//0	13//0	Lat. epicond. humerus	8//0	9//6	11//00

Epiphyseal ossifications for hand, wrist and extremities

*Compiled from the data obtained from the Harvard Growth Study, FELS Institute, BRUSH Foundation, and the University of Colorado, Child Research Council.
I F.P,.1//3 = 1yr 3 months
‡ 50th percentile and mean are approximately the same in most studies.
¶ <term = before term
**s which are most variable time and order of appearance

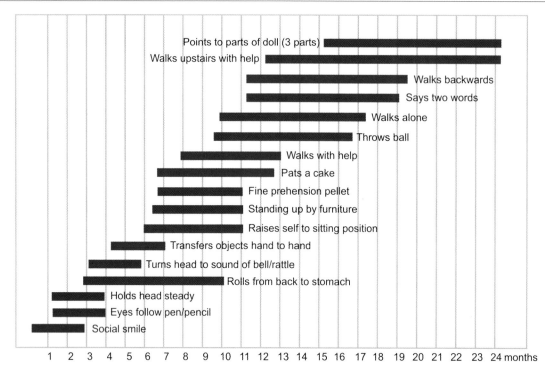

A vertical line is drawn, or a pencil is kept vertically, at the level of the corrected age of the child (in months) being tested. If the child fails to achieve any item that falls short on the left side of the vertical line, the child is considered to have a development delay (for use in 0-2 years old)

Fig. 18.1.1: Thiruvananthapuram developmental screening chart (TDSC).
Based on BSID Baroda norms, MKC Nair, Babu George, Elsie Philip, Indian Peditr, 1991;28:829

That is to say, the child does understand everything but cannot speak out. One can have poor language development, but early speech development. An example is autism where children may speak 3 to 4 word sentences but attribute no meaning to it (echolalia).

vi. Development is influenced by nature (in-born characters) and nurture (environmental influence). The former is the most important factor but the latter can influence and modify it substantially. Hence, the importance of early intervention by way of mother centred stimulation programmes.

vii. Preterm babies must be assessed for development by the corrected age and not the chronological age.

viii. Parental concern on development must not be disregarded even if formal development assessment is normal. After all, it is the mother who spends the maximum time with the child. The best course of action would be to call for frequent re-evaluations.

EARLY DETECTION OF ABNORMALITIES

Examination for assessment should include a formal neurological examination, developmental milestones (mainly from history), primitive reflexes and positional reflexes. Positional reflexes are concerned with spatial orientation and the centre of gravity control.

Rapid assessment of development is possible using charts like Thiruvananthapuram development screening chart (TDSC) (Fig. 18.1.1). Once a delay is noted, a detailed developmental evaluation must be done in each domain of development such as gross motor, fine motor/ adaptive, social and language; and the child may be given a developmental quotient.

Developmental Evaluation

Gross Motor Development

Since most of the information is obtained by history, inquiry should be made on the quality of child's movements. For example, turning around while sitting is a more advanced development than just sitting. Grading of the three cardinal motor developmental milestones pioneered by the child development centre Thiruvananthapuram, comes handy to decide whether a child has actually achieved these milestones. Gross motor skills correlate least with cognitive development or future intelligence. The usual primitive reflexes that are looked for are Moro, tonic labyrinthine, symmetric tonic neck reflex, asymmetric tonic neck reflex, etc. and the postural reflexes. Persistence of primitive reflexes beyond the usual age of disappearance is abnormal. Most of the primitive reflexes like the Moro and the asymmetric tonic neck reflex will have disappeared by 4 to 6 months of age. When an infant is held by axillary suspension, crossing of legs indicates hypertonia (cerebral palsy). Asymmetric leg swinging may indicate a difference in the muscle tone between the two legs. Hand preference before 18 months of age may indicate a weakness of the contralateral side. Persistent fisting at three months of age is abnormal and indicates a cortical functional defect. Rolling prior to three months may indicate hypertonia. Absent head control on slow pulling by hands in supine position but apparently good head control while holding the infant prone indicates extensor hypertonus. Pulling directly to a stand without the development of sitting may indicate hypertonia. Persistent toe walking may indicate hypertonia, the commonest cause of hypertonia is cerebral palsy. Frog leg position and W-sitting may indicate hypotonia. The commonest cause of hypotonia is benign hypotonia and not the big sounding syndromes. Ankle clonus (usually up to 4 months and sometimes, beyond this age) and positive Babinski's sign (till the child walks) are normal during infancy. Once a motor deficit is identified, detailed CNS examination, especially tone and deep tendon reflexes can be used to identify whether it is a pyramidal tract lesion, or spinal cord lesion or a peripheral nerve lesion or a muscle disorder. If it is a CNS dysfunction, the next task is to follow up and see if it is a static lesion (cerebral palsy) or a progressive lesion. Whatever be the type of lesion, stimulation and physiotherapy programmes must be started immediately. It will not help if the lesion turns out to be a progressive one like the metabolic disorders but it does no harm.

Cognitive Development

Language and adaptive abilities are the best assessments of cognitive development and future intelligence.

Receptive skills indicate the ability to understand language. Expressive skills indicate the ability to convey the messages to others. Speech is just one of the ways of expression. A child who has not started speech but conveys messages by gestures or signs has the expressive language developed but the speech delayed. A child with cerebral palsy may have speech delay because of incoordination rather than the lack of intelligence. Devices that help them to express themselves like a computer keyboard may help such children. Always remember that the most common cause of isolated speech delay (with normal adaptive skills) is hearing loss.

Receptive Language

Alerts to sound (one month), turns to voice (5 months), responds to name (10 months), responds to commands with gesture (12 months) or without gesture (15 months). Note that the normal development of receptive language may be possible upto the level of commands with gesture in a hearing impaired child. Points to three body parts on request (18 months). Follows two step commands like fetching the toy and placing it in the bed (24 months).

Expressive Language

Social smile (2 months), laughs aloud (4 months), vocalizes to mirror/speaker/turns to voice/babbles, baba, gaga (6 months). Any delay should alert to hearing deficit. Remember that a child with hearing deficit may also start babbling but it slowly disappears due to the lack of auditory feedback. Mama, dada, bye, etc. with meaning (10 months). 1 to 2 words other than mama, dada (12 months). 10 words (18 months). 2 to 3 words sentences with meaning (24 months). Non-communicative speech is not normal (consider autism). Non-communicative speech means sentences uttered by the child without the purpose of communicating. These children fail to follow simple commands inspite of their ability to speak sentence simply because they do not understand the meaning of what is being spoken to. This is a deviant language development and is not normal.

Adaptive Skills (Problem Solving Skills)

Fixes to face (one month), holds the objects given and takes it to the mouth (4 months), stranger anxiety/transfers objects hand to hand (6 months). It is postulated that the absent stranger anxiety may be due to multiple care givers (e.g. prolonged NICU care). Uncovers hidden object, under the cloth if hidden while the child was watching (10 months). Pincer grasp (12 months). Objects are used as play objects (and not for mouthing) by one year. Persistent mouthing suggests intellectual subnormality. Tower of three cubes (18 months). Matches objects to pictures (e.g. pen in hand and pen in picture/turns pages of a book/draws lines (24 months).

Psychosocial Development

Social smile, prefers human face (2 months). If this is delayed make sure that the vision is normal. If the vision is normal it may mean an attachment problem, child neglect, etc. Happy on sight of food/unhappy if the mother leaves/stranger anxiety (6 months). Responds to no or change in facial expression of the mother (9 months). Solitary play/peek a boo/kiss the parent on request (12 months). Feeds from the cup/helps in dressing (18 months). Removes the clothes (24 months).

Development is greatly affected by the parenting skills. Examples of undesirable parenting styles are over-protective parenting, over-controlling parenting, rejecting parenting, etc.

Learning disability Learning disability must not be diagnosed until the child is in school (5 to 6 years). Learning difficulties are likely before that age as the child is not yet ready for formal education. Usually, the child will have learning disabilities in specific areas like mathematics, language, reading, etc. that can be circumvented by a multisensory approach or other suitable means. For example a child with a reading problem should be read to while he is going through the text. The neurological basis of this may be some dysfunction in cortical information processing.

Every baby follows his or her own unique schedule of development within fairly broad limits. The general developmental competence of an infant can be assessed clinically. Despite the limitations and controversy surrounding the available infant assessment techniques, they continue to have merit as effective means of identifying infants at risk for developmental disabilities later. The score obtained is not an IQ score, but rather a relatively short-term, best estimate of developmental progress, which may prove useful in detecting the precursors of later impairment. The limitations of individual infant assessment techniques, however, must always be taken into account, and attempts to make long-term predictions about individual children are not usually warranted.

Development Assessment Techniques

Developmental Observation Card (DOC)

Using cut off points for four simple developmental milestones, one can identify the large majority of developmental delays.
*   Social smile   Achieved by completed 2 months
*   Head holding   Achieved by completed 4 months
*   Sitting alone   Achieved by completed 8 months
*   Standing alone   Achieved by completed 12 months.

Developmental disabilities are often seen in infants with no apparent risk factors. Hence, it is recommended that the mothers use this developmental observation card (DOC), for detecting problems in their children.

CDC (Thiruvananthapuram)
Grading of Motor Milestones

Since the development is usually history assessed, the achievements of milestones as perceived by different caretakers will affect the assessment. To have uniformity, CDC. Thiruvananthapuram grading of motor milestones is useful. Any child who has grade 3 or more is considered to have achieved that milestone.

a. *Head-holding (normally achieved at completed four months).*

Grade 0	No head holding at all.
Grade I	Momentary head holding.
Grade II	In supine position, lifts the head when pulled up by arms.
Grade III	In prone position, elevates self by chest and arms.
Grade IV	Holds the head steady when the mother moves around.
Grade V	Head is balanced always irrespective of body position.
	This stage is achieved because of development of postural reflexes.

b. *Sitting (normally achieved at completed 8 months).*

Grade 0	No sitting at all
Grade I	Momentary sitting
Grade II	Sits at least for 30 seconds, leaning forward
Grade III	Sits with the child's back straight
Grade IV	While sitting the child can manipulate a toy
Grade V	Raises self to sitting position

c. *Standing (normally achieved at completed 12 months)*

Grade 0	No standing at all
Grade I	Stands holding on to the furniture
Grade II	Takes a few steps with both hands held
Grade III	Stands alone without support

Grade IV   Stands up all alone without support, by throwing weight on arms.

Grade V   Takes a few steps without support.

Thiruvananthapuram Development Screening Chart (TDSC)

This is a simple developmental screening test designed and validated at the Child Development Centre, Thiruvananthapuram for use among children below 2 years of age. There are 17 test items in the chart. The left-hand side of each horizontal dark bar (line) represents the age at which 3% of the children and the right end represents the age at which 97% of children perform the item. A vertical line is drawn or a pencil is kept vertically, at the chronological age of the child being tested. If the child fails to achieve any item whose bar ends on the left side of the vertical line, the child is considered to have a developmental delay. Any obvious asymmetry is also considered abnormal (see Fig. 18.1.1).

Predicted Growth Formulae

a. *Predicted weights from age* If you know the age of a child and want a rough estimate of the weight and height, following formulae will be helpful.

For 3-12 months	: Weight (lb)	= age (mon) + 11
For 1-6 years	: Weight (lb)	= age (yr) × 5 + 17
For 7-12 years	: Weight (lb)	= age (yr) × 7 + 5
For 2-14 years	: Height (in)	= (2½ × age) + 30

b. *Predicted heights from age* The formula of Tanner et al demonstrates that height at age 3 years correlates better with height at maturity than it does at any other age:

Adult height (cm) = 1 .27 × height (at 3 yr) + 54.9 cm (males)

Adult height (cm) = 1 .29 × height (at 3 yr) + 42.3 cm (females)

If you cannot remember these formulae, the commonly accepted statement that the child at age 2 has achieved one-half of his or her final height is quite satisfactory.

Growth Assessment

Essential tools include growth charts and a device to measure standing and sitting height in children and length in infants (under two years of age). Skin-fold calipers, an orchidometer, and a bone-age assessment book are optional extras. When measuring lengths (lying, standing or sitting) ensure that the head is in a standard position with the outer canthus of the eye in the same horizontal plane as the external auditory meatus. The maximum length is obtained by exerting gentle traction on the mastoid processes.

At the clinical consultation the following measurements should be made routinely: height (standing and sitting), parents' heights (first visit), weight, head circumference; and puberty ratings.

Gather birth data on the child and siblings. Then calculate the decimal age and plot data on the appropriate growth charts (NCHS Charts 18.1.1 to 18.1.8).

The skeletal maturity (as assessed by X-ray of the left hand and wrist) will provide an index of how much growth has occurred and how much is to come.

INTRAUTERINE GROWTH RESTRICTION (IUGR)

Measurement of the crown-rump length from 5 to 12 weeks of gestation can provide an estimate of the gestational age accurate to within 3 to 5 days. During the first to third trimesters, measurement of the biparietal diameter of the foetal skull and foetal femur length are useful in estimating gestational age. IUGR may reflect chronic deficiencies in supply of oxygen or nutrients to the foetus. IUGR is defined as foetuses with birth weight and/or length less than 2 standard deviation below the mean or less than 3rd centile or less than 10th centile for gestational age depending upon the study.

Early onset or symmetrical type of IUGR is due to insult beginning early in pregnancy prior to 28 weeks in which head and body is proportional. The ponderal index (wt. for ht.) is normal. Late onset or asymmetrical, head sparing, IUGR begins after 28 weeks. Head is large for the body size. The ponderal index is low and the infants seem long and the growth is late flattening.

Causes of IUGR

The causes of IUGR can be classified according to whether they are foetal, placental or maternal (Table 18.1.3). The growth failure can be classified as 'intrinsic', which implies an abnormality at the time of conception or within the first trimester (foetal and some maternal causes), or 'extrinsic', implying a later onset of growth retardation (placental and some maternal causes).

Intrinsic Foetal Growth Restriction

Early-onset growth restriction, which tends to give rise to a small for gestational age (SGA) infant who is

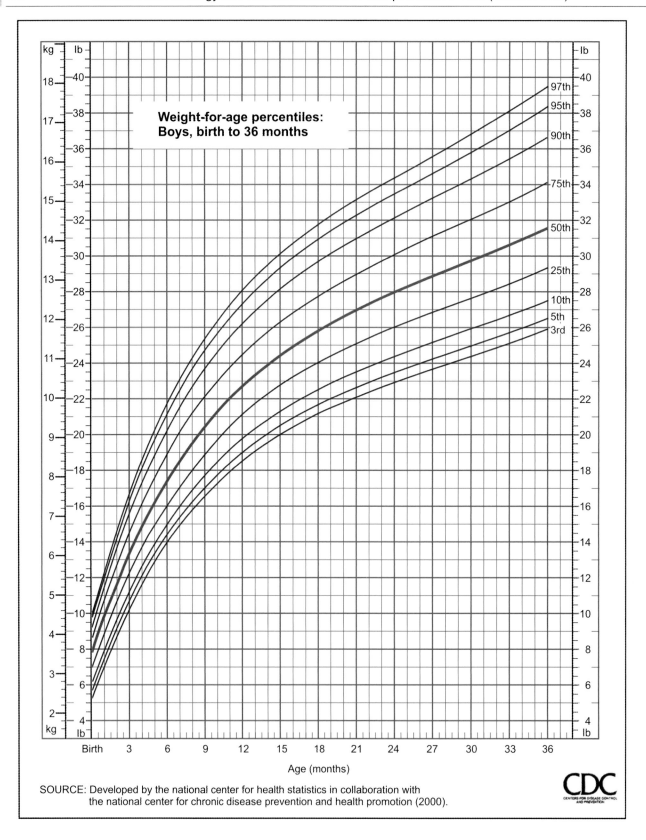

Chart 18.1.1: Weight-for-age percentiles, boys, birth to 36 months, CDC growth chart: United States

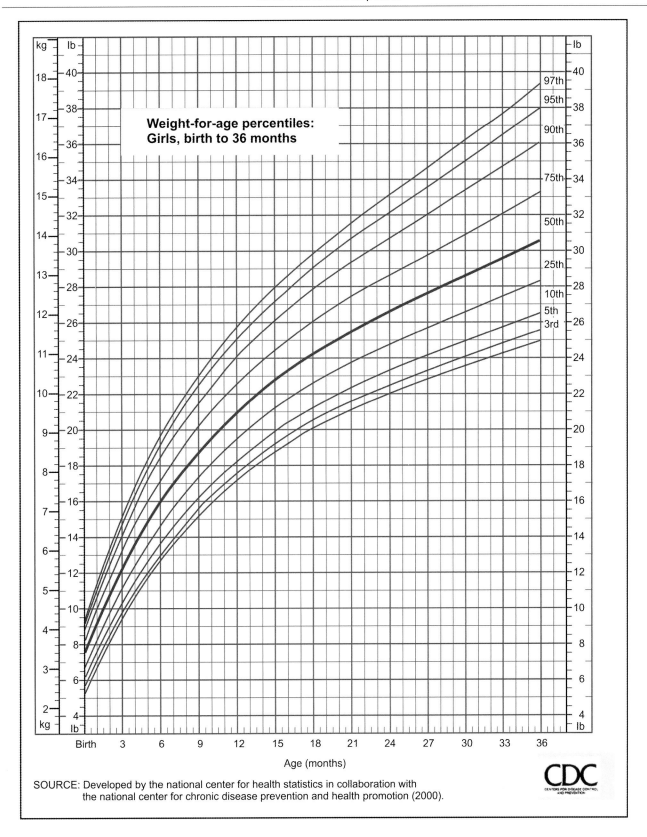

Chart 18.1.2: Weight-for-age percentiles, girls, birth to 36 months, CDC growth chart: United States

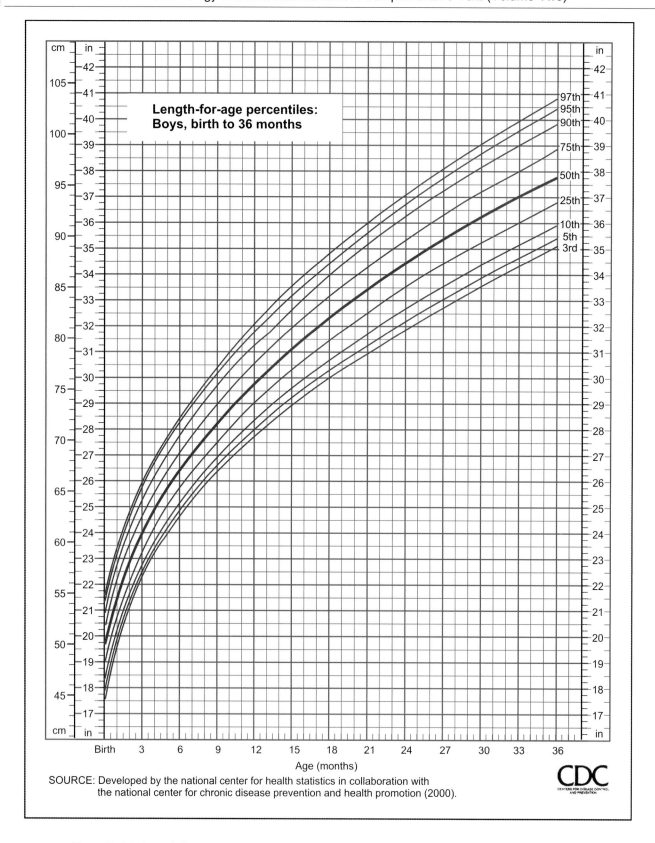

Chart 18.1.3: Length-for-age percentiles, boys, birth to 36 months, CDC growth chart: United States

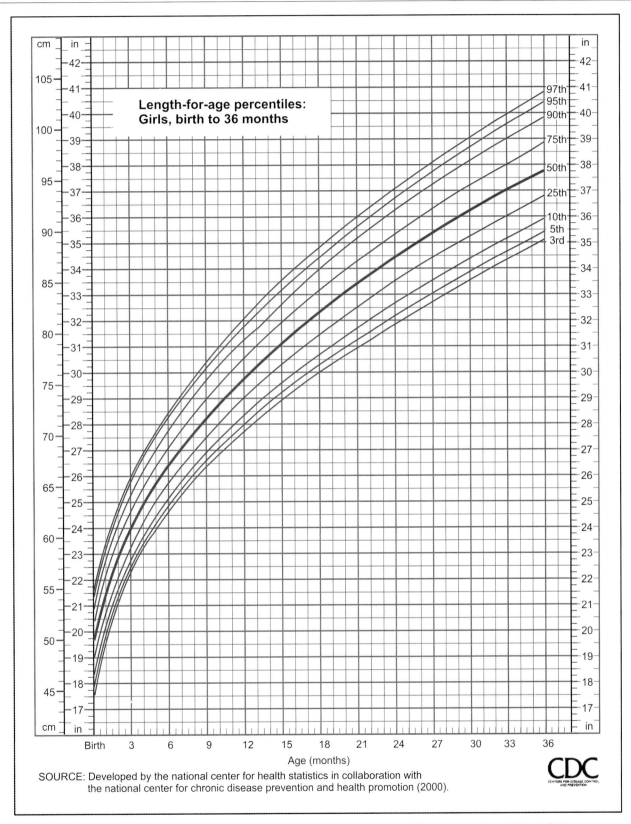

Length-for-age percentiles: Girls, birth to 36 months

SOURCE: Developed by the national center for health statistics in collaboration with the national center for chronic disease prevention and health promotion (2000).

CDC

Chart 18.1.4: Length-for-age percentiles, girls, birth to 36 months, CDC growth chart: United States

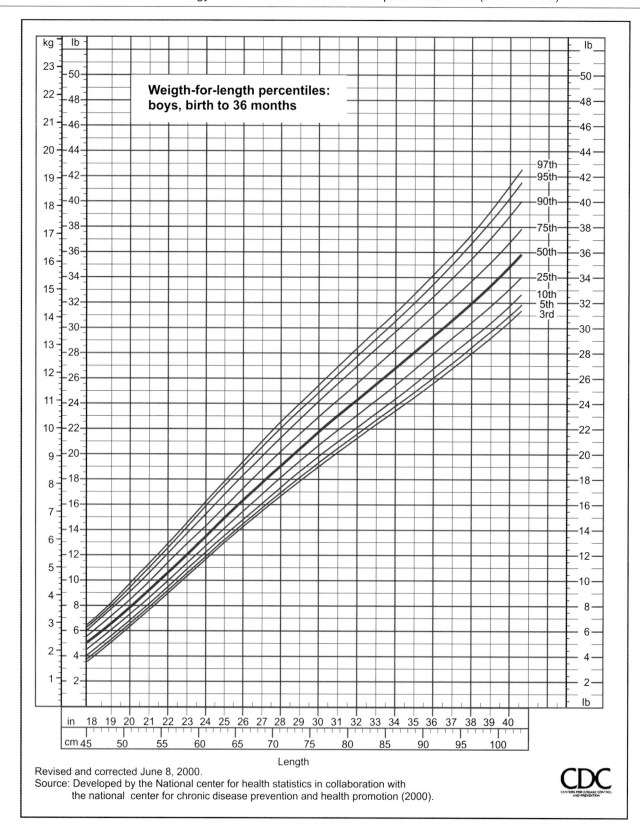

Chart 18.1.5: Weight-for-length percentiles, boys, birth to 36 months, CDC growth chart: United States

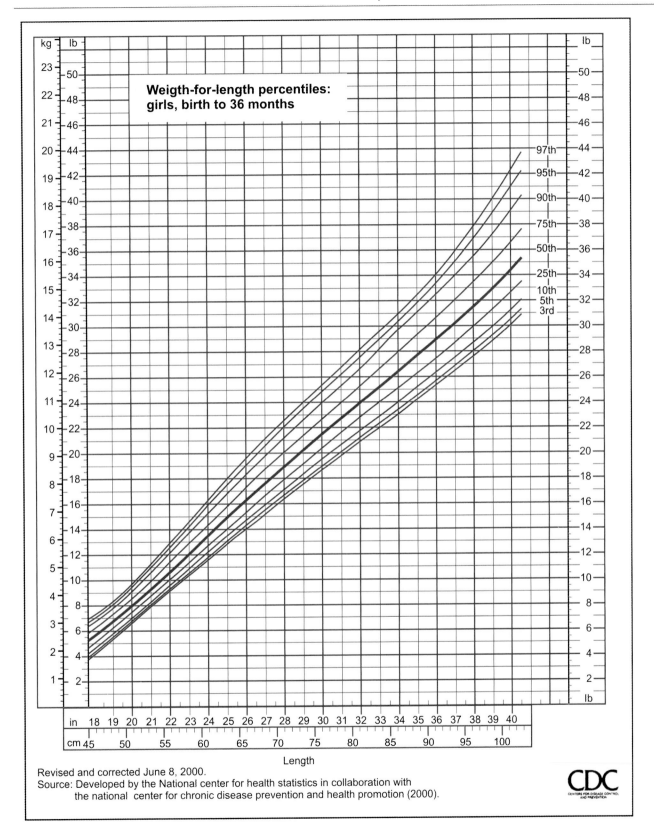

Weigth-for-length percentiles: girls, birth to 36 months

Length

Revised and corrected June 8, 2000.
Source: Developed by the National center for health statistics in collaboration with
the national center for chronic disease prevention and health promotion (2000).

CDC
CENTERS FOR DISEASE CONTROL
AND PREVENTION

Chart 18.1.6: Weight-for-length percentiles, girls, birth to 36 months, CDC growth chart: United States

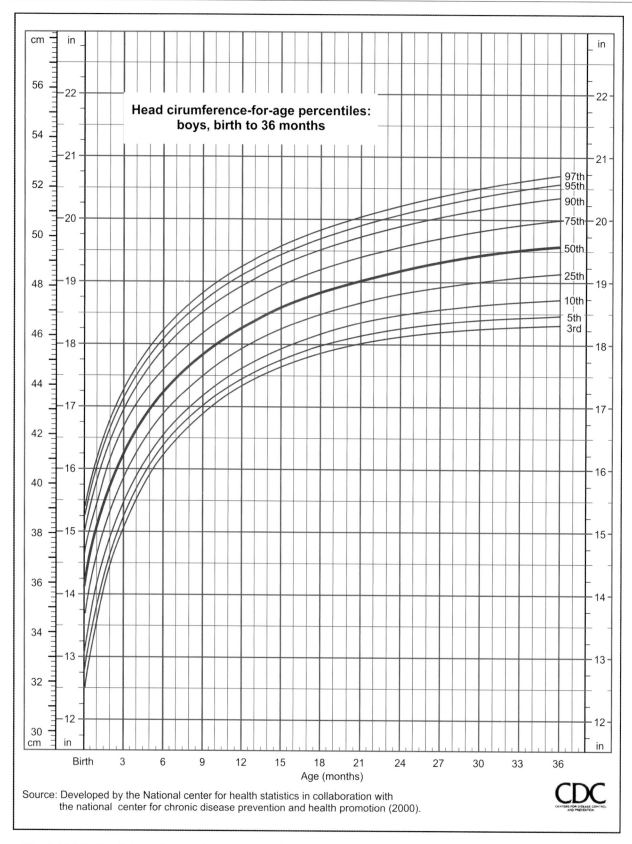

Head cirumference-for-age percentiles: boys, birth to 36 months

Source: Developed by the National center for health statistics in collaboration with the national center for chronic disease prevention and health promotion (2000).

Chart 18.1.7: Head circumference-for-age percentiles, boys, birth to 36 months, CDC growth chart: United States

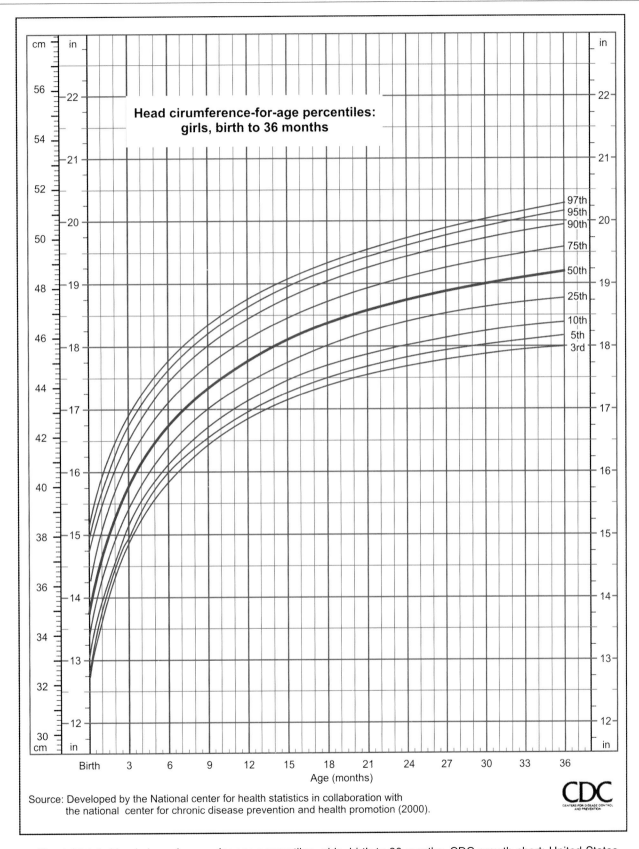

Chart 18.1.8: Head circumference-for-age percentiles, girls, birth to 36 months, CDC growth chart: United States

TABLE 18.1.3

Foetal	Placental	Maternal
Chromosomal abnormalities	Toxaemia of pregnancy	Maternal disease
Prenatal viral infection	Multiple pregnancy	Alcohol
Dysmorphic syndromes	Small placental size	Smoking
X-rays	Site of implantation	Malnutrition
	Vascular transfusion in monochorial twin placentas	Attitude

Causes of intrauterine growth restriction

proportionate, symmetrical, hypoplastic and has a normal placenta, is more likely to have an intrinsic cause of growth failure. During the first trimester, global insults include chromosomal anomalies (e.g. trisomy syndromes), perinatal infections (e.g. toxoplasmosis, other, rubella, cytomegalovirus, herpes simplex type II: TORCH), dwarfing syndromes (e.g. achondroplasia, chondrodystrophic dwarfism, Russell-Silverman syndrome), maternal recreational drug abuse (e.g. alcohol, narcotics, cocaine), exposure to teratogenic drugs and ionizing radiation. Constitutional growth retardation relates to parental stature and racial and ethnic factors. These infants, often referred to as having type-I growth retardation, show symmetrical growth retardation, with similar growth reductions in weight, length and head circumference. They do not exhibit a head-sparing effect and, because of a decreased number of cells, as well as decreased cell size, do not have the potential for normal growth. Fortunately, this group comprises only about 10 to 30% of all SGA babies in modern western societies, but if they are evaluated after the first trimester by ultrasound assessment of biparietal diameter, an inappropriately low assessment of gestational age may result.

Extrinsic Foetal Growth Restriction

Later onset of foetal growth restriction results from disorders of the placenta or from maternal problems. Extrinsic mechanisms operate during the later half of pregnancy and are associated with impaired delivery of oxygen and nutrients from the placenta. These factors may become operative at different times during pregnancy, resulting in less predictable effects on foetal growth. Maternal factors include hypertension (e.g. essential, pregnancy-induced, renal), diabetes mellitus with vascular complications, renal disease, cardiac disease, sickle cell disease and collagen disorders. Maternal smoking, alcohol and narcotic abuse and

maternal hypoxias (e.g. cardiac disease, pulmonary disease, residence at high altitude) may also cause IUGR.

Placental Factors

These all have the common feature of diminished placental blood flow, which may become more severe later in pregnancy. Twins will show a normal rate of intrauterine growth until the demands of the two foetuses outstrip the placental blood supply. This usually occurs at about 32 weeks gestation, and foetal growth rates fall off from this time. Placental disorders associated with IUGR include chronic villitis, haemorrhagic endovasculitis, chorioangioma, chronic abruptio placentae, hydatidiform degeneration, single umbilical artery and twin to twin transfusion syndrome.

Specific Problems of the Growth-restricted Foetus and SGA Infant

When considering the problems of SGA babies, it seems more appropriate to compare them with their gestational age peers rather than with babies of similar birth weight. When IUGR results from restricted nutrient supply, the foetus adapts to maximise the prospect of good outcome by sparing brain growth, accelerating pulmonary maturity and increasing the red cell mass (polycythaemia). These features may initially represent important adaptational strategies, but they later become pathological when deprivation is more extreme and foetal distress supervenes.

The expression of the endowed genetic potential for growth and intelligence is influenced by the interplay of nutritional, environmental and socioeconomic factors, (Fig. 18.1.2). The role of malnutrition in reducing mental development is difficult to separate from the other associated retarding social and environmental factors. Because multideprivations including malnutrition has been identified as the most important constraint in the

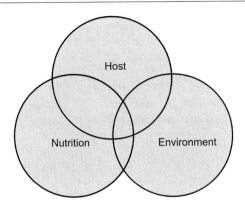

Fig. 18.1.2: Interaction between host, nutrition and environment

total development of children, the mode of treatment has to be multidisciplinary including primary health care, nutritional supplementation, developmental stimulation, psychosocial support and socioeconomic advancement.

A composite stimulation package including nutritional input, developmental stimulation, primary health care and psychosocial support is needed for optimum development and quality of survival.

SUMMARY

The assessment of growth and development in early childhood entails a comprehensive and holistic approach which embraces evaluation of sensory, motor, cognitive and sexual development and anthropometric growth. The ultimate outcome is the result of genetic, environmental and endocrine factors, early detection of an aberration is necessary to offer an appropriate inter-

vention. Therefore, periodic review of the child is essential.

Mothers are advised to use developmental observation card to appreciate the progress in their children while the care provider should refer to CDC Thrivananthapuram for grading of motor milestones for an objective assessment. Various milestones in a child's development, anthropometry charts and relevant formulae for predicted height and weight have been enclosed for ready reference.

FURTHER READINGS

1. Agarwal OK, Agarwal KN, Upadhyay SK, Rai S, Prakash R, Mittal R. Physical and sexual growth pattern of affluent. Indian children from 5-18 years of age. Indian Pediatr 1992; 29(10):1203-82.
2. Agarwal KN, Manwani AH, Khanduja PU, Agarwal DK, Gupta S. Physical growth of Indian school children. Indian Pediatr 1970; 7:146.
3. Gupta M, Agarwal KN. Nutritional status of pre-school children. Indian Pediatr 1973;10:81.
4. A longitudinal study of length, weight, head circumference from birth to 2 years among children of higher socioeconomic urban community in Delhi. Indian Pediatr 1974;II:395-8.
5. Indian Academy of Pediatrics, Parthasarthy, Menon, Nair (Eds). Textbook of Pediatrics 1999.
6. Indian Council of Medical Research Growth and Physical Development of Indian Infants and Children, 1972TRS-18. Part 1-A. ICMR. Growth and development in Indian Children. Tech Rep Ser no 18, 1968.
7. Mehta K, Merchant SM. Physical growth of children in the first year of life in higher and lower socio-economic classes of Bombay city. Indian Pediatr 1972;12; 751-6.
8. Rajashree S, Soman CR. Nutritional status of children in Kerala. Indian Pediatr 1994;31:651-5.

18.2 Normal Growth, Development and Hormonal Interplay

Y Sachdev

INTRODUCTION

The detailed description of normal human growth and development in early childhood has been given in the previous chapter where value of proper assessment and holistic evaluation has been stressed. In this chapter, an attempt is made to recapture the essence of the normal growth process, role of various hormones and discuss disorders of growth and puberty with particular reference to hormonal interplay.

NORMAL GROWTH

Normal human growth in height and body cell size is genetically determined and is influenced by a large number of intrinsic and extrinsic factors. The ultimate height achieved is dependent on the rate of linear growth and its duration. The various factors which influence the growth vary at different stages of growth, e.g.

a. Foetal growth is mainly affected by size of the mother, parity and intrauterine environment.
b. Infancy and early-childhood growth is influenced mainly by the thyroid and growth hormone.
c. Adolescence growth by androgens and oestrogens.

In all these stages, optimal nutritional supply, of course, is essential. While assessing growth, all parameters like height, weight, skeletal proportions, skeletal maturation, dental development (Table 18.2.1) and maturation of facial features must be considered along with cognitive and sexual development.

Foetal Growth

The foetal growth is little affected by the hormonal factors as intrauterine environments are able to overcome the effects of hormonal disorders which if continued later cause stunting of growth. It is a usual clinical experience to see a normal birth size in infants with congenital growth hormone deficiency. Similarly in congenital adrenal hyperplasia where adrenal androgens are present in excess, neither body length nor skeletal maturation are significantly advanced at birth. In congenital hypothyroidism, the birth length is usually normal though the skeletal maturation is markedly delayed. Foetal growth gets affected if there is placental dysfunction or there is, in some way, impairment of intrauterine nutrition. Maternal disease, smoking, uterine size, pre-eclampsia of pregnancy may also reduce the foetal size. Similar reduction in foetal size is seen at high altitude environments. It is seen that many a time temporary interference with foetal growth may cause permanent reduction of body stature.

Growth in Infancy and Childhood

Normally an infant increases its birth length by 50% in the first year and 16% and 10% in the second and third years respectively. Thyroid and growth hormones are essential for the normal growth after birth. If there is temporary interference with growth by infection etc. there is always a compensatory period of 'catch-up' growth. Between 5 and 8 years there is a slight growth spurt. After

TABLE 18.2.1

	Calcification		Eruption*		Shedding	
	Begins at	Completes at	Maxillary	Mandibular	Maxillary	Mandibular
Primary or deciduous teeth						
Central incisors	4-5 foetal months	18-22 months	6-11 months (2)	5-9 months (1)	7-8 yr	6-7 yr
Lateral incisors	5-6 foetal months	18-22 months	8-12 months (3)	7-10 months (2)	8-9 yr	7-9 yr
Cuspids	6-7 foetal months	30-38 months	16-21 months (6)	16-21 months (6a)	11-12 yr	9-11 yr
First molars	5-6 foetal months	24-32 months	10-18 months (5)	10-18 months (3)	9-1 l yr	10-12 yr
Second molars	6-7 foetal months	36 months	22-32 months (7)	22-32 months (7a)	9-12 yr	11-13 yr
Secondary or permanent teeth						
Cental incisors	3-4 months	9-10 yr	7-8 yr	6-7 yr (2)		
Lateral incisors						
Maxilla	10-12 months	10-11 yr	8-9 yr (5)	7-8 yr (4)		
Mandible	3-4 months					
Cuspids	4-5 months	12-15 yr	11-12 yr (11)	9-11 yr (6)		
First premolars	18-24 months	12-13 yr	10-11 yr (9)	10-12 yr (8)		
Second premolars	24-30 months	12-14 yr	10-12 yr (9)	11-13 yr (10)		
First molar	Birth	9-10 yr	5½ -7 yr (1)	5½-7 yr (1a)		
Second molar	30-36 months	14-16 yr	12-14 yr (12)	12-13 yr (12a)		
Third molar						
Maxilla	7-9 yr	18-25 yr	17-30 yr (13)	17-30 yr (13a)		
Mandible	8-10 yr					

Times of calcification and eruption of deciduous and permanent teeth

* Figures in parentheses indicate order of eruption. Many otherwise normal infants do not conform strictly to the stated schedule.

this the growth slows down progressively until the beginning of pubertal growth spurt. During late childhood, it is entirely normal to grow only 3 to 4 cm per year and even as little as 1 to 2 cm per year in later teens.

Growth in Adolescence

The growth spurt is dependent on sex and growth hormones. Androgens in boys and probably in girls are responsible for the adolescent growth spurt. During childhood, the rate of linear growth (height velocity) gradually diminishes and reaches a minimum immediately before the start of the growth spurt. The peak height velocity of the adolescent growth spurt occurs on an average 1 to 2 years earlier in girls than in boys. Boys therefore have 1 to 2 more years of prepubertal growth than girls. Thus the amplitude of their growth is greater.

The normal girls start their adolescent growth spurt with the onset of clinical puberty. Their peak height velocity occurs a year before the menarche. By the time the first menstrual period (menarche) appears, their growth rate has already begun to decelerate. This is primarily due to the fusion of the epiphyses of the long bones of the lower limbs. In normal boys, the adolescent growth spurt is a later event in puberty. Their peak height velocity coincides with the penultimate stage of (stage 4) genital and pubic hair development (Figs 18.2.1 and 18.2.2).

ASSESSMENT OF GROWTH

It involves anthropometric measurements especially height, weight, left midarm circumference, head and chest circumference, upper and lower segments and arms span.

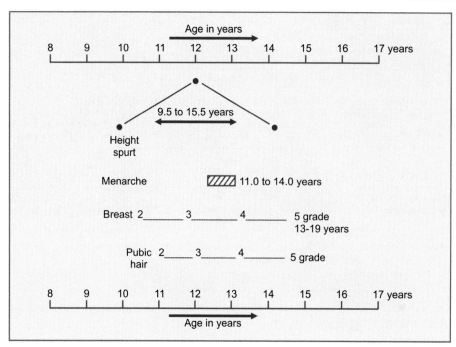

Fig. 18.2.1: Sequence of development events in normal girls (approx. average age)*

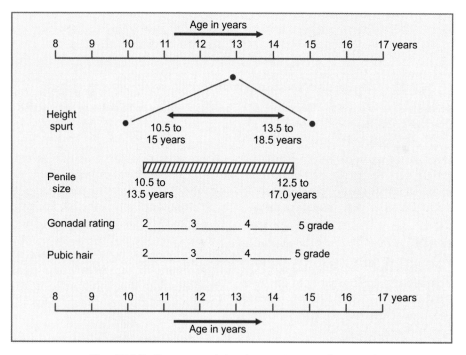

Fig. 18.2.2: Sequence of development events in normal boys (approx. average age)*

* Data based on Indian population

Besides anthropometry, cognitive development, sexual and facial and bone maturation also require to be recorded. Where malnutrition is suspected, skin fold thickness should be recorded.

Measurement of Height

An accurate stradiometer is required for standing height measurement. In infants and younger children supine length is measured. In both cases, gentle upward traction under the jaws is applied to eliminate postural changes. Growth charts, in which, the normal children population is divided into centiles (division of 100) are used to plot the height and height velocity of the patient. Patients whose height falls below the third centile or above the 97 centile will require further observation and evaluation.

Body Weight

The NCHS charts depicting BMI, weight-for-age and length-for-age percentiles for both boys and girls aged 2 to 20 years are enclosed (Charts 18.2.1 to 18.2.8). It is important to remember that these charts should never be interpreted rigidly as there are considerable variations in bone structure and lean body mass. In malnutrition, body weight reduces to a greater extent than the height. Degree of malnutrition is evaluated better by measuring triceps and subscapular skinfold thickness.

Skeletal Proportions

Evaluation of limb growth is obtained by measuring sitting height and subtracting it from the full height. This gives what is called 'subischial leg length.' Standard charts for this are also available. At birth the ratio of upper segment to lower segment is about 1.7:1. Since the limbs grow more rapidly than the trunk, this ratio decreases and by the age of 10 to 11 years it reaches 1:1 and remains so thereafter.

The adolescent growth spurt is predominantly spinal, and patients with delayed puberty have relatively long legs. Same applies to the arms span as arms and legs grow in a similar fashion. In normal adults, the span is equal to the height.

Maturation of Facial Features

Facial features are an important guide to skeletal maturity. The growth of the nasal bridge is retarded in hypothyroidism giving a characteristic immature face to a cretin. Similarly the increase in the length of the jaw and nose that occurs at normal puberty is impaired in hypopituitary dwarfs who retain a somewhat juvenile look.

Bone Maturation

It is another important index of maturity. It is estimated by taking X-ray of the left hand wrist and elbow (irrespective of dominance) and calculating the bone age from the radiographic atlas of skeletal development of the hand and wrist by WW Greulich and SI Pyle (1959). In this, the X-ray films are compared with standard films of healthy children at different ages. The second method is to use Tanner et al (1975) method of 'maturation score' where each bone is given a 'maturation score' compared with X-ray standards. The total score is compared with standard score for age. A skeletal or bone age more than 2 standard deviations from the mean, makes it highly probable that the child is abnormally advanced or retarded.

SHORT STATURE

Definition

Short stature is defined as height or length less than 2 standard deviation below the mean or below the 3rd percentile for that age. An important parameter, that is crucial in the diagnosis of failure to grow, is growth velocity (GV) or growth rate. It involves averaging the growth over a span of time (say 3 to 6 months) and expressing the velocity in cm per year. The expected GV in young children is given in Table 18.2.2.

TABLE 18.2.2

Ages	Growth velocity (GV) cm/year
1 to 6 months	18 to 22 cm/year
7 to 12 months	14 to 16 cm/year
1 to 2 years	11 cm/year
2 to 3 years	8 cm/year
3 to 4 years	7 cm/year
4 to 9 years	5 to 6 cm/year

Expected linear growth velocity rate per year

Factors Affecting Height

The ultimate height an individual achieves is the result of several factors interacting in a complex manner. The more important of these factors are: genetic make up, nutritional intake and assimilation, somatic problems, endocrine status, environmental influences, social interaction and emotional relationship. Secretion like GH, IGF-1, sex steroids, thyroid hormones, paracrine growth factors and cytokines exert a prominent influence on linear growth.

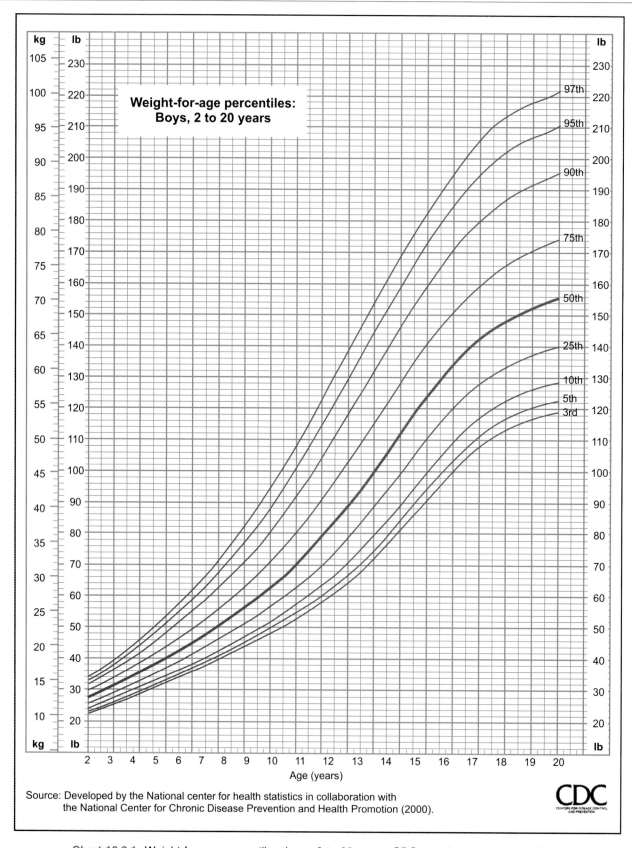

Source: Developed by the National center for health statistics in collaboration with
the National Center for Chronic Disease Prevention and Health Promotion (2000).

Chart 18.2.1: Weight-for-age percentiles, boys, 2 to 20 years, CDC growth charts: United States

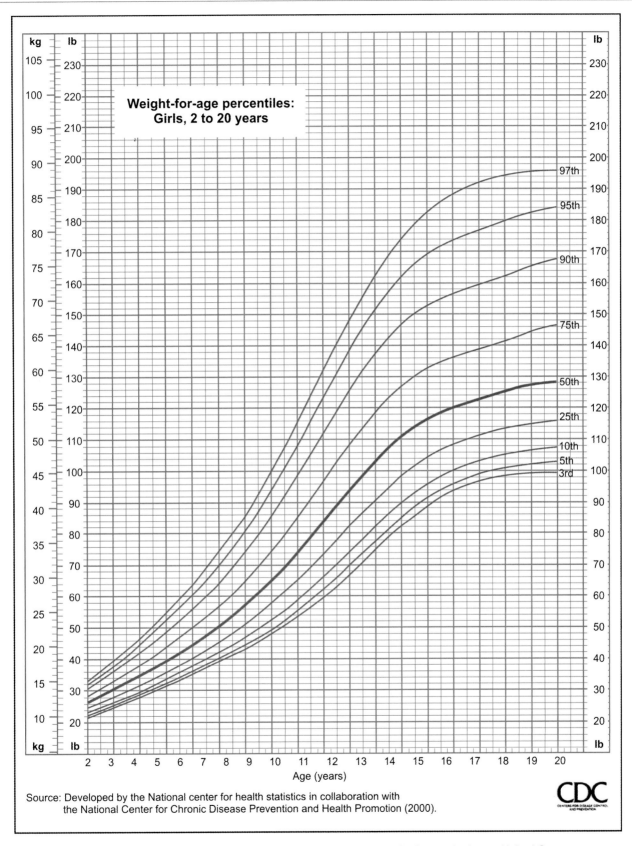

Weight-for-age percentiles:
Girls, 2 to 20 years

Source: Developed by the National center for health statistics in collaboration with
the National Center for Chronic Disease Prevention and Health Promotion (2000).

CDC

Chart 18.2.2: Weight-for-age percentiles, girls, 2 to 20 years, CDC growth charts: United States

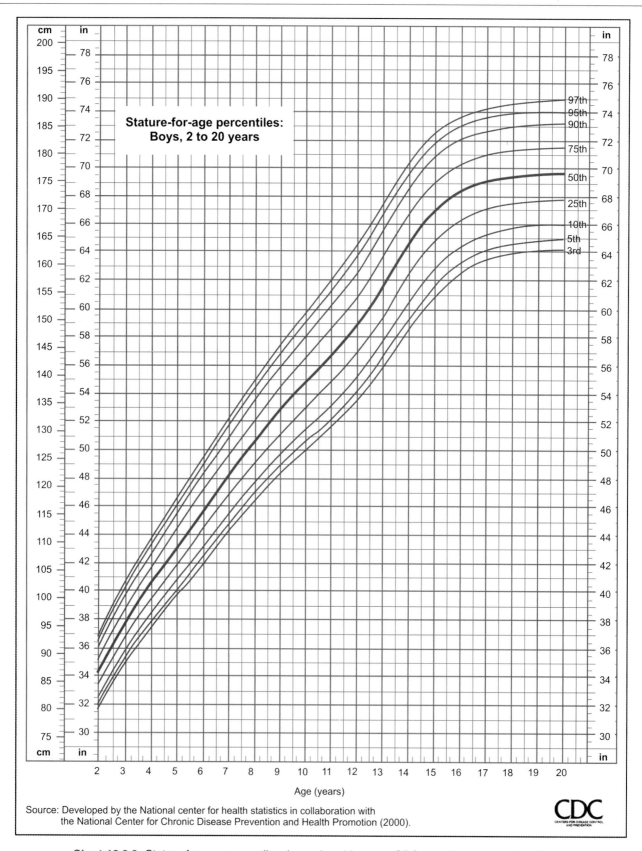

Chart 18.2.3: Stature-for-age percentiles, boys, 2 to 20 years, CDC growth charts: United States

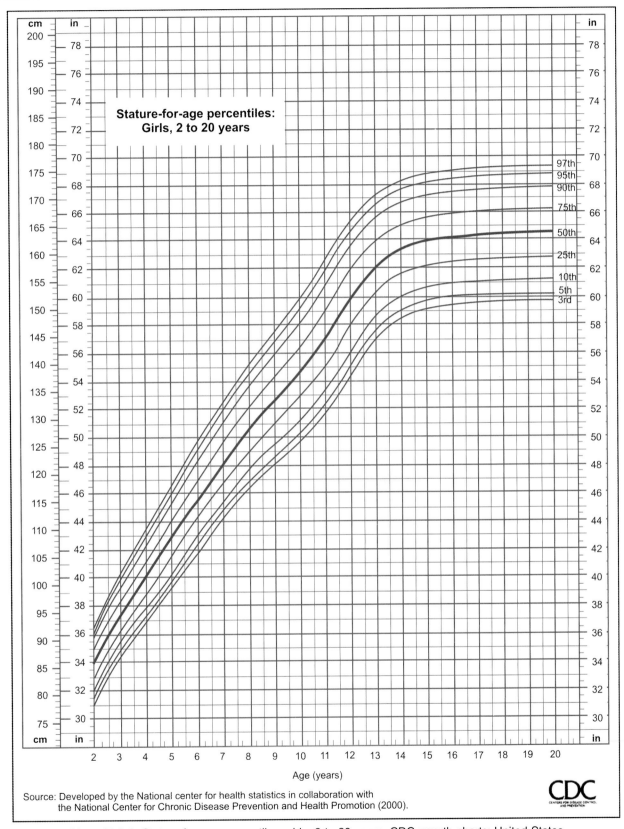

Chart 18.2.4: Stature-for-age percentiles, girls, 2 to 20 years, CDC growth charts: United States

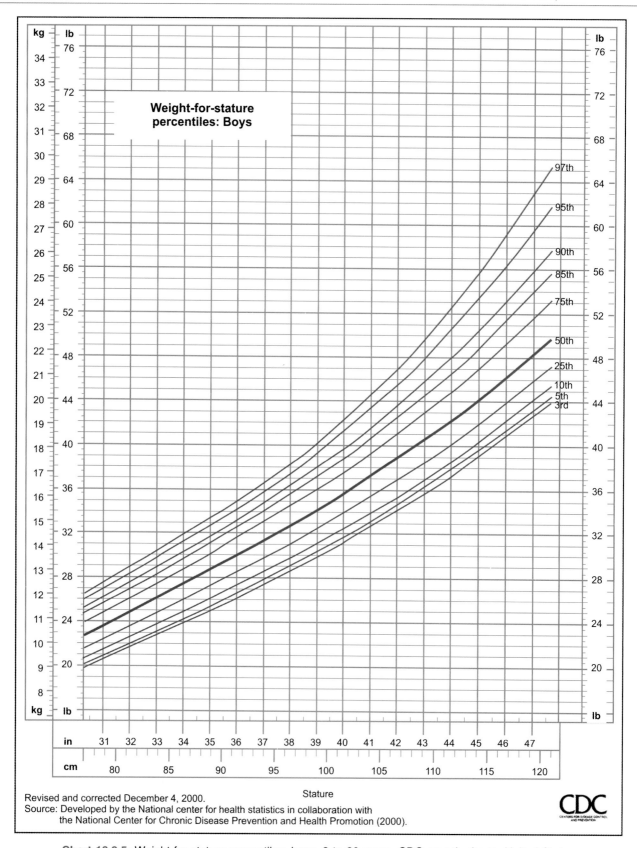

Weight-for-stature percentiles: Boys

Revised and corrected December 4, 2000.
Source: Developed by the National center for health statistics in collaboration with
the National Center for Chronic Disease Prevention and Health Promotion (2000).

CDC

Chart 18.2.5: Weight-for-stature percentiles, boys, 2 to 20 years, CDC growth charts: United States

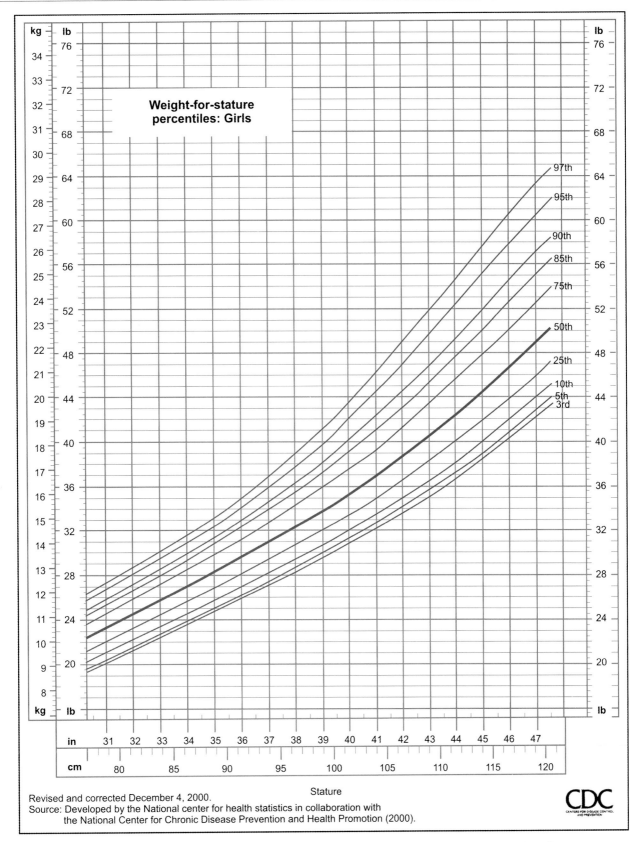

Weight-for-stature percentiles: Girls

Revised and corrected December 4, 2000.
Source: Developed by the National center for health statistics in collaboration with
the National Center for Chronic Disease Prevention and Health Promotion (2000).

CDC

Chart 18.2.6: Weight-for-stature percentiles, girls, 2 to 20 years, CDC growth charts: United States

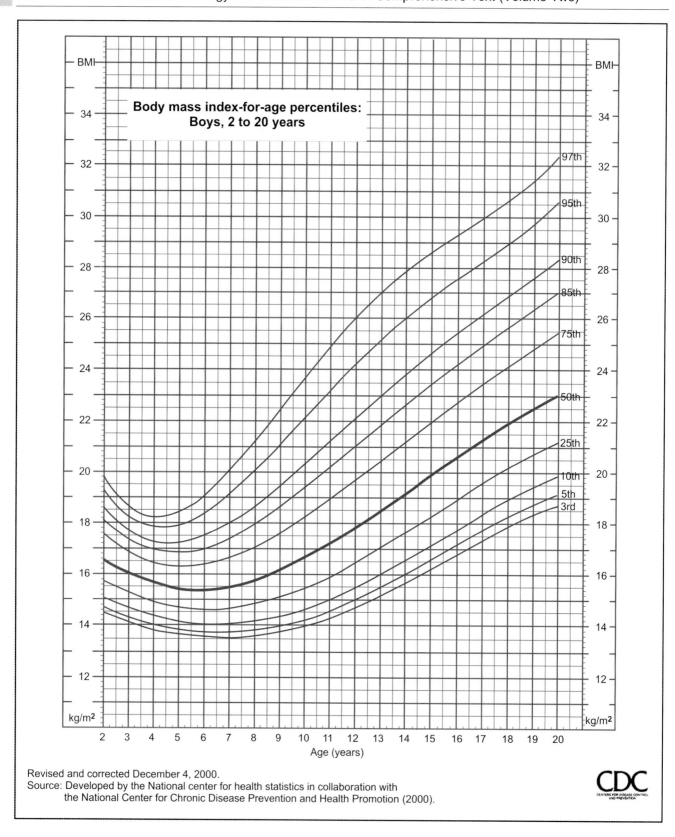

Chart 18.2.7: Body mass index-for-age percentiles, boys 2 to 20 years, CDC growth charts: United States

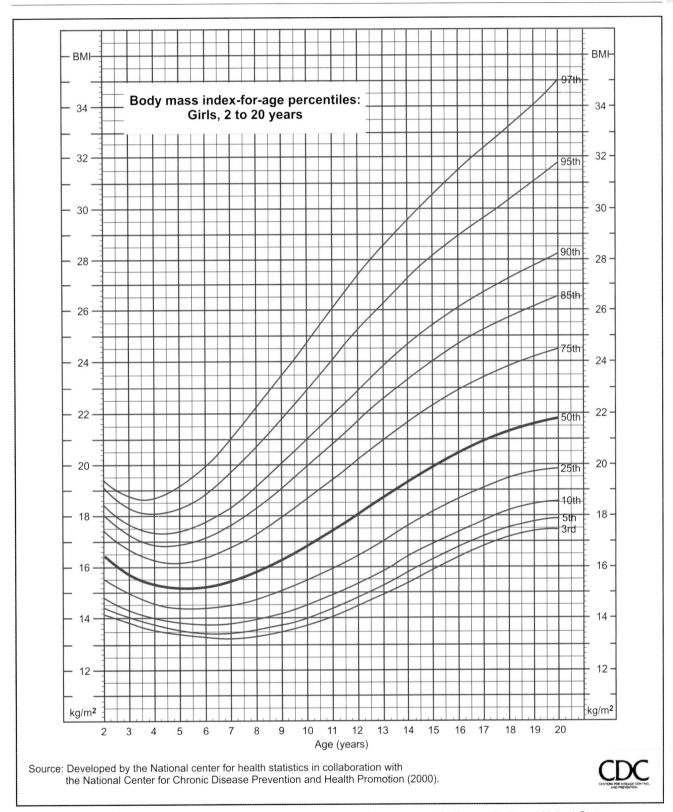

Chart 18.2.8: Body mass index-for-age percentiles, girls 2 to 20 years, CDC growth charts: United States

Clinical Approach

A rational approach to the problem of 'short stature' involves particular attention to the family history of growth and development, patient's birth weight and length, pattern of growth in height, epiphyseal development, facial features maturation, dental development, secondary sex characteristics, body weight, appetite, sleep, chronic ailments and infections. Old medical documents must always be pursued with a critical eye. Every effort must be made to get patient's past growth records and, if possible, accurate heights of parents and first degree relations.

The physical examination should be comprehensive. It must include, besides detailed clinical systematic examination, accurate recording of the standing and sitting height, upper segment, lower segment, arm span, head circumference and body weight. Visual assessment, fundoscopy, Tanner's staging, abnormalities in body configuration like neck webbing, cubitus vulgaris, shortness of the metacarpals, body fat distribution, sexual maturation especially body hair growth, breast, penile and testicular size (by orchidometer) should all be recorded. Growth velocity is assessed from the growth charts, if available. Growth failure is defined as growth velocity less than 2 standard deviation below the mean for chronological age. Upper and lower segments ratio or alternatively the sitting and standing height ratio is useful in detecting disproportionate short stature (e.g. skeletal dysplasias) cases. Nutritional status is assessed by left mid-arm-circumference, skinfold thickness, weight for age and weight for height charts. During the first three years of life, head circumference is an important parameter to be noted. From the above mentioned data, one can easily make an impression whether the short stature of dysmorphic nature (usually with chromosomal abnormalities), disproportionate skeletal dysplasia (achondroplasia, rickets, etc.) or nutritional type. Normal looking children with normal growth velocity are usually normal endocrinologically also. Non-dysmorphic children with poor growth velocity could be due to undernutrition, psychological deprivation, or endocrine disorders.

Laboratory Tests

Initial laboratory tests should include haemogram, stools, urine analysis, blood chemistry (plasma glucose, LFT, BUN, creatinine, electrolytes), X-ray chest, (PA view) and skull (lateral view), and bone age. Karyotype, anti-gliadin antibodies and calcium homeostasis tests, MRI and CT scan may be asked for, if indicated. Endocrine hormonal

TABLE 18.2.3

A. Short stature with abnormal proportions (skeletal disease)

   a. Congenital phocomelia

   b. Hereditary

      i. Primarily affecting bones, e.g. chondrodystrophies (achondroplasia)

      ii. Affecting other tissue as well, e.g. Hurler's syndrome, diastrophic dwarfism, Lawrence-Moon-Biedl syndrome, Ellis-van-Creveld syndrome, pseudo-pseudohypo-parathyroidism

      iii. Vitamin D resistant rickets, hypophosphatasia

B. Short stature with normal proportions

   a. Nonendocrine causes.

      i. Constitutional delay in growth and adolescence

      ii. Familial short stature

      iii. Chromosomal and genetic syndromes: Turner's syndrome, Noonan's syndrome, Russell-Silver syndrome, progeria, Aarskog's syndrome, Bird-headed dwarfs, Leprechaunism (Donahue's syndrome), Silver's syndrome, Cockayne's syndrome.

      iv. Coeliac disease

      v. Low birth weight/shortness of stature

      vi. Chronic ailments: renal disease, hepatic disorders, cardiac disease, pulmonary dysfunction, anaemia, gastro-intestinal disorders, CNS problems, chronic infections

      vii. Malnutrition

      viii. Psychological deprivation

   b. Endocrine causes:

      Hyperthyroidism, glucocorticoids excess-iatrogenic and over-production, adrenal insufficiency, congenital adrenal hyperplasia, hypopituitarism (isolated GH deficiency, panhypopituitarism, craniopharyngioma), hypothalamic hypogonadism, diabetes insipidus

Common causes of short stature

tests include estimation of thyroid hormones, IGF-1, GH, cortisol, LH, FSH and sex steroids.

Classification and Causes

Table 18.2.3 gives the common causes of short stature. Broadly these causes can be divided into:

A. Short stature with abnormal proportions (Short limb dwarfism).

B. Short stature with normal proportions. This could be due to:

- Non-endocrine and
- Endocrine causes.

Short Stature with Abnormal Proportions

This type of shortness of stature is uncommon but may cause severe stunting. Children with milder abnormality are diagnosed only when their standing and sitting height and subischial leg length is compared with Tanner's/NCHS charts. Bone disease, acquired or hereditary, is the main cause of this group. Other tissues may also be involved as in Hurler's syndrome and 'diastrophic dwarfism.' Table 18.2.4 gives salient manifestations of some common types of 'short limb dwarfism.' In Conradi's syndrome there is dotted calcification of the developing cartilage. The Ellis-van-Creveld syndrome is a rare, recessively inherited, condition with chondroectodernial dysplasia and characteristic nails and teeth.

TABLE 18.2.4

Syndromes	Salient manifestations
Achondroplasia	Dominant transmission. Large head, short limbs
Achondrogenesis	Recessive transmission. Grossly deficient calcification, fatal in neonatal period.
Cartilage-hair hypoplasia	Recessive transmission. Fine, sparse, fragile hair, scalloped metaphyses.
Conradi's syndrome	Recessive. Punctate calcification of developing cartilage.
Dystrophic dwarfism	Recessive. Limitation of joints, club foot, scoliosis develops after birth.
Ellis-van-Creveld syndrome	Recessive. IUGR, chondroecto-dermal dysplasia with hypoplastic nails and teeth, short limbs, polydactyly, small thorax, short upper lip, congenital heart disease.
Hypochondroplasia	Dominant, slightly large head, short limbs, lumbar lordosis.
Hypophosphataemic rickets	X-linked dominant, poor renal tubular reabsorption of PO_4. Needs high doses of vit D.
Hypophosphatasia	Recessive. Variable severity, low alkaline phosphatase levels.
Osteogenesis imperfecta (Fragilitas ossium)	Autosomal dominant (mutants). Bowing of legs, pectus excavatum or carinatum, hyperextensible ligaments, kyphoscoliosis, hypoplastic teeth, thin skin, blue sclera, otosclerosis

Some of the common types of short limbed dwarfism

Short Stature with Normal Proportions

Constitutional delay in growth and adolescence: It is a condition seen more in boys than in girls. These patients represent the lower end of the normal distribution curve. Birth weight and length are usually normal, but throughout childhood, the growth velocity is below average and epiphyseal development is retarded. Very often puberty and puberty related growth spurt is delayed. There is a strong family history of delayed growth and adolescence. Such patients usually attain 'normal' height and development without any treatment. In case, delayed growth causes any psychological problem, hormonal treatment to initiate puberty may be justifiable.

In boys, hormonal treatment should preferably be started after 15 years of age. A course of human chorionic gonadotrophins (hCG) in the dose of 1000 IU × twice weekly (Monday and Thursday) for a period of 3 to 6 months is recommended. In girls, cyclical oestrogen/ progesterone treatment may be initiated if the puberty does not start by 14 years. The treatment should be stopped at intervals of 6 months or so, to see if spontaneous development has begun.

Familial short stature: This is common and is not genetic necessarily as environmental factors which affected the parents also affect the children. Before birth, the growth is mainly determined by the intrauterine environments, though the maternal height also affects the foetal growth to some extent. Genetic make up does not appear to have any influence on *in utero* growth of the foetus. However during first two years of life, growth is under genetic control and a child assumes a growth velocity which follows the same curve till puberty.

There is a correlation between a child's height and the mean height of both parents (Midparental height) which can be calculated as per following formula.

$$\text{Boys:} \quad \frac{\text{Father's height} + 13\ cm + \text{Mother's height}}{2}$$

$$\text{Girls:} \quad \frac{\text{Father's height} - 13\ cm + \text{Mother's height}}{2}$$

This formula, provides some general idea of the child's final height but is not an absolutely accurate predictor. In familial short stature, many a time, the birth weight is less than average, but the present weight is appropriate for height. The height curve advances below and parallel to the child centile. Bone age is usually slightly retarded. Usually no treatment is required though assurance and psychological support may be necessary.

Low birth weight and shortness of stature: Most babies born before term but with appropriate weight for their gestational age continue to grow normally after birth and are not short in childhood. Similarly majority of newborns who are underweight at birth for their gestational age tend to reach normal mean weight during childhood. However, some children with low birth weight do continue to stay short and have IGF-I deficiency. This appears to be due to some abnormality of the intrauterine life which has impaired the growth potential like:

i. Intrauterine infections
ii. Placental problems
iii. Autosomal chromosomal anomalies which cause growth retardation with other physical anomalies,
iv. Abnormal pregnancies
v. Recognized and unrecognized genetic syndrome and syndromes with a wide variety of congenital anomalies and stunted growth (Table 18.2.5).

Malnutrition: Optimum nutritional supply is mandatory for the normal growth. It is essential that the food intake is adequate and wholesome; and its absorption and assimilation is not impaired. Kwashiorkor and marasmic children have a reduced growth rate and their growth curves are related to the time of malnutrition and its duration. Bone age is retarded in proportion to the stunting in height. Malabsorption syndromes due to giardiasis, tropical sprue, coeliac disease, non-specific ulcerative colitis, Crohn's disease must be looked for and excluded/treated in ail cases of malnutrition and short stature. In diabetes insipidus, food intake is usually reduced because of impaired appetite resulting from excessive fluid intake. Brain damage and mental retardation may also show similar symptomatology.

Many other inborn errors of metabolism like glycogen storage disease, aminoacidurias have stunting of growth as one of the presenting manifestations.

Caloric deprivation, malnutrition, uncontrolled diabetes mellitus, chronic renal failure, etc. result in abrogated GH receptor function. These conditions also stimulate production of pro-inflammatory cytokines including tumour necrosis factor-α (TNF-α) and ILs which block GH-mediated signal transduction. GH values are elevated as these conditions are associated with growth hormone resistance. This leads to low IGF-I and II values. Rarely, GH receptor antibodies are also formed.

Chronic ailments: Systemic ailments have to be severe and of some duration to affect growth adversely and result in short stature. Congenital heart disease, especially

TABLE 18.2.5

Syndromes	Salient features
Prader-Willi syndrome	Intrauterine and postnatal hypotonia, obesity, mental deficiency, hypogonadism. Small hands and feet, growth retardation may be mild. (Fig. 18.2.4)
Russel-Silver syndrome (Described independently by these two paediatricians in 1950s)	Asymmetry of limbs and body. Small triangular face, big forhead, short incurved 5th finger, renal anomalies, prenatal onset of growth failure (IUGR), mental development usually normal.
Noonan's syndrome	Neck webbing. Low hairline, shield chest, pectus excavatum, congenital heart, mental subnormality, small penis, cryptorchidism. Karyotype normal.
Cornelia de Lange's syndrome	Mental retardation, abnormal lips and mouth, short nose. Anteverted nostrils, thick eyebrows, long curly eyelashes, hypertonicity, abnormal cry
Bird-headed dwarfism (Seckel's syndrome)	Microcephaly. Premature synostosis. Mental subnormality, facial hypophasia, prominent nose, low set ears, cryptorchidism, growth failure.
Progeria (Hutchinson-Gilford syndrome)	Premature ageing. Severe growth failure
Cockayne's syndrome	Mental subnormality. Deafness, peripheral neuropathy, retinal pigmentation, optic atrophy, microcephaly, photosensitive dermatitis, premature ageing.
Leprechaunism	Intrauterine growth retardation. Prominent eyes, thick lips, large ears, large phallus, hyperplastic breasts, hirsutism, islet cell hyperplasia, ↑ insulin, and insulin resistance, severe growth failure.
Aarskog's syndrome	? X-linked. Growth failure. Hypertelorism, broad nasal bridge, short nose, anteverted nostrils, short broad hands and feet, dorsal scrotum fold surrounding penis (Shawl scrotum) cryptorchidism.

Salient features of some of the dysmorphic syndromes

cyanotic variety is usually associated with short stature. Once the defect is corrected, growth velocity improves and a dramatic compensatory growth spurt is seen. Similarly, chronic renal disease, chronic pulmonary infection or obstructive lung disease have growth retardation as one of their components. Mental retardation, severe brain damage, infections of the CNS also impair the growth pattern. The more severe the mental defect, the greater is the shortness of height.

Chromosomal and genetic causes: Many of the sex chromosomes abnormalities are associated with short stature. Turner's syndrome (45 XO) is always accompanied by reduction in linear growth. Many of these syndromes have peculiar chromosomal anomalies while others have metabolic problems. It is important to reach a definite diagnosis and evaluate patient's present and future intellectual ability to plan genetic counselling if needed. Many of the disorders are of unknown aetiology and occur as a result of single or multiple gene defects or environmental insults during embryogenesis. Typically the hormonal values are normal and bone maturation slightly delayed or normal. The Russel-Silver syndrome shows a normal skull circumference for age with some asymmetry of body growth. Noonan's syndrome has clinical features like those of Turner's syndrome (Fig. 18.2.3) but chromosomes are normal. Aarskog's syndrome is also associated with short stature. Progeria patient has alopecia, thin skin, lack of subcutaneous tissue, skeletal hypoplasia, periarticular fibrosis and arthritis. Joints are stiff and swollen and partially flexed. There is premature ageing with atherosclerosis and elevated cholesterol.

The Prader-Willi syndrome has shortness in height, gross obesity, mental subnormality, marked hypotonia small hands and feet and hypoplastic genitalia (Fig. 18.2.4). Later carbohydrate intolerance and diabetes mellitus develop. These children have both gonadotrophin defect and primary hypogonadism. Table 18.2.5 gives salient features of some of the better known dysmorphic syndromes.

Endocrine causes of short stature

i. Hypothyroidism: It is an important cause of short stature in countries where neonatal screening is not practised. The upper and lower segments proportions remain infantile, the naso-labial configuration stays immature and dental development is delayed. Bone age is retarded even more than the height and X-ray of the bones shows disturbed epiphyseal development and epiphyseal dysgenesis. The epiphysis is misshaped with irregular margins and fragmentation. With appropriate treatment, the linear growth rate increases along with bone maturation (Fig. 18.2.5). Usually a 'catch up' growth spurt is seen with treatment. Overtreatment should be avoided by periodic TSH monitoring as it may

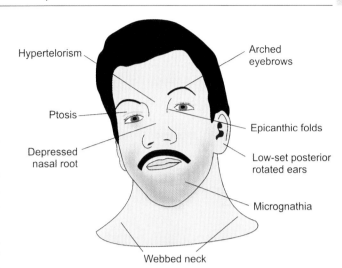

Fig. 18.2.3: Facial features in Noonan's syndrome

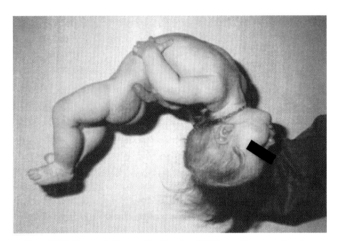

Fig. 18.2.4: An infant with Prader-Willi syndrome showing marked hypotonia

result in disproportionate advancement of bone age.

ii. Growth hormone deficiency: Growth hormone (GH) stimulates growth by initiating the production of insulin like growth factor especially IGF-I. Liver is the main source of circulating IGF-1. Bones and other tissues also make it. IGF-I is a potent growth and differentiation factor. Its effects on peripheral tissues are both dependent on and independent of GH. Both IGF-I and IGF-II are bound to one of the six IGF-binding proteins (IGFBPs). These binding proteins regulate IGF bioactivity.

• IGF-I levels increase during puberty, peak at 16 year and subsequently decline by about 80% during ageing. GH being the major determinant of hepatic IGF-I synthesis, GH synthesis abnormalities reduce IGF-I values.

Derby Hospitals NHS Foundation Trust

Library and Knowledge Service

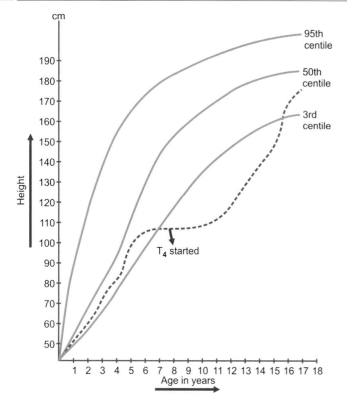

Fig. 18.2.5: Growth curve in a hypothyroid boy diagnosed at 9 years

TABLE 18.2.6

Conginital causes	Acquired causes
1. Genetic	
• Usually autosomal recessive occasionally X-linked or dominant	1. Tumours of the pituitary or hypothalamus, e.g. cranio-pharyngioma, hamartoma, neurofibroma, germinoma
• Familial isolated GH deficiency/panhypo-pituitarism	2. Heart injury or postsurgery
• Transcription factor defects	3. Granulomas, e.g. sarcoidosis, eosinophilic granuloma, post-meningitis especially tuber-culosis
• Mutation of growth related genes	4. Post- irradiation to the head
• Deletion of GH gene	5. Temporary GH failure due to other endocrine problems and emotional deprivation
2. Midline embryonic defects	
• Septaoptic dysplasia	
• Cleft lip and palate	
• Absence or hypoplasia of pituitary	
3. Pygmies	
4. Haemorrhagic infarction at birth, e.g. in breech presentation	

Common causes of growth hormone deficiency/impaired action

• Genetic disorders like pituitary transcription factor defect, mutation in growth related genes may be responsible for GH deficiency. GH deficiency even of the congenital type is often not absolute and such cases may respond to GH deficiency therapy. Laron type of dwarfism is unresponsive to GH therapy and is associated with high circulating levels of GH. In pygmies, the short stature is due to peripheral resistance to IGF-I.

In some patients there is isolated GH deficiency while in others there are multiple deficiencies. Most frequent affected hormones along with GH are gonadotrophins and TSH. Table 18.2.6 gives a list of common causes of GH deficiency/impaired action seen in clinical practice. Growth hormone does not influence *in utero* growth and, unlike hypothyroidism and IUGR, in GH deficiency the growth during the first few months is normal.

In GH deficiency, growth failure may become apparent by 6 months of life though it is often not obvious until 4 to 5 years or when child starts going to school and is evidently shorter than his peers. Rarely a GH deficient child may experience hypoglycaemia and come to the hospital as an emergency. Besides this rare presentation, the condition remains asymptomatic. After 3 years, the annual increment in height is usually less than 3 cm though it may increase to 5 cm per year around puberty which is usually delayed.

Clinically a GH deficient child appears plump with immature facies and genitalia. The limbs are delicate, muscular development is poor, head size is relatively large and dentition is delayed. Intelligence is normal unless hypoglycaemia has been severe and repeated with inadequate treatment. Eyes must be examined carefully for optic nerve dysplasia, atrophy and field defects. Nearly 30% of boys with isolated growth hormone deficiency have a small penis while in other 70%, the genitalia are immature and testes partially descended. All endocrine short statured children should have their skull X-ray for pituitary fossa, CT scan of pituitary and hypothalamus, bone age estimation and complete evaluation of GH and other endocrine gland evaluation.

Treatment: The clinical diagnosis of GH deficiency must always be confirmed by laboratory tests like GH profile during 24 hours or insulin tolerance test, arginine test, etc. At least 2 dynamic tests must be used to confirm GH deficiency. Additional endocrine tests will depend on suspected hormonal abnormalities and may include TSH, cortisol, metyrapone and synacthen stimulation tests.

Recombinant growth hormone (rGH) is recommended as specific replacement therapy in the dose of 0.175 to 0.350 mg/kg/week (or 0.02 to 0.05 mg/kg/day) The dose is better given daily before the child goes to sleep. This therapy is seen to be effective in Turner's syndrome, and chronic renal failure children also where higher dose (0.375 mg/kg/week) is recommended. The focus of treatment is to attain normal growth rates by this therapy.

Initially there used to be scarcity of GH supply as it was extracted from human pituitary glands at autopsy. One gland yielded as much as (7 mg) 14 units of purified hGH. At that time the usual dose could only to be 0.1 units/kg body weight given thrice a week. Now with the availability of recombinant growth hormone (rGH), the optimum dose presently is as recommended above.

With GH therapy, the GH deficient children almost always have an immediate spectacular acceleration in linear growth rate. It is a usual experience to see growth velocity as high as 15 to 16 cm/year during the first 3 months of treatment. Younger children respond better than adolescents. Similarly obese respond better than the thin, and severely deficient children respond better than those with partial deficiency. With treatment, invariably there is decline in growth response and after 2 to 3 years growth velocity declines and may even fall below normal. If this happens it may be advisable to stop therapy for 6 to 8 months. A renewed growth response is seen with resumption of therapy. Treatment should be continued as long as there is satisfactory growth response and reasonable adult height is reached (Figs 18.2.6 and 18.2.7).

Circulating antibodies to GH develop to a variable extent during GH therapy depending upon the preparations used. It could be in as low as 5 to 10% and as high as 60% of patients. Antibodies usually appear within the first few months of therapy and may persist as long as therapy is continued. If these antibodies attenuate growth, change of preparation sometimes is helpful. It is always advisable to check serum TSH and cortisol as GH therapy sometimes may produce hypothyroidism and/or hypo-adrenocortical state. Hormonal replacement may be

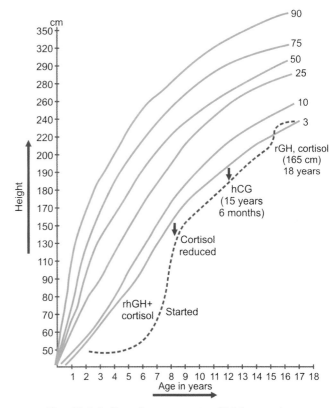

Fig. 18.2.6: Growth response to rGH therapy in a hypopituitary boy having multiple hormonal deficiencies

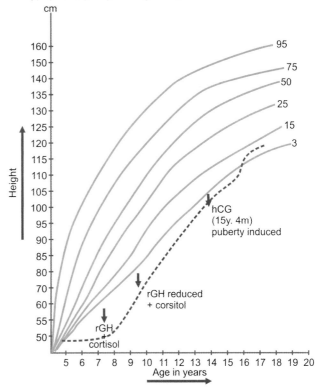

Fig. 18.2.7: Growth response to rGH therapy in a hypopituitary boy with GH deficiency

required in such cases. Another method to attain greater height in hypopituitary children is to use analogues of gonadotrophin releasing hormone (GnRH analogue) so as to delay the onset of puberty while GH therapy is continued.

Side effects of a rhGH are few. Pseudotumour cerebri, leukaemia especially in Down's syndrome, intracranial tumours have been reported in some patients with limited substantial evidence. Slipped capital femoral epiphyses and scoliosis have been reported.

It is advisable to continue rhGH therapy for 4 to 6 months even when growth ceases as the GH supports normal gonadal function and helps attain normal bone density.

There are several preparations of rhGH available in the market like serostim, nutropin, genotropin, humaprope, saizen, etc. All these preparations have similar effect. Nutropin depot is a long-acting preparation and its administration is recommended once or twice a month.

WHO rhGH reference reagent 88/624 for somatotrophin is 3 IU/mg.

iii. *Hypercortisolism:* Chronic elevated levels of circulating cortisol may be due to overactivity at pituitary or adrenal cortex, malignant disease or by exogenous cortisol administration. It is always associated with growth retardation in children. Both linear and skeletal growth are affected. High cortisol level reduces GH release and impairs its peripheral action.

iv. *Congenital adrenal hyperplasia (CAH)* Excess of androgens seen in CAH causes increased linear growth and skeletal maturation after birth. Ultimate height is usually reduced. The treatment of this condition is aimed at reducing ACTH production and thereby excess androgen production. This definitely slows down the skeletal growth, though rarely average height is achieved.

v. *Sexual precocity* In both, true precocious puberty as well as due to androgen secreting tumours, excessive skeletal growth and maturation is seen. This reduces the final height and juvenile body proportions with relatively short legs may be seen.

vi. *Psychosocial or emotional deprivation* Psychosocial and emotional deprivation is yet another important cause for short stature. Emotional deprivation leads to temporary hypothalamic disturbances with impaired release of GH and at times even corticotrophin. The child may refuse to eat or may develop a voracious appetite, thirst and pass large offensive stools with undigested food particles. In such cases,

the condition may have to be differentiated from the malabsorption syndrome.

Bone age is retarded proportional to the reduced height. Facial appearance is immature and so are the intellect and behaviour, GH and ACTH response to stimuli is blunted. Social history and interrelation assessment reveals gross incompatibility and disorder of the family relationship and environments.

Once the child is removed to secure atmosphere, the growth pattern gradually becomes normal. Many a time, parents also need psychological and social assistance.

Most of these children do not require any hormonal therapy as social and psychological help suffices.

Treatment of Short Stature

It depends when the underlying causative factor. Hypothyroid children attain their full height if the treatment is started in time (refer Fig. 18.2.5). Growth hormone deficient children respond very well to GH replacement therapy. In GH resistance/insensitivity syndrome, IGF-1 therapy (obtained by recombinant DNA technique) in the dose of 50 to 150 µg/kg/day is recommended. It is more expensive than GH therapy. There are some indications, though not totally substantiated, that IGF-1 therapy could be a cancer risk. Correction of congenital cardiac problem, treatment of chronic renal failure, malnutrition and care of the emotionally deprived children leads to attainment of a normal height in course of time.

In constitutional or familial delayed puberty, no therapy may be required. Sometimes, however, if puberty does not start in boys even by 15 to 16 years, there is a possibility of causing adverse psychological effects. In such cases judicious use of human chorionic gonadotrophin (hCG) is recommended. Similarly in girls if puberty does not set in by 14 to 15 years, oestrogen-progesterone therapy may be indicated. The therapy should be withdrawn after 3 to 6 months as usually it is followed by spontaneous menstruation.

For congenital short statured children, there is no ideal therapy though at times some response to GH therapy may be seen. Androgens and anabolics do not help much to increase the ultimate height as they accelerate skeletal maturation.

In our country adequate intake of wholesome nutrition, prevention of water borne diseases and timely treatment of infections is the core issue in most of the short statured children.

LINEAR CATCH-UP GROWTH

The concept of 'catch up growth' was first introduced in 1908 and the term was coined in 1963 by Prader et al. It is defined as height velocity above statistical limits of normality for age and/or maturity during a defined period of time, following a transient linear growth inhibition. It is supranormal linear growth which continues till the child has caught up with its pre-illness normal growth. The capacity to catch up is variable in different phases of growth. It differs from person to person and in the same person at various stages of development. Three types of catch up growth are usually described:

Type 1: In infancy and childhood, the catch-up growth is swift and may be 4 times the normal velocity.

Type 2: In adolescence, the catch-up growth is less dramatic and persists for a longer duration. The growth velocity may show no or very small increase.

Type 3: In this type, the catch-up growth has characteristics of both type 1 and type 2. In other words there is some increase in height velocity as well as delay and prolongation of growth.

It is observed that catch up growth is more intense at younger age and is favourable if the period of growth arrest is short. Immediate and absolute removal of growth inhibitory-condition (malnutrition, malabsorption, hypercortisolism, etc.) and initiation of appropriate therapy leads to complete catch up growth and attainment of potential target height.

Repeated episodes of growth inhibitory condition will result in lower catch-up rates in the subsequent periods and extremely delayed growth may not reach an appropriate final height. Availability of GH and IGF-I are essential for this phenomenon of catch-up growth to occur.

TALL STATURE

Most children with tall stature do not suffer from any detectable endocrine disease. They usually represent the upper end of the normal distribution of height. Very often there is family history of tallness in the parents. Table 18.2.7 enumerates the common causes of tallness or statural overgrowth.

TABLE 18.2.7

Causes	Salient manifestations
1. Constitutional or familial	Family history of tallness
2. Non-endocrine pathological causes	Systematic clinical examinations normal, no endocrinopathy:
a. Overnutrition and exogenous obesity	a. Gross weight gain accelerated linear growth.
b. Perinatal brain damage	b. History of difficult labor birth trauma, brain damage, mental subnormality.
c. Cerebral gigantism (Soto's syndrome)	c. Large elongated head, large ears and jaw, accelerated growth, early puberty.
d. Beckwith-Wiedemann syndrome	d. Newborn with macrosomia, macroglossia, hypoglycaemia, advanced bone age.
e. Arachnodactyly (Marfan's syndrome)	e. Long limbs, span > height, connective tissue defects.
f. Homocystinuria	f. Span > height, mental subnormality, excess homocystine in urine, thromboembolic disease.
g. Chromosomal syndrome	
i. Klinefelter's syndrome (47 XXY)	Eunuchoid proportions small testes, gynaecomastia.
ii. XYY karyotype	↑ testosterone, sometimes impaired intellect, and deviant behaviour, hairy ears.
3. Endocrine causes	
a. Gigantism (due to excess GH)	a. Eosinophilic or chromophobe tumours, Sella may be normal.
b. Sexual precocity	b. Early height increased, final height reduced
c. Eunuchoidism	c. Increased height due to delayed epiphyseal fusion
d. Total lipodystrophy	d. Absence of adipose tissue, muscular hypertrophy. Enlarged genitalia, Hyperlipidaemia. May be present ↑ GH and acanthosis nigricans
e. Hyperthyroidism	e. Modest acceleration of growth

Common causes and clinical manifestations of tall stature

Common Causes

Constitutional or Familial Tall Stature

This represents normal variant of the normal growth pattern and reflects the more complete realization of genetic potential. There is a strong family history of tallness in one or both parents and/or some of the first degree relatives. Children with constitutional advanced growth have increased growth hormone secretion as seen during sleeping hours. The final height can be predicted by the assessment of bone age. If the bone is advanced then the final height may not be excessive.

Overnutrition

Overnutrition leads to weight gain and obesity. Obese children are often taller than average for their age. Bone maturity is also advanced. Occasionally even puberty may occur earlier. Most of these obese children have normal birth weight. With the weight loss, the bone growth and maturity slow down.

Neonatal Brain Damage

Some children are overweight at birth and continue to grow rapidly in height. Their skeletal maturation lags behind only slightly. These children are the products of difficult labour and birth trauma. Some of them may even be subnormal mentally. It is postulated that probably growth aberration is also the result of brain damage.

Cerebral Gigantism (Soto's Syndrome)

In this syndrome, the growth is rapid for the first 5 to 6 years of life and then gradually slows down and becomes normal. The syndrome is characterised by the presence of gigantism, large head, prognathism, mental subnormality, high arched palate, frontal bossing, hyperteleorism, anti-mongoloid slant of the palpebral fissure and various neuromuscular disorders. These disorders manifest in ataxia, clumsy movements and an awkward gait. The lateral and third ventricles are usually dilated. Convulsions may appear. EEG is often abnormal. If the increase in growth occurs *in utero*, delivery may be difficult. Such children are above 90th centile for length and weight at birth. Endocrine parameters are normal and aetiology of the syndrome is unknown. Bone age is usually advanced and puberty occurs early. Therefore ultimately these individuals may not be noticeably tall as adults.

Beckwith-Wiedemann Syndrome

The newborns with this syndrome exhibit marked macrosomia, macroglossia, omphalocoele, and hypoglycaemia.

The hypoglyaemia is associated with islet cell hyperplasia and hyperinsulinism. It disappears during infancy. Accelerated growth continues. Skeletal maturation is advanced. In later life these patients exhibit a tendency to develop tumours. Hyperinsulinism is blamed for this syndrome. IGF-I is high normal or elevated.

Arachnodactyly (Marfan's Syndrome)

These patients usually have above average height and are not out of normal range. High arched palate, subluxated lens, myopia, tendency to retinal detachment valvular lesion, long fingers and narrow hands, long patellar ligaments, hyperextendable joints and kyphoscoliosis are some of the other prominent features of this syndrome. Arm span is longer than the height and lower segment is longer than upper segment. The increased length of the metacarpals has been used to calculate metacarpal index.

$$\frac{\text{Length}}{\text{Width}} = > 8.4 \text{ is abnormal}$$

Arachnodactyly is a congenital and often familial anomaly and it usually manifests at an early age. Death usually occurs in adult life due to aortic aneurysm which is rarely present in childhood.

Chromosomal Syndromes

Children with some chromosomal anomalies like XXY or XYY may have above average height. In XXY anomaly, the androgen deficiency is partly responsible for the tall stature.

Gigantism

Gigantism in childhood or adulthood is due to excess of circulating growth hormone. Besides elevated GH, these children demonstrate insulin resistance and even carbohydrate intolerance. Elevated GH is usually associated with chromophobe or eosinophilic adenoma. The pituitary fossa is not always enlarged. The clinical findings are classical and rarely pose any diagnostic difficulty. Both GH and IGF-I are elevated. Other endocrine hormones may also be affected if the tumour compresses the normal pituitary gland.

Sexual Precocity

Over production of sex hormones in a precocious child leads to accelerated linear growth and bone maturation. This results in above average early height but the final height is always reduced.

Eunuchoidism

Hypogonadism from any cause produces an increase in the linear growth due to delayed fusion of epiphyses. This will happen only if the GH secretion is not impaired.

Hyperthyroidism

Hyperthyroidism due to any cause and overtreatment of hypothyroidism with thyroxine leads to an increase in growth rate along with advanced bone age. Premature fusion of skull sutures with raised intracranial tension is also known to result due to a prolonged overtreatment with thyroxine.

Treatment of Tall Stature

It depends on the cause. Endocrine causes like excess of GH, thyrotoxicosis, hypogonadism require urgent appropriate treatment. Constitutional and familial tall stature rarely require any therapeutic intervention in boys. In girls sometime treatment is sought as too much height may lead to psychological problems. It is generally accepted that if a girl's final height is predicted to be in excess of 175 to 180 cm, hormonal intervention is justifiable, provided the girl and parents agree. Treatment is effective if it is started before the menarehe and before the bone age of 11.5 to 12 years. The safe and most acceptable treatment is to administer Ethinyl oestradiol 200 µg daily for 24 days along with norethisterone 5 µg daily from 15 day onwards for 10 days. The cycle is repeated after one week or after withdrawal bleeding has ceased. Treatment is continued until the growth curve has leveled off, bone age of 15 years achieved and epiphyses of the knee have united. Once the treatment is withdrawn, the menstruation proceeds in a normal cyclic manner. There are no long-term hazards of this therapy.

FURTHER READING

Normal Growth

1. Cole TJ. Secular trends in growth. Proc Nutr Soc 2000;59:117.
2. He Q, Karlberg J. BMI in childhood and its association with height gain, timing of puberty, and final height. Pediatr Res 2001;49-244-51.
3. Moggi-Cecchi J. Questions of growth. Nature 2001;414:595-7.
4. Tanner JM, Whitehouse RH, Marshal WA, et al. Assessment of skeletal maturity and prediction of adult height. TW2 Method, New York. Academic Press 1975.
5. Tanner JM. A history of the study of human growth. Cambridge University Press 1981; 286.
6. Wright CM, Cheetham TD. The strenghths and limitations of the parental heights as a predictor of attained height. Archives of Dissease in Childhood 1999; 8'(3): 257-60.

Short Stature

7. Soliman AT, Darwish A, Alsalmi I, Asfour M. Defective growth hormone secretion and hypogonadism in the new syndrome of congenital hypoparathyroidism, growth failure and dysmorphic features. Ind Jour Padiatr 1996; 63(5):679-82.
8. Krishna J. A rational approach to short stature: focus on use and abuse of growth hormone. Ind Journ Pediatr 1997;64(2):145-52.
9. Petry A, Richton S, Sy JP, Blethen SL. The effect of growth hormone treatment on stature in Aarskog syndrome. Jr Pediatr Endocrinology Metab 1999;12(2):161-5.
10. Rosenbloom AL. 1GF-1 deficiency due to GH receptor deficiency. Hormone and Metabolic Research 1999;31(2-3),161-7.
11. Haffner D, Schaefer F, Nissel R, Wuhl E, Tonshoff B, Mehls O. Effect of growth hormone treatment on the adult height of children with chronic renal failure. NEJM 2000;343(13):923-30.
12. Cutfield W, Lindberg A, Albergtsson Wikland K, Chatelain P, Ranke MB, Wilson P. Final height in idiopathic growth hormone deficiency: the Kigs experience. Kigs International Board. Acta Paediatrics 1999; 88(428): 72-5.

Linear Catch-up Growth

13. Prader A, Tanner JM, von Harnack GA. Catch-up growth following illness or starvation. An example of development canalization in man. J Pediatr 1963;62(2):646-81.
14. Williams JPG. Catch up growth. J Embryol Exp Morph 1981; 65(suppl);89.
15. Saxena Anita, Phadke R Shubha, Aggarwal SS. Ind Jr Pediatr 2000;67(3):225-30.

Tall Stature

16. Greulich WW, Pyle SI. Radiographic atlas of skeletal development of the hand and wrist. 2nd edition OUP London 1959.

18.3 Puberty and its Disorders

Y Sachdev

- Puberty and Hormonal Interplay, Stages of Puberty
- Disorders of Puberty:
  - Precocious Puberty: Central, Peripheral or Pseudo, Partial (Thelarche, Adrenarche, Menarche), Clinical Features, Management

- Deficient or Delayed Puberty: Constitutional, Hypothalamic Anterior Pituitary Dysfunction, Primary Gonadal Failure, Isolated Gn Deficiency (Kallmann's Syndrome), Isolated LH Deficiency or Fertile Eunuch Syndrome, Management

INTRODUCTION

Puberty is that stage of human growth and development which is characterised by a spurt in height and sexual development. Both these components of pubertal growth are accompanied by a distinct surge in the level of circulating growth and sex hormones and a change in the social outlook. Normal pubertal growth in both boys and girls is for about 2 to 3 years.

HORMONAL INTERPLAY

The normal growth in height and size is the result of interplay between hypothalamus, anterior pituitary and gonads. In the prepubertal child, very small amounts of gonadal steroids are able to suppress the gonadotrophin releasing activity of the hypothalamus and the anterior pituitary. However, a year or so before the onset of puberty, the suppressive effect of gonadal steroids starts waning and low levels of plasma luteinizing hormone (LH) become demonstrable during sleep. The average age of onset of puberty in boys is 11 to 12 years and in girls 10 to 11 years. Table 18.3.1 enumerates the various endocrine glands and their hormones affecting puberty.

The sleep-entrained LH (and to a lesser extent FSH) secretion occurs in a pulsatile fashion and reflects the endogenous episodic discharge of hypothalamic gonadotrophin/LH-releasing-hormone (GnRH/LHRH). Nocturnal pulses of LH continue to increase in frequency and amplitude as clinical puberty approaches. By mid puberty, LH pulses become evident even before sleep and occur at 60 to 120 minutes interval. It is the pulsatile secretion of gonadotrophin (Gn) that provides the initial stimulation for gonadal maturation. The major drive to the pituitary is pulsatile LHRH from the hypothalamic neurones, and their associated afferent inputs. This neurosecreting unit is known as the 'LHRH pulse generator.' Pineal melatonin has an inhibitory effect on LHRH pulses. At puberty, there is qualitative as well as quantitative change in LH and the ratio between bioactive and immunoreactive LH increases. Both FSH and LH act synergistically to promote changes in gonads at puberty (Fig. 18.3.1). A second critical event seen in girls at middle or late adolescence is the development of a positive feedback mechanism whereby rising oestrogen levels in midcycle cause a distinct increase of LH (Fig. 18.3.2). Prior to mid-adolescence, this ability of

TABLE 18.3.1

Endocrine gland	Hypothalamus	Anterior pituitary	Adrenal cortex	Testes	Ovaries
Hormones	Gonadotrophin releasing hormone (GnRH)	Luteinizing hormone (LH) and follicle stimulating hormone (FSH)	Androgen	Testosterone	Progesterone and oestrogen
Actions	Stimulates the anterior pituitary to secrete LH, FSH	LH controls the testosterone production from the testes. In girls, LH triggers ovulation and controls menstrual cycle. FSH controls spermatogenesis in boys and ovulation in girls.	Responsible for growth of axillary hair independent of other hormones.	Controls sexual development and maturation and functions of spermatozoa	Control the menstrual cycle along with LH, FSH. Oestrogens also control sexual development in girls

Endocrine glands and hormones affecting puberty

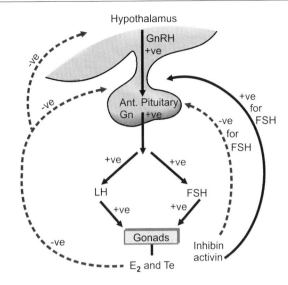

Fig. 18.3.1: LH, FSH feeback mechanism

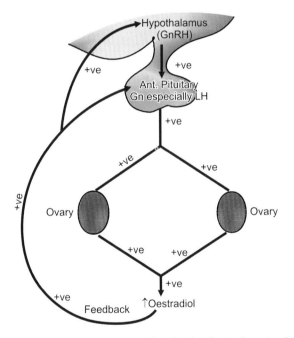

Fig. 18.3.2: Midcycle positive feedback effect of oestradiol on hypothalamic-anterior pituitary axis

oestrogens to release LH is not found. Adrenocortical androgens also play a role in pubertal maturation (adrenarche).

Dehydroepiandrosterone (DHEA) and dehydro-epiandrosterone sulphate (DHEAS) begin to rise around 6 years age-well before the increase of gonadotrophin, testosterone and oestrogens. This rise is more rapid in girls than in boys. Perhaps, there is an adrenal androgen stimulating factor other than ACTH which initiates adrenarche.

STAGES OF PUBERTY

The onset of puberty is more closely correlated with osseous maturation than chronological age.

In girls the breast is the first sign of puberty (10 to 11 years). Pubic hair growth begins within 6 months of breast bud. In some, pubic hair may appear first or simultaneously with the breast. Menarche appears 1 to 1½ years later (sometimes even 5 to 6 years later). In India mean age of menarche is 11.5 years. Axillary hair usually appears one year after pubic hair. Peak height velocity always precedes menarche and is attained 2 years earlier in girls than in boys. Wide variations, however, are seen in the sequence of changes involving growth spurt, appearance of breast bud, pubic hair and genital development. Genetic and environmental factors play a dominant role in this. Athletes, swimmers, runners and sports women demonstrate marked delay in attaining puberty and menarche.

In boys, the growth of the testes is the first sign of puberty (11½ to 12 years) followed by pigmentation of the scrotum and growth of the penis. Pubertal testicular size is 3 mm or >2.5 cm in length. Pubic hair then appears. Appearance of axillary hair usually marks the mid-point puberty. The voice deepens, acne and frequent erections occur and linear growth is accelerated. The growth acceleration in boys begins when puberty is well underway and is maximum from 14 to 16 years. Growth may continue well beyond 18 years. Figures 18.3.3 and 18.3.4 give the changes seen in growth of pubic hair. Figures 18.3.5 and 18.3.6 represent stages of breast development in girls and genital development in boys respectively.

DISORDERS OF PUBERTY

Precocious Puberty

Precocious puberty is difficult to define as marked age variations when normal puberty begins are seen. This is more so in the boys. However, it is generally accepted that if the onset of secondary sexual characteristics is before 8 years in girls and 9 years in boys, it may be considered precocious.

Precocious pubertal development is classified as:
a. True (central) precocious puberty.
b. Peripheral precocious puberty
    i. Isosexual
    ii. Heterosexual
c. Partial or incomplete precocious puberty
    i. Precocious or premature thelarche
    ii. Precocious or premature adrenarche
    iii. Precocious or premature menarche.

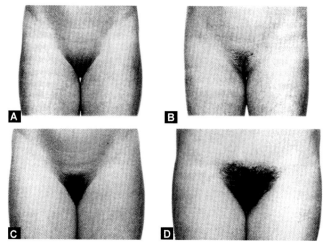

Figs 18.3.3A to D: Stages in normal female pubic hair development

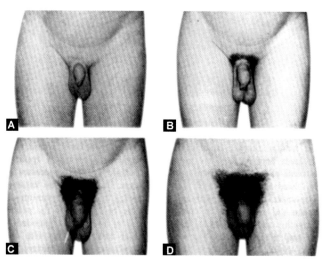

Figs 18.3.4A to D: Stages in normal male pubic hair growth

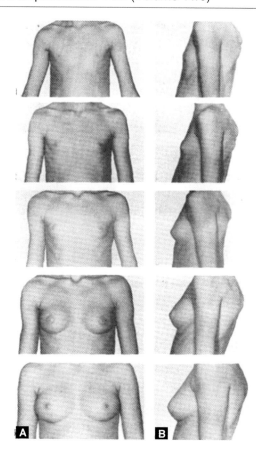

Figs 18.3.5A and B: Stages in normal female breast development [front (A) and lateral view (B)]

Table 18.3.2 enumerates the common conditions causing precocious puberty.

a. True (Central) Precocious Puberty

It is the result of premature activation of the hypo-thalamic-anterior pituitary-gonadal axis. The pubertal growth may or may not proceed in an orderly manner. It is the common form of puberty (>50%) and is much more common in girls. The precocity involves not only secondary sexual characteristics but also an increase in the size and activity of gonads including spermatogenesis in boys. The classical picture is always appropriate for the sex of rearing (isosexual). GnRH and gonadotrophin are elevated.

b. Pseudo (Peripheral) Precocious Puberty

It is not the result of premature activation of the hypothalamic-pituitary-gonadal axis. Gonads do not mature and only secondary sexual characteristics appear. If due to an ectopic hCG-producing tumour, then the condition may still be Gn-dependent. Tumours of adrenal, ovary and testes cause increased steroid secretions and signs of puberty which may be isosexual or heterosexual. Familial Gn-dependent puberty known as 'testotoxicosis' is a disorder with single base mutation in one of the transmembrane helix of the LH receptor. This change increases cAMP production, provides autonomy to Leydig cell and raises testosterone levels causing pseudo-precocious puberty. It is inherited as an autosomal dominant sex-linked fashion, but it can also occur sporadically. Carrier women can transmit the disease without manifesting any features.

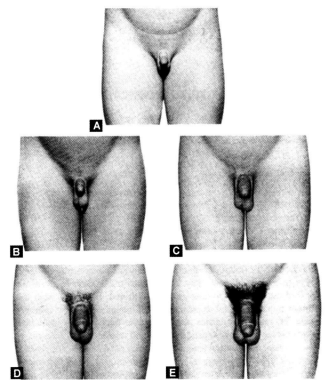

Figs 18.3.6A to E: Stages in normal male genital development

Incomplete or Partial Precocious Puberty

Precocious Thelarche

It is an early development of breast tissue in girls without other signs of puberty. Usually, it is unilateral or asymmetrical mostly seen between 1 to 2 years but may occur at any age. In some infants it is present at birth and persists. It may be a precursor of precocious puberty. Therefore such children must be kept under periodic observation. It may also be the result of exogenous exposure to oestrogens or associated with oestrogens-producing ovarian cysts/tumours. Benign thelarche may disappear spontaneously, fluctuate in size or persist till normal onset of puberty. Serum oestradiol and gonadotrophin levels are invariably low. Occasionally basal FSH is elevated and an exaggerated response to GnRH may be seen. In true precocious puberty LH secretion is predominant. Occurrence of thelarche in children after 2 years of age is usually due to some other cause than mere benign precocious thelarche. Exceptions to this, however, are there.

Precocious Adrenarche

It is an early development of pubic and axillary hair without other evidence of maturation. It is more common

TABLE 18.3.2

1. True (central) Precocious Puberty
   - Idiopathic (Constitutional, Functional) Male, Female
   - Central nervous system lesions
     Hypothalamic hamartoma, brain tumours, malformations, hydrocephalus
     Brain trauma, post-encephalitic scaring, prolonged untreated hypothyroidism, treatment of congenital adrenal hyperplasia, McCune-Albright-syndrome (late), administration of gonadotrophins
2. Pseudo (Peripheral) Precocious Puberty
   a. Females
      i. Isosexual: ovarian tumours, granulosa-theca cell tumours, teratoma, chorioepithelioma, autonomous ovarian cyst, McCune-Albright syndrome (early), adrenocortical tumours, exogenous administration of oestrogens
      ii. Heterosexual: Congenital adrenal hyperplasia, adrenocortical tumours, androgen producing tumours, testosterone producing tumours, exogenous administration of androgens
   b. Males
      i. Isosexual: Male-limited autosomal dominant precocious puberty, congenital adrenal hyperplasia, adrenocortical tumours, Leyding cell tumours, teratoma with adrenocortical tissue, hCG secreting tumours, hepatoblastoma, mediastinal tumours
      ii. Heterosexual: Adrenocortical tumour, exogenous administration of oestrogen, Sertoli cell tumour, sex-cord tumour with annular tubules
3. Incomplete or Partial Precocious Puberty
   Premature thelarche, adrenarche, menarche

Common conditions causing precocious puberty

in girls where it may be confined to pubic or labial hair growth alone (Pubarche). Hair appears first on labia majora and slowly spreads to the pubic region and finally it appear in the axilla. Affected children are mildly advanced in height and osseous maturation. DHEAS, androstenedione, 17-hydroxyprogesterone are higher as compared to age matched controls and are in the prepubertal range. This confirms that premature adrenarche is simply early maturational event of adrenal androgen production. Possibility of late onset of congenital adrenal hyperplasia and virilising adrenal tumours must be considered in this condition especially when it is associated with clitoral enlargement, acne and advanced bone age (>3SD above mean).

Premature Menarche

Isolated menses without other evidence of sexual development is less frequent. The majority of affected girls have a few (1 to 3) episodes of bleeding and puberty occurs at the usual time. Gn are normal and oestrogen is elevated. Local vaginal causes and ovarian follicular cysts must be rued out.

CAUSES OF PRECOCIOUS PUBERTY

True or Central Precocious Puberty

Some of the common conditions leading to true precocious puberty are described below.

Idiopathic (or Constitutional/Functional) Precocious Puberty

It is Gn-dependent and isosexual. There is no demonstrable anatomical intracranial lesion. It is common in girls (65%) and is usually sporadic. Sexual development is usually seen at very early age, between 4 to 8 years. Sometimes it may start even in infancy. It follows the same orderly sequence of events seen in normal puberty. The clinical course however is variable - may be rapid or slow, may stay static or even regress to resume development later. In both boys and girls, the height, weight and osseous maturation are advanced. Dental and mental development are usually normal. LH, FSH are usually elevated but may be normal. Serial blood estimations, however, reveal well defined pulsatile secretion of gonadotrophins especially during sleep with LH secretion predominating. There is brisk pubertal response to LHRH test. Abdominal ultrasonography reveals pubertal size enlarged ovaries. Testosterone in boys and oestrogen in girls are raised to pubertal range.

Precocious Puberty due to CNS Lesions

About 40 percent of boys and 10 per cent of girls with true precocious puberty have an intracranial tumour. As some grow slowly, there may be no neurological deficit. In others neuroendocrine manifestations may be present for 1 to 2 years before tumour is detected radiologically. Rapidly progressive sexual precocity in very young children suggests the likelihood of hamartoma of tuber cinerium. Hamartomas are developmental malformations consisting of ectopic hyperplastic neural tissue where the neurones secrete GnRH which activates the pituitary gonadal axis. Hamatomas do not grow and donot become maliganat. Tumours in the pineal region (germinoma, astrocytoma, etc.) cause precocious puberty in boys by secreting hCG which stimulates Leydig cells of the testes. Hypothalamic hamartoma is the most common tumour causing precocious puberty in boys. These tumours may be associated with gelastic seizures (uncontrolled crying/laughing). Other causes include

meningitis, encephalitis, cerebral abscess, neural tube abnormalities, tuberculosis and head trauma. All these conditions exert an adverse effect on the tonic control of GnRH secretion which normally operates in infancy and childhood. Postencephalitic scars, optic gliomas, ependymomas and neurofibromas may also result in precocious puberty. Hydrocephalus due to aqueduct stenosis even after successful surgery in infancy may lead later to precocious puberty. Similarly children with spina bifida sometimes develop early puberty. Irradiation to CNS is another factor which can lead to precocious or delayed puberty.

In all these conditions, the sexual precocity is always isosexual. Hypothalamic signs and symptoms like diabetes insipidus, adipsia, hyperthermia, obesity and cachexia may also be seen in some case. Precocious puberty has also been seen in young girls aged 4 to 9 years adopted from developing countries. This appears to be due to the rapid repair of undernutrition with increased production of free active steroid hormones, which could, in turn, stimulate hypothalamic pituitary gonadal axis.

Precocious puberty and hypothyroidism Onset of puberty in untreated hypothyroid children is usually delayed until epiphyseal maturation reaches 12 to 13 years. Precocious puberty in an untreated hypothyroid child however is not uncommon and presents with an unphysiological association of hypothyroid clinical picture, prepubertal bone age, and precocious puberty.

Affected children are usually severely hypothyroid for a long period. Sexual development in girls is primarily in the form of breast development and menstrual period. Boys show enlargement of testes without signs of virilization. Sella may be enlarged. Sometimes, there may be even suprasellar extension of the pituitary. Plasma levels of TSH, prolactin, FSH and LH are elevated. There appears to be preferential secretion of FSH over LH. This appears to be secondary to elevated TRH. As a result of this, there is testicular enlargement with no Leydig cell stimulation in boys. In girls, there is increased oestrogen secretion from the ovaries but there is no concomitant increase in androgens. This hypothyroid-associated precocious puberty is an incomplete form of Gn dependent puberty. Appropriate treatment of hypothyroidism corrects the clinical and biochemical manifestation.

Gonadotrophin-secreting tumours There are hCG producing hepatoblastomas, teratomas and germinoma in the pineal body and hypothalamus area. They stimulate premature maturation of the testes and cause precocious puberty in males. The reason appears to be a cross reaction between hCG and LH. Plasma levels of hCG and alpha-fetoproteins are usually elevated in hepatic tumours and are useful markers to assess the effects of treatment. Intracranial hCG producing tumours are not common in girls and rarely produce precocious puberty. This probably is due to the fact that complete ovarian function cannot occur without FSH priming.

Adrenal Causes of Precocious Puberty

Adrenal tumours or adrenal hyperplasia due to 21 or 11 beta-hydroxylase enzyme deficiency result in virilization. Generally these conditions are associated with small (appropriate for the age of the child rather than its apparent pubertal status) testes. In females, genitalia at birth are ambiguous. Late onset adrenal hyperplasia females present with hirsutism, irregular menses and infertility. Androstenedione, DHEA, and other adrenal androgens are elevated. Bone age is advanced. Treatment with appropriate doses of glucocorticoids, combined with mineralocorticoids, if necessary, is very effective. Some patients may progress to true precocious puberty when androgen concentration is reduced to normal. In such cases GnRH agonist therapy is useful.

Ovarian Causes of Precocious Puberty

In girls, ovarian cysts and tumours may cause signs of pseudo-precocious puberty. Simple follicular cysts may occasionally secrete sufficient oestrogen to promote breast development and vaginal bleeding. Granulosa and theca cell tumours are the most likely ovarian tumours to cause endocrine disturbances in girls. Ingestion of oestrogens and use of oestrogen containing creams cause breast development and withdrawal vaginal bleeding.

Testicular Causes of Precocious Puberty

Testicular tumours and testicular adrenal rests may result in precocious puberty. This is due to direct synthesis of androgens or oestrogens from the tumour or production of hCG which stimulates sex steroids secretion. Prepubertally the precocity is isosexual while in adult males features of feminisation with gynaecomastia may be seen due to imbalance of androgen/oestrogen ratio. Treatment is dependent on the type of the tumour and consists of surgical removal, irradiation to areas of lymphatic drainage and chemotherapy. Fragile X-syndrome causes macro-orchidism.

McCune-Albright Syndrome

It is a specific syndrome associated with:
a. Precocious puberty
b. Neck and back cafe-au-lait skin pigmentation and
c. Polyostotic fibrous dysplasia of the bones.

The skin lesions are brown, non-elevated and pigmented. They correspond usually to the same side as bone lesions and rarely cross the midline. The syndrome is common in girls who may present with vaginal bleeding and other secondary sex characteristics before other signs of puberty. The average age of onset is about 3 years, though it may be seen as early as 4 to 6 months. Ovarian cysts are often palpable on rectal examination and are visualized on ultrasonography examination of the pelvis. Autonomous hyperfunctional states of extragonadal endocrines like hyperprolactinaemia, hyperthyroidism, acromegaly and Cushing's syndrome may also be associated. Precocity is due to functioning luteinized follicular cysts of the ovary independent of gonadotrophins. It is believed that the disorder is caused by somatic mutation in a gene that encodes the α subunit of protein Gs which stimulates adenylate cyclase. This increases cyclic AMP resulting in precocious gonadal steroid production. The change in protein Gs also modifies the ion channels and calcium pump modulation, producing effects in other systems.

LH, FSH values are suppressed and there is no response to LRH stimulation. Oestradiol levels vary from the normal to markedly elevated (>900 pg/ml) levels. LHRH agonists do not help. Later on when pubertal age is reached true precocious puberty (Gn-dependent) may supercede the antecedent pseudo-puberty (Gn-independent), menstrual periods become regular and even fertility has been documented. Many a time functioning ovarian cysts disappear spontaneously and rarely need aspiration/surgery.

Affected boys may have asymmetrical enlargement of the testes in addition to the signs of sexual precocity. Repeated fractures may result from bony lesions. The associated hyperthyroidism usually has a multinodular goitre while the Cushing's syndrome is characterised by bilateral adrenocortical nodular hyperplasia.

CLINICAL FEATURES OF PRECOCIOUS PUBERTY

The development of a breast bud or an increase in the testicular volume are the first signs of puberty in girls and boys respectively. Idiopathic true puberty in girls usually follows the same orderly sequence of events characteristic of normal puberty. Vaginal bleeding may be the presenting feature in the McCune-Albright syndrome. When precocious puberty is idiopathic, the presenting age is usually between 4 to 8 years at times it may start even in infancy. Sometimes tall stature, increased growth velocity and advanced bone age may be the only presenting features in a girl. Although serum gonadotrophin levels are within the pubertal range, the progression through all definitive stages may not be seen. Boys with penile enlargement, pubic and axillary hair growth, acne, increased muscle development and small testes have pseudo precocious puberty. The likely cause is an adrenal tumour or congenital hyperplasia.

MANAGEMENT OF PRECOCIOUS PUBERTY

A detailed clinical examination including age of onset of precocity, perinatal and family history, anthropometry, evidence of congenital anomalies, blood pressure reading, fundi, visual fields, galactorrhoea, grades of pubertal growth, mental, dental and bone age must be documented. Bone age is usually advanced by 4 to 5 years except in hypothyroidism where it is delayed. Ovarian mass may be felt per abdomen or by rectal examination. Investigations include evaluation of colour of the vaginal mucosa and discharge, skull X-ray to rule out intracranial space occupying lesion, estimation of hormones include testosterone, oestrogen, hCG, and GnRH test. Sex hormones are elevated in true precocious puberty. A peak serum LH level >10 IU/L following GnRH test is a reliable evidence of central precocious puberty. Plasma 17-hydroxyprogesterone and 11-deoxycortisol are elevated in 21 and 11β hydroxylase enzyme deficiencies respectively. Dehydroepiandrosterone and androstenedione are markedly elevated in androgen secreting adrenal tumours. Elevated LH value with normal FSH values, particularly in a boy is a pointer to hCG secreting tumour and must be confirmed by specific βhCG radioimmunoassay. If gonadotrophin are low but sex steroid are raised then gonadal or adrenal autonomous source is to be suspected.

CT scan/MRI and ultrasonography of abdomen and pelvis may be required to evaluate ovarian, uterine and adrenal status. Skeletal survey is useful when McCune-Albright syndrome is suspected.

If bone age is not advanced and there is no hypothyroidism, probably it is a case of early normal puberty. Such children should have a close follow-up every 3 to 6 months. In other cases, treatment should be definitive wherever possible. An underlying cause must be excluded particularly in boys. Surgical removal of CNS, adrenal and gonadal tumours and predunculated hypothalamic hamartomas wherever feasible is recommended. Some of the tumours are radiosensitive, Unpedunculated hypothalamic hamartomas do better with medical treatment (GnRHa) and surgical intervention is almost never necessary. Hypothyroidism is treated with appropriate thyroxine replacement.

Symptomatic treatment aims to stop further pubertal growth, promote regression of existing signs and reduce the acceleration in growth velocity and skeletal maturation.

Therapeutic agents used inhibit Gn secretion and in turn sex steroids formation. They are:

Long-Acting Agonists of GnRH

The GnRH agonists are synthetic analogues of the natural decapeptide. Chemical substitutions at positions 6 and 10 of the GnRH molecule increase the resistance to enzymatic degradation and improve the affinity to the receptor on pituitary gonadotrophs. Some GnRH analogues have upto 200 times, the potency of the natural hormone, with prolonged action and low toxicity.

Continuous stimulation of the pituitary gland by GnRH agonists suppresses the pulsatile LH and FSH releases with subsequent decrease in gonadal steroid and gametogenesis.

There are various commercial forms of GnRH analogues with different administration routes.

a. Nasal treatment (Nafarelin and buserelin) is not as effective as long-term IM or SC treatment. The nasal therapy has to be repeated twice or thrice daily.

b. The long acting depot preparations most frequently used are
   - Leuprolide depot
   - Triptorelin and
   - Goserelin

They are administered IM (gluteal region) or SC. The recommended dose is (140 to 300 µg/kg) 3.75 mg every 21 to 28 days or 11.25 mg every 3 months. A special preparation of long-acting goserelin (10.8 mg biodegradable depot) is administered every 10 to 12 weeks. Histrelin (8 to 10 µg/kg/day) and leucoprolide (20 to 50 µg/kg/day) are also available in short acting subcutaneous formulations for daily doses.

In short statured patients GnRHa may be combined with rhGH 0.1l U/kg/day subcutaneous 6 days a week for 2 to 3 years to achieve normal height. GnRHa is also recommended in cases of congenital adrenal hyperplasia (CAH) and McCune-Albright syndrome (MAS) to delay the onset and progression of true precocious puberty. Adrenal androgens production is not suppressed by GnRH analogues.

Progestational Agents

These were the mainstay of treatment before GnRHa therapy. They are:
   a. Medroprogesterone acetate 10 to 20 mg daily orally or IM depot injections 100 to 200 mg × every 2 weeks and

b. Cyproterone acetate 100 to 150 mg daily orally. Its use is also recommended in the early stages of treatment with GnRHa as initially there might be accleration of puberty.

Progesteronal agents stop breast development and menses in girls. Cyproterone acetate has both anti-androgenic and anti-gonadotrophic activity. It reduces testicular size and aggressive behaviour in boys and pubic hair regresses. However, neither drug is effective in halting skeletal maturation. Side effects are weight gain and adrenal suppression.

(i) Traditionally, the girls with MAS are managed with aromatase inhibitors like adrenal testolactone (23 mg/kg/day) which stops the conversion of testosterone to oestradiol and androstenedione to oestrone. Sometimes, the effect of testolactone wanes after a few years. Progestational agents are the second choice and have also been used. The results with progestational agents have been disappointing.

(ii) Testotoxicosis is managed with ketoconazole, an imidazole derivative, which inhibits testicular and adrenal steroidogenesis by blocking the P-450 enzyme, $CYPH_{11}A$, that stops the 20, 22 desmolase activity, responsible for conversion of cholesterol to pregnanolone. Progestational agents have also been used but are not more effective.

DEFICIENT OR DELAYED PUBERTY

Some children fail to register a normal spurt of growth with sexual development at the usual time (13 in the girls and 14 in the boys) but eventually undergo puberty by 16 years or later. Thereafter, adolescence may progress rapidly or at a slower pace when growth may continue until 20 to 22 years of age. It is advisable to see an endocrinologist if there are no signs of puberty by 14 years in girls and a 14½ years in boys. There are three main causes of delayed puberty:
a. Constitutional delayed puberty
b. Hypothalamic-anterior pituitary dysfunction
c Primary gonadal failure.

Constitutional Delayed Puberty

These children probably represent the lower end of the normal distribution curve. Most of the short stature children coming for consultation belong to this group. The weight usually remains normal throughout childhood, however, the height is below average and epiphyseal development is retarded. Puberty and its attendant growth spurt are delayed. The growth is prolonged because of the late epiphyseal fusion. Such patients usually attain normal height and development without treatment.

Sometimes, there are psychological disturbance because of delayed puberty, specially so if a younger sibling forges ahead. In such cases it is justified to initiate pubertal growth by hormone therapy. In boys, a course of hCG is given by IM injections in a dose of 500 to 1000 IU twice a week for 3 to 6 months. Alternatively, testosterone enanthate, 100 mg is given IM once a month for 3 to 6 months. This should not be started before 14 to 15 year, oral testosterone is less reliable. In case the main concern is the short stature and not lack of sexual characteristics, a growth spurt can be started by using low dose (½ or 1 tablet of oxandrolone every day for 3 to 4 months. In girls, ethinyl oestradiol 5 to 10 µg or conjugated oestrogen 0.3 mg/daily is given for about 3 to 6 months but not before 13 to 14 years age. If and when breakthrough bleeding occurs, progesterone (5 mg daily for the last 10 days) is added cyclically. The treatment is interrupted at intervals of 3 months or so to see if spontaneous development has begun. It has been seen that children with extremely delayed puberty may not reach a final height appropriate for their parental height. In many such cases this is associated with poor or inadequate growth of the spine and may lead to osteoporosis in later life. Such children are another indication for treatment. Table 18.3.3 compares the clinical features of some of the common causes of delayed puberty.

Delayed Puberty due to Hypothalamic-anterior Pituitary Dysfunction

This could be the result of craniophyrangioma, germinoma of CNS, panhypopituitarism due to various causes, extra pituitary disorders or known syndromes like Prader-Willi syndrome (obesity, mental retardation, hypotonia, delayed puberty), Laurence-Moon-Biedl syndrome (obesity, mental retardation, polydactyly, retinitis pigmentosa, delayed puberty) and chronic systemic infections/diseases. Delayed puberty may also be due to isolated Gn deficiency.

Isolated Gn Deficiency or Kallmann's Syndrome

It is also known as idiopathic hypogonadotrophic hypogonadism. This uncommon disorder was originally described as a familial syndrome associated with anosmia. It occurs both in familial and sporadic forms with or without anosmia. The term 'Kallmann's syndrome' is used to refer to both the sporadic and familial forms with or without anosmia. The syndrome is suspected because of failure to undergo puberty. In

TABLE 18.3.3

Clinical features	Constitutional delayed puberty	Growth hormone deficiency	Isolated gonado-trophin deficiency (Kallmann's syndrome)	Gonadal dysgenesis	Coeliac disease
Family history	Positive	Usually positive	May be positive or negative	Usually negative	Occasionally positive
Birth weight and height	Normal	Normal	Normal	Slightly reduced	Normal
Pattern of growth	Slow from birth	Slow from few months after birth	Normal	Slow from birth	Slow from introduction of cereals
Epiphyseal development	Moderate retardation	Progressive retardation	Usually retarded	Normal but wide variations	Progressive retardation
Features	Immature initially, normal later	Immature	Multiple associated anomalies	Often characteristic features	Immature
Puberty	Late but eventually normal	Usually delayed unless solitary GH deficiency	Delayed	Usually delayed unless mosaic	Delayed
GH level	Normal	Low	Normal	Normal	Normal
Gn level	Normal	Low unless solitary GH deficiency	Low	Raised	Normal

Clinical features of common cause of delayed puberty

childhood it is suspected if there is microphallus and/or cryptorchidism. Growth pattern in childhood is normal, bone age is usually retarded. Some patients, particularly of familial form, have congenital midline facial and head structure defects, besides microphallus and cryptorchidism. Cleft palate, harelip, cranio-facial asymmetry, mental subnormality, syndactyly, short 4th metacarpal, colour blindness, nerve deafness and renal anomalies are the other congenital defects which may be present. The syndrome is more common in males and is due to GnRH deficiency. LH, FSH are low but show a normal response to GnRH. In females it presents as primary amenorrhoea and sexual infantilism. Inheritance is either X-linked or autosomal dominant or autosomal recessive. More than one mutant gene appear to be responsible. Diagnosis is confirmed when clomiphene citras fails to stimulate a normal rise in FSH, LH or testosterone but a normal response is seen to GnRH administration. Treatment ideally is episodic administration of LHRH. Recommended initial dose is 25 ng/kg given S/C every 2 hours through an infusion pump. Testosterone (Te), LH and FSH are monitored and GnRH dose is increased till testosterone value reaches midnormal range. LHRH therapy recreates the pattern of hypothalamic pulse generator. It should be reserved in those cases where infertility is the main problem. Long-acting testosterone or hCG therapy alone works well to promote penile size and pubertal changes. Without treatment, the patient remains eunuchoid, impotent and infertile.

Isolated LH Deficiency or Fertile Eunuch Syndrome

These eunuchoid patients have normal FSH and spermatogenesis (usually oligospermia) but low or undetectable LH. LH probably is enough to allow spermatogenesis but is not sufficient for full development of secondary sex characteristics. Testosterone therapy may be necessary for sexual maturation. hCG may be required to improve semen volume and sperm count.

Primary Gonadal Dysfunctions Leading to Delayed Puberty

Testicular Failure

Nearly all testicular disorders (development defects, sex chromosomes abnormalities with gonadal dysgenesis (Klinefelter's syndrome), local trauma, infections, systemic disease) can lead to partial or total failure of puberty. Gn are elevated while testosterone is diminished.

Ovarian Failure

This could be due to hypoplasia, gonadal dysgenesis, chromosomal abnormalities with gonadal dysgenesis (Turner's syndrome), ovarian autoimmune disease, irradiation or surgical removal of ovaries. Primary or secondary amenorrhoea are the usual presenting features. Hyperandrogenism due to CAH, polycystic ovary syndrome or androgen producing ovarian tumours may be associated with failure of sexual maturation or its regression. Effective treatment of the primary condition results in normal puberty.

SUMMARY

Growth and development is a dynamic continuous process which starts in-utero. The foetal growth is mainly dependent on maternal, placental and foetal factors. Hormones have a marginal effect only. Infancy and childhood growth is essentially dependent on thyroid and growth hormones; in the adolescence, growth is gonadal whereas growth hormones play the pivotal role during puberty. There is an intricate interplay of various hormones like GnRH, gonadotrophins, gonadal secretions, adrenocortical hormones especially androgens.

A defect in chromosomal, genetic, endocrinal, environmental, nutritional and emotional sphere can play havoc with this normal process of growth and development resulting in short or tall stature, precocious or deficient puberty. The various conditions, syndromes and dysfunctional states responsible for these abnormalities are discussed with their clinical manifestations and management.

FURTHER READING

Puberty

1. David R. Beier, Robert G Dluhy. Bench and bedside—The G protein coupled receptor GPR54 and puberty. N Engl J Med 2003; 349:1589-92.
2. Drife JO. Breast development in puberty. Ann NY Acad Sci 1986; 464: 58-65.
3. Grumbach MM. Onset of puberty. In Berenberg SR (Ed): Puberty: Biologic and Social Components Leiden. HE stanfort. Kroese 1975; pi.
4. Lee PA, GUO SS, Kulin HE. Age of puberty: data from the United States of America. APMIS 2001;109:81-8.
5. Marshall WA, Tanner JM. In Flanker F, Tanner JM (Eds): Puberty: Human Growth. New York Plenum 1986;171.
6. Rosenfield RL. Puberty and its disorder in girls. Endocrinology and Metabolism Clinics of North America. Puberty and its Disorders 1991 (March): 15-42
7. Schmidt U, Evans K, Tiller J, Treasure J. Puberty, sexual milestones and abuse: how are they related to eating disorders in patients. Psychological Medicine 1995;25 (2):413-7.
8. Stephanie B Seminara, Sophie Messager, Emmanovella E, Chatzidaki et al. The GPR54 Gene as a regulator of puberty. N Engl J Med 2003;349:1614-7.
9. Styne DM. Childhood and adolescent obesity. Prevalence and significance. Pediatr Clin North Am 2001;48:823.
10. Styne DM, Grumbach MM. Puberty in boys and girls in PFAFF DW (ed): Hormone, Brain and Behaviour. Philadelphia: Elsevier 2002, 661-716.
11. Sachdev YR. Disorders of puberty. In Siddharth N Shah (Ed): API Textbook of Medicine 2003;1089-92.
12. Tanner JM. Growth at adolescence. Springfield III, Charles C, Thomas 1962.
13. Wu FCW, Buttler GE, Kelnar CJH, Huhtaniemi I, Veldhuis JD. Ontogeny of pulsatile gonadotrophin releasing hormone secretion from mid childhood, through puberty, to adulthood in the human male: a study using deconvolution analysis and an ultrasensitive immunofluorometric assay. J Clin Endocrinol Metab 1996; 81:1798-1805.

Precocious Puberty

14. Paasquino AM, Pucarelli I, Roggini M, Segni M. Adult height in short normal girls treated with gonadotrophin-releasing hormone analogs and growth hormone. The Clinical Endocrinol and Metab 2000; 85 (2): 619-22.
15. Kaplan SL, Grumbach MM. Clinical review 14: Pathophysiology and treatment of sexual precocity. J Clin Endicrinol Metab 1990; 71 :785-9.
16. Kappy MS, Ganoung CS. Advances in the treatment of precocious puberty. Advances in Pediatrics 1994; 41:223-59.
17. Lee PA, Advances in the management of precocious puberty. Clin Pediatr 1994;33: 54-61.
18. Fahmy JL, Kaminsky CK, Kaufman F, Nelson MD Jr, Paris MT. The radiological approach to precocious puberty. Br J Radiology 2000;73 (869):560.

Delayed Puberty

19. Rosenfield RL. The diagnosis and management of delayed puberty. J Clin Endocrinol Metab 1990;70:559-62.
20. Ranke MB, Guilband O, Lindberg A, Cole T. Prediction of growth response in children with various growth disorders treated with growth hormone. Analysis of data from the Kabi Pharmacia International Growth Study. Acta Pediatr (Suppl) 1993; 391:82-8.
21. Prader A. Delayed adolescence. Clin Endocrinol Metab 1975; 4: 143-55.
22. Shah Nalini. Delayed puberty. Ind J Pediatr 1997;64:159-64.
23. Brook CG. Treatment of late puberty. Hormone Research 1999; 51(SuppJ 3): 101-4.

18.4 Turner's Syndrome

Y Sachdev

INTRODUCTION

Turner's syndrome is a common chromosomal disorder (1 in 2000 live born phenotypic females) that is not diagnosed frequently till adolescence or adulthood. Early recognition of the syndrome ensures timely initiation of therapy to promote growth and normalize secondary sexual development. An early diagnosis also helps in child and family counselling.

DEFINITION

It was Henry Turner who in 1938 reported seven phenotypic females with short stature, sexual infantilism, webbing of the neck, low posterior hairline, and increased carrying angle of the elbows. In 1930, Ullrich had retrospectively described similar clinical features in an 8-year-old girl while Bonnevie had observed sex related congenital anomalies in mice. Thus, the syndrome has also been called Bonnevie -Ullrich or Ullrich-Turner syndrome.

AETIOLOGY

The chromosomal pattern in Turner's syndrome is characterized by an abnormality of one of the X chromosomes. These errors include:
a. Total absence of one X chromosome (45 XO).
b. Structural abnormality in one of the X chromosomes.
c. Mosaicism with at least one cell line that has an abnormal X chromosome.

In the characteristic karyotype of a patient with 45 XO Turner's syndrome, the abnormality may arise from meiotic non-disjunction due to failure of a pair of sister chromatids to separate during anaphase. The resulting egg (or possibly, sperm) has 22 chromosomes, but no sex chromosome. This aneuploidy may also result from anaphase lag, in which a chromosome is lost from a cell during cell division. Typically, the 45 X karyotype is associated with the absence of the Barr body. Nearly 60%

of Turner's syndrome patients have 45 X karyotype while in 20% there are structural abnormalities of one of the X chromosomes. The remaining 20% of patients with Turner's syndrome have a mosaic pattern.

INCIDENCE

The incidence of this syndrome in India is not known. In USA, it is estimated to be 1 in 2000 live-born plenotypic females. A large number of Turner's syndrome foetuses do not survive beyond 28 weeks of gestation, contributing nearly 6 to 7% of all spontaneous abortions.

CLINICAL FEATURES (Figs 18.4.1 and 18.4.2)

The clinical manifestations are variable and many of the classical features like webbing of the neck and low posterior hairline may be absent. Table 18.4.1 represents the major clinical features of the syndrome whereas Table 18.4.2 addresses the chronological presentation. It is important to appreciate that it is not usual to find all features of the syndrome in one individual patient.

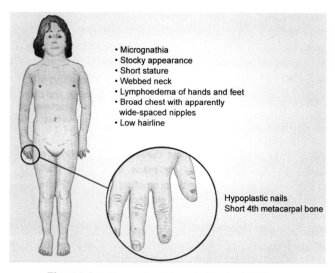

- Micrognathia
- Stocky appearance
- Short stature
- Webbed neck
- Lymphoedema of hands and feet
- Broad chest with apparently wide-spaced nipples
- Low hairline

Hypoplastic nails
Short 4th metacarpal bone

Fig. 18.4.1: Turner's girl and classical features

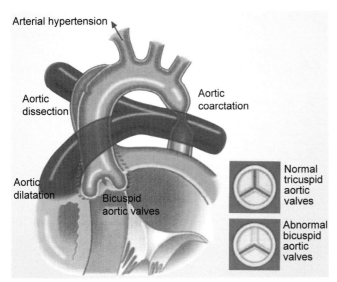

Fig. 18.4.2: Some other features of Turner's syndrome

TABLE 18.4.1

Skeletal growth:
    Short stature (100%), short neck (40%), abnormal upper/lower segment ratio (97%), cubitus valgus (47%), short metacarpals (37%), scoliosis (13%) genu valgum (85%), characteristic facies (micrognathia) 60%, high arched palate (38%)

Face and neck:
    Webbed neck (25%), low posterior hairline (42%), rotated ears (common), oedema of hands and feet (22%), nail dysplasia (13%), typical dermatographics (35%)

Germ cell defects:
    Gonadal failure (96%); infertility (>99%)

Miscellaneous defects:
    Strabismus (18%), Ptosis (11%), multiple pigmented naevi (26%), cardiovascular abnormalities (55%), hypertension (7%), renal and renovascular abnormalities (39%)

Associated disorders:
    Carbohydrate intolerance (40%), Hashimoto's thyroiditis (34%), hypothyroidism (10%), alopecia, vitiligo (rarely)

Clinical features in Turner's syndrome

Endocrine Profile

Elevated LH, FSH even in infancy is usually seen. In late childhood and adolescence, values may be normal. FT_3, FT_4, TSH and microsomal (TPO) antibodies should be estimated in view of high incidence of autoimmune thyroiditis.

Growth

Short stature is the most common clinical finding. Children with Turner's syndrome tend to deviate progressively from the normal height percentile until the

TABLE 18.4.2

Newborn: 10 to 25% of Turner's patients present in the immediate newborn period, typically with lymphoedema of the hands and feet, redundant skin folds in the back of the neck and webbing of the neck.

Infant: The diagnosis of the Turner's syndrome is occasionally made in the evaluation of an infant with a heart murmur resulting from coarctation of the aorta or aortic stenosis.

Child: From infancy until early adolescence, the most common clinical sign is short stature. Because the phenotypic presentation of Turner's syndrome is so highly variable, the diagnosis of Turner's syndrome must be considered in any girl with unexplained short stature. Epicanthal folds, ptosis, lowset ears and micrognathia are other facial features commonly seen in Turner's syndrome.

Early adolescence: The diagnosis of Turner's syndrome must be considered for any girl with delayed puberty (failure to achieve early breast development by the age of 13 years) or arrested puberty. Appearance of sparse public or axillary hair resulting from adrenal androgen production may be observed in girls with Turner's syndrome and does not constitute evidence of normal ovarian development.

Late adolescence: Girls with Turner's syndrome may present between the ages 13 and 18 years for evaluation for primary amenorrhoea. When delayed menarche is observed in combination with short stature, the diagnosis of Turner's syndrome must be seriously considered. Recurrent otitis media ± conductive hearing loss.

Adulthood: On those occasions when early puberty has appeared, with or without menarche, the diagnosis of Turner's syndrome may be missed. Such patients may present in adult life with infertility, menstrual irregularities, or short stature.

Common clinical presentation of Turner's syndrome

age of 14 years: thereafter they tend to approach the normal percentile as their growth, though gradual, gets prolonged due to delayed epiphyseal fusion. Final height is around 146 to 150 cm. Several distinct phases in growth of Turner's syndrome girls have been recognized:

- Mild intrauterine growth retardation
- Normal mean height gain from birth to 3 years
- Progressively decline thereafter till 14 years
- A prolonged adolescent growth with partial return to normal height

Short stature and sexual infantilism are invariable features of Turner's syndrome. The short stature is due to loss of a homeobox-containing gene located in the pseudoautosomal region (PAR) of the short arms of the X (Xp22) and yp 11,3 chromosomes which encodes an osteogenic factor. The gene is called SHOX (short stature homeobox-containing gene or PHOG (pseudo autosomal homeobox-osteogenic gene).

MANAGEMENT

It depends upon early diagnosis, and recognition of the various ramifications of the syndrome. The diagnosis and its implications must be discussed with the parents as well as the child when she is old enough to understand. It needs to be stressed that the child is definitely female and if managed properly is capable to normal sexual maturity, functioning to lead a productive happy life.

Hormonal Therapy for Gonadal Failure

The initiation of oestrogen therapy should be delayed till the child has maximized the height. As such we usually do not prescribe it till the age of 15 to 16 years. Conjugated oestrogens (initially as low as 0.3 mg/day) in a cyclic manner with progestational agent (medoxy-progesterone 5 to 10 mg/day from 17 to 26 day) is started and continued for a period of 3 to 6 months and gradually increased to 0.625 mg and 1.25 mg a day. Alternatively ethinyl oestradiol 5 to 10 μg/day which can be gradually increased to 20 μg/day (with progesterone) may be used. Lowest possible dose compatible with breast development is recommended. Regular periodic breast and pelvic examinations are mandatory.

Hormonal Therapy for Growth Failure

The data from various studies go to prove the beneficial effects of GH therapy used singly or with oxandrolone or ethinyl oestradiol. There are three different ways to stimulate growth:

a. Androgens and anabolic steroids. The most commonly used anabolic steroids are
   i. Oxandrolone 0.05 mg to 0.1 mg/kg/day, and
   ii. Fluoxymesterone 2.5 mg/day.

   The treatment should be individualized. Usually it is started at about 11 years of age. Every patient must be carefully observed for any evidence of androgenization such as acne, deepening of the voice, rapid appearance of pubic or body hair and clitoral enlargement. Liver function must be monitored periodically and bone age must be monitored at 6 to 12 months interval to monitor for rapid skeletal maturation.

b. Low dose oestrogen treatment (ethinyl oestradiol 100 ng/kg/day) may stimulate growth and cause only modest advancement of puberty.

c. GH therapy alone or with oxondrolone given daily at night results in significant growth acceleration. It

is recommended to start GH therapy at an early age (about 7 years), escalate the GH dose to over come the warning effect of GH treatment, and to initiate oestrogen therapy to induce pubertal changes after a minimum period of 4 to 4½ years of GH treatment. This ensures a normal final height in majority of Turner's girls.

Other Endocrine Deficiencies and Associated Disorders

Structural anomalies in the renal tract, cardiac evaluation for asymptomatic/symptomatic cardiac lesions, bacterial endocarditis, aortic aneurysm and audiometry for hearing loss may be required, if such symptomatology demands it.

SUMMARY

A patient of Turner's syndrome rarely shows all manifestations of the syndrome. It is a common chromosomal disorder which if diagnosed early and managed judiciously can result in the affected child leading a useful social, sexual and productive married life.

FURTHER READING

1. Clement-Jones M, Schiller S, Rao E, et al. The short stature homeobox gene SHOX is involved in skeketal abnormalities in Turner syndrome. Hum Mol GENET 2000; 9:695-702.
2. Ellison JW, Wardak, Young MF et al. Phog, a candidate gene for involvement in the short stature of Turner's syndrome. Herm Molec Genet 1997; 6(8):1341-7.
3. Uppe BM. Primary ovarian failure. In Kaplan SA (Ed): Clinical Pediatric and Adolescent Endocrinology. Philadelphia: WB Saunders 1982;275.
4. Takano Kr, Smizume Hibi. Treatment of 46 patients of Turner's syndrome with recombinant human growth hormone (YM-17798) for three years a multicentre study. Acta Endocrinol (Copenh) 1992;124 (4): 296-302.
5. Rosenfeld RG, Frane J, Attie KM Brasel JA. Six years results of a randomized, prospective trial of human growth hormone and oxandrolone in Turner syndrome. Paediat J 1992;121(1):49-55.
6. Rongen-Westerlaken C, Witz M. Dutch growth hormone working group. Growth hormone treatment in Turner's syndrome accelerates growth and skeletal maturation. Eur J Paedtr 1992; 151(7), 477-81.
7. Rosenfeld RG. Update on growth hormone therapy in Turner's syndrome. Acta Paediat Scand (Suppl) 1989;356,103-8.
8. Rosenfeld RG. Nonconventional growth hormone therapy in Turner's syndrome: The United States experience. Horm Res: 1990;33(2-4)127.

18.5 Germinoma Syndrome

Y Sachdev

INTRODUCTION

Germinoma is a rare suprasellar midline tumour resembling testicular seminoma or ovarian dysgerminoma. The terms germinoma, pinealoma, ectopic pinealoma and atypical teratoma are used for midline suprasellar central nervous system (CNS) tumours which resemble morphologically testicular seminoma or ovarian dysgenesis. The germ cell neoplasms of the CNS are classically associatd with a syndrome—germinoma syndrome.

The classical features of this syndrome are diabetes insipidus, hypofunction of the anterior pituitary and visual field defects. In addition, there are many other diverse clinical signs and symptoms which include hypodipsia and adipsia, polyuria, hypernatraemia, profound muscle weakness and hyperlipidaemia.

The germinoma syndrome is a progressive disease process. If untreated, it results in progressive endocrine and neurologic dysfunction and finally death. Even with appropriate treatment (radiotherapy), the pre-existing visual field defects and diabetes insipidus are rarely reversed. The positive effect of radiotherapy is that further tumour progression and its consequences are halted. Hence, an early diagnosis is crucial. A combination of surgery (wherever, and if possible), radiation, gamma knife/chemotherapy has been reported to give long-term palliation. A reliable biochemical marker of the tumour would be of utmost importance in reaching an early diagnosis.

Reports that such tumours produce melatonin, foeto-proteins and chorionic gonadotrophin (hCG) raise the possibility of looking for their presence in blood or CSF as tumour markers. A few patients that author has seen and followed up did not live up to this expectation. Cytological examination of the CSF is helpful especially when ventricular fluid is analyzed. CT scan/MRI are most helpful in delineating the extent of the tumour.

Limited surgical intervention for biopsy is recommended to reach a firm diagnosis, when other diagnostic modalities have failed. However, this is highly hazardous when the tumour is deep seated in the posterior part of the third ventricle. In such cases perhaps it is better to start radiotherapy and follow the response/dissolution of the tumour.

Surgical management is recommended where there is severe hydrocephalus. Surgical decompression of the optic chiasma is successful if it is a compression effect. Its use is debatable when chiasma is involved by direct infiltration.

Histologically, the tumour consists of two cell types:
a. A large polygonal cell with prominent nucleoli, eosonophilic cytoplasm and evidence of mitosis
b. A small cell which appears to be identical with a lymphocyte.

The large cells, unlike mature pineal cells, donot stain with silver and blempharoplast-like inclusions are absent. The tumour may be encapsulatd or infiltrating into surrounding structures.

The initial symptom is nearly always diabetes insipidus. Other endocrine defects (GH, TSH. ACTH. ADH, LH, FSH) may be present in varying grades. According to our experience GH deficiency is most common followed by TSH/ACTH and Gn deficiencies.

The most frequent visual defect is bitemporal hemianopia. Occasionally, it may be centripetal constriction and rarely irregular shaped defects. A less discrete visual defect is more characteristic of infiltrative lesion.

Hypothalamic manifestations include obesity, emaciation, hyperprolactinaemia, somnolence, unconsciousness, and disturbances in thermoregulation.

In children there may be growth retardation, failure to develop secondary sex characters and precocious puberty.

After definitive treatment (radiotherapy/surgery/chemotherapy) appropriate hormone replacement therapy ensures a useful and comfortable life span.

SUMMARY

Germinoma is a rare supresellar tumour. Classical symptoms of germinoma syndrome are diabetes insipidus, various anterior pituitary hormone deficiencies and visual defects. Radiotherapy appears to be the best treatment available while surgery has a limited role.

FURTHER READING

1. Dohlborg SA, Petrillo A, Crosse J R, et al. The potential for complete and durable response in nonglial primary brain tumors in children and young adults with enhanced chemotherapy delivery. Cancer J Sci Am 1998;4:110-24.
2. Howowitz MB. Central nervous system germinomas: a review. Arch Neurol 1991;48:652-7.
3. Sachdev Y, Hall R. Germinoma syndrome. JAPI 1987;36:530-2.
4. Sklar Charles A, Grumbach Melvin M, Kaplan Selna L, ConteFelix A. Hormonal and metabolic abnormalities associated with central nervous system germinoma in children and adolescents and the effect of therapy. Report of 10 patients. Jr Clin Endocrinol and Metab 1981; 52:9-16.

SECTION

19

HYPO- AND HYPERTHYROIDISM IN CHILDREN

19.1 Hypothyroidism in Children

YC Mathur, RC Mathur

FOETAL THYROID DEVELOPMENT AND HORMONE SYNTHESIS

The thyroid tissue develops from distribution and fragmentation of the thyroglossal duct by the second month of conception. Cells of the lower portion of the duct differentiate into thyroid tissue forming the pyramidal lobe of the gland. Thyroglobulin (Tg) synthesis occurs as early as the 29th day of gestation, iodine trapping by 8 to 10th week, and the production of thyroxine (T_4) and to a lesser extent T_3 occurs by 12th week of gestation.

Hypothalamic neurones synthesize thyrotrophin-releasing hormone by 6 to 8 week, the pituitary portal vessel system development begins by 8 to 10 weeks and TSH secretion is seen by 10 to 12 weeks of gestation. Maturation of the hypothalamo-pituitary-thyroid axis occurs in the second half of gestation, but normal feedback relationship is not mature until approximately 3 months of postnatal life. From the clinical viewpoint, several developmental defects could be noted. In rare circumstances thyroid and its remnants could remain at the base of the tongue or thyroid tissue progenitors may migrate into the mediastinum.

THYROID PHYSIOLOGY

The main function of the thyroid gland is to synthesize T_3 and T_4 (Fig. 19.1.1). The formation of normal quantities

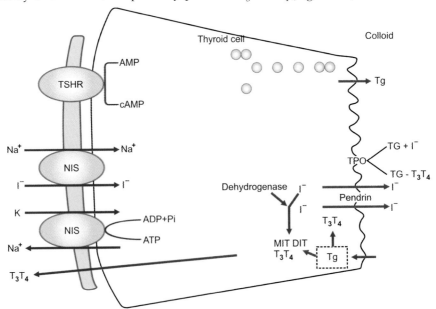

Fig. 19.1.1: Thyroid hormones synthesis (TSHR—Thyrotrophin receptor; Tg—Thyroglobulin; AMP—Adenosine monophosphate; NIS—Sodium iodide symporter; TPO—Thyroidal peroxidase; MIT—Mono-iodotyrosine; DIT—Di-iodotyrosine)

of thyroid hormones requires the availability of adequate supply of exogenous iodine. The recommended daily allowance of iodine is more than 30 µg/kg/day for infants and 90 to 120 µg/day for older children and 150 µg/day for adolescents. Iodine taken orally is converted to iodide and is trapped, transported and concentrated in the follicular lumen for synthesis of thyroid hormone. Iodine transport is carried out by the sodium-iodide symporter (NIS). It is an active process depending upon the presence of sodium gradient. Absence of iodide concentrating mechanisms is associated with congenital hypothyroidism and goitre. A second thyroid cell protein involved in iodide metabolism is pendrin. It is expressed in the apical border of the thyroid cell and is required for iodide transport across the apical membrane of the thyrocyte into the follicular lumen where it is then oxidised and coupled to tyrosine.

Iodide is oxidised using thyroidal peroxidase (TPO). Organification of tyrosine forms monoiodotyrosine and diiodotyrosine. The rate of organic iodination depends upon the degree of thyroid stimulation by TSH. Then coupling of these forms gives rise to T_3 and T_4.

Thyroglobulin (Tg)

T_3 and T_4 are bound with thyroglobulin in the lumen of the follicle (colloid) until ready to be delivered to the body cells. T_3 and T_4 are liberated from the thyroglobulin by the activation of proteases and peptides.

The metabolic potency of T_3 is 3 to 4 times that of T_4. Only 20% of the circulating T_3 is secreted by the thyroid gland, the remainder is produced by deiodination of T_4 in the liver, kidney and other tissues. The free hormones enter cells where T_4 may be converted to T_3 by deiodination. Intracellular T_3 then enters the nucleus, where it binds to the thyroid hormone receptors. There are four different forms of thyroid hormone receptors ($\alpha_1, \alpha_2, \beta_1$ and β_2), Binding of T_3 activates the thyroid hormone receptor element resulting in production of encoded mRNA and protein synthesis of secretions specific for the target cell. Thyroid hormone increases oxygen consumption, influences growth and differentiation, affects carbohydrate, lipid and vitamin metabolisms. About 70% of the circulating T_4 is firmly bound to thyroxine binding globulin (TBG). Less important carriers are thyroxine binding prealbumin (Transthyretin) and albumin. Only 0.03% of T_4 in serum is not bound and comprises free T_4.

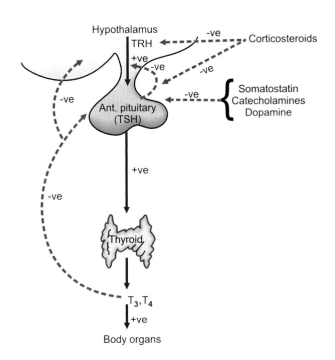

Fig. 19.1.2: Regulatory factors for TSH synthesis

Thyroid Regulation (Fig. 19.1.2)

TSH from the anterior pituitary regulates the thyroid gland. TSH activates the thyroid gland to affect release of thyroid hormones. TSH synthesis and release are stimulated by TSH releasing hormone (TRH), which is synthesised in the hypothalamus and secreted into the pituitary. The level of thyroid hormones has a negative feedback on the release of TSH and TRH, except in neonates where TRH is low. In addition there is an inverse relationship between the glandular organic iodine level and the rate of hormone formation.

Thyroid Function in the Foetus and Newborn

Throughout gestation, serum TSH values are greater than those present in maternal circulation and higher than would be expected in the mother with normal thyroid function. Circulating T_3 levels remain low in contrast to the foetal free T_4.

After delivery the neonatal TSH levels increase rapidly and return to normal after 48 hours. The surge in TSH is due to marked reduction of environmental temperature. After delivery, T_3 and T_4 and Tg in the circulation increase rapidly in the first 24 hours. By the 10th day, serum T_3 and T_4 are lower but exceed normal adult values. Premature infants have an immature hypothalamic-pituitary-thyroid axis with low levels of T_3 and T_4 and TSH. There is a surge of TSH after birth but it is small.

HYPOTHYROIDISM

Hypothyroidism results from deficient production of thyroid hormone or a defect in the hormonal receptor. The disorder may manifest at birth or later, after a period of normal function. The late onset type may be due to either an acquired cause or a delayed manifestation of deficiency. Based on the aetiology, the hypothyroidism is of two types: congenital or acquired. Table 19.1.1 enumerates some of the congenital causes of hypothyroidism.

CONGENITAL HYPOTHYROIDISM

Congenital hypothyroidism (CH) is the commonest treatable and preventable cause of mental retardation.

TABLE 19.1.1

A. Primary hypothyroidism

  a. Defect in thyroid development—Agenesis, hypoplasia, ectopia

  b. Defect in thyroid hormone synthesis (inborn errors)—Thyroid oxidase mutations
  - Iodide transport defects
  - Thyroid peroxidase defect
  - Thyroglobulin synthesis defect
  - Deiodination defect

  c. Iodine deficiency—(endemic goitre) Neurogenic type, myxoedematous type

  d. Maternal antibodies—Thyrotrophin receptor-blocking antibody

    Maternal drugs—Radioiodine, antithyroid drugs, amiodarone

B. Central hypothyroidism

  POU1F1 mutations—deficiency of thyrotrophin, growth hormone, prolactin

  PROP1 mutations—deficiency of thyrotrophin, GH, prolactin, LH, FSH+/– ACTH

  TRH deficiency—isolated or multiple endocrine deficiency

  TRH hyporesponsiveness—TRH receptor mutation

  TSH deficiency—β-chain mutation or multiple pituitary deficiency

  Thyrotrophin unresponsiveness—Gsα mutation, mutation of TSH receptor

Aetiologic classification of congenital hypothyroidism

Worldwide the most common cause of CH is iodine deficiency affecting approximately a billion people. Congenital causes of hypothyroidism may be sporadic or familial, goitrous or non-goitrous. The time of manifestation depends on the severity of the disease. In the west the prevalence rate is 1 in 4000, whereas in India the prevalence is about 1 in 2000 infants. Female children are affected more than males in a ratio of 2:1.

The commonest cause (75 to 80%) of congenital hypothyroidism is thyroid dysgenesis; nearly 10 to 15% are due to inborn errors of thyroxine synthesis (dyshormonogenesis) and 5 to 10% are the result of transplacental maternal TSH receptor blocking antibodies. 98% dysgenesis is sporadic while only 2% are familial. The exact cause of thyroid dysgenesis is not known. It is well documented that three transcription factors TTF-1, TTF-2 and PAX-8 are concerned with thyroid morphogenesis and differentiation. Besides these factors, maternal thyroid antibodies (IgG type) which can cross the placenta, thyroid growth blocking antibodies and cytotoxic antibodies also play a pathogenetic role.

TSH deficiency is usually a part of multiple pituitary hormones deficiency and presents with hypoglycaemia, persistent jaundice, micropenis, septo-optic dysplasia, midline cleft lip, midface hypoplasia and other midline facial anomalies.

Pit-1 mutation results in combination of TSH, GH and prolactin deficiency. Failure of prolactin response to TRH test should prompt examination of pit-1 gene.

Screening for Congenital Hypothyroidism

In iodine deficient and iodine sufficient areas, early diagnosis helps in eradicating mental retardation. Neonatal screening programme have been introduced in various parts of the world with good cost-benefit ratio.

If infant is discharged before 48 hours, take the blood sample before discharge. In home deliveries, take it within 7 days of birth. In mothers who have undergone treatment for thyroid disease, cord blood should be collected to expedite treatment.

Measurement of TSH or T_4 should be done on a filter paper with whole dried blood on days 1 to 4 of life. Babies whose initial TSH > 50 mU/L are more likely to have permanent congenital hypothyroidism, whereas a TSH between 20 and 49 mU/L is frequently a false-positive and represents transient hypothyroidism. Transient hypothyroidism may be due to transplacental passage of maternal thyrotrophin receptor-blocking antibodies and is rare.

A primary TSH estimation will detect frank and compensated hypothyroidism but will miss secondary or tertiary hypothyroidism, a delayed TSH rise, TBG deficiency. On the other hand, a primary T_4 estimation will detect primary, secondary or tertiary hypothyroidism but will miss TBG deficiency. It is a good policy to check both FT_4 and TSH when suspicion of hypothyroidism is very strong while in cases where hypothyroid is unlikely but is to be excluded, to check only TSH. In the very premature infants, T_4 concentrations are lower and the incidence of transient hypothyroidism is much higher than full term babies.

Primary Causes

Thyroid Dysgenesis

The most common (75 to 85%) cause of non-endemic congenital hypothyroidism is thyroid dysgenesis. Out of this, 98% is sporadic, while 2% is familial. Thyroid dysgenesis may be due to complete absence of thyroid tissue (agenesis) or it may be partial (hypoplasia) which is usually associated with failure to descend into the neck (ectopy). Ectopic thyroid tissue (lingual, sublingual, and subhyoid) may produce adequate hormone for many years or may fail in early childhood. This usually becomes clinically evident as a mass at the base of the tongue or midline of the neck, usually at the level of the hyoid. Occasionally, it is associated with thyroglossal cyst. Removal of the ectopic thyroid will lead to hypothyroidism as there is no other thyroid tissue. Genetic and environmental factors have been implicated in the aetiology of thyroid dysgenesis but the cause is unknown in most cases. There is an increased incidence in babies with Down's syndrome. The transcription factors (TTF1, TTF2 and PAX8), which are important for thyroid morphogenesis and differentiation are candidate genes in the aetiology of dysgenesis. These defects have been found in some of the affected patients.

Inborn Errors of Thyroid Hormonogenesis

Inborn errors of thyroid hormonogenesis are responsible for 10 to 15% of congenital hypothyroidism. Defects include decreased TSH responsiveness, failure to concentrate iodide, defective organification of iodide due to an abnormality in the TPO enzyme or in the H_2O_2 generating system, defective Tg synthesis or transport and abnormal iodotyrosine deiodinase activity.

These defects are transmitted as autosomal recessive disorders due to a single gene mutation. Mutations have been observed in the genes for TSH receptor, NIS, TPO

and Tg. When the defect is incomplete, compensation occurs and the onset is delayed. A goitre is almost always present and this will aid in detection.

Iodide transport defect It is very rare and has been reported in few Japanese children. It involves a defect in the gene encoding for the sodium iodine symporter (NIS). Uptake of radioiodine is low in these children. A large dose of Iodine and thyroxine therapy is used for the treatment.

Defects in organification and coupling These defects are the most common of the thyroxine synthesis defects. The defect could be in the generation of H_2O_2, thyroid peroxidase and cofactor hematin. The characteristic finding in all patients with this defect is a marked decrease in thyroid radioactivity when perchlorate or thiocyanate are administered two hours prior to radioiodine .The association of an organification defect with sensory neural deafness is known as Pendred's syndrome. This has been shown to be due to a defect in pendrin gene, which has a similar sequence to sulphate transporters of both thyroid and cochlea.

Defects in Tg synthesis These occur due to a point mutation for the gene for Tg. This is characterised by elevated TSH, low T_4 and absent or low Tg.

Defects in deiodination There is a deficiency of the deiodinase enzyme in the thyroid or in the periphery. These children have large losses of iodine in the urine in the form of iodinated tyrosines.

Thyrotrophin receptor blocking antibody (TRab or thyroid binding receptor immunoglobulin) (Fig. 19.1.3) These maternal antibodies pass through the placenta and inhibit the binding of TSH to its receptor. The mother usually has autoimmune thyroid disease. They also may have TPO antibodies and cytotoxic antibodies which may have a pathogenetic role.

Maternal antithyroid medication Transient neonatal hypothyroidism and goitre may develop in babies whose mothers are being treated with antithyroid medications for Graves' disease. This resolves spontaneously with the clearance of the drug from the babies circulation. Hypothyroidism has also been reported as a result of inadvertent administration of radioiodine during pregnancy.

Iodine deficiency and iodine excess Iodine deficiency or endemic goitre is the most common cause of congenital hypothyroidism in India and worldwide. Endemic goitre almost always occurs in areas of environmental iodine deficiency. This condition is estimated to affect more than 200 million people throughout the world. It is most

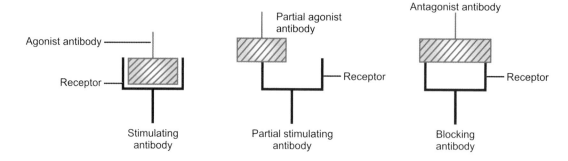

Fig. 19.1.3: Thyroid receptor blocking antibodies

common in the mountainous areas such as Himalayas and its plains owing to the depletion of iodine, consequent to the persistent glacial run off from these regions. The occurrence of endemic goitre can be patchy even within an area of known iodine deficiency; the role of dietary minerals or naturally occurring goitrogens have been suggested in instances of this type. Most abnormalities in iodine metabolism in patients with endemic goitre are consistent with the expected effects of iodine deficiency. The absolute iodine uptake is normal or low. In areas of moderate deficiency the serum T_4 level is usually in the lower range of normal and is below normal in severe deficiency. Nevertheless most patients in these areas do not appear to be hypothyroid because of an increase of more efficient T_3 at the expense of T_4. In the absence of hypothyroidism the effect of goitre is mainly cosmetic. The goitre may become nodular, haemorrhagic or produce compression symptoms on the surrounding trachea, oesophagus and laryngeal nerves. Administration of iodine causes the regression of early hyperplastic goitre but it has little effect on a long-standing goitre. Thyroxine should be given for hypothyroidism.

Endemic cretinism Endemic cretinism is a developmental disorder that occurs in regions of severe endemic goitre. Both parents of an endemic cretins are usually goitrous. In addition to features of sporadic cretinism, endemic cretins often have deaf mutism, spasticity, motor dysfunction and abnormalities in the basal ganglia.

Central Causes

Thyrotrophin Deficiency

Deficiency of TSH usually occurs in association with defects of the pituitary and or hypothalamus. Children with TSH deficient hypothyroidism have multiple pituitary deficiencies and may present within the newborn period with persistent jaundice, hypoglycaemia, and micropenis in association with septo-optic dysplasia

and midline facial abnormalities. TSH deficiency could be a part of the POU1F1 mutation, isolated deficiency of TSH or a mutation in the TSH receptor gene. Failure of prolactin response to TRH test is a pointer to examination of pituitary 1-gene. Isolated TSH deficiency is a rare autosomal recessive disorder.

Thyrotrophin Hormone Unresponsiveness

It is caused by the genetic deficiency of the guanine nucleotide regulatory protein Gs. There have also been reports of isolated TSH unresponsiveness due to mutation in TSH receptor gene.

Thyotrophin Releasing Hormone Abnormality

The TRH receptor abnormality results in TSH and prolactin deficiency and hypothyroidism. This defect is caused by a mutation in the gene coding for the TRH receptor, which leads to the failure in TRH binding to its receptor.

Thyroid Hormone Unresponsiveness

Unresponsiveness can be for both exogenous and endogenous thyroxine. They have goitre and the levels of T_3 and T_4 are elevated and they are clinically euthyroid. TSH is elevated or normal inappropriate to the T_4 levels. It is inherited as an autosomal dominant disorder. Treatment is needed if skeletal and growth retardation occurs.

National Goitre Control Programme

The programme was introduced as part of the 20-point programme of the Prime Minister in 1984. It has three components: (a) survey to identify endemic areas, (b) compulsory fortification of edible salt with iodine, (c) resurvey after 5 years to assess the impact of the measures. The programme is discussed elsewhere in this book.

Clinical Manifestations

Clinical evidence of hypothyroidism is usually difficult to appreciate in the newborn period as the features are not evident due to transplacental passage of moderate amounts of maternal T_4 which provides approximately 30% of T_4 that is normally measured at birth, nonspecific signs that suggest the diagnosis of congenital hypothyroidism are given in Table 19.1.2.

Many of the classic features develop during the following months. In general, the extent of the clinical findings depends on the cause, severity and duration of the hypothyroidism. Babies in whom severe foetomaternal hypothyroidism was present *in utero*, tend to be the most symptomatic at birth. Similarly babies with complete block in thyroid hormonogenesis tend to have more signs and symptoms at birth. However, if the diagnosis is delayed, subsequent linear growth is impaired. The growth is stunted, extremities short and the head size normal or increased. The eyes appear apart and the nose bridge depressed. The palpebral fissures are narrow and eyelids swollen .The mouth is kept open and the tongue protrudes out (Figs 19.1.4A and B). The dentition is delayed. The neck is short and thick and there may be fat deposition at the nape of the neck and above the clavicle. The hands are short and stubby. The skin is dry, scaly with little perspiration. Myxoedema may also be seen in the skin of the eyelids, back of hands and external genitalia. Carotenaemia may cause yellowish discoloration of the skin. Hair are coarse, brittle and scanty. The hairline reaches far down on the forehead. Hypothyroid infants appear lethargic and are slow learners. The voice is hoarse and they do not learn to

TABLE 19.1.2

Clinical signs	Scores
Feeding problem	1
Constipation	1
Inactivity	1
Hypotonia	1
Umbilical hernia	1
Enlarged tongue	1
Skin mottling	1
Dry skin	1.5
Open posterior fontanelle (>0.5 cm)	1.5
Typical oedematous fades	3.0
Total	13.0

Quebec Neonatal Hypothyroid Index   (Daussault JH 1983)

Score of 4 is suspicious of congenital hypothyroidism

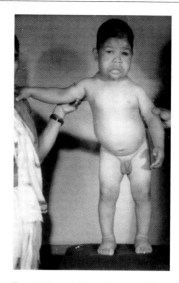

Fig. 9.1.4A: Front view of an 8-year-old cretin with grossly stunted growth, short extremities, protuberant abdomen and coarse facial features

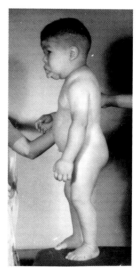

Fig. 9.1.4B: The lateral view of the same boy showing thick enlarged tongue, supraclavicular fat and a big head. The serum TSH was > 120 mU/L and IQ < 25%

talk. Sexual maturation may be delayed or absent. Muscles are usually hypotonic (Fig. 19.1.5) except in rare instances where pseudohypertrophy occurs especially in the calf muscles (Kocher-Debre-Semelaigne syndrome).

Laboratory Evaluation

The diagnosis of congenital hypothyroidism is confirmed by the demonstration of a decreased level of T_4 and an elevated TSH (>20 mU/L). Infants with permanent thyroid abnormalities have a much higher TSH

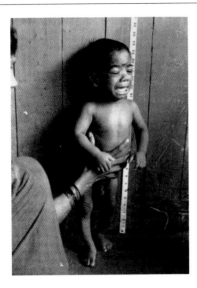

Fig. 9.1.5: A 4½-year-old hypothyroid child with stunted growth, delayed milestones and poor musculature was unable to stand without support. His TSH was > 90 mU/L

concentration. Measurement of T_3 is of little value in the diagnosis. The normal value of T_4 in the first 2 months of life is 6.5 to 16.3 μg/dl. Serum levels of Tg are usually low in infants with thyroid agenesis or defects in Tg synthesis or secretion, but may be increased with ectopic glands and other inborn errors of thyroxine synthesis. In babies with low T_4 unaccompanied by TSH elevation, a free T_4 should be measured and TBG concentration evaluated. The finding of a low T_4 in the presence of a normal Tg may suggest the diagnosis of secondary or tertiary hypothyroidism. In these cases TRH testing will distinguish whether the abnormality is pituitary or hypothalamic. Pituitary function testing and brain imaging should also be performed in these infants. In premature, low birth weight or sick babies in whom a low T_4 and normal TSH is found, the free T_4 is frequently not as low as the total T_4. In these infants the TSH should be measured every 2 weeks until the T_4 is normal because of the rare occurrence of delayed TSH rise. Similarly any baby suspected of being hypothyroid clinically should have repeated thyroid function tests.

Bone development is delayed in a third of the congenitally hypothyroid infants and the degree of affection determines the duration and severity of the hypothyroidism *in utero*. The earliest sign in the newborns is the absence of distal femoral epiphysis. In untreated children there is epiphyseal dysgenesis (multiple foci of ossification), deformity of the lower thoracic and lumbar vertebrae. The gap in the chronological age and bone age increases. X-rays of the skull shows wormian bones, large open fontanelles.

A radionucleotide scan can identify the underlying cause in infants with congenital hypothyroidism. By using either ^{123}I or ^{99m}Tc pertechnetate, the location, size and trapping ability of the gland can be assessed. Ectopic glands can be identified. A normally situated thyroid with a normal uptake of the radionucleotide indicates a defect in the hormone biosynthesis. Scintigraphy with ^{123}I is usually preferred because of greater sensitivity and since it is organified it allows quantitative uptake measurements and tests for both iodine transport defects and thyroid oxidation defects.

Ultrasound is helpful to confirm the absence of thyroid tissue when there is no uptake on thyroid imaging. It is also useful in confirming the presence of a ectopic thyroid gland if transient abnormality is suspected.

In late cases ECG may show low voltage P and T waves with diminished amplitude of QRS complexes, which indicates a poor ventricular function and pericardial effusion.

Treatment

The treatment of congenital hypothyroidism consists of replacement with oral L-thyroxine in a single daily dose of 10 to 15 μg/kg/day. The total replacement dose may be used at the onset of therapy unless there is evidence of cardiac disease. Thyroxine should not be given with substances that interfere with its absorption, such as iron, soya or fibre. The goal of the therapy includes maintenance of T_4 levels in the upper half of the normal range for age. The serum concentrations normalize in most infants within one week and the TSH in a month. In primary hypothyroidism several months of therapy may be necessary before TSH normalizes. Current recommendations are to repeat T_4 and TSH at 2 and 4 weeks after initiation of treatment, every 2 months in the first year of life; every 3 months in the next three years; and then every year. After a dose modification, reevaluation should be done after 4 to 6 weeks of therapy.

If transient hypothyroidism is suspected, reevaluation can be done at around 3 years of age. The therapy must be stopped for two months before reevaluation.

Iatrogenic thyrotoxicosis in infants and children may advance bone maturation, accelerate bone suture closure, reduce bone mineralisation and produce neuropsychiatric abnormalities. Occasionally intracranial hypertension develops soon after initiation of therapy. In such children a low starting dose followed by gradual increment every 4 to 8 weeks should be done until normal serum concentrations are attained.

Prognosis

With prompt and adequate treatment children with congenital hypothyroidism have the potential to have normal somatic, intellectual growth and development. Higher intelligent quotients are attained when treatment is started before two weeks of age. If left untreated, mental retardation, neurological dysfunction manifested as ataxia, attention deficits, abnormal muscle tone and speech defects may develop.

ACQUIRED HYPOTHYROIDISM (JUVENILE HYPOTHYROIDISM)

Aetiology

The causes of hypothyroidism after the neonatal period are listed in Table 19.1.3. Some of these conditions are described in brief.

Chronic Lymphocytic Thyroiditis (CLT)

It is the most frequent cause of hypothyroidism after the neonatal period. It is chacterised by lymphocytic and cytokine mediated thyroid destruction. Goitrous

TABLE 19.1.3

Autoimmune
- Chronic lymphocytic thyroiditis
  - Hashimoto's thyroiditis—goitrous
  - Primary myxoedema—atrophic
  - Polyglandular autoimmune syndromes I, II and III

Congenital abnormality
- Thyroid dysgenesis
- Dyshormonogenesis

Iatrogenic
- Antithyroid drugs, iodide, lithium, anticonvulsant
- Goitrogens—cabbage, sweet potatoes, cassava, cauliflower, broccoli, soyabeans
- Irradiation
- Radiographs of neck/whole body
- Radioiodine
- Thyroidectomy

Systemic
- Cystinosis
- Histiocytosis X

Central causes
- Hypothalamic or pituitary tumour
  (especially craniopharyngioma)/surgery/irradiation

Aetiology of acquired hypothyroidism

(Hashimoto's thyroiditis) and non-goitrous (Primary, myxoedema) variants have been identified. The disease has a predilection for females and there is a positive family history of autoimmune thyroid disease in approximately 25 per cent of the cases.

It can also occur as part of an autoimmune polyglandular syndrome (APS). There is an increased incidence of CLT in patients with Down's, Turner's, Klinefelter's and Noonan's syndromes. Antibodies to Tg and TPO antibodies are found in patients with CLT.

Thyroid Dysgenesis and Dyshormonogenesis

Occasionally they escape detection in the newborn period and present later in the childhood with non-goitrous hypothyroidism or as an enlarged mass at the base of the tongue or along the course of the thyroglossal duct. Similarly children with dyshormonogenesis may present later in childhood as goitre.

Consumptive Hypothyroidism

The term has been used for hypothyroidism seen in infants (and adults) with visceral haemangiomas and related tumours.

Clinical Features

The earliest signs of hypothyroidism in a child are slowing of linear growth rate, delayed bone age and delayed puberty. Other features depend on the circulating levels of the hormone (Table 19.1.4).

TABLE 19.1.4

- Delayed puberty
- Dry, coarse skin
- Hoarse cry
- Macroglossia
- Pseudomuscular hypertrophy
- Growth retardation
- Delayed skeletal maturation
- Delayed tooth eruption
- Myopathy
- Constipation
- Generalised myxoedema
- Deceleration of linear growth
- Galactorrhoea

Clinical features of acquired hypothyroidism

Laboratory Evaluation

Measurement of TSH, T_4 and T_3 should be done for the diagnosis of hypothyroidism. Chronic lymphocytic thyroiditis (CLT) is diagnosed by the elevated levels of Tg and /or TPO antibodies.

Treatment

The aim of the treatment is to ensure normal growth and development and maintain FT_4 value in the upper half of the normal range. Rapid replacement of thyroxine is not essential in the older children, especially in those with a long standing severe hypothyroidism as it may result in side effects like poor school performance, short attention span, hyperactivity, insomnia and behaviour problems. The typical replacement dose of L-thyroxine in childhood is 4 to 6 µg/kg for children 1 to 5 years of age, 3 to 4 µg/kg for those of age 6 to 10 years and 2 to 3 µg/kg for those 11 years or older. After the child has received the recommended dosage for at least 8 weeks, T_4 and TSH should be measured. Once they have attained euthyroid state patients should be monitored every 6 to 12 months. Growth and bone age should also be regularly monitored.

If in a pregnant woman, ultrasonography reveals foetal goitre, foetal hypothyroidism must be considered and blood samples collected by cordocentesis (if expertise is available) and intra-amniotic T_4 should be given 250 to 500 µg per week for 2 to 4 weeks.

SUMMARY

The thyroid hormone deficiency may be either congenital or acquired. The commonest cause (78 to 85%) of congenital hypothyroidism is thyroid dysgenesis, nearly 10 to 15% are due to inborn errors of thyroxine synthesis (dyshormonogenesis) and 5 to 10% are the result of transplacental TSH receptor blocking antibodies (TSHRB Ab). Acquired hypothyroidism particularly in the presence of goitre usually results from deficiency of dietary iodine or due to chronic lymphocytic thyroiditis. Of the genetically determined enzymatic defects that cause hypothyroidism iodide organification defects have distinguishing clinical features. Goitrogens in the form of drugs and foods cross placenta and produce goitres. Several rare thyroid hormone resistance syndromes have been identified. The severity of the symptoms and signs depend on the age of onset and the degree of deficiency. Even with congenital absence of the thyroid gland, the first finding may not appear for several days to weeks. Evaluation of T_3, T_4, and TSH forms the basis of diagnosis and follow-up. Congenital hypothyroidism should be diagnosed by neonatal screening within 30 days of birth to give a good therapeutic prognosis. A daily single dose of L-thyroxine is the mainstay of treatment. Periodic regular monitoring of hormone levels is essential. Endemic goitre should be treated with addition of oral iodine. Growth monitoring is important to assess effects of therapy, ensure normal intellectual development and avoid iatrogenic thyrotoxicosis.

FURTHER READING

1. Donaldson MDC. Neonatal screening for congenital hypothyroidism. Sem in Neonatal 1998;3:35-47.
2. Fisher DA. Management of congenital hypothyroidism. J Clin Endocrinol Metab 1991;72:523.
3. Foley TP. Disorders of the thyroid in children. Pediatric endocrinology. Ed MA Sperling, WB Saunders & Co. 1996;170-94.
4. Toft AD. Drug therapy. Thyroxine therapy. N Engl J Med 1994;331:174.
5. American Academy of Pediatrics. Newborn screening for congenital hypothyroidism. Recommended guidelines. Pediatrics 1993;91:120-3.
6. Desai MP, Karandikar S. Autoimmune thyroid disease in childhood. A study of children and their families. Indian Pediatr 1999;36(7): 659-68.
7. Desai M. The profile of congenital hypothyroidism in India. Indian Pediatr 1989;26(3):207-11.
8. Desai M, Colaco MP, Sameul AM, Vas FE. Etiology of childhood hypothyroidism. Indian Pediatr 1989;26(3):212-22.

19.2 Hyperthyroidism in Children

Y Sachdev

AETIOLOGY

Hyperthyroidism in children can occur at any age. It is almost always (>95%) due to Graves' disease. The other causes like transient hyperthyroidism of thyroiditis, hyperactive adenoma, McCune-Albright syndrome, iodine-induced hyperthyroidism and TSH excess, etc. are rare (<5 %). During infancy, hyperthyroidism is usually transient; though at times it may be more persistent.

NEONATAL GRAVES' DISEASE

It is uncommon and forms less than 1% of paediatric Graves' disease patients. Both boys and girls are affected. There are two distinct forms of neonatal Graves' disease.

a. Mild and self-limiting form. It becomes evident at or soon after birth and is seen in neonates born of mothers with active or recently active Graves' disease. Commonly spontaneous recovery starts well within six weeks though sometimes it may be delayed till 3 months. The infant is asymptomatic by 6 months.

b. Less commonly, the disease may not appear at birth and onset may be delayed till one year. In such children, the mother may not be a patient of Graves' disease though a positive history of thyroid disease may be present in many family members. The disease is more severe, persists for longer periods, is difficult to control and even may recur. In such infants, late sequelae like advancement in bone age, premature fusion of the cranial sutures, microcephaly, mental retardation, acropachy, learning disorders and short stature may be seen.

Clinical Features

The clinical manifestations are similar in both forms though they may differ in severity. Neonate may be premature or a low birth weight baby. Goitre is almost always present and may cause cyanosis or respiratory distress. The infant looks anxious, is restless, irritable and fussy. Appetite is voracious and there may be feeding difficulties due to goitre. Skin is flushed and coarse. Fever may be present, eye signs like a stare, periorbital oedema, lid retraction, proptosis, etc. are always present. Other signs include tachycardia, cardiomegaly, heart failure and arrhythmias. Jaundice, hepatomegaly, thrombocytopenia and upper respiratory tract infection are observed in some of these infants.

Care of the Foetus and Newborn of the Mother with Graves' Disease

a. Maternal hyperthyroidism particularly in the early stages, is difficult to diagnose during pregnancy as symptoms like apprehension, nervousness, irritability, increased sweating and appetite are not unusual during first trimester of pregnancy. Suspicion will be aroused if she has family history of thyroid disorder, tachycardia, palpable/visible thyroid gland, systolic hypertension and marginally elevated FT_3, FT_4. It is advisable to carry out TRab estimation in all such cases to determine if the foetus is at risk for Graves' disease *in utero*. Once the diagnosis is confirmed, mother is treated on the standard lines as discussed earlier.

b. The evaluation of the foetal thyroid status *in utero* in done as outlined below:
   - Determine foetal growth at each clinical visit of the mother by careful measurement of the uterine fundus.
   - Serial foetal measurement by ultrasonographic examination
   - Assessment of foetal heart rate by auscultation or external monitoring (normally it is between 120 and 150 beats/minute). Tachycardia beyond 180/

minute or bradycardia (if mother is on antithyroid drug therapy) needs modification in maternal treatment.

c. *Evaluation at birth*
- Clinical examination for intrauterine growth retardation, goitre, exophthalmos, tachycardia, bradycardia, anterior fontanelle size, synostosis, congenital abnormalities require to be recorded.
- Clinical review of the gestational age by dates, ultrasonography during pregnancy.
- Plotting the intrauterine growth by gestational age
- Detailed neurological examination
- Bone age (left knee)
- Cord blood for FT_4, TSH, TRab.

d. *Evaluation of the infant 2 to 7 days*
- Clinical examination
- FT_3, FT_4, TSH, TRab
- Thyroid scan, if hypothyroid is suspected
- Initiate appropriate treatment

e. *Long-term assessment of children with abnormal thyroid function in utero or neonatal period will include*
- Periodic growth and development evaluation,
- Neurological assessment including auditory and visual evoked potentials
- Bone age (left knee)
- X-ray skull if marked frontal bossing, large/small anterior fontanelle, synostosis is present
- Serum FT_3, FT_4, TSH every week/fortnight/month depending upon holistic assessment.

GRAVES' DISEASE IN CHILDHOOD

It is seen in all ages. The incidence increases with age and the peak is reached at adolescence. Nearly 70% patients belong to 10 to 15 years age group. Girls are affected more than boys (4 to 6:1). The clinical picture is same as seen in adults. The onset of the disease is usually insidious manifesting over months or even years. In some, however, the onset may be acute and rapid. In insidious cases, the diagnosis may be difficult and symptoms like emotional lability, hyperactivity, restlessness in a child who is active, alert and eating well may be attributed to family or school tension and maladjustment. It is seen that some children who are previously quiet and easily manageable become restless, never sit still and are constantly on the move. They have rapid mood changes-periods of exuberance, unhappiness and tears.

A hyperthyroid child may be too demanding, impatient and rebellious. She may be unable to perform previous tests despite excessive energy expended. She lacks tidiness in appearance and her personal effects. There may be some alterations in sleep habits. She is unable to fall asleep. There may be complete disruption of bed covers, bed tossing, bed wetting, nightmares, crying out during sleep and falling out of bed. The child may adopt awkward positions while reading, writing or TV watching and she tries repeatedly to seek more comfortable postures without much success. The parents and teachers confirm a decline in school performance. There is obvious weight loss or failure to gain weight. Menstrual disturbances and accelerated linear growth with advanced epiphyseal maturation are usually present.

The thyroid gland is firm, nontender with diffuse enlargement and well defined borders. The presence of local bruit or thrill indicates increased blood supply to the gland. Eye signs are similar to those seen in the adult Graves' disease.

The clinical diagnosis is confirmed by estimation of FT_3, FT_4, TSH and in some cases TRH test. Elevated microsomal and thyroglobulin antibodies are a pointer towards Hashimoto's disease (Hashi-thyrotoxicosis). Treatment is by pharmacotherapy, RAI, surgery or combination of these. Drug therapy is easy to administer, is cheap, safe in vast majority and effective. However on withdrawal of medication, relapses are liable to occur. In some children compliance also becomes a problem.

RAI is also a safe, reliable and simple alternative. However, it takes a long time (a few years) to act and hypothyroid does result in the long run. Moreover enhanced risk of malignancy and genetic damage go against its use in childhood and adolescence. Surgery on the other hand is quick, safe and radical method but is expensive. Relapses are also known. Therefore, the management has to be individualized and with the consensus of the patient and her parents. The usual recommendations are:

a. Drug therapy for children with mild thyrotoxicosis and serological evidence of Hashimoto's.
b. Surgery for a large goitre and severe thyrotoxicosis and those who object to RAI and drug therapy.
c. RAI[131] for recurrent thyrotoxicosis after surgery or thyrotoxicosis in Down's syndrome.

The drug used are:
a. Propylthiouracil 5 to 10 mg/kg ÷ 8 hourly or Methimazole/carbimazole 0.5 µg to 1 mg/kg ÷ 8 hourly with
b. Lugol's solution (5 to 10 drops) or 10% KI solution (1 to 2 drop × 8 hourly). Continue both for 24 to 48 hours. Increase the dose if necessary. Thereafter, use
c. Propranolol 1 to 2 mg/kg/day to control tachycardia and sympathetic overactivity.

d. Phenobarbitone 8 mg × BD to control irritability
e. Digoxin elixir if heart failure (0.05 mg per ml) is present.

Adjust above mentioned treatment as perclinical response.

Medication may be withdrawn in 2 to 3 months time when complete recovery takes place.

SUMMARY

The commonest cause of childhood hyperthyroidism is Graves' disease. Other causes are rare (<5%). Neonatal Graves' disease forms less than 1% of paediatric hyperthyroidism. The section deals with the care and management of the foetus and the neonate born to a Graves' disease mother. It also discusses its treatment among children and adolescent.

FURTHER READING

1. Collen RJ, Landaw EP, Kaplan SA, Lippe BM. Remission rates of children and adolescents with thyrotoxicosis treated with antithyroid drugs. Pediatrics 1980;65:550.
2. Gruters A. Treatment of Graves' disease in children and adolescents. Horm Res 1998;49(6):255-7.
3. Hamburger JI. Management of hyperthyroidism in children and adolescents. J Clin Endocrinol Metab 1985;60:1019.
4. Hanna CE, La Franchi SH. Adolescent thyroid disorders. Adolescent Medicine 2002;131(1):13-36.
5. Kraiem Z, New Field RS. Graves' disease in childhood. J Pediatr Endocrinol Metab 2001;14:229-43.
6. Rapopert B, Melachlan S. Endocrine updates Graves' disease. Kluwer Academic Publisher. The Netherlands 2000.
7. Weetman AP. The immunomodulatory effects of antithyroid drugs. Thyroid 1994;145-6.

SECTION

20

CONGENITAL ADRENAL HYPERPLASIA

RG Holla

Congenital Adrenal Hyperplasia (Adrenogenital Syndrome, Adrenal Virilism)

RG Holla

BACKGROUND

Congenital Adrenal Hyperplasia (CAH) refers to a group of diseases comprising several autosomal recessive disorders that share complete or partial deficiency of enzymes involved in cortisol and aldosterone biosynthesis. Since the earliest case reported by De Crecchio in 1865, a number of enzymatic defects have been described. The genetic defect results in a relative or absolute deficiency of the respective hormone and accumulation of hormones preceding the blocked enzymatic step.

BIOSYNTHESIS OF STEROID HORMONES

The adrenal gland synthesizes three main classes of hormones: Mineralocorticoids, glucocorticoids and androgens. The biosynthetic pathway utilized by the adrenal cortex, and gonads involves a number of steps as shown in Figure 20.1. The pituitary regulates adrenal steroidogenesis via adrenocorticotrophic hormone (ACTH), which, in turn, is controlled by corticotrophin releasing hormone (CRH) from the hypothalamus. Stress and diurnal rhythms mediate the release of ACTH.

Many of the enzymes involved in cortisol and aldosterone syntheses are cytochrome P450 proteins designated CYP, The first reaction in converting cholesterol to C_{18}, C_{19} and C_{21} steroids involves the cleavage of a 6-carbon group from cholesterol and is the principal committing, regulated, and rate-limiting step in steroid biosynthesis. The enzyme system that catalyzes the cleavage reaction is known as P450-linked side chain cleaving enzyme (P450 scc) or desmolase, and is found in the mitochondria of steroid-producing cells, but not in significant quantities in other cells. The product resulting from the mitochondrial activity of P450ssc, pregnenolone, moves to the cytosol, where it is converted either to androgens or to 11-deoxycortisol and 11-deoxycorticosterone by enzymes of the endoplasmic reticulum. The latter two compounds then re-enter the mitochondrion, where the enzymes are located for tissue-specific conversion to glucocorticoids or mineralocorticoids, respectively. Zona glomerulosa cells lack the P450c18 that converts pregnenolone and progesterone to their C_{17} hydroxylated analogues. Thus, the pathways to the glucocorticoids (deoxycortisol and cortisol) and the androgens (dehydroepiandrosterone (DHEA) and androstenedione) are blocked in these cells. Zona glomerulosa cells are unique in the adrenal cortex in containing the enzyme, P450c18 or 18α-hydroxylase, also called aldosterone synthase, responsible for converting corticosterone to aldosterone, the principal and most potent mineralocorticoid. The result is that the zona glomerulosa is mainly responsible for the conversion of cholesterol to the weak mineralocorticoid, corticosterone and the principal mineralocorticoid, aldosterone. Cells of the zona fasciculata and zona reticularis lack aldosterone synthase and thus these tissues produce only the weak mineralocorticoid corticosterone. However, both these zones do contain the P450 c17 missing in zona glomerulosa and thus produce the major glucocorticoid, cortisol. Zona fasciculata and zona reticularis cells also contain the $C_{17,20}$ lyase, whose activity is responsible for producing the androgens, dehydroepiandrosterone (DHEA) and androstenedione. Thus, fasciculata and reticularis cells can make corticosteroids and the adrenal androgens, but not aldosterone.

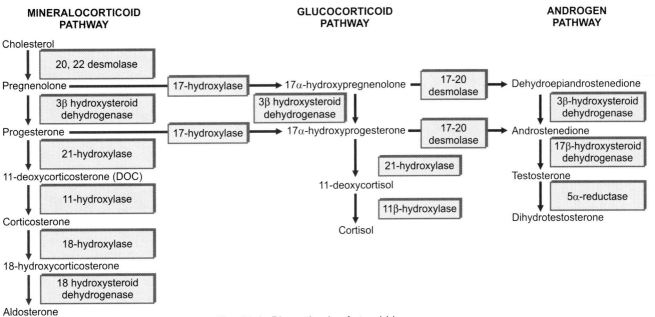

MINERALOCORTICOID PATHWAY

Cholesterol
↓ 20, 22 desmolase
Pregnenolone —————→ 17-hydroxylase ———→ 17α-hydroxypregnenolone
↓ 3β hydroxysteroid dehydrogenase
Progesterone —————→ 17-hydroxylase ———→ 17α-hydroxyprogesterone
↓ 21-hydroxylase
11-deoxycorticosterone (DOC)
↓ 11-hydroxylase
Corticosterone
↓ 18-hydroxylase
18-hydroxycorticosterone
↓ 18 hydroxysteroid dehydrogenase
Aldosterone

GLUCOCORTICOID PATHWAY

17α-hydroxypregnenolone — 17-20 desmolase →
3β hydroxysteroid dehydrogenase
17α-hydroxyprogesterone — 17-20 desmolase →
↓ 21-hydroxylase
11-deoxycortisol
↓ 11β-hydroxylase
Cortisol

ANDROGEN PATHWAY

Dehydroepiandrostenedione
↓ 3β-hydroxysteroid dehydrogenase
Androstenedione
↓ 17β-hydroxysteroid dehydrogenase
Testosterone
↓ 5α-reductase
Dihydrotestosterone

Fig. 20.1: Biosynthesis of steroid hormones

PATHOPHYSIOLOGY

The hypothalamic-pituitary-adrenal feedback system is controlled by the levels of cortisol in the serum. An enzyme deficiency acts as a dam behind which steroid precursors accumulate. Any condition that decreases cortisol secretion results in increased ACTH secretion. This translates clinically as symptoms related to the deficient hormone as well as to those of the accumulating precursor. In 21-hydroxylase deficiency, for example, the aldosterone and cortisol pathways are blocked and the androgen pathway, which does not involve 21-hydroxylation, is over-stimulated. The characteristic virilisation results from excessive secretion of adrenal androgens. A similar state exists in the deficiency of 11β-hydroxylase, with decreased cortisol synthesis and consequent overproduction of androgens. However, an additional finding of hypertension usually, but not always coexists. This occurs due to accumulation of the aldosterone precursor, deoxycorticosterone (DOC), a steroid with salt retaining activity. The phenotype, therefore, has a wide spectrum of presentation and depends on which particular protein is affected and the severity of the mutation or degree of deletion of the particular gene encoding for the protein involved in steroidogenesis. The phenotype can vary from clinically inapparent disease (occult or cryptic adrenal hyperplasia) to a mild form of disease, which is expressed in adolescence or adulthood (non-classical adrenal hyperplasia), to severe disease resulting in adrenal insufficiency in infancy, with or without virilisation and salt wasting (classical adrenal hyperplasia).

Disorders of adrenal steroidogenesis have been described in association with deficiencies of the enzymes 21-hydroxylase, 11β-hydroxylase, 3 β-hydroxysteroid dehydrogenase, cholesterol desmolase and 17-hydroxylase.

21-Hydroxylase Deficiency

The deficiency of this enzyme causes 90% of all cases of CAH and is related to a partial mutation or deletion of the CYP21 gene. The 21-hydroxylase gene lies on chromosome 6p21.3 in the HLA major histocompatibility complex. An inactive pseudogene (CYP21P, CYP21A), located close to the CYP21 is thought to predispose to crossovers in meiosis between CYP21 and CYP21P, resulting in loss of gene function. This recombination accounts for approximately 95% of the cases. Other defects occur because of gene deletions or mutations. Both classic and non-classic forms of 21-hydroxylase deficiency are inherited in a recessive manner as allelic variants. The phenotype depends on the function of the less severely affected allele because that determines the level of enzyme activity. Since the enzyme activity required for aldosterone synthesis is less than that required for cortisol synthesis, only patients with the most severe loss of CYP21 function have salt wasting symptoms. Characteristic combinations of HLA alleles

TABLE 20.1

Deficiency syndrome	Genital ambiguity	Postnatal virilisation	Salt metabolism	Diagnostic hormones
21 hydroxylase				
a) Classic				
i) Salt wasting	Female	Yes	Salt wasting	17 hydroxyprogesterone
ii) Simple virilising	Female	Yes	Normal (high renin)	17 hydroxyprogesterone
b) Non-classic	No	Yes	Normal	17 hydroxyprogesterone
3β hydroxysteroid dehydrogenase				
a) Classic	M (±F)	Yes	Salt wasting	17 hydroxyprogesterone, dihydroepiandrostenedione
b) Non-classic	No	Yes	Normal	17 hydroxyprogesterone, dihydroepiandrostenedione
11β-hydroxylase				
a) Classic (hypertensive CAH)	F	Yes	Salt wasting	Deoxycortisol 11-deoxycortisol(S)
b) Non-classic	No	Yes	Normal	S ± deoxycortisol
17α-hydroxylase	M	No	Salt retention	Deoxycortisol, corticosterone (B)
20,22-desmolase	M	No	Salt wasting	None
Corticosterone methyl Oxidase type II	No	No	Salt wasting	18-hydroxycorticosterone
17,20 Lyase	M	No	Normal	None

Clinical and laboratory features of disorders of adrenal steroidogenesis

or haplotypes are associated with different forms of 21-hydroxylase deficiency. HLA-B47; DR7 is observed in an increased frequency in the classic form of the disorder, while HLA-B14; DR1 is associated with the non-classic variety.

There is decreased production of aldosterone and cortisol. The levels of hormones proximal to the block, namely progesterone, dehydroepiandrosterone (DHEA) and androstenedione increase (see Table 20.1 for metabolic abnormalities). DHEA is a weak androgen. Because adrenocortical function starts in the third month of gestation, a foetus with 21-hydroxylase deficiency is exposed to oversecreted adrenal androgens at the critical time of sexual differentiation, leading to masculinisation of the female foetus. The internal genitalia (i.e. uterus and fallopian tubes), which arise from the Mullerian ducts are normal because the foetus does not possess testes, the source of mullerian inhibiting factor. Boys with 21-hydroxylase deficiency do not manifest genital abnormalities at birth. Urinary metabolites of these precursors (17-ketosteroids and pregnanetriol) are raised. The decreased secretion of aldosterone results in salt loss with hyponatraemia and hyperkalaemia and plasma renin activity is elevated. In partial enzyme deficiencies,

the aldosterone deficiency is not expressed, and patients remain normovolaemic with normal sodium and potassium levels.

The incidence of classic 21-hydroxylase deficiency ranges from 1/10,000 to 1/15,000 live births. The disease occurs in all races and both sexes are affected equally. The frequency of non-classic form is considerably higher.

Clinical Features

The clinical features can be broadly divided into the classic and the non-classic (or milder) variety (Table 20.2).

Classic 21-hydroxylase Deficiency

Female neonates with the classic disorder are recognized at birth due to ambiguity of the genitalia, which may range from mild clitoral hypertrophy with partial fusion of the labial folds to complete labial fusion and a penile urethra. The vagina has a common opening with the urethra (urogenital sinus). The clitoris may be so enlarged that it resembles a penis, and because the urethra opens below the organ, a mistaken diagnosis of hypospadias with cryptorchidism is sometimes made (Fig. 20.2).

TABLE 20.2

S. no.	Features	Classic	Non-classic
1.	Prenatal virilisation	Females	Nil
2.	Postnatal virilisation	Males and females	Variable
3.	Salt wasting	75% of cases	Nil
4.	17-hydroxy progesterone levels after ACTH challenge	Extreme elevation (>20,000 ng/ml)	Moderate elevation (2000 to 15,000 ng/ml)
5.	Genotype of CYP 2IB	Both alleles severely affected	One or both alleles mildly affected
6.	Associated HLA haplotype	B47; DR7	B14; DR1

Comparison of classic and non-classic varieties of 21-hydroxylase deficiency

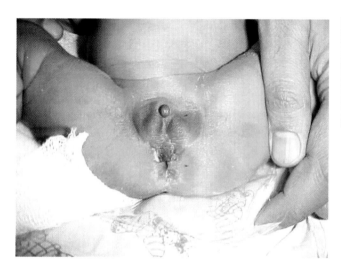 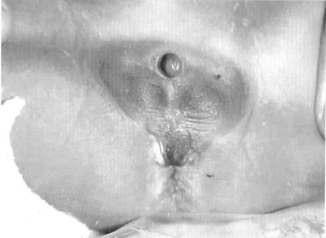

Fig. 20.2: A newborn with ambiguous genitalia
(A result of classic 21-hydroxylase deficiency. Management approach is outlined in the text)

After birth, there is premature development of axillary and pubic hair, acne and a masculine voice. Height and bone age are advanced. Although the internal genital organs are those of a normal female, menstruation and breast development do not occur unless the excessive androgen production is suppressed by treatment.

Male neonates have normal genitalia and are usually not diagnosed immediately at birth. Signs of sexual and somatic precocity appear within the first six months of life or develop more gradually, becoming evident at about 4 to 5 years of age. There is enlargement of the penis, scrotum, prostate, and general musculature. The testes are prepubertal in size and contrast with the enlarged penis. Pubic hair and acne appear and the voice deepens. The bone age is advanced for the chronological age. Adult stature, despite accelerated growth during early childhood is stunted due to premature closure of the epiphyses. About three quarters of the patients of the classic variety have salt wasting syndrome.

In most patients treated adequately from early life, the onset of puberty in both boys and girls with classic CAH occurs at the expected chronological age, with age appropriate gonadotrophin response to gonadotrophin-releasing hormone (GnRH). Precocious puberty (super-imposed 'true precocious puberty') may, however occur, especially if the bone age is 12 years or more, due to a hypothalamic gonadotrophin response to decreasing sex steroid levels following glucocorticoid therapy. Menstrual irregularity and amenorrhoea may occur in post-mencheal girls, related to either under- or over-treatment, the former being due to interference by adrenal androgens, and the latter due to excessive gluco-corticoid treatment. Successfully treated male patients with 21-hydroxylase deficiency have normal pubertal development, testicular function and spermatogenesis. However, persistence of small testes and aspermia have been reported in patients with inadequately treated disease.

Non-classic 21-hydroxylase Deficiency

An attenuated, late-onset (non-classical) form of adrenal hyperplasia occurs due to a partial deficiency of 21-hydroxylase and results in normal or near normal appearance at birth. This disorder is among the most frequent human autosomal recessive disorders. The symptomatology is variable and may present at any age. Female patients may present with premature pubarche, accelerated skeletal growth, clitoromegaly and early or abnormal appearance of facial and body hair. Severe cystic acne, male pattern baldness and hirsutism, delayed menarche, secondary amenorrhoea, and oligo-menorrhoea are some of the other features seen in female patients. Male patients may show early beard growth, acne, growth spurt and features of adrenal (as opposed to testicular) androgen excess viz. presence of pubic hair, enlarged penis and relatively small testes. An asymptomatic subset of non-classic 21-hydroxylase deficiency may be detected during the evaluation of incidental adrenal masses.

Salt Wasting Syndromes in CAH

Patients with various forms of CAH can manifest with salt wasting crises:

a. Seventy five per cent of infants with 21-hydroxylase deficiency come to medical attention at a few weeks of life with salt wasting.
b. Patients with 3β-hydroxysteroid dehydrogenase are usually salt-losers but are less virilised.
c. Males or females with 11β-hydroxylase deficiency may present in early infancy (second or third week of life) with a salt loss crisis. This occurs because of the relative inability of the elevated 11-DOC levels to replace the defective levels of aldosterone.
d. Infants with 20,22 desmolase deficiency (lipoid adrenal hyperplasia) usually have signs of adrenal insufficiency and salt wasting. Males with this form of adrenal hyperplasia have female or ambiguous genitalia. Females have normal female genitalia. Salt wasting results from inadequate secretion of salt retaining steroids, particularly aldosterone. In addition, hormonal precursors may act as mineralocorticoid antagonists in the marginally competent sodium conserving mechanism of the immature newborn renal tubule. Symptoms begin at a variable period after birth with failure to regain birth weight, inappropriate natriuresis, progressive weight loss, and dehydration. Disturbances in cardiac rate and rhythm may occur with cyanosis and dyspnoea. Without treatment, collapse and death may occur. Salt wasting forms of adrenal hyperplasia are accompanied by low

serum and urinary aldosterone concentrations, hyponatraemia, hyperkalaemia, and elevated plasma renin activity indicating hypovolaemia.

The frequency of unexplained deaths of male infants in families later recognized to be at risk for CAH demonstrates the risk of death from adrenal crisis in newborns with CAH. A differential diagnosis of pyloric stenosis, intestinal obstruction, heart disease, cow-milk protein intolerance, inborn errors of metabolism and other causes of failure to thrive must be kept in mind.

In the hypotensive patient, 0.9% sodium chloride (normal saline) must be given (450 ml/m^2 or 20 ml/kg IV) rapidly over the first hour, followed by a continuous intravenous infusion of 3200 ml/m^2/day or 200 ml/kg/100 cal of estimated resting energy expenditure as normal saline or half normal saline to restore intravascular volume. Dextrose also must be provided.

If the patient is hypoglycaemic, 2 to 4 ml/kg of 10% dextrose will correct the hypoglycaemia. 5% dextrose must be provided to prevent further hypoglycaemia or prevent hypoglycaemia from occurring if the patient is not hypoglycaemic. Potassium is not needed for patients with salt wasting forms of adrenal hyperplasia because these patients usually are hyperkalaemic. Once appropriate diagnostic studies are obtained or the results are known, glucocorticoid and/or mineralocorticoid therapy may be instituted. In patients who are sick and have signs of adrenal insufficiency, therapy should consist of stress doses of hydrocortisone (50 to 100 mg/m^2 or 1 to 2 mg/kg intravenously as an initial dose followed by 50 to 100 mg/m^2/day intravenously in four divided doses). Comparable stress doses are 10 to 20 mg/m^2 of methylprednisolone and 1 to 2 mg/m^2 of dexamethasone. Methylprednisolone and dexamethasone have negligible mineralocorticoid effects; thus, if the patient is hypovolaemic, hyponatraemic, or hyperkalaemic, large doses of hydrocortisone (double or triple the stress doses mentioned above) are preferred.

Diagnosis

In an infant with ambiguous genitalia, the diagnosis of congenital adrenal hyperplasia should be suspected and an early diagnosis followed by appropriate therapy and counselling is of paramount importance (Table 20.3). The distinguishing characteristic of 21-hydroxylase deficiency are a very high serum concentration of 17-hydroxyprogesterone (usually exceeding 1000 ng/dl), Δ^4-androstenedione, dehydroepiandrosterone and urinary pregnanetriol (metabolite of 17-hydroxyprogesterone) along with diminished levels of cortisol and aldosterone.

TABLE 20.3

S. no	Features	Defects
1.	Ambiguous genitalia in females	21-hydroxylase defieciency 11 β-hydroxylase deficiency 3 β-hydroxysteroid deficiency
2.	Males with ambiguous or female genitalia	20,22 desmolase deficiency Classic 3 β hydroxysteroid deficiency 17 hydroxylase deficiency
3.	Hypertension	11 β-hydroxylase deficiency 17 hydroxylase deficiency

Typical clinical features of certain forms of congenital adrenal hyperplasia

Salt wasting forms of adrenal hyperplasia are accompanied by low serum aldosterone concentrations, hyponatraemia, hyperkalaemia, and elevated plasma renin activity indicating volume contraction.

The genotype of the 21-hydroxylase deficiency can be assessed by the measurement of 17-hydroxyprogesterone level 60 minutes after intravenous administration of a bolus of ACTH (0.25 mg). The results are compared with a nomogram which provides hormonal standards for assignment of the 21-hydroxylase genotype.

Neonatal Screening

Neonatal screening for 21-hydroxylase deficiency is possible by evaluating levels of 17-hydroxyprogesterone from heel blood samples collected on filter paper on day 2 to 5, permitting early identification of this disorder and prevention of salt wasting. False-positive results (less than 0.2%) are usually associated with prematurity, with severe illness, age less than 24 hours and technical problems. Currently, 13 countries screen neonates for this disorder. This approach permits early identification of newborns and helps prevent salt wasting crises in males who are unrecognized at birth, identification of completely virilised females who may be mistaken for males with cryptorchidism, and the identification of patients of both sexes with simple virilising adrenal hyperplasia, which enables early treatment before undue advancement in skeletal maturation.

Treatment

Medical management: The goals of medical treatment of CAH are:
  i. Optimal gender assignment in newborns with genital ambiguity.
  ii. Appropriate replacement of inadequately produced adrenal and gonadal steroids.

The aim of endocrine therapy is to replace the deficient hormones. This corrects the deficiency and suppresses ACTH overproduction. Proper replacement therapy also prevents excessive stimulation of the androgen pathway, preventing further virilisation and allowing normal growth and a normal onset of puberty. A variety of glucocorticoids and dosage schedules have been used for the treatment of this condition. The effective and convenient drug therapy involves the use of hydrocortisone (Cortisol 10 to 20 mg/m^2/24 hours) administered orally in two or three divided doses. Infants usually require 2.5 to 5 mg two to three times a day and children 5 to 10 mg two to three times a day. Patients with disturbances of electrolyte regulation (salt wasters) and elevated plasma renin activity require a mineralocorticoid and sodium supplementation in addition to the glucocorticoid. Maintenance therapy with 9α fludrocortisone (0.05 to 0.3 mg daily) and sodium chloride (1 to 3 grams daily) is usually sufficient to normalise plasma renin activity. Although aldosterone levels are not deficient in simple virilising form of 21-hydroxylase deficiency, plasma renin, a product of the renin-angiotensin-aldosterone axis is commonly elevated in the simple virilising and the salt wasting form as well. It has been demonstrated that addition of a salt retaining hormone to the glucocorticoid replacement therapy in the simple virilising form improves the hormonal control of the disease. Normalisation of plasma renin activity is associated with fall in the ACTH levels, improved statural growth and allows a decrease in glucocorticoid dosage.

Doses are individualised by monitoring growth, osseous maturation and hormonal levels. Plasma levels of 17-hydroxyprogesterone, androstenedione, testosterone and renin measured preferably at 9:00 am, usually provide adequate indices of control. The administration of hydrocortisone must be continued life-long in all patients. Augmentation of dosage is indicated during periods of stress such as infection or surgery or during periods of decreased salt intake.

Surgical management: Surgical treatment of infants born with ambiguous genitalia has evolved continuously since Hendron and Crawford described the management of adrenogenital syndrome in 1969. Several types of repair exist. The exact method of reconstruction depends on the anatomy of the patient. When a child is born with ambiguous genitalia, a multidisciplinary approach to diagnosis and management is essential because the clinical issues have much wider social and medical significance. Urologic and endocrine consultation should be obtained immediately. The actual gender assignment must be reserved until adequate biochemical and anatomical information is obtained.

In ambiguous genitalia caused by congenital adrenal hyperplasia, appropriate surgical repair may be made once a sex- assignment has been made based on a reliable diagnosis of the underlying enzyme disorder. The aim of surgical repair is to remove redundant erectile tissue, preserve the sexually sensitive glans clitoris and provide a normal vaginal orifice that functions adequately for menstruation, intromission and delivery. A good age for surgery is 6 to 12 months. The clitoris is freed and repositioned beneath the pubis with preservation of the glans, corporal components and all neural and vascular elements. The parents should be reassured that complete sexual function can be restored.

11β-Hyproxylase Deficiency

An enzymatic deficiency of 11β-hydroxylase results in decreased cortisol synthesis with consequent overproduction of cortisol precursors and androgens. Thus, 11β-hydroxylase deficiency shares the clinical features of virilisation with the 21-hydroxylase disorder. The disease accounts for 5 to 8% of cases of adrenal hyperplasia.

The gene for 11β- hydroxylase (CYP11B1) resides on chromosome 8q22. There is no pseudogene and no known HLA associations exist. The enzyme acts at both the glucocorticoid and mineralocorticoid pathways catalyzing the conversion of 11-deoxycortisol to cortisol and of deoxycorticosterone (DOC) to corticosterone respectively. The gene that codes for aldosterone synthetase (CYP11B2), which converts corticosterone to aldosterone in the zona glomerulosa is located nearby and shares 95% homology with the CYP11B1 gene. Mutations and deletions of CYP11B2 gene result in diminished aldosterone synthesis.

Female infants, with the most severe form, present in the newborn period with sexual ambiguity. Hyper-

tension, seen in both sexes, is a distinctive clinical feature but is absent in the first few years of life. The hypertension is thought to derive from excessive levels of DOC, a steroid with 3 to 5 per cent of the activity of aldosterone's salt retaining property. Males or females with 11β-hydroxylase deficiency may rarely present in early infancy (second or third week of life) with a salt loss crisis. This is explained by the relative inability of the elevated 11-DOC levels to replace the defective levels of aldosterone, a phenomenon that disappears with the progression of age and the gradual decreased dependency of the infant from aldosterone. Salt wasting can (uncommonly) occur after institution of glucocorticoid therapy because levels of DOC decrease and aldosterone levels remain inadequate for normal salt balance.

The electrolyte abnormalities include hypernatraemia, hypokalaemia and metabolic alkalosis. 11β-hydroxylase deficiency is indicated by basal or ACTH stimulated elevations of 11-deoxycortisol and desoxycorticosterone or by an elevation in the ratio of 24-hour urinary tetrahydrocompound S (metabolite of 11-deoxycortisol) to tetrahydrocompound F (metabolite of cortisol). Both are accompanied by elevated 24-hour urinary 17-ketosteroids, the urinary metabolites of adrenal androgens.

Therapy consists of glucocorticoid replacement. Hypertension gradually subsides after this treatment. Adequacy of therapy is monitored by following the levels of 11-deoxycortisol, renin and androgens, as well as the growth rate, bone age and pubertal development.

3β-Hydroxysteroid Dehydrogenase Deficiency

Congenital deficiency of 3β-hydroxysteroid dehydrogenase occurs in fewer than 5% of patients with congenital adrenal hyperplasia, causes a severe depletion of steroid formation, and is frequently lethal in early life. The classical form of this disease includes the association of severe salt-losing adrenal insufficiency and ambiguity of external genitalia in both sexes.

3β-hydroxysteroid dehydrogenase is a bifunctional enzyme that catalyzes the conversion of Δ^5 steroids (pregnenolone, 17-hydroxypregnenolone, and dehydroepiandrosterone) to Δ^4 steroids (progesterone, 17-hydroxyprogesterone and androstenedione). Deficiency of the enzyme results in decreased synthesis of cortisol, aldosterone and androgens. The gene is located on chromosome Ipl3.1 and encodes a 371 amino acid protein. Inherited adrenal and gonadal 3β-hydroxysteroid dehydrogenase deficiency is most likely caused by a mutation of the type II β-hydroxysteroid gene.

Two tissue forms 3 β-hydroxysteroid dehydrogenase have been described. Type I occurs primarily in the adrenal and gonad, while type II occurs primarily in the placenta and liver. The genes for both forms reside on chromosome Ip13. The classic form of 3 β-hydroxysteroid dehydrogenase deficiency results from mutations or deletions in the gene for the adrenal form of the enzyme.

In the classic form of the disease, there is often a salt wasting crisis in the newborn period, boys are incompletely virilised and have hypospadias and girls are mildly virilised. The virilisation is thought to occur due to increased precursor steroid formation; that is, the increased amount of DHEA is probably converted by peripheral 3 β-hydroxysteroid dehydrogenase in the liver, skin and other biochemically active androgens that induce mild masculinisation of the female foetus. Some patients appear to have the nonclassic forms of this disease as evidenced by symptoms and signs of virilisation later in life. These symptoms include oligomenorrhoea and infertility. These patients have not been shown to have mutations or deletions of any of the genes that code for adrenal 3β-hydroxysteroid dehydrogenase. The molecular basis for this disorder remains undefined. Considerable overlap between this condition and polycystic ovary disease exists in clinical and hormonal findings. Some of the patients with polycystic ovary disease benefit from suppression of adrenal steroidogenesis with dexamethasone. 3β-hydroxysteroid dehydrogenase deficiency is indicated by an abnormal ratio of 17-hydroxypregnenolone to 17-hydroxyprogesterone and dehydroepiandrosterone to androstenedione.

20,22 Desmolase (Cholesterol Desmolase) Deficiency or Steroidogenic Acute Regulatory Protein (StAR) Deficiency or Lipoid Adrenal Hyperplasia

The cholesterol side chain cleavage enzyme P-450scc is responsible for the first step in steroidogenesis. Its deficiency results in impaired synthesis of all adrenal and gonadal steroids. In this rare but serious disorder, a large number of patients die within the first few months of life. The disease occurs due to the autosomal recessive inheritance of the abnormality (mutation) in the steroidogenic acute regulatory protein (StAR) gene and not due to any abnormality of the P-450scc gene. This protein appears to be involved in the transport of cholesterol across the mitochondrial membrane where it can be acted upon by P-450scc, which converts cholesterol to pregnenolone and then is processed in the various steroidogenic tissues into cortisol, aldosterone, or sex steroids. Thus, a deficiency of StAR results in a global steroid deficiency state.

Histological examination reveals enlarged, lipid laden adrenal glands, giving the name lipoid adrenal hyperplasia. A similar picture is seen in the testes and leydig cells. Wolffian duct development may occur in some males, presumably resulting from partial testicular production of testosterone. Biochemically, there are decrease or absent levels of all adrenal and sex steroids and an accumulation of cholesterol and its esters in the adrenal gland and the gonads.

The clinical course is stormy with development of severe adrenal insufficiency, severe salt wasting and often hypoglycaemia. Due to the absence of androgens, males have female or ambiguous genitalia while females have normal female genitalia. Hyperpigmentation and respiratory problems are frequent. 20, 22 desmolase deficiency should be considered in all cases of adrenal insufficiency, hyperpigmentation and genital ambiguity in XY males. Hormonal studies and imaging demonstrate the deficiency of glucocorticoids, mineralocorticoids and androgens. Females with adrenal insufficiency and no genital abnormalities may be differentiated from those having congenital adrenal hypoplasia by demonstrating the presence or absence of the adrenal gland.

Treatment, which should be aggressive, particularly during infancy, includes glucocorticoid, mineralocorticoid and salt replacement therapy, as outlined for 21-hydroxylase deficiency. Growth, ACTH levels and plasma renin activity are used to monitor therapy. Sex steroid replacement is required during puberty.

17α-Hydroxylase Deficiency

17α-hydroxylase deficiency (P-450c17) manifests clinically as hypertension and hypogonadism. The defect results in the impaired conversion of pregnenolone and progesterone to its 17α-hydroxy product. The consequent decreased production of cortisol and androgens leads to ACTH induced overstimulation of the 17-deoxysteroid (mineralocorticoid) pathway in the zona fasciculate and zona reticularis to produce increased DOC, corticosterone and 18-hydroxycorticosterone. The low-renin hypertension which results is frequently associated with hyperkalaemic alkalosis and hypernatraemia. Adrenal insufficiency does not develop. The XX females have normal genitalia at birth but fail to undergo secondary sexual development at puberty. 46, XY males have phenotypically female or variably masculinised genitalia, often with a distal vagina, variable testicular descent and frequent occurrence of inguinal hernias. Apart from incomplete wolffian duct development, the internal genital development is appropriate for gender.

A single CYP17 gene on chromosome 10 encodes P-450c17 for the adrenals and gonads. One or more additional CYP17 genes are also present in the human genome, possibly encoding enzymes in peripheral tissues. The defect results from mutation in the CYP17 gene.

The diagnosis is based on the finding of low cortisol with elevated DOC and corticosterone levels. Serum levels of progesterone are sometimes raised. Serum levels of testosterone remain low and respond poorly to hCG stimulation. Therapy with cortisol reverses the hypertension and biochemical abnormalities.

PRENATAL MANAGEMENT

Prenatal diagnosis for certain forms of CAH (21-hydroxylase deficiency and 3 β-hydroxysteroid dehydrogenase deficiency) is possible by amniocentesis or chorionic villus biopsy if a sibling with a known mutation/deletion has preceded the pregnancy. These disorders are consistent with normal development and survival if treated, and therefore the choice of terminating an affected pregnancy is rare. The mother is treated with dexamethasone (20 μg/kg/day divided in 3 doses) as soon as the pregnancy is recognized in an attempt to suppress foetal ACTH secretion and prevent the foetal adrenal gland from overproducing adrenal androgens. Once diagnosed antenatally, prenatal treatment of CAH appears to be somewhat successful in preventing the virilisation of a female foetus from 21-hydroxylase deficiency.

Dexamethasone treatment is discontinued if chorionic villus sampling (at 8 to 12 weeks) or amniocentesis (at 18 to 20 weeks) indicates that the foetus is male or if genetic analysis indicates that the foetus is unaffected. Because only the female foetus is at risk of disfigurement from virilisation, this strategy results in unnecessary treatment of 7 out of 8 foetuses. However, because virilisation occurs within the first 12 weeks of gestation, if one waits until the sex and diagnosis of the foetus are known, the virilisation of an affected female foetus already will have occurred. So far, this strategy has not resulted in an increase in foetal wastage or congenital malformations in treated pregnancies. It is, however, associated with considerable maternal adverse effects during the pregnancy. Long-term follow-up studies are ongoing and are required to determine whether dexamethasone treatment in early pregnancy results in any long-term adverse effects.

SUMMARY

Genital ambiguity and abnormalities of sexual development are clinical hallmarks of congenital adrenal hyperplasia, especially when combined with salt wasting syndrome or hypertension. These can be traced to discrete defects in the steroidogenic pathway which are inherited in an autosomal recessive manner. 21 hydroxylase deficiency accounts for nearly 90% of CAH cases. 75% of its classic variety have salt wasting syndrome while its non-classic variety may manifest in late childhood. A subset of non-classic 21 hydroxylase deficiency may be detected only during evaluation of incidental adrenal masses. Neonatal screening, early diagnosis and institution of appropriate treatment ensures normal development.

FURTHER READING

1. Carlson AD, Obeid JS, Kanellopoulou N. Congenital adrenal hyperplasia: update on prenatal diagnosis and treatment. J Steroid Biochem Mol Biol 1999;69(1-6):19-29.
2. Dahms WT, Danish RK. Abnormalities in sexual differentiation. In Fanaroff AA, Martin RJ (Eds): Neonatal Perinatal Medicine (7th edn), Mosby 2002;1416-68.
3. Garner PR. Congenital adrenal hyperplasia in pregnancy. Semin Perinatol 1998;22(6):446-56.
4. Rapaport R. Disorders of the gonads. In Behrman RE, Kleigman RM, Jenson HB (Eds): Nelson Textbook of Pediatrics (17th edn), Saunders 1921-47.

Part 4

IMAGING AND RADIODIAGNOSIS IN ENDOCRINOLOGY

Section 21
Imaging in Endocrinology

Section 22
Mammography and Imaging

SECTION

21

IMAGING IN ENDOCRINOLOGY

MN Sree Ram

Imaging of the Endocrine System

MN Sree Ram

INTRODUCTION

Endocrine system is one of the two important systems which control the functioning of the body; the other being nervous system. The diagnosis of the endocrine system disorder is usually based on the clinical presentation which is further confirmed by assay of the appropriate hormone. However, imaging findings are of importance in certain cases where the clinical and laboratory findings are equivocal. The degree of severity does not correlate with that of the size of the lesion in the endocrine disease. Production of the ectopic hormone further adds to the challenge for the radiologist. With the availability of various cross-sectional imaging modalities and with use of interventional procedures to assess the functional capability of the affected organ, no endocrine gland remains out of the purview of a radiologist.

The human body consists of following endocrine glands:
1. Hypothalamus
2. Pituitary gland
3. Adrenals
4. Thyroid gland
5. Parathyroid glands
6. Pancreas—islet of Langerhans
7. Ovaries
8. Testes.

HYPOTHALAMUS AND PITUITARY GLAND

HYPOTHALAMUS

It is situated behind the optic chiasm between the optic tracts and anterior mammillary bodies. It weighs around 4 grams. It is divided into four regions with arbitrary margins. These include:
* Preoptic region
* Supraoptic region

* Tuberal or infundibular region
* Posterior or mammillary region
  It can also be divided longitudinally into:
  * Medial
  * Lateral zones.

Preoptic Region

This region contains various nuclei and is thought to be of importance for temperature regulation through various mechanisms like sweating.

Supraoptic Region

This area also contains various important nuclei which produce various hormones regulating diverse metabolic functions and hormone secretion of pituitary gland and its target organs.

Tuberal/Infundibular Region

It is intermediate in location between supraoptic region anteriorly and mammillary body caudally. It mainly controls food and water intake.

Posterior/Mammillary Body Region

It is situated behind tuberal region. The exact function of this part is not well defined.

PITUITARY GLAND

This gland derives its name from the Greek word *pituo* means 'to split' and the Latin *pituita* means 'mucus' which reflects the early belief that this organ was to siphon fluid from brain and excrete it into nose. This weighs approximately 0.5 to 0.9 grams and is heavier in females especially during lactation and pregnancy.

Adenohypophysis

The pituitary gland lies in sella turcica of the sphenoid bone. It consists of two portions, the adenohypophysis (anterior lobe) and the neurohypophysis (posterior lobe), which are attached to the hypothalamus by the pituitary stalk.

The adenohypophysis can be further divided into:
- *Pars tuberalis:* This is a delicate layer of pituitary tissue applied to the median eminence and permeated by numerous capillary loops of hypophyseal pituitary axis; occasionally a site of origin of adenomas and acts as residual pituitary tissue that functions after hypophysectomy.
- *Pars intermedia:* Largely vestigial in function although it is prominent in foetal life and during pregnancy.
- *Pars distals:* Forms the principal mass of the intrasellar adenohypophysis; lactotrophs and somatotrophs lie predominantly in the wings where as thyrotrophs and gonadotrophs lie in the medial third. The characteristic location of these functional cell types correlates well with various types of adenomas recovered at the surgery.

Neurohypophysis

It comprises of posterior hypophyseal lobe, infundibular stem and median eminence. This part is responsible for secretion of ADH and oxytocin which in turn are secreted by hypothalamus.

Figure 21.1 represents the gross appearance of the pituitary gland.

VASCULAR SUPPLY

Both pituitary and hypothalamus are supplied primarily by:
- Superior hypophyseal artery ⎱ From internal
- Inferior hypophyseal artery ⎰ carotid artery

The adenohypophysis does not have a direct arterial supply but it receives its blood supply from the hypophyseal portal system. This pathway also serves as conduit for transport of the hypothalamic hormones. The venous drainage of the pituitary gland is into the cavernous sinus which subsequently drains into the petrosal system. The importance of such vascular supply includes:
- Since adenohypophysis lacks a direct blood supply it is potentially prone to ischaemia which explains the postpartum necrosis.
- This lack of direct arterial blood supply is reflected in the contrast enhanced MRI or CT scan obtained in the dynamic mode.

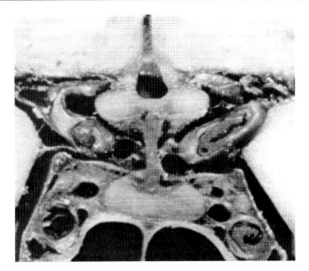

Fig. 21.1: Gross specimen showing the pituitary gland

- The relatively predictable ipsilateral venous drainage of each half of the gland allows reliable sampling of the hormones from the petrosal sinuses.
- Trans-sellar venous channels provide a route for shunting of the arterial blood in the carotico-cavernous and carotico-dural fistulas.

Imaging Modalities

Plain X-ray

In the present era of imaging, this modality has a few takers; however, it can be utilized as preliminary modality to evaluate crudely the size of sella turcica.

CT Scan

Although served as the main modality of the investigation during eighties for evaluating the sellar and parasellar region, it has now given way to MRI.

MRI

Owing to its precise detailed imaging as compared to CT scan it is, at present, the preferred method of investigation. It has a higher SNR, greater spatial resolution in addition to multiplanar capability and absence of ionizing radiation. The intrinsic anatomy of hypothalamic nuclei cannot be identified. The anterior margin of hypothalamus is formed by optic chiasm and its posterior extent formed by the mammillary bodies can be delineated. The pituitary on the other hand can be delineated easily due to higher signal intensity of the posterior pituitary lobe on T1WI. This signal intensity is

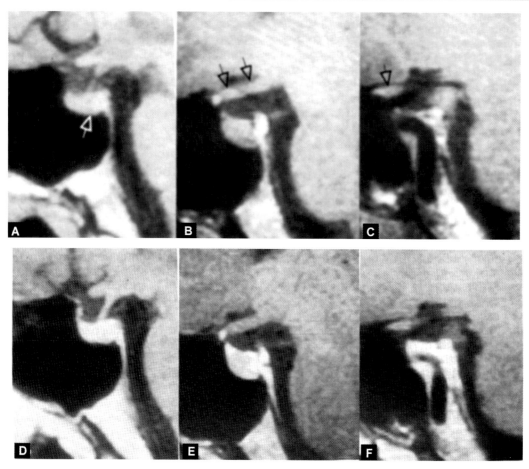

Figs 21.2A to F: Precontrast MR images of pituitary gland (A-F)

due to phospholipids and neurosecretory granules. The anterior lobe has similar signal characteristics that of the white matter. With high resolution technique the diaphragma sellae appears as a band of low signal intensity which allows identification of intrasellar and suprasellar regions. Lateral dural reflections of cavernous sinus can be seen as a band of low signal intensity. The thin medial dura cannot be visualized. The appearances of gland vary in different age groups. In neonates the gland is convex in shape with higher signal intensity than that of the brain stem on T1WI. After two months, infant pituitary signal changes to that of the pons with a flat superior surface. In childhood the upper surface of the pituitary gland is flat with a height of 2 to 6 mm without any sex difference. The pituitary stalk increases during childhood. During puberty there is a dramatic change in the size of the gland. In females it may swell up to 10 mm while in males it may reach 7 to 8 mm. Physiologic enlargement of the gland occurs during pregnancy and MR has shown a linear increase in the height of the gland throughout pregnancy. An increase in the signal intensity

similar to the neonates maybe seen on T1WI. During immediate postpartum period the gland may measure 12 mm in size. Figures 21.2A to F show MR images of the pituitary gland.

MR Protocol

The success of MR imaging depends upon a balance between spatial resolution, image contrast and imaging time. High spatial detail requires the use of slices < 3 mm, a fine matrix (256 × 256) and a small FOV (16 to 20 cm). On routine imaging SE T1 and T2 WI in all planes are obtained. The use of contrast agents like paramagnetic substances DTPA enhances the areas of absent blood brain barrier or the area which is not well developed. (Figs 21.2 G to L).

PET

This imaging modality uses 11-methionine and helps in distinguishing viable tissue from fibrosis, cyst and necrosis.

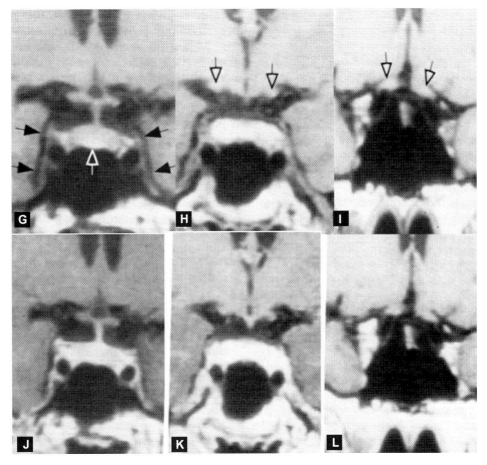

Figs 21.2G to L: Postcontrast images of pituitary gland

Diseases

Pituitary Adenoma

This is a benign neoplasm which generally involves the anterior lobe of the gland. They constitute 10 to 15% of all the intracranial neoplasms. These are classified by their size and function.

a. Microadenoma : < 10 mm in size
b. Macroadenoma: > 10 mm in size.

Imaging

i. *MRI:* It is the modality of choice for detection of pituitary adenomas. Microadenomas are relatively hypointense to the normal gland on unenhanced T1WI. Dynamic scans are obtained using a fast multiplanar spoiled gradient recall sequences. Coronal images are obtained at four locations within the sella using a flip angle of 45 degrees two excitations, slice thickness of 3 mm, 128 × 192 matrix with a TR/TE of 52/4 ms (Fig. 21.3). Images obtained at 20 to 30 seconds after rapid injection of the contrast shows earliest enhancement in the

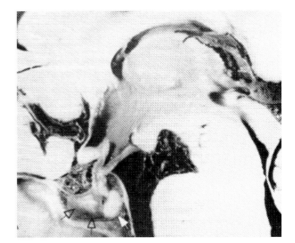

Fig. 21.3: Coronal section showing the parts of pituitary gland

infundibulum of the gland followed by gradual enhancement in the anterior lobe which occurs after about 80 seconds of contrast injection. The normal gland enhances earlier than that of the adenomatous part. The adenomas appear slightly hypointense as

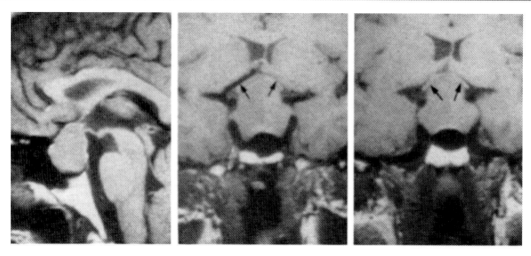

Fig. 21.4: Pre- and postcontrast MR images of pituitary macroadenoma

compared to the contrast enhanced normal gland. Peak enhancement in the adenoma varies from 60 to 120 sec after contrast injection (Fig. 21.4). Micro-adenomas are best visualized during earlier phases of contrast enhanced dynamic scans. Delayed scans after 30 to 60 min may either mask the normal difference of the gland and adenoma or there may be reversal of the pattern the adenomas giving a higher signal as compared to the gland. Micro-adenomas situated in the lateral lobe can cause shift of the pituitary stalk. The small microadenomas when invade cavernous sinus are difficult to discern as the dural reflection on the medial aspect of this sinus is very thin. The lateral wall of the cavernous sinus is seen on MR imaging, and if tumour extends to this site, invasion of the cavernous sinus can be picked up easily. The normal flow voids of intra-cavernous part of internal carotids can be seen easily and encasement of the vessel by the tumour, though rare can be picked up. However, constriction or occlusion of the intracavernous part of the internal carotid is rare. The adenomas may rarely extend below to involve the sphenoid sinus. Tumours of size more than 10 mm are prone to apoplexy. In subacute phases, haemorrhage, which contains extracellular methaemoglobin will be seen as hyperintense lesion on T1 and T2WI. In acute phase the haemorrhage appears as isointense on T1WI and hypointense on T2WI. The cystic degenerations within the tumour are seen as hypointensity on T1WI and hyperintensity on T2WI. There may be fluid level present within the gland. Figures 21.5 to 21.7 show the MR and CT images of pituitary adenomas.

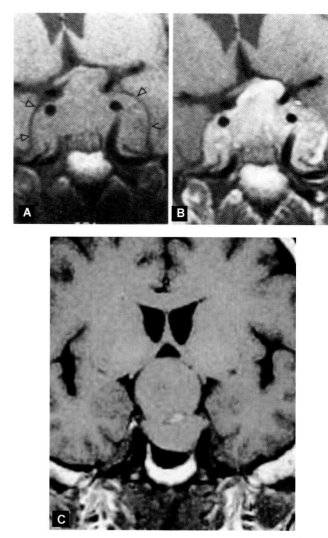

Figs 21.5A to C: MR images of pituitary macroadenoma

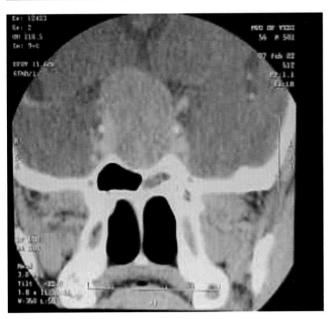

Fig. 21.6: CT images of pituitary macroadenoma

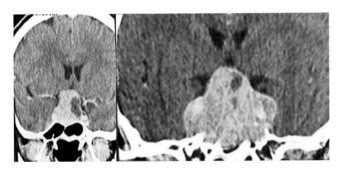

Fig. 21.7: Coronal CT images of pituitary macroadenoma

ii. *Interventional radiology:*
   • *Petrosal sinus sampling:* Inferior petrosal sinus sampling can be done to detect small tumours.
iii. *Plain X-ray:* This modality as described earlier is used only for screening purpose. However, in case of the hyperfunctioning of the somatotroph adenoma manifesting before closure of the epiphysis, it gives rise to features of gigantism and after closure of the epiphysis gives rise to acromegaly. The key imaging plain X-ray findings include the following.

Gigantism

Large stature with increase in the length and diameter of the bone.

Acromegaly
• Enlargement of acral (extremity) parts (hands and feet)

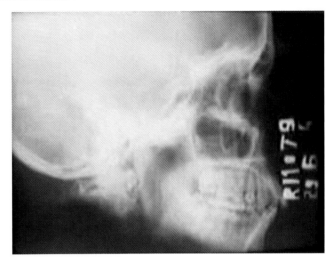

Fig. 21.8: Plain X-ray image showing acromegalic skull

• Enlargement of sella
• Enlargement of frontal and maxillary sinus.
• Enlargement of mandible (Fig. 21.8)
• Increase in the heel pad thickness of more than 21 mm in males and 19.5 mm in females
• Spade like appearance of terminal phalanges
• Increase in sesamoid index (> 40 in males and > 32 in females)
• Articular cartilage hypertrophy with osteoarthritis.
• Scalloped vertebral bodies
• Normal to increased bone density.

Metastases

Symptomatic metastasis is rare as the patients die of primary malignancy before the pituitary manifestations. Most commonly secondaries from lung, leukaemia, lymphoma and breast are seen in the pituitary and diabetes insipidus is the earliest manifestation. It frequently involves the pituitary stalk and hypothalamus. It shows rapid growth as compared to that of the adenomas.

Imaging

On MR imaging these lesions are seen as enhancing lesions in the gland (Fig. 21.9).

Meningioma

These lesions arise most commonly from diaphragma sellae or posterior clinoid process and may project into the sella turcica. In case there is suprasellar extension these lesions resemble adenomas. Rarely a sub diaphragmatic intrasellar meningioma has been described.

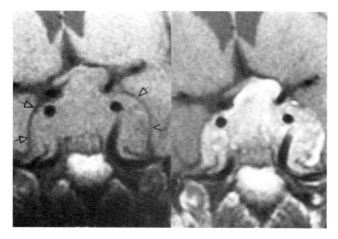

Fig. 21.9: MR images of metastasis to pituitary

Imaging

On MR imaging a prominent intra- or suprasellar mass is seen which shows prominent uniform enhancement after contrast administration (Fig. 21.10).

Craniopharyngiomas

These lesions originate from squamous epithelial cells of Rathke's pouch or cleft in pars tuberalis. These are benign in nature, slow growing tumours and may have solid or cystic components. There is a bimodal pattern seen. The first peak is in childhood around 5 to 10 years and the second peak is seen in the sixth decade. The incidence is more in females as compared to the males. They are seen in both intra- and suprasellar location.

Clinical Presentation

Their presentation differs as per the age group. They present as raised intracranial tension in children and as

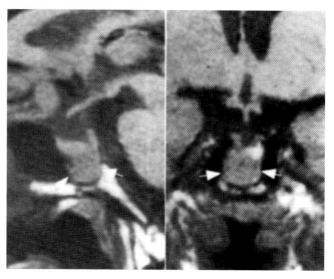

Fig. 21.10: MR images of meningioma of pituitary gland

pituitary insufficiency in adults due to compression of the normal gland. There may be visual disturbances due to optic nerve involvement. In children calcification may be seen within the tumour.

Imaging: The cysts within tumour may contain cholesterol, keratin, proteinaceous fluid, haemorrhage and necrotic debris. On MR imaging the solid portion of the tumour appears hypointense on T1WI and hyperintense on T2WI. The cystic portion of the tumour may show a low signal on T1WI but higher than CSF. Increased signal intensity may be seen if protein concentration is more than 90 gm/L or there is presence of met-Hb. The solid portion of tumour may contain calcium and may give rise to mottled appearance with low signal intensity (Figs 21.11 to 21.13).

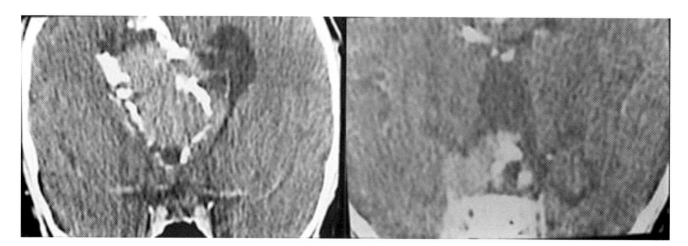

Fig. 21.11: CT scan showing craniopharyngioma

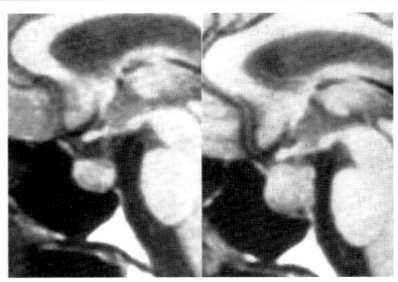

Fig. 21.12: MR images of craniopharyngioma

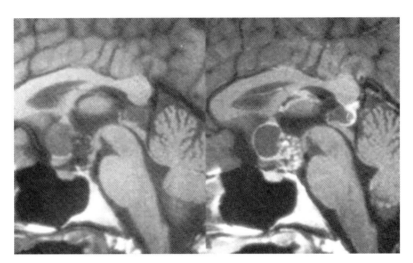

Fig. 21.13: MR images of intrachiasmal craniopharyngioma

Rathke's Cleft Cyst

These lesions are thought to arise from epithelium of Rathke's cleft. The presentation may be that of headache, galactorrhoea, visual field defects or hypopituitarism if the cyst is large enough to compress the adjacent structures.

Imaging: On MR imaging the cyst tends to be discrete and well defined (Fig. 21.14). The lesion may be purely intrasellar or with suprasellar extension. There may be a small intrasellar region which appears hyperintense on T1WI. Larger cysts containing serous fluid may appear as isointense to CSF on all sequences. These cysts do not enhance and hence, are differentiated from cranio-pharyngiomas.

Arachnoid Cysts

Their location may be juxta or suprasellar and hence, giving the endocrinological manifestations. Of all the cases, 15 per cent may be parasellar in location.

Imaging: On MR imaging they appear as smooth, well marginated masses isointense to CSF on all sequences. The differential diagnosis remains that of ependymoma, parasitic granuloma or Rathke's cleft cyst.

Histiocytosis

These lesions present with classic triad of diabetes insipidus, exophthalmus and lytic bone lesion. They are characterized by proliferation of histiocytes. In unifocal type of the disease the pituitary hypothalamus axis is spared while a multifocal type involves the axis.

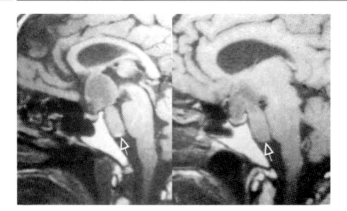

Fig. 21.14: MR images of Rathke's cleft cyst

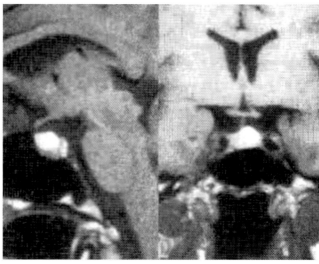

Fig. 21.15: MR images of histiocytosis

Imaging: On MR imaging the pituitary stalk is enlarged symmetrically with homogenous contrast enhancement. There may be absence of the high signal intensity of the posterior lobe. The involvement of temporal bone supports the diagnosis (Fig. 21.15).

Hamartoma of Tubercinerium

It is made of neural tissue similar to that of the hypothalamus and hence, not considered to be a neoplasm. They hardly grow or invade the tissues. The general manifestations are of precocious puberty, gelastic

seizures with episodes of uncontrollable laugh or hyperphagia.

Imaging: On MR imaging a sessile pedunculated mass of variable size is noted in the region of tuber cinerium. These lesions are generally isointense to grey matter on T1WI and iso- to hyperintense on T2WI. These lesions do not show post contrast enhancement with gadolinium (Fig. 21.16).

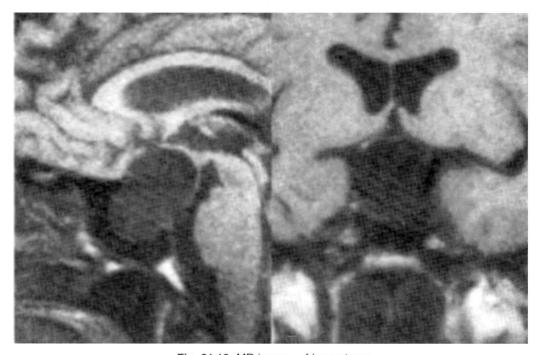

Fig. 21.16: MR images of hamartoma

Germinoma/ Teratoma

These are of germ cell origin. Germinomas are least differentiated of all the germ cell tumours while teratomas differentiate in all the cell lines. About 20% of these tumours are seen in the sellar or suprasellar region. These tumours do not have any sex predominance. The earliest symptom is that of diabetes insipidus due to involvement of hypothalamus.

Imaging: On MR imaging the germinomas are isointense to brain on both T1 and T2WI but may have slightly increased T2 signal intensity. They are homogenous and rarely have cystic appearance. They demonstrate marked contrast enhancement and the normal posterior pituitary hyperintensity is lost. The teratomas on the other hand show mixed signal intensity due to their heterogeneous composition. There may be fat/calcification noted within.

Dermoid/Epidermoid Tumours

Their main presentation is due to compression of the adjacent neural structures. They may present like other pituitary tumours with diabetes insipidus, visual disturbances or hypopituitarism. Dermoids may occur in the paediatric age group and located in the midline most commonly in the fourth ventricle or vermis. The cyst wall of these lesions may contain dermal appendages like hair follicle, sebaceous cysts and sweat glands. The epidermoid tumours are seen in the fourth to fifth decades of life. They are found in basal cisterns, CP angle and parasellar region. The contents are usually waxy material containing desquamated keratin products and cholesterol crystals.

Imaging: On MR imaging the dermoid give heterogeneous signal intensity due to their mixed composition. They may show high signal intensity on T1WI due to high fat content and there may be presence of a fat-fluid level. In case there is rupture of the cyst there may be ventriculitis or meningitis giving increased signal on T1WI. The epidermoid tumour appears slightly hyperintense to CSF on T1 and T2WI. On PD sequences these lesions appear slightly hyperintense to brain and CSF. At times they may give heterogeneous signal intensity due to their varied contents. Post-contrast images do not show any enhancement (Fig. 21.1.17).

Infections

Infections of the pituitary gland are rare. Tuberculosis and syphilis are two main diseases which affect the gland. The bacterial infections become apparent when

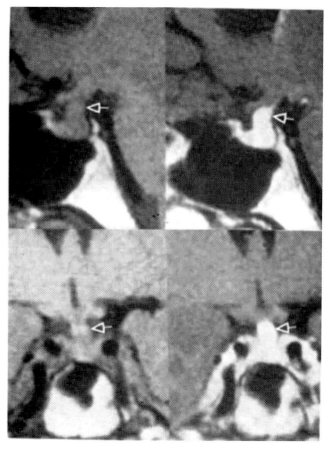

Fig. 21.17: MR images of dermoid

pituitary abscess is present. There may be manifestations of non functioning of the gland.

Imaging: On MR imaging the lesion is indistinguishable from normal gland. However, post-contrast images showing enhancement of the lesion (Fig. 21.18).

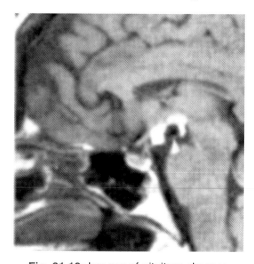

Fig. 21.18: Images of pituitary abscess

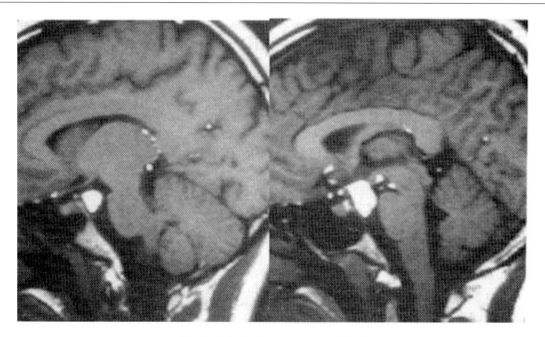

Fig. 21.19: MR image of sarcoidosis

Sarcoidosis

It is of unknown aetiology and when involves pituitary it presents as diabetes insipidus or as a case of panhypopituitarism.

Imaging: On MR imaging the stalk of pituitary may be thickened. On post-contrast images there is ill defined enhancement seen in the basal meninges (Fig. 21.19).

Miscellaneous Disorders

This group includes lesions like haemochromatosis. This is due to excess iron overload in the form of ferritin and haemosiderin in the pituitary gland along with other organs in the body. The gonadotrophic cells are more susceptible. On MR imaging the gland appears abnormally dark on T2WI.

SUMMARY

- Hypothalamus and pituitary gland remains the most obscure glands in the body with varied manifestations.
- Modern imaging modalities like MRI and CT scan have given access to both of these glands.
- Pituitary micro- and macroadenomas are commonest disease process and have manifestations as per the cells involved.
- MRI remains the primary modality of investigation.

ADRENAL GLAND

INTRODUCTION

Cross-sectional imaging techniques, especially CT and MRI visualize adrenal glands with a resolution and clarity unimagined even 20 years ago. But such images provide no information about excessive or insufficient elaboration of steroid or catecholamine hormones, which is the basis of all diagnostic and therapeutic decisions in adrenal endocrinologic problems. Interpretation of adrenal images should never be attempted without the knowledge of the patient's pertinent clinical information and hormonal status.

ANATOMY OF ADRENAL GLANDS

These glands lie anterosuperior to the upper part of each kidney. They are somewhat asymmetrical yellowish in colour, and lie within their own compartment of renal fascia. Suprarenal gland is an alternative name. Right adrenal gland is pyramidal in shape while left is crescentic (Fig. 21.20).

Blood Supply

Both glands receive blood from three sources:
1. Superior adrenal arteries descend from interior phrenic arteries on each side.
2. Middle adrenal arteries arise directly from aorta.

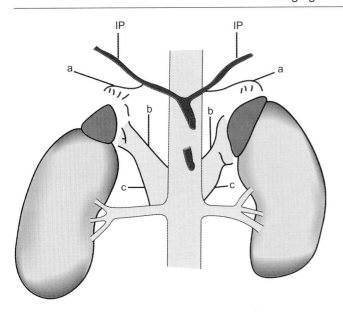

Fig. 21.20: Vascular anatomy of adrenals

(IP—Inferior phrenic artery; a—branch from IP, b—branch from aorta, c—branch from renal artery)

3. Inferior adrenal arteries ascend from ipsilateral renal arteries.

In contrast there is usually a single vein. The right vein is only a few millimeters long and enters the vena cava; the left vein is longer and enters the left renal vein.

Lymph Drainage

The adrenals drain to para aortic nodes.

Nerve Supply

The main supply is by myelinated preganglionic sympathetic fibres from the splanchnic nerves via the coeliac plexus; the fibres synapse directly with medullary cells. Blood vessels in all parts receive the usual postganglionic sympathetic supply, although cortical control is not neural but by ACTH from the anterior pituitary.

Cross-sectional Anatomy

Both glands lie in the upper retroperitoneal region on either side of spine and consist of medial and lateral limbs that tend to diverge inferiorly (Figs 21.21A and B).

Right Adrenal Gland

It lies above the upper pole of right kidney; its medial and lateral limbs join anteriorly in the configuration of inverted 'V'. The medial limb lies lateral and parallel to the crus of the diaphragm; the more interior lateral limb extends horizontally often parallel to the posterior surface of the inferior vena cava. Proximity to the cava accounts for the short course of the right adrenal vein, which drains directly into the posterior wall of the inferior vena cava. The medial limbs of the normal right adrenal gland

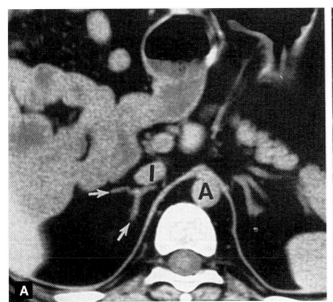
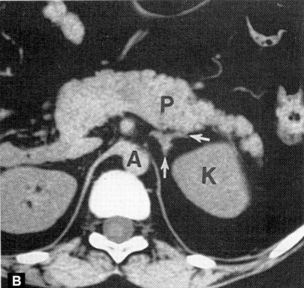

Figs 21.21A and B: Cross-section CT anatomy
(A—aorta, K—kidney, P—pancreas, I—IVC, arrows—adrenals)

averages 3 to 4 mm in thickness and never exceeds 5 mm. It can be compared with adjacent right diaphragmatic crus for presence of hyperplasia.

Left Adrenal Gland

It lies at a lower level than right gland medial to the upper pole of left kidney. Its medial and lateral limbs are shorter and their confluence thicker, thus giving the gland an arrowhead appearance. Left adrenal vein is a longer vessel. Anomalous venous drainage may be present on right side in 3 to 5% of cases, draining to adjacent hepatic veins. It is rare on the left side.

With modern cross-sectional imaging techniques, there is never an indication of performing diagnostic retrograde venography. Careful evaluation of the size and imaging characteristics (radiodensity on CT or changes in signal intensity on inphase/out-of-phase MRI) of an incidental adrenal mass, coupled with patient's clinical and biochemical findings, should precede aspiration biopsy and often justifies follow-up by serial imaging (Fig. 21.22).

PHYSIOLOGY

The adrenal gland has an outer yellow cortex completely enclosing a much thinner grey medulla.

Adrenal Cortex

Its principal products are cortisol, aldosterone, androgens and related hormones. It consists of three zones: Zona glomerulosa (outermost), fasciculata and zona reticularis (innermost).

Adrenal Medulla

It has larger cells secreting the catecholamine adrenaline (80%) and noradrenalin (20%) and some dopamine. Many of the medullary cells exhibit the chromaffin reaction. Dilated capillaries are usually prominent in the medulla and not in the cortex.

IMAGING TECHNIQUES

X-ray

Conventional radiology helps in detecting mass or calcification. A mass may displace the kidney. This can be better appreciated by performing intravenous urography , which differentiates a mass in the upper pole of kidney and the one in adrenal. Second abnormality that can be seen on X-ray is calcification in the adrenal area. Calcification can occur in granulomatous diseases

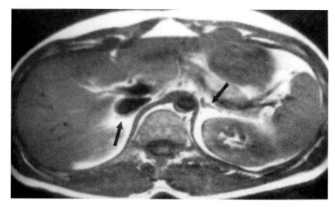

Fig. 21.22: MR anatomy (arrows—adrenals)

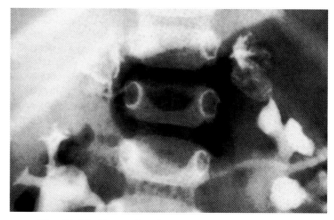

Fig. 21.23: X-ray showing calcification of adrenals

like tuberculosis, in carcinomas, in adrenal haemorrhage, cysts, Wolman's disease or may be idiopathic (Fig. 21.23).

Retroperitoneal Air Insufflation

This technique is no longer used now as better imaging modalities have come up.

Phlebography

This technique has been superseded by CT but is still used for venous sampling of adrenal hormones (Fig. 21.24).

Computed Tomography

CT has revolutionized the imaging of adrenal glands and is the modality of choice. With modern CT scanners, normal adrenals are imaged in practically 100% of patients. Five sections 3 mm in thickness are optimal when searching for small masses such as aldo-steronomas. CT examinations should always extend several centimeters above and below the visualized limits of both glands because exophytic masses arising from

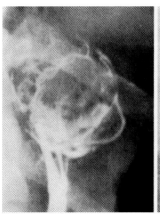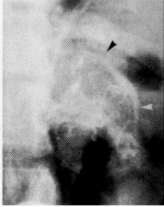

Fig. 21.24: Phlebography of adrenals

the medial or the lateral limb of the gland are not unusual. Adrenal masses >10 cm can be difficult to distinguish from masses of the upper pole of the kidney (bilateral) or masses of hepatic origin (right side). This is particularly true for adrenal carcinomas and cysts. It is crucial under such circumstances to detect the connective tissue planes separating adrenal masses from the upper pole of the kidney or from the under surface of the liver because adrenal cancers seldom invade these adjacent organs directly. USG and MRI are better in demonstrating planes between large adrenal masses and adjacent organs.

CT scan distinguishes non-hyperfunctional adrenal adenomas (incidentalomas) from metastasis by measuring decreased signal intensity (HU) in adenomas as a result of their lipid content. HU values < 10 suggest that the adrenal mass is adrenocorticoid in origin and should be monitored by serial imaging. If HU>10, then it suggests metastasis and therefore biopsy is to be done. If unenhanced studies are not available to measure the lipid content, then tracking the clearance of contrast by taking a post-30-minute scan discriminates adenoma from metastasis as contrast is cleared from adenomas faster than from metastasis.

Magnetic Resonance Imaging

Despite the spatial resolution being inferior to CT, MRI has definite contribution to adrenal imaging by virtue of its improved tissue contrast and its ability to image in multiple planes. In addition, analysis of MRI signal intensities may provide a clue to the histology of the adrenal mass.

On spin echo T1 weighted MRI, adrenal glands have low signal intensities than liver and are clearly outlined by bright retroperitoneal fat. On T2 weighted images, normal and hyperplastic adrenals show low signal intensity (similar to liver) as do masses of benign cortical tissues such as non-hyperfunctioning adenoma or so called incidentalomas. Adrenal cortical adenomas differ from all other endocrine adenomas which are bright on T2 weighted MRI. Adrenocortical carcinomas and metastasis have increased signal intensity relative to liver. Phaeochromocytomas have bright or light bulb appearance.

Arteriography and Venous Sampling

Arteriography is seldom indicated in the investigation of adrenal masses. The complex arterial supply, non-specificity of appearances, risk of catecholamine release during arteriography of phaeochromocytomas and development of superior cross-sectional imaging techniques have eliminated the role of arteriography.

Venous sampling is not to define anatomy but to lateralize functioning tumours by measuring differential hormone levels in both adrenal veins.

Symptomatic cortisol producing adenomas and phaeochromocytomas are always larger than 1.5 cm and easily visualized on CT.

Adrenal venous sampling is not indicated in Cushing's syndrome or phaeochromocytomas.

It is critical that various samples be obtained simultaneously from right and left adrenal veins because of periodicity of hormonal secretion. Left adrenal veins can be successfully catheterized in all patients because of its greater length and predictable drainage into posterior wall of IVC between right renal vein and diaphragm and occasional drainage into hepatic vein.

Ultrasonography

Although the adrenal glands can be visualized by USG, CT and MRI have largely replaced USG in evaluation of functional adrenal disease. USG can be used to demonstrate planes between adrenocortical carcinoma and ipsilateral kidney and liver preoperatively to evaluate resectability. Otherwise, it plays a minor role in adrenal imaging (Fig. 21.25).

Scintigraphy

Scintigraphy, like adrenal venous sampling, evaluates gland function rather than anatomy.

Scintigraphy imaging of adrenal cortex is based on administration of 6B-^{131}I-iodomethyl-19-norcholesterol (NP-59), which is incorporated into the intraglandular biosynthesis of cholesterol. This occurs over a period of

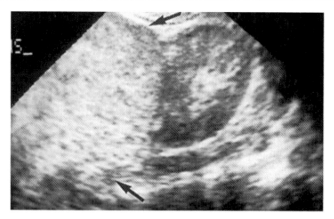

Fig. 21.25: USG showing neuroblastoma

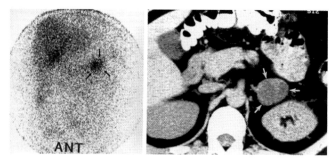

Fig. 21.26: NP-59 scintigraphy and CT scan—adrenal adenoma

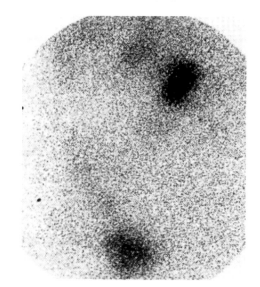

Fig. 21.27: MIBG scan—phaeochromocytoma

several days, so repeated scintigraphic studies must be obtained from days 2 to 6 after administration to allow radioactive background counts to decline. Normal glands are not imaged.

In Cushing's syndrome, bilateral uptake suggests an ACTH dependent disease or less commonly an ACTH independent bilateral adrenal cause such as primary pigmented nodular adrenal disease (PPNAD) or ACTH-independent macronodular adrenal hyperplasia (AIMAH).

Unilateral uptake is suggestive of autonomous cortisol producing adenomas. In primary hyper-aldosteronism, dexamethasone suppression should precede scanning. Unilateral uptake suggests aldosteronoma and bilateral uptake indicates idiopathic hyperplasia.

Thyroid gland should be blocked by administering iodide solution several days before scanning and continued throughout the study.

Significant radiation to the adrenals (15 to 30 rad/mCi of tracer) plus 3 to 5 days duration of study limits the use of radio iodinated cholesterol imaging to specific problems (e.g. Hypercortisolaemic children with normal glands by CT and suppressed ACTH levels).

^{131}I-metaiodobenzylguanidine (^{131}I-MIBG), an analogue of guanidine, located in adrenergic vesicles can be used to image intra-adrenal or extra-adrenal phaeochromocytomas (Figs 21.26 and 21.27).

After intravenous administration of 0.5 mCi ^{131}I-MIBG, normal adrenal medullary tissue is not visualized, but the isotope is retained in phaeochromocytomas for several days. CT is a less expensive, simpler technique for imaging and localization of intra-adrenal phaeo-chromocytomas. ^{131}I-MIBG is useful for screening for ectopic phaeochromocytomas and for detecting metastatic disease.

DISEASES OF THE ADRENAL CORTEX

Cushing's Syndrome

Adrenal imaging has little impact on work-up of patient with ACTH dependent hypercortisolaemia. The most common cause of ACTH independent hypercortiso-laemia is an adrenocortical adenoma. Such tumours are 1.5 cm or larger in diameter and are readily visualized in a fat filled retroperitoneum (Figs 21.28 and 21.29).

When an adrenal mass measures >6 cm in diameter, is inhomogeneous (suggesting necrosis) or when it contains calcification, a functioning adrenal carcinoma must be considered (Figs 21.30A and B).

When carcinoma is suspected, T2 weighted MRI would show increased signal intensity in comparison to benign adenoma.

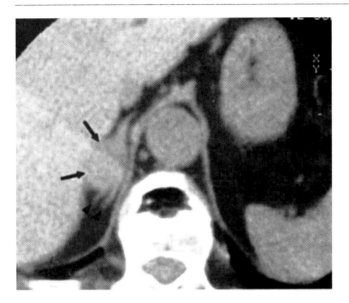

Fig. 21.28: CT scan showing right adrenal adenoma

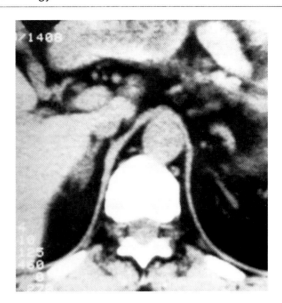

Fig. 21.29: Bilateral adrenal hyperplasia

Adenomas show unilateral uptake on NP-59 scintigraphy but radionuclide studies are seldom necessary.

Steroidogenesis is less efficient in carcinomas and they may not demonstrate uptake on NP-59 scintigraphy.

In the presence of an obvious unilateral adrenal tumour, it is essential to carefully inspect the ipsilateral uninvolved and contralateral gland. The limbs of the adrenal gland that contains an autonomous adenoma should be of normal thickness or atrophic. Similarly, the contralateral gland should appear normal or less commonly atrophic, a reflection of suppressed ACTH levels. If the ipsilateral uninvolved or contralateral gland is hyperplastic, the possibility of ACTH dependent macronodular hyperplasia with a unilateral dominant nodule should be considered.

In primary pigmented nodular adrenocortical disease (PPNAD), CT sections 3 mm thick can detect subtle nodularity or lumpiness of affected glands even in the presence of sub centimetre nodules. This unique and pathognomonic finding results from atrophy of internodular adrenocortical tissues, which leads to a "string of beads" appearance that is normally never seen in adrenal glands of patients younger than 20 years (Figs 21.31A and B).

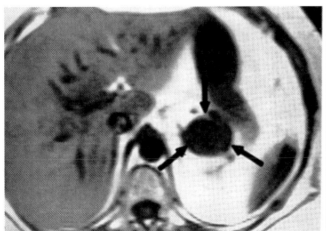

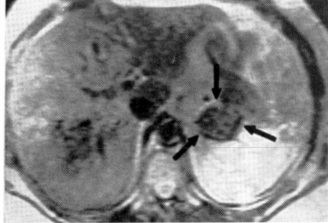

Figs 21.30A and B: MRI showing (A) adenoma, and (B) carcinoma

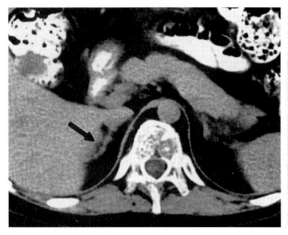
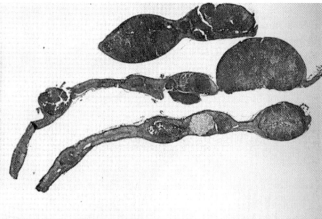

Figs 21.31A and B: CT scan showing PPNAD with a characteristic "string of beads" appearance

Imaging features of systemic effects of Cushing's syndrome are osteoporosis leading to vertebral collapse and spontaneous rib fractures. Ischaemic necrosis of femoral heads may also occur.

Primary Aldosteronism

Role of imaging is to separate surgically remediable unilateral aldosteronoma from bilateral hyperplasia.

After clinical diagnosis of primary hyperaldosteronism, CT should be the first imaging study. Most aldosteronomas are smaller than cortisol secreting tumours. CT sections 3 mm thick should be taken. This is to avoid "geographic misses" or misregistration. It is now avoided by newer spiral CT scanners, where intra-adrenal masses as small as 5 to 7 mm are imaged.

Aldosteronomas have lower CT density than cortisol producing adenomas, density approaching retroperitoneal fat. Care must be taken not to misinterpret adenoma as an angiolipoma.

When a unilateral adrenal tumour and a normal contralateral gland are demonstrated by CT with other tests supporting diagnosis of aldosteronoma, adrenal venous sampling is not indicated.

As imaging techniques improve, the demonstration of small incidental adrenal nodules in the middle aged population has increased and is compromising the diagnosis of primary hyperaldosteronism secondary to hyperplasia based on imaging findings alone. Some investigators have recently recommended adrenal venous sampling as a critical study in hyperaldosteronism (Fig. 21.32).

NP-59 scintigraphy shows unilateral uptake in 75 to 80% patients with surgically proven aldosteronoma.

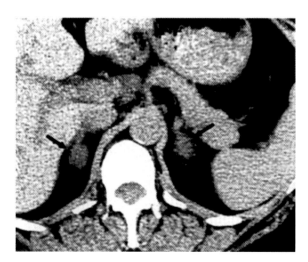

Fig. 21.32: CT scan showing Conn's syndrome (arrows—enlarged adrenals)

However, due to high radiation dose, CT is the preferred first study.

Adrenal Insufficiency

Adrenal insufficiency results from inadequate secretion of cortisol and/ or aldosterone. It is potentially fatal and notoriously variable in presentation.

Adrenal insufficiency is most commonly due to auto-immune atrophy, which may be part of polyendocrine deficiency syndrome. CT demonstrates miniscule glands bilaterally.

When granulomatous disease like tuberculosis and histoplasmosis are suspected causes of adrenal insufficiency, CT provides clinically useful information within a few months of onset of adrenal insufficiency from granulomatous adrenalitis.

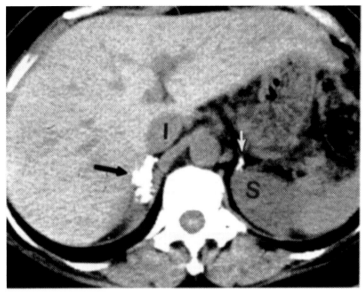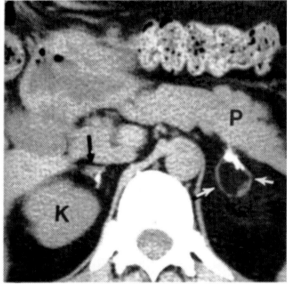

Figs 21.33 A and B: CT scan showing adrenal calcification in a chronic granulomatous disease
(I—IVC, S—spleen, P—pancreas, K—kidneys)

When large glands are demonstrated bilaterally having inhomogeneous texture, it suggests caseous necrosis.

When adrenal insufficiency is due to granulomatous disease of more than one-year duration, then atrophic glands having calcification are seen and no visible glandular tissue is present (Figs 21.33A and B).

Primary/secondary haemochromatosis causes mild adrenal insufficiency from iron deposition in pituitary gland as well as adrenals. Adrenal imaging demonstrates small, dense glands of normal configurations (Fig. 21.34).

Imaging findings in adrenal insufficiency associated with AIDS and antiphospholipid antibody syndrome are nonspecific (enlarged, normal or atropic glands).

Demonstration of bilaterally dense adrenal masses in presence of acute adrenal insufficiency is diagnostic of haemorrhage. Adrenal imaging is not indicated in congenital adrenal hyperplasia. Depending on adequacy of steroid replacement normal to diffusely hyperplastic glands are found. Because of chronically elevated levels of ACTH, congenital sets of adrenal tissue in the testis may undergo hyperplasia and lead to testicular masses, pain and infertility. Hyperplastic adrenal sets appear as low intensity foci with bright testis with MRI. USG demonstrates bilateral masses.

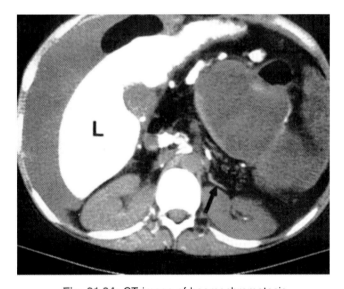

Fig. 21.34: CT image of haemochromatosis

DISEASES OF ADRENAL MEDULLA

Phaeochromocytomas

An 85% of the phaeochromocytomas are intra-adrenal; therefore, radiologic investigations should begin with CT of adrenal glands. Symptomatic phaeochromocytomas are always 2 cm or larger. Many phaeochromocytomas

Derby Hospitals NHS Foundation
Trust
Library and Knowledge Service

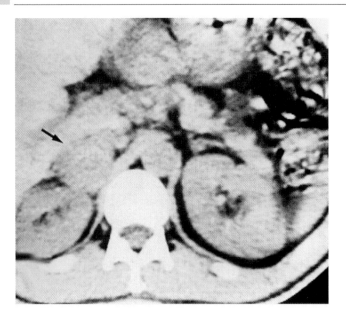

Fig. 21.35: CT scan image of right phaeochromocytoma

are inhomogeneous on CT because of areas of necrosis (Fig. 21.35). They may also contain calcification.

Phaeochromocytomas are extremely bright on T2 weighted images, but MRI adds little to a CT diagnosis of an intra-adrenal phaeochromocytoma.

Unlike adrenocortical carcinomas, the size of the phaeochromocytomas does not always determine their malignant potential. Tumour less than 5 cm may be malignant and metastasize, whereas some of the largest phaeochromocytoma have been benign and totally

resectable. MRI does not distinguish benign from malignant phaeochromocytomas because both are bright on T2 weighted images.

A number of hereditary disorders are associated with bilateral phaeochromocytomas like MEN-2A (Sipple syndrome) and 2B, familial progangliomatous, neuro-fibromatoses, von Hippel-Lindau syndrome. In these groups of disorders, an asymptomatic lesion less than 2 cm in size is seen and appearance of high signal intensity on T2 weighted images suggests the presence of asymptomatic phaeochromocytomas (Figs 21.36A and B).

MRI has advantage of scanning in coronal plane because most ectopic phaeochromocytomas occur in intrarenal paravertebral region, T2 weighted coronal MRI of abdomen and pelvis is helpful in screening for ectopic phaeochromocytomas (Fig. 21.37).

With fat suppressed T1 weighted sequences, Gd DTPA can be helpful.

Only necrotic adrenal metastasis and adrenal cysts have comparably high signal intensity on T2 weighted imaging and cannot be differentiated from phaeo-chromocytomas on MRI.

Up to 15% of phaeochromocytomas are ectopic and under such circumstances both MRI and ^{131}I-MIBG scanning are helpful. ^{123}I-MIBG is replacing ^{131}I-MIBG scanning because the shorter half-life allows a high dose of ^{131}I and permits single photon emission CT scanning (Fig. 21.38).

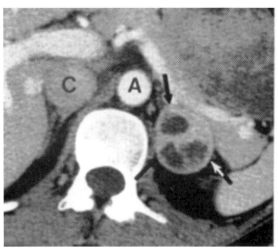
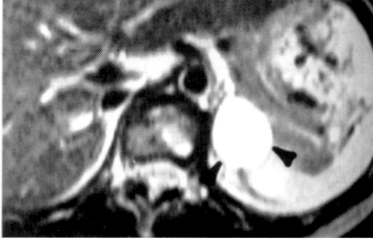

Figs 21.36A and B: (A) T1W and (B) T2W MR image of phaeochromocytoma (A—aorta, arrows—enlarged gland)

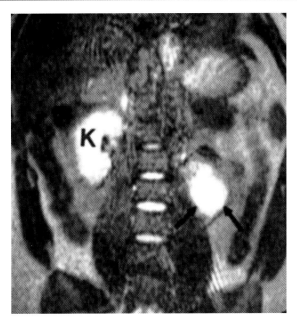

Fig. 21.37: MR image showing characteristic light bulb effect in a case of phaeochromocytoma (K—kidney)

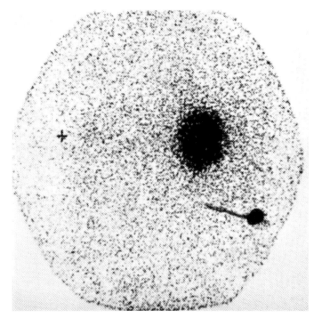

Fig. 21.38: MIBG scan showing increased uptake in case of phaeochromocytoma

Adrenal Masses

CT or MRI examination in a patient without evidence of adrenocortical or medullary dysfunction demonstrating an adrenal mass is commonly referred to as "incidentaloma".

They occur in 3% of all patients undergoing abdominal CT. Some masses (adrenal cyst, myelolipoma), by virtue of pathognomonic imaging characteristics are diagnosed by CT findings alone, but homogeneous unilateral or bilateral masses of soft tissue density in the 2 to 3 cm range require further workup. Even though most eventually prove to be non-hyperfunctioning adrenocortical adenomas, a careful history, physical examination, and few simple laboratory studies usually exclude adrenocortical hyperfunction or insufficiency as well as phaeochromocytoma.

Metastasis from a known or an occult primary cancer is more difficult to exclude.

Imaging can often provide clues that permit fairly confident diagnosis of adenoma and a recommendation for a non-invasive follow-up study.

Non-hyperfunctioning adrenocortical adenomas are homogeneous, smoothly outlined tumours upto 5 cm in diameter. Many appear radiolucent on CT. Differential diagnosis of adrenal masses may be based on their measured CT density. Relatively lucent adrenal masses (< 10 HU) are always non-hyperfunctioning adenomas (i.e. less than water CT density denotes lipid content which is specific for adrenocortical tissue) (Fig. 21.39) When adrenal mass is of soft tissue density (>10 HU), then it suggests cortical adenomas, phaeochromocytomas or metastases. These cannot be differentiated.

MRI may help distinguish carcinoma, metastases or silent phaeochromocytoma. Non-hyperfunctioning adenomas have low signal intensity similar to liver on T2 weighted images. Mass liver ratios <1:2 indicate adenoma, ratios greater than 1:4 indicate metastases or

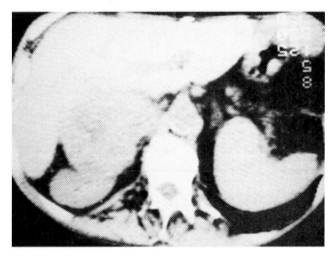

Fig. 21.39: CT scan image of right adrenal metastases

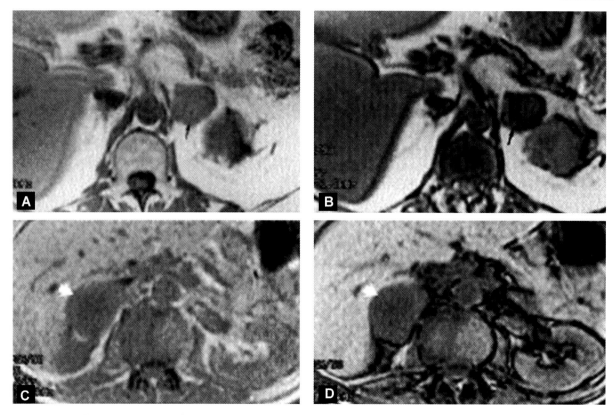

Figs 21.40A to D: Chemical shift imaging (CSI) showing difference between an adrenal adenoma and an adrenal carcinoma

adrenal carcinomas and ratios greater than 3:1 indicate phaeochromocytomas.

Scintigraphy with NP-59 may also distinguish non-hyperfunctioning adenomas from metastases. Non-hyperfunctioning adenomas frequently take up iodo-cholesterol, often with suppression of uptake in the contralateral gland. The presence of iodocholesterol uptake in an adrenal mass excludes metastases.

Chemical shift MRI helps in distinguishing adrenal adenoma from metastases. Loss of signal intensity on out-of-phase images indicates the presence of lipid containing adrenal adenoma (Figs 21.40A to D).

Thus CT, scintigraphy and MRI, are all useful in distinguishing an incidentally discovered, non-hyperfunctioning adenoma from more serious pathology in patients without obvious endocrinologic abnormalities.

For summary of preferred imaging modalities in adrenal conditions see Table 21.1.

TABLE 21.1

Conditions	Preferred imaging modalities
Adrenal adenoma	CT
Adrenal carcinoma	CT or MRI
Pigmented primary nodular adrenal disease (PPNAD)	
> 10 years	CT
< 10 years	Adrenal scintigraphy
ACTH-independent macronodular adrenal hyperplasia (AIMAH)	CT
Primary hyperaldosteronism	CT
Adrenal insufficiency	CT
Phaeochromocytomas	CT MRI (adds little to what CT has shown) (helpful in screening for ectopic phaeochromocytomas) [131]I—MIBG scan

Adrenal conditions and preferred imaging modalities

THYROID GLAND

INTRODUCTION

The thyroid gland is situated in front and the sides of the midline of the neck. The normal function of the gland is directed to the secretion of L-thyroxine (T4) and 3, 5, 3-triiodo-L-thyronine (T3), the active thyroid hormones that influence diverse metabolic processes. Diseases of the thyroid are manifested by qualitative and quantitative alterations in the hormone secretion, enlargement of the thyroid or both. Insufficient hormone secretion results in hypothyroidism or myxoedema, in which decreased calorie expenditure (hypometabolism) is a feature.

ANATOMY

Each lobe of the gland is conical in shape with the apex directed upwards. It extends above up to the junction of the middle and lower 1/3rd of the oblique line of thyroid cartilage and below up to 5th or 6th tracheal ring.

True capsule is formed by the fibrous part of the gland and false capsule by the pre-tracheal layer of the fascia.

Isthmus is the part connecting the two lobes of the gland. It is situated in front of the 2nd, 3rd, 4th tracheal ring with a length of 1.25 cm and breadth 1.25 cm.

Pyramidal lobe is situated above the isthmus and is said to be the third lobe of the thyroid gland (Fig. 21.41).

Accessory thyroid is present as the vestiges of the thyroglossal duct at foramen caecum of the tongue (lingual thyroid) or in the thorax (retrosternal thyroid).

Microscopically the gland is made up of a number of closed vesicles lined by cubical epithelium, containing a thick homogeneous semifluid called 'colloid.' Each vesicle forms a gland unit. Each vesicle is separated from each other by septum, which is formed by the prolongation of the true capsule.

Vascular Supply

Arterial Supply

The gland is mainly supplied by superior thyroid artery, which is a branch of external carotid artery and inferior thyroid artery, which is a branch of thyrocervical trunk. Occasionally a small supply may come from arteria thyroidea ima, which is a branch of arch of aorta.

Venous Drainage

Veins starts from a plexus within the true capsule of the gland. Veins follow the arteries. Superior and middle thyroid veins drain into the internal jugular vein. Inferior thyroid vein drains into the subclavian or brachiocephalic vein.

Lymphatic

They start as a plexus on the wall of the gland. From it lymph vessels form a plexus on true capsule. Main lymphatics from it form ascending and descending lymph trunks. Ascending lymph vessels drain into prelaryngeal and deep cervical lymph nodes. Descending lymph vessels drain into pre- and paratracheal lymph nodes and into thymus.

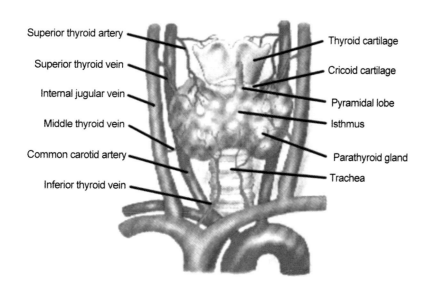

Fig. 21.41: Anatomy of thyroid and parathyroid

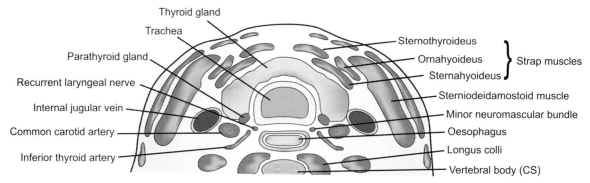

Fig. 21.42: Cross-sectional anatomy

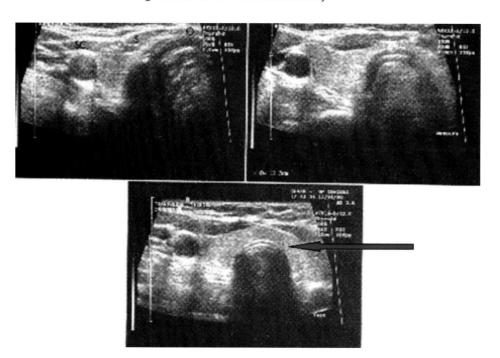

Figs 21.43A to C:Transverse images of normal thyroid gland (Arrow—thyroid gland)

Cross-sectional Anatomy

Ultrasonography enjoys the distinction of the most commonly used imaging modality for evaluation of thyroid gland. On USG thyroid has a fine homogeneous echotexture. It is more echogenic than the adjacent muscles. Echotexture is interrupted by vascular structures. Thyroid capsule appears as a thin echogenic line surrounding the gland. It may show areas of calcification within.

On colour Doppler imaging the superior and inferior thyroid arteries are well seen at the periphery. However, minimal flow is seen within the gland.

Dimensions of the gland vary significantly with age and body habitués. The normal measurements seen in adults are as follows:

- Length—4 cm (< 5 cm)
- Width—2.5 cm
- AP diameter—2.5 cm

If the AP diameter is greater than 2.5 cm on a longitudinal scan it is suggestive of enlargement. In thin subjects the length may reach up to 7 cm, but the depth usually remains within the range of 0.7 to 1 cm (Figs 21.42 to 21.45).

IMAGING MODALITIES

Conventional

Plain film study has a minor role in the imaging of thyroid gland and a subsidiary to clinical investigation. A anteroposterior or lateral projection of the neck may show a thyromegaly with indention or compression of the air passages.

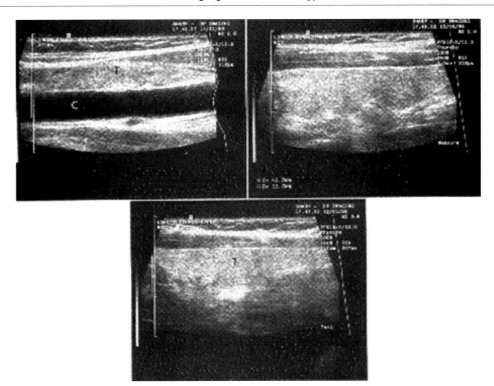

Figs 21.44A to C: Longitudinal images of normal thyroid gland (C–carotid, T–thyroid)

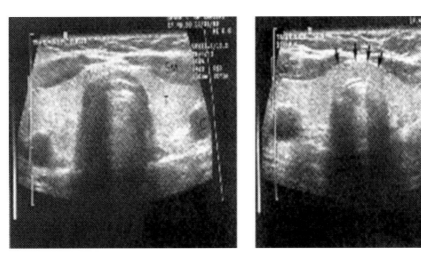

Figs 21.45A and B: (A) Both lobes of thyroid, (B) isthmus (shown by arrows)

Ultrasound Including Doppler

Ultrasound is considered the imaging modality of choice because of the following reasons:

The location of the gland is in a favourable position in front of the neck for USG examination. High incidence of thyroid abnormalities that can be picked up with the use of high frequency probe. Sonography is definitely more helpful than palpation for detecting thyroid nodules. Diagnostic accuracy is also very high. Low cost and fast examination time has made it readily available. No use of ionizing radiation and no requirement of patient preparation are some of the inherent advantages associated with it. The status of the surrounding organs can be assessed very easily. It is particularly valuable in serial follow up of patients with thyroid disorders noninvasively. Interventional procedures, like fine needle biopsy of the gland are commonly undertaken with ultrasound guidance.

Colour Doppler study is used to assess the vascularity of a lesion, though not very helpful in characterization of a lesion. The vascularity depends on the size of the lesion rather than the histological nature. Doppler indices show considerable overlap between the benign and malignant lesions. However, malignant lesions, particularly papillary carcinoma shows hypervascularity in about 90% of the cases.

The use of ultrasound contrast agents may be helpful in differentiating benign from malignant lesions. The time intensity curves and washout curves are studied. Benign nodules usually show a regular and monophasic pattern of washout while malignant nodules show irregular polyphasic pattern. Overall ultrasound has a sensitivity of 63 to 87%, specificity 61 to 95% and accuracy of 80 to 94% in detecting thyroid abnormalities.

Computerized Tomography (CT) Scan

The thyroid gland is well seen on CT due to its higher than average soft tissue attenuation, caused by the physiologically high iodine content of the gland.

Thyroid adenomas and carcinomas are seen as soft tissue masses within the gland; calcification and cyst formation is seen in both types of lesion and CT cannot readily distinguish benign from malignant thyroid masses unless metastatic disease, bone or cartilage destruction or neurological involvement is identified in the latter.

Iodine containing contrast enhancement may prevent subsequent radioactive iodine treatment of thyroid gland for up to 6 months. CT is therefore not recommended for staging of thyroid carcinoma.

Thyroid carcinoma or lymphoma may be seen as an infiltrating soft mass extending from the thyroid. Retrosternal extent of thyroid can be demonstrated.

Magnetic Resonance Imaging

MRI has acknowledged advantages over CT for detecting neck masses and is now the imaging modality of choice; but careful assessment and use of needle biopsy should avoid the use of MRI for inflammatory and simple nodules of the thyroid. MRI shows clearly the major vessels of the neck without added contrast. T1- weighted sequences have the best spatial resolution and give a strong signal of fat in the tissue planes. However, T2-weighted protocols are most useful for showing muscle invasion (Figs 21.46A and B).

Image degradation by movement and failure to depict calcification or fine bone details are disadvantages of MRI. Evaluation of cervical lymphadenopathy for the staging of metastatic disease is best done by contrast enhanced CT at the present time. Ring enhancement, capsular penetration, and extranodal spread into the fat are well shown by CT but MRI appears promising in distinguishing end stage fibrosis from recurrent tumour. Neither technique can differentiate with certainty nodal neoplasia from inflammatory hyperplasia.

Scintigraphy

The ability of the thyroid gland to trap iodine or iodine analogues such as ^{99m}Tc pertechnetate forms the basis of a large number of thyroid function tests, as well as of thyroid scanning. The isotopes commonly used are:

i. ^{131}I: The biophysiological properties of ^{131}I make it unsuitable for general diagnostic works, but it is valuable therapeutic agent.

ii. ^{123}I: This is the most suitable radionuclide physically, mainly for its γ-energy (159 KeV) which is ideal for gamma camera. It has a short half-life and a low radiation dose.

iii. ^{99m}Tc : The pertechnetate ion is trapped in a similar fashion to iodine as they are analogues. But, it does

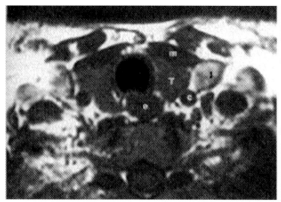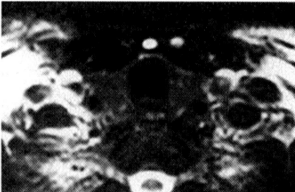

Figs 21.46A and B: MR images of thyroid (T–thyroid, C–carotid, J–internal jugular vein)

not take part in any further synthesis and this is a relative disadvantage.

iv. Thalium-201: This radioisotope shows uptake in various thyroid disorders including cancers. Main application is in patients with residual or recurrent thyroid cancers with raised thyroglobulin and negative ^{131}I body survey.

v. ^{99m}Tc MIBI: It is seen to have better resolution and easier to interpret with higher sensitivity and specificity. However, they have considerable hepatic and abdominal activities. (These agents do not require withdrawal of thyroid suppressive treatment).

vi. Gallium-67: It is mainly used to study inflammatory conditions of the gland.

vii. ^{123}I MIBG and pentavalent ^{99m}Tc DMSA are used in the investigation of the medullary carcinoma of the thyroid.

The principal application of radionuclide study is to classify thyroid nodules. Hot nodule is seen in autonomous thyroid tissue and in hyperfunction of normal thyroid tissue. Cold nodule is detected in neoplastic conditions like adenomas and carcinomas (Figs 21.47 to 21.49).

They are also helpful in detection of ectopic thyroid gland and to differentiate a retrosternal goitre from any other superior mediastinal mass. A well differentiated carcinoma can be separated from a poorly differentiated carcinoma. However, they have no importance in diagnosis of inflammatory conditions of the gland due to varied uptake pattern.

Interventional Radiology

The primary role of intervention in thyroid pathologies is ultrasound guided fine needle aspiration cytology and biopsy (FNABC) for histological diagnosis of a lesion. Newer techniques like, US guided percutaneous ethanol injection or US guided laser photocoagulation are directed towards palliative reduction of tumour bulk and thus relief of symptoms in surgically inoperable cases. Evaluation of lymphatic drainage of a lesion with intra-tumoural injection of ^{99m}Tc nanocolloid is a recent addition in interventional procedures.

Ectopic Thyroid

Imaging: Scintigraphy is the modality for convincingly localizing the ectopic thyroid. A lateral scan may be the best way of showing the upper part of the neck and the region of the foramen caecum, for normal salivary gland activity may cause problem of interpretation (Fig. 21.50).

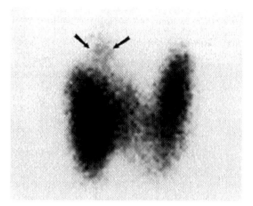

Fig. 21.47: ^{131}Iodine scan in a patient of Graves' disease

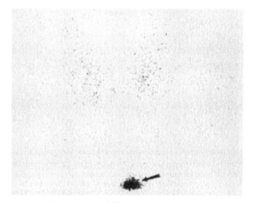

Fig. 21.48: ^{123}Iodine sialography in a patient of thyroiditis

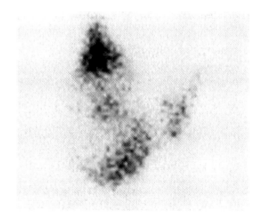

Fig. 21.49: ^{99m}Tc pertechnetate scan in a patient of multinodular goitre

Retrosternal Thyroid

Imaging

i. Conventional chest radiograph—will show a superior mediastinal mass.

ii. Ultrasonography—with a suprasternal approach will be able to localize the lesion.

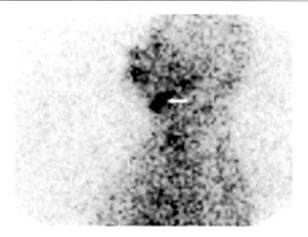

Fig. 21.50: Lingual thyroid

Interventional procedures, like fine needle biopsy of the gland is done with USG guidance.

iii. Scintigraphy—A positive radionuclide scan is the simple and discriminatory test.

CT of the chest and neck is the best in demonstrating the retrosternal extension of the gland and also the encroachment on the surrounding structures (Figs 21.51 A and B).

Thyroid Nodule

Imaging

i. Conventional radiography—has a limited role in detection of thyroid nodules. Radiograph of neck may show an enlarged gland with evidence of microcalcification. Chest radiograph may be helpful in evaluating metastatic disease from a malignant thyroid nodule.

ii. Ultrasonography—high resolution small part scanners can now resolve small colloid nodules in

up to 25% of the cases. The sequence of events in the information of colloid goitre is initially colloid accumulation within the thyroid cells leading to necrosis and confluence with the formation of solid colloid nodules. Haemorrhage, cyst formation, fibrosis, scarring and calcification all occur in advanced disease, together with overgrowth of residual thyroid parenchyma. The USG appearance varies significantly with the stage of the disease but the typical appearance is that of a poorly echogenic nodule, a lobular contour, foci of increased echogenicity representing fibrosis and linear or curvilinear anechoic degenerative areas and small cysts occurring within and between nodules.

Features on USG that point towards a benign lesion are, a sharp well marginated hypo- to hyperechoic lesion, presence of anechoic halo and fine calcification (Fig. 21.52). Malignant nodules are denoted by predominantly hypoechoic, poorly marginated lesion, a thick incomplete halo, and scattered calcification.

Colour Doppler helps in assessing the vascularity of a lesion and thus helps in better characterization of a lesion.

iii. Scintigraphy—in a 'hot nodule', the activity is greater than the surrounding normal tissue and there may be clinical signs of thyrotoxicosis. It may be due to hyperfunction of a gland that has been previously damaged by surgery or irradiation. It is very rare for carcinoma to accumulate as much activity as the surrounding tissue.

A 'cold nodule' is one in which there is defect of activity corresponding to the palpable nodule. The common possibilities are adenoma, which may be cystic or solid and carcinoma. Other causes of cold nodules are focal thyroiditis, abscess and parathyroid adenoma.

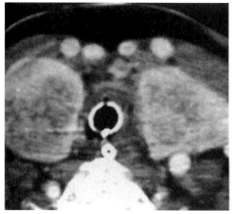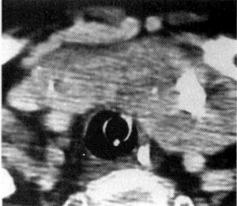

Fig. 21.51A: CT scan showing multinodular goitre with substernal extension

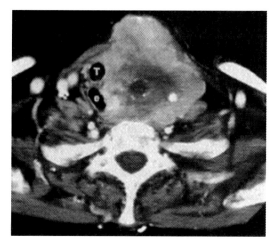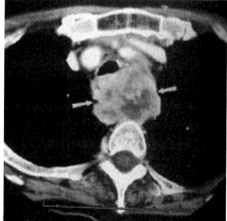

Fig. 21.51B: CT image of multinodular goitre with substernal extension and compression of trachea

Cross-sectional imaging has a very limited role in evaluation of thyroid nodules.

Interventional radiography is directed towards confirmation of diagnosis by biopsy of a nodule, which is usually done under the guidance of USG.

Hashimoto's Thyroiditis

Imaging: Conventional radiography may show a soft tissue swelling in the neck.

Ultrasonographic appearance is that of multiple, ill-defined hypoechoic areas separated by thick fibrous stand. Overall the gland appears hypoechoic with coarse echotexture. Normal parenchyma may not be identified (Figs 21.53A and B).

On scintigraphy the scan appearance may vary from absent uptake to diffusely increased uptake.

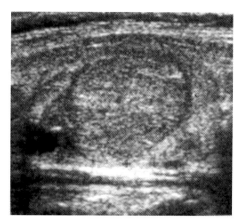

Fig. 21.52: Sonography of a palpable thyroid nodule with a sonolucent halo suggestive of benign lesion

Riedel's thyroiditis is a rare condition and may mimic carcinoma.

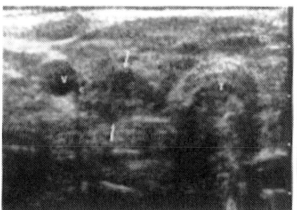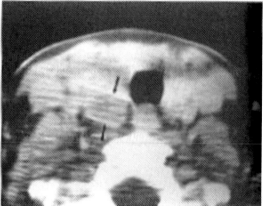

Figs 21.53A and B: Hashimoto's thyroiditis

Acute and subacute thyroiditis is usually diagnosed clinically and scan appearances are not important.

Graves' Disease (Diffuse Toxic Goitre)

Imaging: Plain radiography detects the thyromegaly.

On ultrasonography it appears as a diffusely enlarged hypoechoic gland with echotexture more inhomogeneous than in goitre. Contour of the gland shows lobulation without palpable nodule.

On colour flow imaging it shows a marked increase in vascularity, which is typically described as 'thyroid inferno.' The intrathyroid vessels show an increased flow velocity with a turbulent pattern of flow. Arteriovenous shunts may also be seen within the gland (Fig. 21.54).

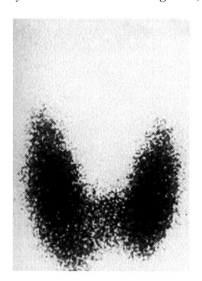

Fig. 21.54: Graves' disease

Scintigraphy shows a pattern of diffuse increase in uptake. Incidental nodules may get superimposed on pre-existing adenomatous goitre.

De Quervain Thyroiditis

Imaging: On ultrasound the affected gland segment is enlarged with ill-defined, irregular margins and show reduced echogenicity. On colour Doppler the vascularity of the gland is reduced.

Scintigraphy shows low radioiodine uptake with poor visualization of thyroid initially. Multiple hypofunctional areas may be visible. Increased uptake is seen during the phase of hypothyroidism.

Thyroid Adenoma

Imaging

Ultrasound: The characteristic ultrasound finding is a very thin smooth halo around the lesion. It is less than 1 mm in thickness and represent the thyroid capsule. The internal feature of thyroid adenoma depends very much on the size of lesion and presence of degeneration. Approximately 60% contain a central cystic cavity. Occasionally, the cyst may grow so large so as to compress to a thin rim beneath the capsule. Blood clot is commonly seen within the cyst. The echogenicity of the thyroid adenomas varies considerably but majority are more echogenic than the normal thyroid tissue

Follicular adenomas and follicular carcinomas cannot be differentiated on USG. Thyroid adenomas are rarely multiple but may reach a very large size (Figs 2.55A and B).

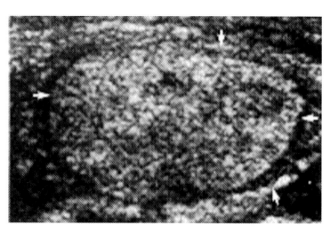

Fig. 21.55A: Ultrasonography showing adenoma

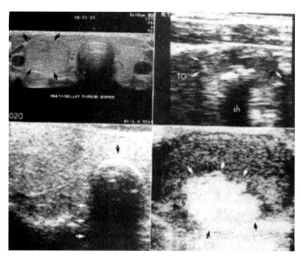

Fig. 21.55B: Sonographic variations of adenoma

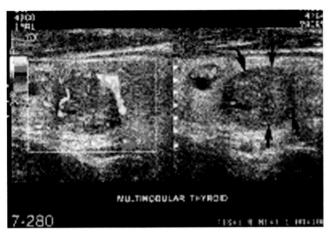

Fig. 21.56: CDI—Increased vascularity

USG guided biopsy helps in giving histopathological diagnosis.

On colour Doppler study blood vessels are characteristically seen extending from the periphery to the centre giving the 'spoke and wheel' pattern (Fig. 21.56).

Scintigraphy: Adenomas appear as cold nodule; however, the radioisotope uptake pattern varies considerably.

CT and MRI scans are particularly helpful in characterization of this lesion and to differentiate from malignant conditions.

Thyroid Carcinoma

Papillary carcinoma

Imaging: Conventional radiograph shows enlarged gland with punctate/psammomatous calcification at the tumour periphery.

Ultrasound: They appear as solid, hypoechoic lesions. There may be cystic changes with intracystic septa showing blood flow within. Punctate calcification is highly suggestive of papillary carcinoma (Figs 21.57A and B). Cervical lymphadenopathy is a common feature which is seen either due to primary disease or as postoperative spread. Nodes often resemble the primary lesion with microcalcification seen within.

On colour Doppler the lesion gives the appearance of a chaotic vascularity.

Follicular Carcinoma of Thyroid

Imaging: Conventional radiography is helpful in detecting metastases into the lung and also bony metastases.

Ultrasound: The lesion appears as a predominantly solid, homogeneous hyperechoic mass. It has a thick irregular capsule with extracapsular spread being common. On Doppler examination tortuous perinodular and intranodular blood vessels are seen.

Anaplastic Carcinoma

Imaging:
i. *Ultrasound:* The lesion appears diffusely hypoechoic with areas of necrosis. Dense amorphous calcification is seen within the lesion. Distant or nodal metastases are seen in 80% of the cases. It characteristically has an irregular margin with early invasion into the capsule and into the surrounding structures (Fig. 21.58).
ii. *CT:* It appears as a mass of inhomogeneous attenuation. The areas of necrosis, calcification and

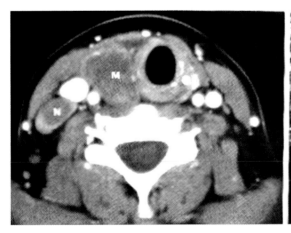
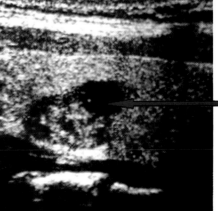

Figs 21.57A and B: Papillary carcinoma thyroid (M–mass, N–nodes, arrow–hypoechoic malignant lesion)

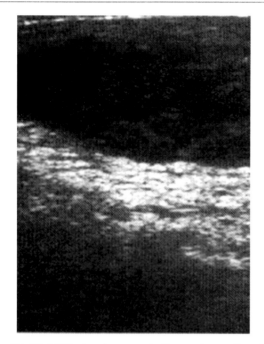

Fig. 21.58: USG showing anaplastic carcinoma thyroid

Scintigraphy of thyroid carcinomas: Over half of the thyroid carcinomas produce a cold nodule on a scan and carcinoma is the commonest cause of such a nodule. Thus scan is not an absolute discriminator of carcinoma of thyroid but helps to determine the probability, especially if the nodule is cold. [131]I scanning is very helpful in detecting metastasis from known thyroid cancer, depending on its activity for iodine. Serial body scans are used to locate metastases, determine the activity required to treat them and follow the response to treatment.

Skeletal Features of Hypothyroidism

Conventional radiography: In children skeletal maturation is delayed and growth is retarded. Epiphyses are late in appearing and fragmented; although when they do appear the sequence is normal. Deformity is seen in the hip joint. Wormian bones are seen in the skull, and sella is either small or bowel-shaped or of large rounded 'cherry sella' appearance. The paranasal sinuses are underdeveloped. In the spine, bullet shaped vertebral

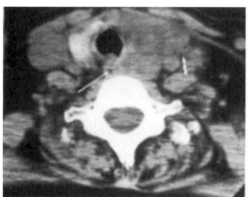
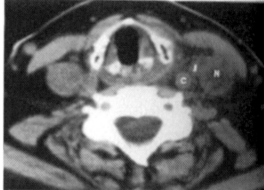

Figs 21.59A and B: CT showing anaplastic carcinoma thyroid

regional lymphadenopathy are better appreciated as well as invasion into internal carotid artery/jugular vein/larynx is clearly detected (Figs 21.59 A and B).

Medullary Carcinoma

Imaging

  i. *Ultrasound:* The lesion appears hypoechoic, lobulated, avascular with areas of necrosis within. The surrounding parenchyma is heterogeneous with encasement of the great vessels (Fig. 21.60).
 ii. *CT:* They appear as masses of low attenuation (no iodine concentration) (Fig. 21.61).

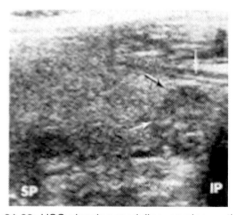

Fig. 21.60: USG showing medullary carcinoma thyroid

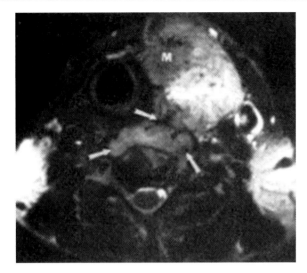

Fig. 21.61: CT showing vertebral extension of medullary carcinoma thyroid

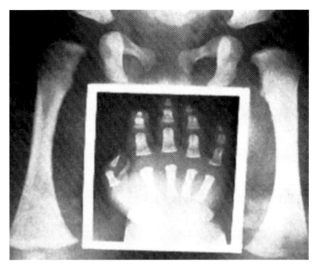

Fig. 21.62: Plain X-ray showing skeletal changes of cretinism (short tubular shape of the long bones)

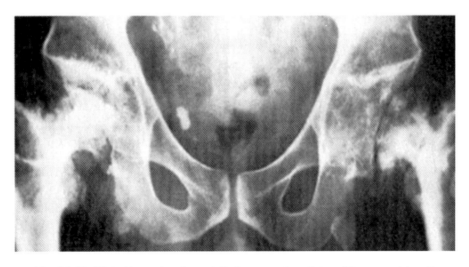

Fig. 21.63: Plain X-ray showing adult changes of cretinism (Narrow pelvis with fragmented femoral epiphysis)

bodies is seen, especially at the thoracolumbar region, where kyphosis may appear. All the long bones are short. In the pelvis the incidence of slipped capital femoral epiphysis is increased, and the pelvis itself is often narrow, with coxa vara deformities. In the adult the changes are exaggerated (Figs 21.62 and 21.63).

SUMMARY

i. Sonography is an integral imaging study in evaluation of thyroid pathology.

ii. Sonography with FNAC highly effective in the diagnosis of questionable thyroid nodules

iii. Sonography useful in the evaluation of diffuse thyroid disease.

iv. Colour flow imaging is a useful addition to real time studies.

v. Radioisotopes are mainly helpful in classification of thyroid nodule.

vi. Cross sectional imaging is mainly helpful in assessing metastatic lymph nodes and invasion of surrounding structures in malignancy and thus staging of cancers.

PARATHYROID GLAND

ANATOMY

Superior parathyroid is developed from the 4th pharyngeal pouch.

Inferior parathyroid is developed from the 3rd pharyngeal pouch.

Hence, developmentally inferior parathyroid is superior and superior parathyroid is inferior (Figs 21.64 to 21.68).

1. *Superior parathyroid:* It is constant in position within the true capsule and embedded in the substance of the thyroid gland. It is situated at the middle of the posterior border of the thyroid gland where lies the anastomotic artery connecting the superior with the inferior thyroid arteries. It lies usually dorsal to the recurrent laryngeal nerve.
2. *Inferior parathyroid:* It is inconstant in position. It may lie in one of the following positions:
   a. Near the lower pole of the thyroid gland, outside or inside the false capsule or within the substance, above or below the inferior thyroid artery.
   b. In the thorax, alongwith the thymus, ventral to the recurrent laryngeal nerve.

Arterial Supply

   i. Branches from the inferior thyroid artery.
   ii. Branches from the anastomosis between the superior and inferior thyroid artery.

Cross-sectional Anatomy

With the newer imaging techniques it is now increasingly possible to localize the gland. The techniques which are commonly employed are:
a. Ultrasonography with a sensitivity rate of 75%.
b. Scintigraphy.
c. Magnetic resonance imaging—with a sensitivity of 88%.

Most adults have four parathyroid glands (two superior and two inferior), each measuring 5 mm by 3 mm by 1 mm and weighing on an average 35 to 40 mg. Supernumerary 5th gland is present in up to 13% of the population and may result from the separation of the parathyroid remnants during development. These supernumerary glands are often adjacent to the thymus in the anterior mediastinum, suggesting a relationship in their development with the inferior parathyroid glands.

The normal parathyroid gland varies from a yellow to red-brown colour, depending on the parenchymal yellow fat and chief cell content. It is generally oval or bean shaped but may be spherical, elongated or lobulated. Normal glands can be seen occasionally with high frequency ultrasound, especially in young patients, but sonographic visualization of a normal parathyroid gland in a patient without hyperparathyroidism is not an indication for surgery.

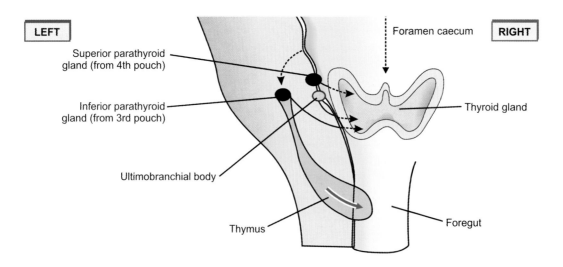

Fig. 21.64: Schematic representation of development of parathyroid gland

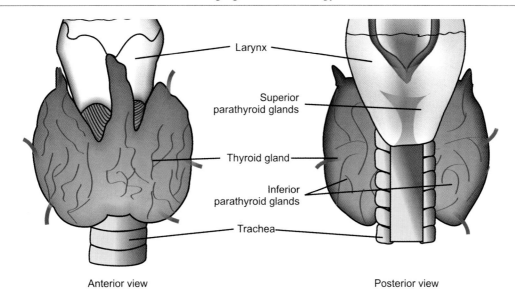

Fig. 21.65: Gross anatomy of parathyroid glands

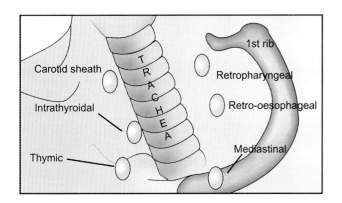

Fig. 21.66: Various position of parathyroid

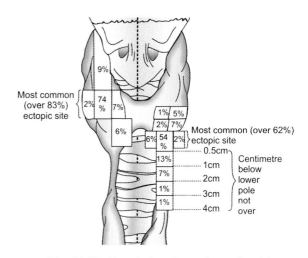

Fig. 21.67: Ectopic locations of parathyroid

IMAGING MODALITIES

Conventional Radiography

It has a very limited role in the detection of the primary pathology in the gland. However, plain radiograph still remains an excellent means of detecting and localizing the characteristic bony lesions associated with the hypo- or hypersecretion of the gland. Calcification in different organs including renal stone formation can be easily detected with the use of conventional techniques like, intravenous urography. Measurement of bone density is important in detecting the severity of the disease.

Ultrasonography

Both superior and inferior parathyroid glands have long vascular pedicle. The upper glands are found 2 cm below the upper margin of the thyroid contiguous to its posterior surface. With adenoma formation the pedicle may lengthen and migration behind the oesophagus or ventral to the thyroid or into the superior mediastinum is relatively common.

Adenomas are poorly echogenic when small and are separated from the thyroid by a thin echogenic line, which represents the encasing fascia and associated fat. If the tumours grow to over 2 cm in diameter, degenerative changes are common and the appearance is similar to that of thyroid adenoma. Differentiation is done by FNAB and PTH assay.

Hyperplasia is difficult to detect unless marked. With current equipment approximately 70% of parathyroid adenomas are found by USG.

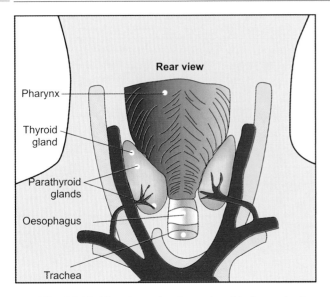

Fig. 21.68: Blood supply of parathyroids (rear view)

Parathyroid carcinoma is rare usually non-functioning and indistinguishable from thyroid scan.

Intraoperative sonography occasionally is a useful adjunct in the surgical detection of parathyroid adenoma, particularly in the reoperative setting. It is best suited for localization of inferior and intrathyroid abnormal parathyroid glands. The technique reduces the operation time.

Sonography guided percutaneous biopsy is being used with increasing frequency for preoperative confirmation of suspected abnormal parathyroid gland. This technique has increased the specificity of sonography by permitting reliable differentiation of parathyroid adenomas with other conditions, such as thyroid nodules and cervical lymph nodes.

Percutaneous ethanol ablation—sonography has been used for percutaneous injection of ethanol into abnormally enlarged parathyroid glands for chemical ablation.

Scintigraphy

Primary hyperparathyroidism is nearly always due to solitary adenoma and very rarely due to adeno-carcinoma. Very rarely there is hyperplasia of all parathyroid glands, which may be associated with multiple endocrine neoplasia syndrome. Secondary hyperparathyroidism is due to severe chronic renal disease which may give rise to autonomous hyperplasia or tertiary hyperparathyroidism.

Thallium subtraction scanning is the most widely used imaging technique, although its sensitivity lies between 72 to 92%, depending on the size of the adenoma and it may fail to identify ectopic tumours, especially if they are retrosternal. In this test, thallium 201 chloride is taken up by thyroid and parathyroid and the thyroid component is subtracted by doing a ^{99m}Tc scan, leaving parathyroid activity.

The best result has been recorded in primary hyperparathyroidism due to adenoma or carcinoma (specially, if the gland is ectopic) and in recurrent secondary hyperparathyroidism. The results are more disappointing in parathyroid hyperplasia. A false-positive result may arise from thyroid neoplasm producing a cold nodule, nodular colloid goitre, and adjacent lymph node pathology, all of which may accumulate thallium but not technetium.

Technetium-99m sestamibi has a specificity of 88 to 100% in detection of smallest adenomas (Figs 21.69 and 21.70).

Computerized Tomography (CT)

Parathyroid adenomas can be localized on CT, but this is usually only required after neck exploration has failed to find an expected adenoma. CT can identify ectopic parathyroid in the neck or upper mediastinum (Fig 21.71).

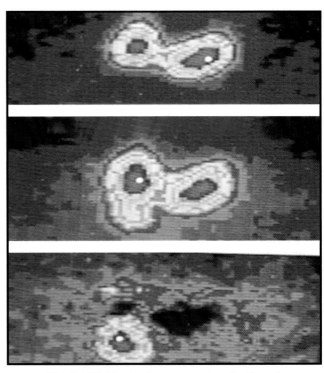

Fig. 21.69: Technetium scan—localization of parathyroid adenoma

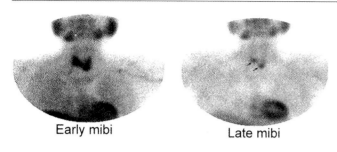

Early mibi   Late mibi

Fig. 21.70: *Early MIBI:* Shows increased activity in thyroid as well as parathyroid adenoma in the lower pole of left lobe of thyroid gland. *Late MIBI:* Shows persistent activity region in the lower pole of left lobe of thyroid (parathyroid adenoma). The activity over the thyroid gland has nearly washed out

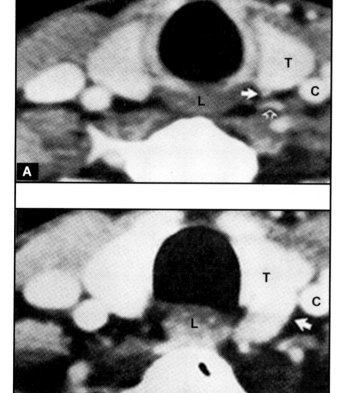

Figs 21.71A and B: Axial CT section of the neck showing parathyroid adenoma (T–Thyroid, C–Carotid, E–Oesophagus, Arrows–adenoma)

Magnetic Resonance Imaging (MRI)

MRI technique using fat suppression is becoming the method of choice for detecting thyroid adenoma, although it may overlook small lesions, particularly those in hyperplasia.

Interventional Radiography

Procedures like, angiography and venous sampling are more invasive, more expensive and are more technically demanding than the other modalities. These procedures can be associated with an unacceptably high incidence of complications and are being used in a decreasing number of centres.

Hypoparathyroidism

Imaging: Imaging modalities have got very limited role in the detection of the primary pathology in the gland, however they are highly sensitive in detection of the secondary effects of hypofunctioning of the gland and the low level of calcium in the ECF.

Conventional radiography shows osteosclerosis, particularly of the pelvis, inner table of the skull, proximal femur and vertebral bodies, as well as abnormal tooth development in hypoparathyroidism.

Pseudohypoparathyroidism and pseudopseudo-hypoparathyroidism shows short metacarpals particularly the fourth and the fifth. Abnormal dentition is also seen, with hypoplasia and cranial defects and there may be calcification in the connective tissues of the skin, ligaments, tendons and facial planes. Coxa vara, coxa valga, cone-shaped epiphyses and bowing of long bones are reported.

Ultrasonography is insensitive in detecting an atrophic gland. However, peroperative sonography can be useful in detecting the absence or reduced size of the gland.

CT scan is superior in detecting bony lesions (Fig. 21.72). Basal ganglia calcification is seen. Bone density measurements are commonly carried with the use of CT. CT is also helpful in detecting associated abnormalities.

MRI appreciates intracranial lesions better.

Interventional procedures have a very limited role.

Hyperparathyroidism

Imaging: Conventional radiography is most helpful in detecting bony lesions. Bone resorption is seen. Bone mineral content measurements confirm bone mineral loss in approximately 50% of cases. More advanced cases may show ground glass appearance.

Subperiosteal erosion of bone, particularly along the radial aspect of the middle and index finger is virtually

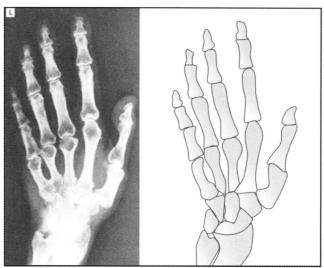

Fig. 21.72A: Short 4th and 5th metacarpal bones are seen. Although not specific for pseudohypoparathyroidism, this is a characteristic finding

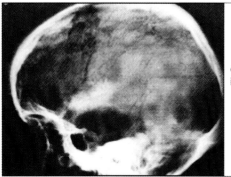
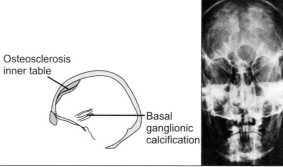

Osteosclerosis inner table

Basal ganglionic calcification

Fig. 21.72B: Osteosclerosis inner table and basal ganglia calcification are seen. Basal ganglia calcification is more common in pseudohypoparathyroidism than in idiopathic hypoparathyroidism

Fig. 21.72: Bony lesions of pseudohypoparathyroidism

pathognomonic (Fig. 21.73). Other sites are medial aspect of proximal tibia, femur, humerus and the ribs (Fig. 21.74). Loss of lamina dura along the teeth occurs (Figs 21.75 and 21.76).

Subchondral bone resorption is another common occurrence, being found in the distal and sometimes proximal end of the clavicle, symphysis pubis and sacroiliac joints (Figs 21.77 and 21.78). Disc herniation is seen at vertebral end plates.

Intracortical bone resorption gives rise to small oral or cigar shaped lucencies within the cortex. Loss of corticomedullary junction may occur with a 'basket work' appearance to the cortex.

The skull give rise to so called 'pepper pot' or 'salt and pepper' appearance (Fig. 21.79).

Brown tumours are locally destructive areas of intense osteoclastic activity. They present as a lytic lesion, which may be expansive and may destroy the overlying cortex (Fig 21.80). Pathological fracture may occur. Nephrocalcinosis may also be seen (Fig. 21.81).

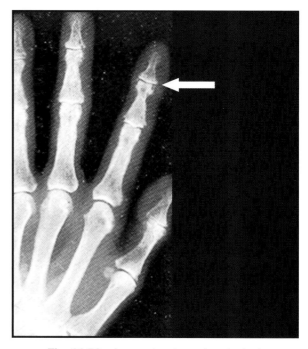

Fig. 21.73: Arrow showing subperiosteal resorption of bone

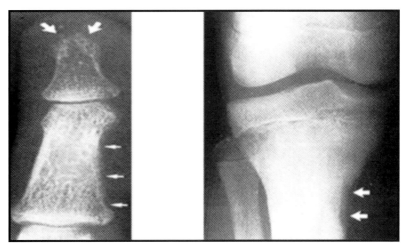

Fig. 21.74: Site of subperiosteal resorption. Plain X-ray showing skeletal changes in hyperparathyroidism

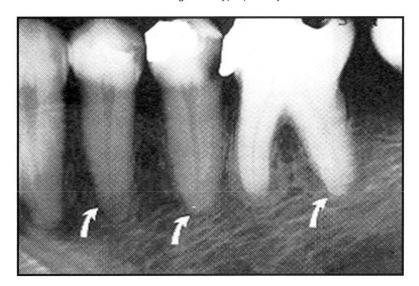

Fig. 21.75: Loss of lamina dura is seen

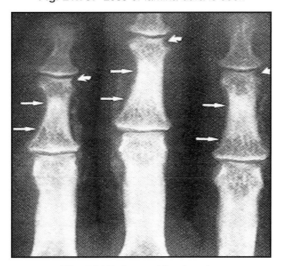

Fig. 21.76: Loss of lamina dura

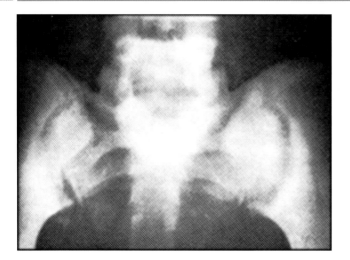

Fig. 21.77: Bone resorption

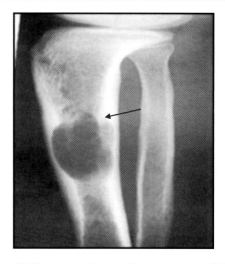

Fig. 21.80: Arrow showing brown tumour of tibia

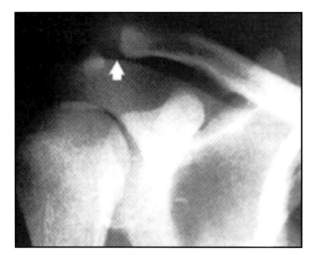

Fig. 21.78: Subchondral resorption

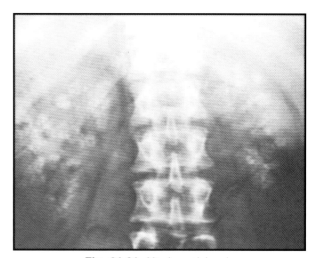

Fig. 21.81: Nephrocalcinosis

Renal calculi have been reported in as many as 50% of patients.

Ultrasonography adenomas: They are usually oval in shape. They dissect between the longitudinal muscle planes and acquire a characteristic oblong shape. There is often symmetry in the enlargement. The uniform hypercellularity of the gland gives a hypoechoic appearance and the echogenicity is usually less than the thyroid glands. The adenomas are homogeneously solid. 2% cases show internal cystic appearance. The lengths of the adenomas vary from 0.8 to 5 cm.

Sonography is reliable in detecting adenomas in typical locations. However ectopic parathyroid adenomas, like retrotracheal, mediastinal, intrathyroid and in the carotid sheath are difficult to detect with ultrasonography (Figs 21.82 to 21.91).

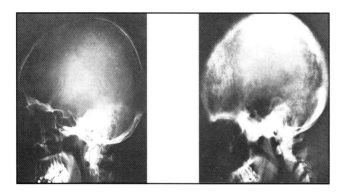

Fig. 21.79: 'Pepper pot' skull or salt and pepper' skull. There are multiple characteristic lucencies throughout the skull

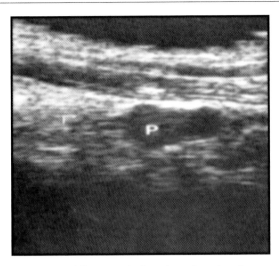

Fig. 21.82: Ultrasound of neck region showing parathyroid adenoma (P)

Colour Doppler study of an enlarged gland may demonstrate a hypervascular pattern with prominent diastolic flow. A vascular arc enveloping between 90 and 270 degrees of the mass, arising from the inferior thyroid artery branches, has also been described as a typical finding in parathyroid adenoma.

Carcinoma

Sonographically carcinomas are larger than adenomas. They frequently have a lobulated margin, heterogeneous internal architecture, and internal cystic components. Gross invasion of the surrounding structures, such as vessel or muscle, is the only reliable preoperative criterion for diagnosis of malignancy but this is an uncommon finding.

Scintigraphy: The best result of subtraction scan has been recorded in primary hyperparathyroidism due to adenoma or carcinoma (specially, if the gland is ectopic) and in recurrent secondary hyperparathyroidism. There is a host of conditions that may mimic the condition including thyroid nodule and enlarged lymph node. Figure 21.92 shows a classical picture of parathyroid hyperplasia.

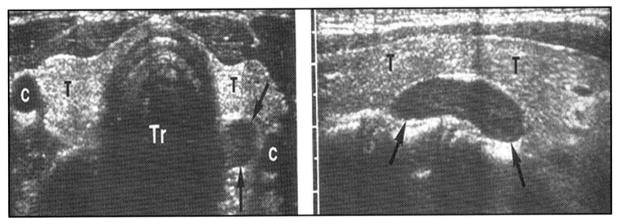

Fig. 21.83: USG parathyroid adenoma (T–thyroid, Tr–trachea, C–carotid, Arrow–parathyroid)

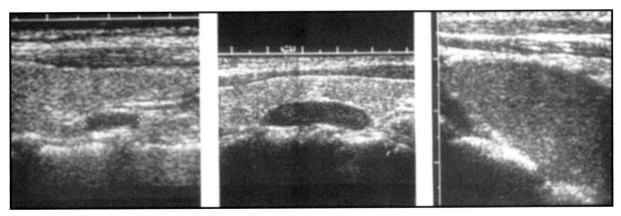

Fig. 21.84: USG showing spectrum of adenoma in respect to its size

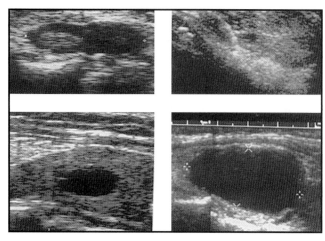

Fig. 21.85: USG showing adenoma in respect to its echogenicity

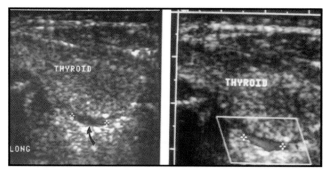

Fig. 21.86: Colour Doppler of adenoma

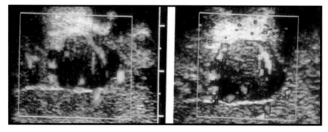

Fig. 21.87: Increased vascularity parathyroid adenoma

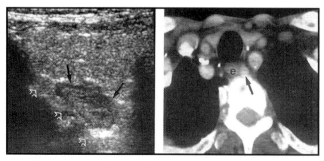

Fig. 21.88: USG and CT scan of ectopic location of adenoma, tracheo-oesophageal groove

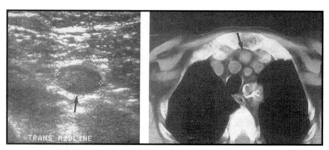

Fig. 21.89: USG and CT scan of ectopic location of adenoma, antero-superior mediastinum

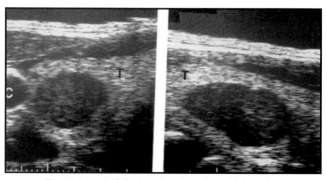

Fig. 21.90: USG showing intrathyroid location

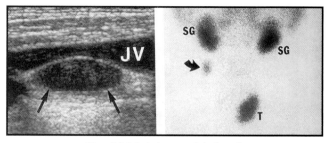

Fig. 21.91: Intracarotid sheath
(JV–jugular vein, SG–salivary glands, T–thyroid)

Technetium-99m sestamibi has a specificity of 88 to 100% in detection of smallest adenomas.

CT is mainly indicated when other methods fail to localize the gland or its enlargement. The effects of hyperparathyroidism, particularly the bony lesions are better evaluated with CT as well as the intracranial complications.

MRI of the neck with fat suppression is superior to other modalities for detection of parathyroid adenomas. However, it is usually used in very doubtful cases.

Interventional radiology has a very limited role in evaluation of hyperparathyroidism. Ultrasound guided biopsies are performed for preoperative histological diagnosis of parathyroid enlargement.

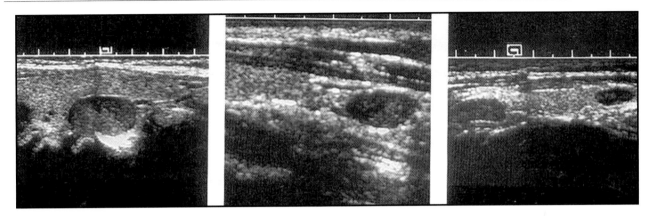

Fig. 21.92: Parathyroid hyperplasia

SUMMARY

a. Imaging of parathyroid pathology is used as an adjunct to biochemical examination.
b. Imaging is more sensitive in detection of the effects of disorders of PTH secretion rather than identifying the primary pathology.
c. Commonest cause of hyperparathyroidism is parathyroid adenoma.
d. Ultrasound is the most commonly used modality for detecting primary pathology.
e. Scintigraphy is primarily used to differentiate lesions of the gland and to detect ectopic glands.
f. Cross-sectional imagining is used for characterization of lesions as well as to detect invasion into surrounding structures.

IMAGING OF PANCREAS

INTRODUCTION

In the not so recent past of radiography, the pancreas was a hidden structure seen only indirectly through studies exploring the surrounding organs such as barium examination of upper GI tract.

The current armamentarium of non-invasive radiographic imaging of pancreas, i.e. ultrasound (USG), computerized tomography (CT), magnetic resonance imaging (MRI) and magnetic resonance cholangiopancreatography (MRCP) have markedly improved the diagnosis of pancreatic disease based on specific changes in the pancreatic parenchyma, duct, and vessels in addition to changes affecting the neighbouring organs.

CROSS-SECTIONAL ANATOMY

The pancreas lies in the most anterior of the three retroperitoneal compartment, the anterior pararenal space. Ventrally this is bounded by the posterior parietal peritoneum. Dorsally the space is bounded by the anterior renal or Gerotas fascia and more laterally by the lateral conal fascia.

Other structures occupying the pararenal space on either side include the duodenal loop and ascending and descending colon. The pancreas is surrounded by retroperitoneal fat (Figs 21.93 to 21.95).

VASCULAR SUPPLY

Arterial

The head of the pancreas is supplied by the superior and inferior pancreaticoduodenal arteries. The body and tail of the pancreas is supplied by branches of splenic artery, the main being 'arteria pancreatica magna'.

Venous Return

The head drains into the superior and inferior pancreaticoduodenal veins which in turn drains into the portal vein and the superior mesenteric veins. Rest of the pancreas drain into the splenic vein.

IMAGING MODALITIES

Conventional Radiographs

Includes plain radiographs and barium studies.

Plain Radiographys

- The sensitivity and specificity of conventional radiographs are low.
- Pancreatic calcification may be picked up (Fig. 21.96).
- Large pancreatic masses may be seen as soft tissue masses displacing gas shadows of stomach.
- Various findings and signs have been enumerated in case of pancreatic pathology such as:

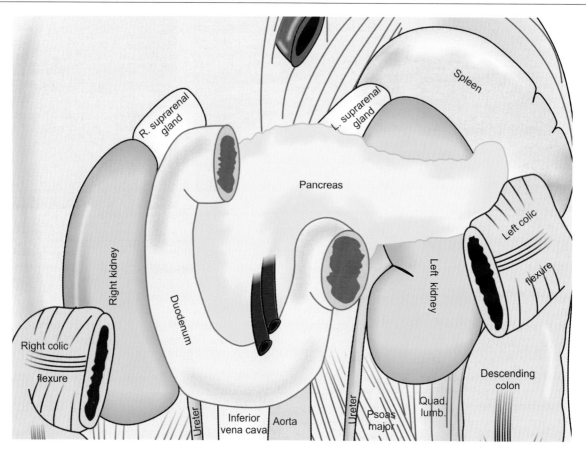

Fig. 21.93: Gross anatomy of pancreas

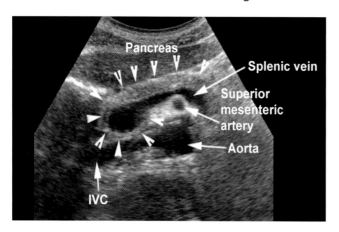

Fig. 21.94: Ultrasound anatomy

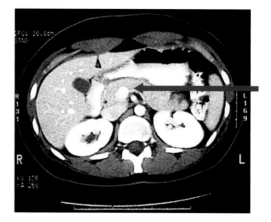

Fig. 21.95: Anatomy (arrow representing the pancreas)

- Sentinel loop—dilated gas filled duodenum or jejunal loops
- Colon cut off sign—sharp limitation of gas shadow at splenic flexure (Fig. 21.97)
- Obliteration of left psoas shadow
  The above mentioned signs are seen in 10 to 55% cases of acute pancreatitis.

However, they are of low sensitivity and specificity.
- Radiograph chest must be done to look for any pleural effusion.

Barium Studies

Provide indirect evidence of pancreatic pathology due to their effect on surrounding bowel loops.

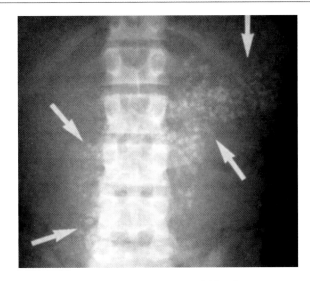

Fig. 21.96: Pancreatic calcification

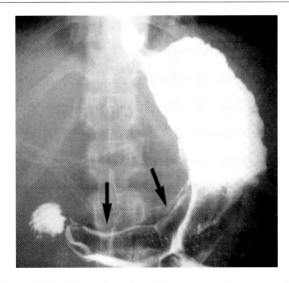

Fig. 21.98: Thickening of gastric rugae–acute pancreatitis

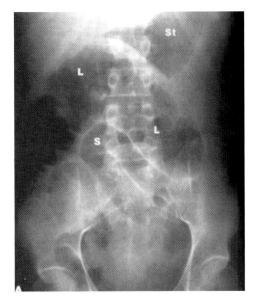

Fig. 21.97: Colon cut-off sign—acute pancreatitis
(L–large bowel, S–small bowel)

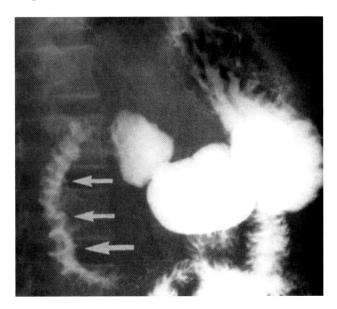

Fig. 21.99: Widening of the C-loop of duodenum

Findings seen in pancreatic pathology are as listed below:
- Tumour or pseudocyst arising in the tail of pancreas may cause elevation of the intra-abdominal oesophagus.
- Stomach may be displaced superiorly and anteriorly with widening of the retrogastric space by a large pancreatic mass (Fig. 21.98).
- Lesions in the head affect the pyloric antrum and duodenal loop, i.e. enlargement of duodenal loop is described as the Frostberg's 'reverse 3' sign (Fig. 21.99).

- Lesions in the body of pancreas may cause mucosal oedema or irregularity in the distal duodenum, duodenojejunal flexure and body of stomach.

Ultrasonography (USG)

- It is an excellent modality for demonstrating bile duct dilatation which could be of value in assessing pancreatic lesions.
- Fluid in and outside the pancreas is well demonstrated by ultrasound.

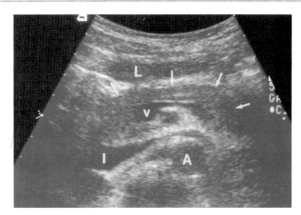

Fig. 21.100: Sonogram of normal pancreas
(A–aorta, V–portal vein, L–liver)

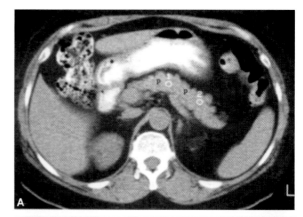

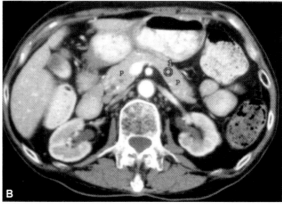

Figs 21.101A and B: Normal CT (P—pancreas)

- Small pancreatic tumours that do not alter the contour of pancreas, particularly functioning islet cell adenomas are better demonstrated by USG than computed tomography (Fig. 21.100). Intraoperative ultrasound has been used for such lesions to delineate the lesion better during surgery.
- Overall it is an effective screening modality for pancreatic diseases.

Disadvantages

- Highly operator dependent.
- Limited use in obese patients and patients having gas distended abdomen.
- Pancreatic tail difficult to demonstrate.
- Assessment of retroperitoneum by ultrasound is limited.

Computed Tomography (CT)

a. Method of choice for assessment of pancreas
b. Only modality that can consistently provide accurate information on status of pancreas.
c. Superior to US in demonstrating pancreatic neoplasm, of retroperitoneum and provides higher anatomic resolution of tumour beyond its margins (Figs 21.101A and B).

Technique

- Dynamic spiral scanning during a single breath hold is the optimum method.
- Intravenous contrast agents should be used
- Region from 3rd part of duodenum extending cranially to end at the superior margin of the liver should be included in the scan.
- Whenever possible oral contrast materials should also be administered to avoid confusion of nonopacified bowel loops.

Magnetic Resonance Imaging (MRI)

Role of MRI in pancreatic disease is yet to be established. However, technical advances have allowed considerable improvement in the quality of pancreatic imaging by MRI.

Constraints of MR Imaging

a. Pancreas on T1 and T2 weighted sequences are often indistinguishable from surrounding loops of small bowel.
b. Breathing artefacts, vascular motion, bowel peristalsis and lack of intraluminal contrast impairs visualization of pancreas.
c. Problem is magnified further in patients with only small amounts of retroperitoneal fat.

Technical Advances in MRI

a. Gradient echo imaging allowing breath hold acquisition.
b. Dynamic studies with gadolinium enhancement.
c. Fast spin echo imaging have shortened acquisition time and has improved signal to noise ratio.

d. Use of frequency selective fat saturation and phased array surface coils have further improved image quality.

e. Use of organ specific contrast agents.

Technique

- Parenchyma of normal exocrine pancreas shows a characteristically bright signal on T1WI, however fat surrounding the pancreas also produces a high signal on T1, therefore fat suppression is helpful to define margins of gland.
- Spin echo imaging allows better signal to noise ratio than breath hold gradient image, but the latter are required for dynamic sequential acquisition during gadolinium enhancement. T2 weighted image is required for detection of suspected islet cell tumour but is less sensitive than T1 imaging in detecting small pancreatic carcinoma.
- T2 imaging is also helpful in distinguishing between fluid and solid component of exudate and pseudocyst.
- For detection of either diffuse or focal pancreatic disease transverse images are used.
- For demonstrating the relation of tumours to portal vein, superior mesenteric and splenic veins, direct coronal or oblique coronal views are helpful.
- Demonstrating the relation of pancreatic lesions to the stomach and duodenum require the use of oral contrast agents.

MR Cholangiography and Pancreaticography (MRCP)

a. An effective noninvasive method of demonstrating biliary tree and pancreatic duct.
b. Extreme T2 weighting effectively eliminates signals from all tissue except stationary free water protons so that images display only those structures containing localized fluid collection.
c. As far as possible gastric and duodenal contents must be excluded from image volume.

Advantages

- Noninvasive
- Pancreatic duct anatomy can be shown in patients with tight strictures or total obstruction of main duct where ERCP is unsuccessful
- Suitable in patients who have undergone gastric or pancreatic surgery rendering endoscopic approach impracticable.

Disadvantages

- Does not offer opportunity to carry out therapeutic maneouvres
- Image disturbances may be produced by stents, metal clips at the site of previous surgery
- Relatively lower resolution which limits the demonstration of branched ducts.

Endoscopic Retrograde Pancreaticography (ERP)

Even with the availability of better non-invasive imaging modalities ERP continues to play a role in diagnosis and guiding further management in patients with pancreatic disease.

The uses of ERP in pancreatic disease are the following:
a. Assessment of complications of acute pancreatitis (Abscess and pseudocyst)
b. Definition of ductal anatomy in chronic pancreatitis for planning surgery (Resection or drainage)
c. Further investigation or assessment of pancreatic abnormality in cases of suspected pancreatic disease where findings in USG or CT have been negative or equivocal.
d. Prelude to interventional procedures.

Interventional Procedures

Radiologists have a vital role to play in the management of patients with pancreatic diseases in addition to their ability to image pancreas.

Biopsy of Pancreatic Lesions

Focal pancreatic masses should be biopsied so that benign lesions can be distinguished from malignant ones.

Almost all pancreatic masses can be biopsied under USG or CT guidance.

USG guided biopsy is usually performed using anterior approach, CT guided biopsy can be done using anterior, posterior or lateral approach.

FNAB using 20 to 22 guage needle may be performed or cutting needle 18 to 20 guage can be used to produce a core of tissue.

Accuracy of pancreatic biopsy is between 86.7 and 93% and complication rates are very low (3 to 4%).

Drainage of Pancreatic Fluid Collection

Percutaneous drainage in acute pancreatitis is done to assess whether a fluid collection is infected or not and to drain the collection if infected or an abscess has formed.

Large catheter 12F is used to drain abscesses with cure rates of up to 86%.

Other Inteventional Radiographical Procedures

- Percutaneous access into dilated pancreatic ducts for balloon dilatation or stenting and benign pancreatic duct strictures.
- Percutaneous cystogastrostomy—the creation of a communication between a pancreatic pseudocyst and the stomach by a percutaneous insertion of drainage catheter between the cyst and the stomach.

DISEASE ENTITIES

Pancreatic Divisum

Results when the ductal systems of the dorsal and the ventral buds fail to join or join incompletely. Usually patient is asymptomatic but it may play a role in the pathogenesis of acute recurrent idiopathic pancreatitis.

Imaging Findings

1. US AND CT—May be completely normal or show a pseudomass in the head and uncinate process of pancreas.
2. MRCP AND ERCP (Fig. 21.102). Reliable method of diagnosis showing a short and thin duct of Wirsung, the duct of Santorini draining most of the pancreas.

Annular Pancreas

Uncommon congenital anomaly in which a ring of normal pancreatic tissue circles the 2nd part of duodenum. This may be associated with Down's syndrome, CHD and malrotation. Occurs due to the failure of the ventral bud to rotate around the duodenum. It causes obstructive vomiting in neonate.

Imaging Findings

1. *Plain radiograph:* May show dilated air filed stomach and duodenum with little or no gas shadow in the distal bowel—the double-bubble sign.
2. *Barium studies:* Double contrast studies of the UGI tract shows eccentric narrowing and lateral notching, with medial retraction of the duodenal sweep at the level of the annulus.
3. *CT:* Shows enlarged pancreatic head and occasionally a peninsular protrusion of tissue into the duodenal lumen.
4. *ERCP:* Is diagnostic in 85% cases in whom the annular duct opens into the main pancreatic duct.

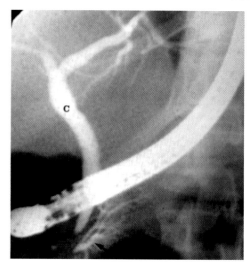

Fig. 21.102: ERCP—chronic pancreatitis with pancreas divisum

Acute Pancreatitis

Image Findings

Plain radiograph of abdomen
a. Sentinel loop secondary to adynamic ileus may be seen.
b. Duodenal ileus is considered fairly specific.
c. Abdomen may be gasless due to persistent vomiting.
d. *Colon-cut-off sign* where the dilated transverse. Colon becomes abruptly gasless in the splenic flexure.
e. There may be obliteration of (left) psoas shadow and fat.
f. Necrosis sign may be present.

Plain radiograph of chest
Left sided pleural effusion, elevated diaphragm and atelectasis should be looked for. Signs of pulmonary infarction and ARDS may be seen.

Contrast studies
a. Thickening of gastric rugae folds especially along the posterior aspect and lesser curvature of stomach maybe seen.
b. Displacement of stomach, widening of C sweep and Frostberg's inverted 3 sign may be seen.
c. Poppel's papillary sign due to enlarged papilla of vater may be present.
d. Non-specific oedema or mucosal thickening, most prominent in proximal jejunum may be seen.

Ultrasonography (Figs 21.103 and 21.104)
a. Abnormal USG is seen in 33 to 90% of the cases. Interstitial oedema results in a diffuse enlarged and hypoechoic gland with irregular contour.

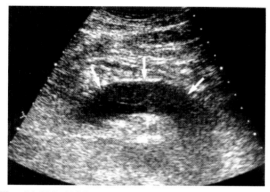

Fig. 21.103: USG appearance of acute pancreatitis

b. Maximal decrease in the echogenicity occurs 2 to 5 days after initial episode of pain.
c. Dilatation of pancreatic duct may be observed (Normal—2 mm, > 3 mm is significant).
d. Intrapancreatic abnormalities like fluid collection, phlegmon or haemorrhage can be seen as focal changes.
e. Perivascular cloaking seen as hypoechoic inflammatory changes around PV and SMV may be seen.
f. Extrapancreatic spread of inflammation and fluid collection involving the lesser sac, anterior pararenal space may be identified.
g. Pseudocyst can be identified as an anechoic, well defined fluid collection.

Computed Tomography (CT) (Figs 21.104A to C)

• Due to its superb capacity for demonstrating early inflammatory changes, extrapancreatic fluid collection and pancreatic necrosis, it is the imaging modality of choice.
• CT is indicated if patient has 2 or more Ramson's signs or if clinical symptoms do not resolve in 24 to 48 hours
• Shows sensitivity of 77 to 92% and specificity close to 100%.

Diagnostic Indicators

a. Diffuse enlargement of gland.
b. Extension of inflammation to surrounding peripancreatic fat will increase the attenuation values of surrounding peripancreatic fat (hazy density).
c. Pancreas becomes heterogeneous and extrapancreatic fluid collection may be seen.
d. Pancreatic necrosis, a hallmark of acute pancreatitis presents on CT as an area of no enhancing parenchyma (< 30 HU) larger than 30% of pancreatic volume (Fig. 21.105).
e. Acute fluid collection, intra- or extrapancreatic will appear as low attenuation, poorly defined homogeneous or heterogeneous collections (Figs 21.106A and B).

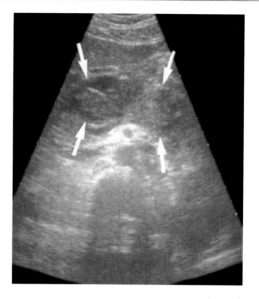

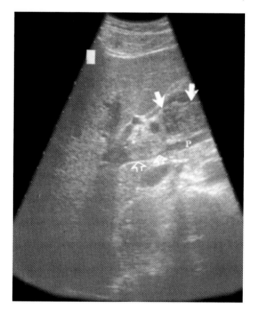

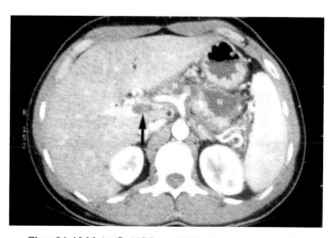

Figs 21.104A to C: USG and CT of acute pancreatitis

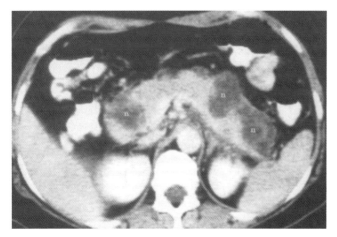

Fig. 21.105: Pancreatic necrosis

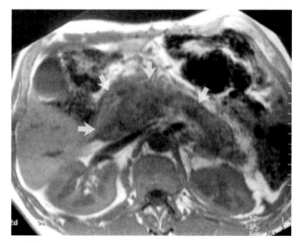

Fig. 21.107: MR picture of acute pancreatitis

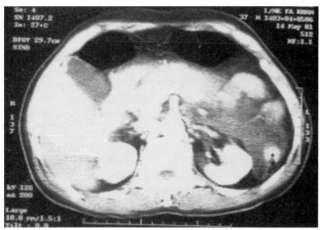

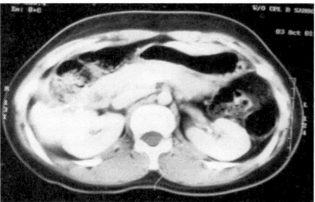

Figs 21.106A and B: Acute pancreatitis

Magnetic Resonance Imaging (Fig. 21.107)
a. Oedema causes diffuse signal reduction on T1 images and reduced enhancement after IV enhancement.
b. Dynamic post-Gad acquisition is sensitive for demonstrating the presence and extent of necrosis.

c. Exudates and fluid collections can be seen on T1, but are also well shown on T2 images.
   T2 images give a clear distinction between fluid and solid component.
d. Haemorrhagic component of acute pancreatitis can be detected by gradient echo images.

Chronic Pancreatitis

Imaging Findings

Plain Radiograph/Barium Studies
a. Pancreatic calcification are a hallmark and are seen in 75 to 90% of chronic pancreatitis patients. Calcification is small in size and irregular.
b. Atrophy of the whole gland is a common consequence; however, enlargement of the gland may also be seen in the form of mass effect on surrounding bowel as mentioned earlier.

Ultrasonography
a. Alteration in pancreatic size and echotecture may be seen.
b. Focal mass, calcification, pancreatic duct dilatation and pseudocyst formation may be visualized on ultrasonography (Fig. 21.108).

Role of Endoscopic Ultrasonography
- Has been used to diagnose chronic pancreatitis
- Pancreas may appear shrunken or enlarged with a heterogeneous appearance
- Hyper echoic foci with shadowing (calcification) may be seen
- Wall of MPD may be thickened and show increased echogenicity.

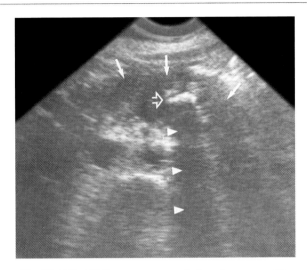

Fig 21.108: USG appearance of chronic pancreatitis

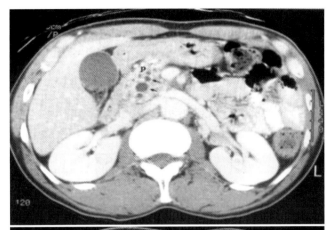

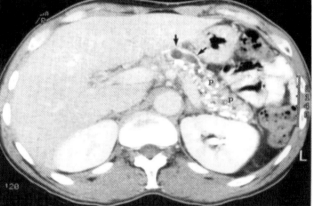

Figs 21.109A and B: CT of chronic pancreatitis

Computed Tomography (CT)
a. Diagnosis based on:
   - Assessment of pancreatic size
   - Dilatation and shape of pancreatic duct.
   - Presence of calcification.
b. Has a sensitivity of 50 to 90% and specificity of 55 to 85%
c. Gland is considered enlarged when AP diameter exceeded 3 cm in head and 2.5 cm in body or tail or the pancreaticovertebral ratio exceeded 1 and atrophied when AP diameter in the region of the head <1.5 cm and <1 cm in the body or tail and pancreatico-vertebral ratio of < 0.5 cm (Figs 21.109A and B).

ERCP
   i. Indications
      - To establish diagnosis
      - Assess anatomy for presurgical evaluation
      - To perform endoscopic therapy such as stone removal, stenting and stricture dilatation.
   ii. Normal measurements:
      - 6.5 mm within head
      - 5 mm within body
      - 3 mm within tail
   iii. Changes in chronic pancreatitis
      - Dilatation, contour irregularity and stenosis of 1st and 2nd order branches may be seen
      - As disease progresses MPD dilatation, irregularity and loss of normal tapering is seen
      - Dilatation of side branches gives the characteristic "chain of lakes appearance"
      - Strictures can also be observed within the CBD resulting in the double duct sign (Fig. 21.110).

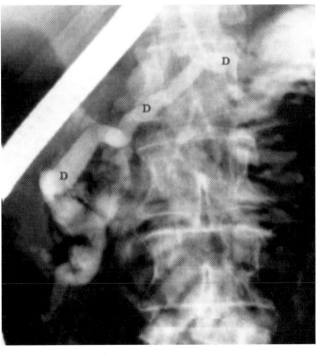

Fig. 21.110: ERCP chronic pancreatitis

Magnetic Resonance Imaging (MRI)

a. Loss of functioning acinar tissue accounts for diffused reduction in signals from gland on suppressed T1 weighted images.

b. Generalized or localized dilatation of pancreatic duct and pseudocysts are shown as areas of low signal on T1 and high signal on T2 weighted images.

c. Although it lacks sensitivity to detect calcification it is more sensitive to detect fibrosis.

d. MRCP is helpful as non-invasive modality to detect ductal changes (agreement between ERCP and MRCP in case of ductal dilatation 83 to 92%, 70 to 92% in ductal narrowing and 92 to 100% in cases of intra-luminal filling defect) (Fig. 21.111).

IMAGING OF PANCREATIC NEOPLASM

- Ultrasonography is often used as the initial screening method.
- CT is the modality of choice due to its superb spatial resolution.
- MRI has several potential advantages due to high tissue contrast, ability to visualize and assess vessel patency and multiplanar imaging. However, potential superiority of MRI over CT has not yet been realized as MRI takes twice as long and is more expensive.
- Endoscopic ultrasonography is helpful in detection of small pancreatic tumours.

NON-ENDOCRINE TUMOURS OF PANCREAS

Pancreaticoblastoma is the commonest pancreatic tumour in childhood and has an increased incidence in Beckwith-Wiedemann syndrome. This is an autosomal dominant disease with hemihypertrophy and a 10% incidence of malignant tumours.

Adenocarcinoma of the Pancreas

- Commonest pancreatic neoplasm.
- 60% of these tumours arise in the head of the pancreas.
- Usually present with symptoms of epigastric discomfort, anorexia, weight loss and jaundice.
- Very low survival rate of 25%.

Imaging Findings

Conventional Radiography

a. Will show mass effect in the form of displaced, widening of C sweep of duodenum.

b. Invasion of tumour may show mucosal irregularities and ulceration of surrounding bowel loops resulting in abnormal peristalsis and rarely obstruction.

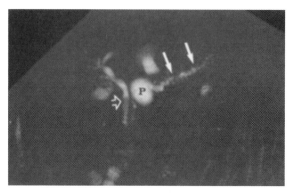

Fig. 21.111: MRCP chronic pancreatitis (P—pancreas, white arrows—pancreatic duct, open arrow—CBD)

c. Apart from upper bowel, the tumour may also invade the transverse and descending colon resulting in mucosal irregularities, nodularity of folds and localized strictures.

Ultrasonography

a. The neoplasm may be seen as local or diffuse pancreatic mass which is hypoechoic relative to the parenchyma.

b. Dilatation of the pancreatic or biliary ducts can be seen.

c. Associated findings such as obstructed MPD, pseudocyst formation, splenomegaly due to tumour invasion of splenic or portal vein and spread to local lymph nodes and metastatic spread to liver may be detected.

d. Ultrasound is accurate in evaluation of tumour involving pancreatic head; however, it is less effective in assessing body and tail lesions and in demonstrating spread of malignant process into the abdomen and retroperitoneal tissues. Endoscopic ultrasound may overcome some of these limitations (Fig. 21.112).

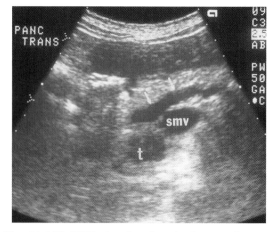

Fig. 21.112: USG showing ductal adenocarcinoma

Computed Tomography (Figs 21.113 to 21.115)

a. CT with contrast enhancement is the most effective technique for diagnosis and staging of pancreatic carcinomas.

b. The tumour mass may not be visible on a preliminary enhanced image but, because the tumour is less vascular than surrounding normal pancreatic parenchyma, it will be seen as a poorly enhancing focal area within the densely enhancing normal pancreatic tissue on dynamic contrast enhanced CT (large volumes of IV contrast is given and helical scanning is used in arterial phases with a delay of 20-40 s from start of injection).

c. Ancillary findings on CT are local tumour, tumour extension (loss of fat planes surrounding superior mesenteric artery), and invasion of neighbouring organs and vessels or metastatic disease.

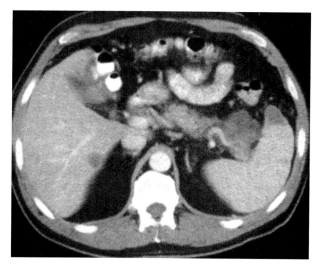

Fig. 21.114: CT scan showing carcinoma of tail of pancreas

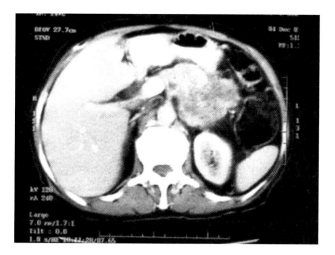

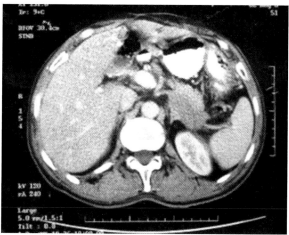

Fig. 21.113: Carcinoma—tail of pancreas

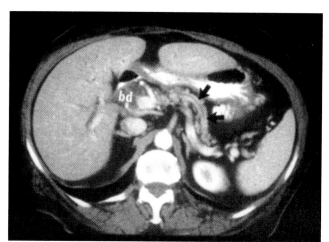

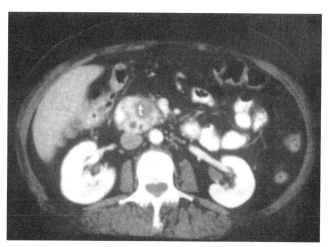

Figs 21.115A and B: Adenocarcinoma of head of pancreas (bd—bile duct, t—tumour, arrows—pancreatic duct)

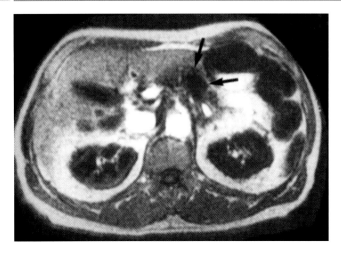

Fig. 21.116: MRI—carcinoma of pancreatic body

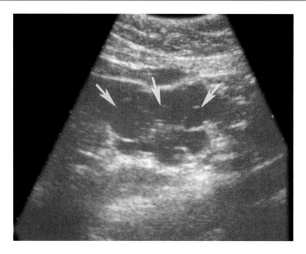

Fig. 21.117: Cystic tumour

Magnetic Resonance Imaging (Fig. 21.116)

a. Tumour seen as area of low signal on fat suppressed T1 images. Signal intensity in tumour is less than that seen in chronic pancreatitis.
b. On T2WI the tumour is often hyperintense, but may be of variable signal intensity.
c. Involved lymph nodes show increased signal on T2 weighted images as do liver metastases.

ERCP

a. Most specific modality as 90% of pancreatic tumours arises from pancreatic duct.
b. ERCP is particularly helpful in distinguishing pancreatic neoplasm arising from head from surrounding tissue or organs and in distinguishing pancreatitis from neoplasms.

Cystic Neoplasms of Pancreas

• Constitute about 5% of pancreatic tumours
• They are classified into 2 main groups—serous cystic neoplasm and mucinous cystic neoplasm
• Serous cystic neoplasms are always benign
• Mucinous cystic neoplasms are potentially malignant.

Imaging Findings

Conventional Radiography

a. Usually small tumours and rarely show evidence of mass effect on surrounding bowel loops.
b. Dystrophic calcification is seen in 10 to 20% of cases which is usually peripherally located.

Ultrasonography

a. Cysts are usually too small to be resolved by USG. However mucinous cysts, which usually are greater than 20 mm in diameter, may be seen as anechoic lesion.

b. Calcification may be picked-up as echogenic foci with posterior shadowing.
c. Large cyst, which may be rarely seen, can be differentiated from pseudocysts (Fig. 21.117).

Computed Tomography

a. CT is helpful in differentiating between serous and mucinous tumours.
b. Criteria on CT for differentiating between the two are:
   • Serous cystic tumours
      Number of cysts within tumour > 6
      Diameter of cyst < 2 cm
      Calcification is more common.
   • Mucinous cystic tumours (Fig. 21.118)
      Number of cysts < 6
      Size > 2 cm.

Magnetic Resonance Imaging

a. With advances in technology, MRI is a better imaging modality for cystic neoplasm than CT as septa, shape and wall thickness of lesion are better demonstrated.
b. Also the outer contour of lesion is well demonstrated on MRI and differentiation between serous and mucinous compartments is possible on T2 imaging.

ISLET CELL TUMOURS

• The islet cells are the endocrine cells of the pancreas.
• Over 80% of these tumours lie in the triangle bordered by the confluence of the cystic and common hepatic duct superiorly, the junction of the second and third parts of duodenum inferiorly and the head and body of pancreas medially.
• Insulinoma is the most frequent accounting for 60% of all islet cell tumours. It is usually solitary and small

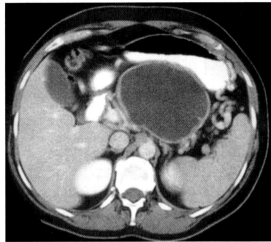

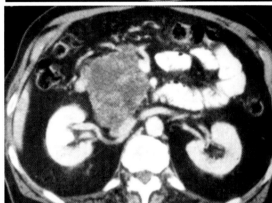

Figs 21.118A and B: Mucinous cystic neoplasm

(< 2 cm). However, malignant insulinomas tend to be larger (2.5 to 12 cm).

- Gastrinomas are the second most common functioning islet cell tumours accounting for 18%. They give rise to Zollinger-Ellison syndrome, which comprise increased gastric acid secretion, diarrhoea and peptic ulceration. They tend to be small and frequently multiple calcification is seen in 25% and have a coarse nodular pattern which invariably indicates malignancy.
- Glucagonomas cause non-ketogenic diabetes mellitus and a characteristic migrating, necrolytic venous thrombosis. The tumours have an average diameter of 4 to 7 cm and are malignant in approximately 60% of the cases.
- VIPOMAS produce watery diarrhoea, hypokalaemia and achlorhydria. The site of tumour is intra-pancreatic in 90% of cases, with the remainders originating in the sympathetic chain and adrenal medulla. 50% of pancreatic vipomas are malignant.
- Somatostatinomas are very rare and slow growing and produce clinical triad of gallstones, diabetes

mellitus and steatorrhoea. These tumours arise from pancreas in 50% and duodenum in 50%.
- Pancreatic polypeptide is often secreted in association with other hormones and isolated secretion is very rare.

IMAGING FINDINGS

Transabdominal Ultrasound (Fig. 21.119)

a. It is generally the first line investigation.
b. Islet cell tumours are usually seen as cell circum-scribed mass that is hypoechoic in relation to surrounding pancreatic parenchyma.
c. There may be a hyperechoic rim and larger tumours may show evidence of necrosis and calcification.
d. Few lesions, especially gastrinomas may be hyperechoic.
e. In young patients tumour may be iso or hyperechoic, probably because normal pancreas is less echogenic in younger patients.

Endoscopic Sonography

a. Allows use of high frequency probes (7.5 to 12 MHz) to be placed in close proximity to pancreas and duodenum.
b. Detects approximately 80% of small endocrine tumours not detected on TAS or non-helical CT.

Intraductal Sonography

a. Makes use of a 30 MHz transducer mounted on the tip of a 135 cm 4.3 Fr probe inserted into biopsy channel of gastroscope at time of ERCP.
b. So far only limited experience and studies are available as to success of this method.

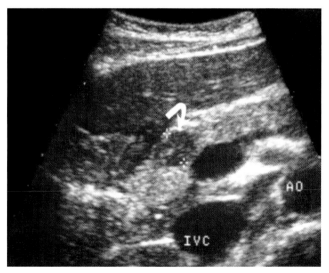

Fig. 21.119: USG of insulinoma

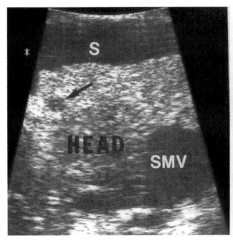
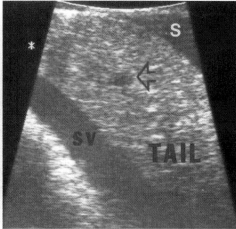

Fig. 21.120: Intraoperative USG showing insulinoma of head and tail of pancreas (arrow marks)

Intraoperative Ultrasound (Fig. 21.120)
a. Provides high resolution images with 7.5-10 MHz probes.
b. Improves detection of small masses and clarifies relationship of the mass to pancreatic and bile ducts.
c. Tumours as small as 3 mm may be identified.

Computed Tomography (Figs 21.121 and 21.122)

a. Most widely used method for localizing islet cell tumours.
b. Most islet cell tumours are isodense on unenhanced CT and will not be seen, as they are rarely large enough to deform the pancreatic outline.
c. Islet cell tumours typically enhance distinctly but briefly and their appearance is often subtle.
d. Sensitivity of CT is 50 to 80%.
e. Central necrosis may be seen in large lesions and calcification may be picked-up.

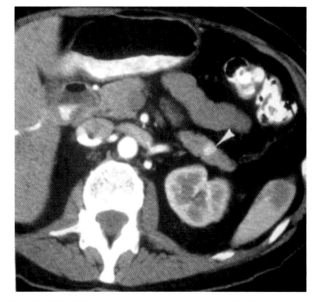

Fig. 21.121: CT scan showing insulinoma of tail of pancreas

Magnetic Resonance Imaging

a. Increasingly being used in the localization of islet cell tumours.
b. Due to their highly vascular nature they produce marked reduction in signals on T1 and increased signals T2 weighted images.
c. Lesions enhance post gadolinium, but the enhancement is transient, so rapid sequential images are essential.
d. The relatively high content of free water protons in these lesions may account for them being more apparent on FSET2 as a result of magnetization transfer effect and reduced T1 contribution associated with FSE.

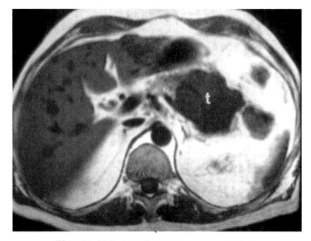

Fig. 21.122: Insulinoma pancreatic tail

e. Liver metastases from these tumours are hyper-vascular and show increased signal intensity on early post-gadolinium images.

Arteriography (Fig. 21.123)

a. Remains an important tool in localizing endocrine tumours.
b. Unless super selective studies are performed the tumour may be missed.
c. Islet cell tumours typically appear as well circum-scribed blush in the capillary and early venous phase. Abnormal feeding vessels may be seen in large tumours.
d. Angiographic features of malignant lesions include tumour irregularity, marked tortuosity of bleeding vessels, arterial encasement and venous obstruction.
e. Sensitivity of this procedure in detecting insulinomas is 54 to 89% and gastrinomas are 64 to 100%.

Transhepatic Portal Venous Sampling (TPVS)

a. TPVS is performed by transhepatic catheterization of right portal vein with a SF catheter.
b. Samples for hormonal analysis are obtained from splenic vein, superior mesenteric vein, portal vein and pancreatic veins.
c. TPVS only localizes the tumour to a region of pancreas and exact location of tumour cannot be pinpointed. Also problems of interpretation may arise when there are multiple tumours or if the hormone gradient is low.

Arterial Stimulation and Venous Sampling (ASVS)

a. In this selective pancreatic arterial injections of a secretogogue (calcium for insulinomas and secretin

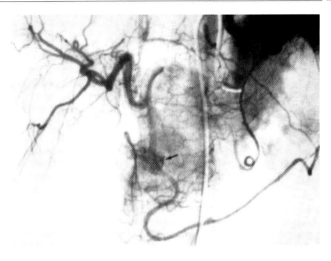

Fig. 21.123: Selective angiogram showing insulinoma

for gastrinoma) are made and hepatic venous outflow is sampled.
b. When arteries supplying the tumour are injected there is a rise in hepatic venous hormone concentration.
c. It is a very sensitive preoperative test for localization of insulinomas with sensitivity of 80 to 90%.

Scintigraphy

a. Useful for neuroendocrine tumours of the pancreas and bowel and is performed using radiolabelled somatostatin analogues and vasoactive intestinal peptide (^{123}I- VIP).
b. The main advantages of scintigraphy are its ability to image the whole body and to detect tumours or their metastases as small as 1 cm in diameter.
c. Also useful in monitoring the effects of therapy (Fig. 21.124).

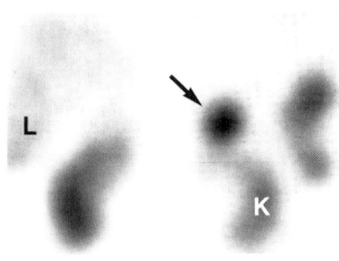
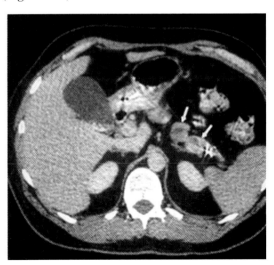

Fig. 21.124: Radionucleotide and CT scan—glucagonoma

SUMMARY

Conventional Radiography

- Low sensitivity and specificity.
- Calcification and indirect evidence in the form of mass effect and invasion into surrounding bowel loops may be obtained.

Ultrasonography

- Modality of choice for screening pancreas.
- However have drawbacks for imaging of body and tail of pancreas and the retroperitoneum.

Computed Tomography

- Modality of choice in pancreatic imaging.
- Dynamic spiral scanning during a single breath hold is the optimal method.
- Provides high anatomic resolution and helps in better evaluation of retroperitoneum and vasculature.

Magnetic Resonance Imaging

- Modality of the future.
- Presently role limited to MRCP imaging of suspected islet cell tumours and as an adjunct to other imaging modalities.

Scintigraphy

Role limited to evaluation of neuroendocrinal tumours of pancreas.

Interventional Radiology

- Have both a diagnostic role, and a therapeutic role.
- Helpful in diagnosis of endocrine cell tumours by techniques such as arteriography, TPVS and ASVS.
- Therapeutic role in the form of guided biopsies, drainage procedures, balloon dilatation of duct strictures, stenting and procedures like percutaneous cyst gastrostomy.

IMAGING OF TESTES AND OVARIES

INTRODUCTION

Endocrine disorders of testes and ovaries are seen commonly in neoplastic disorders. Testicular neoplasms constitute 1 to 2% of all malignant neoplasms in men and are more common in young males. The most common risk factor for developing testicular malignancy is cryptorchidism; other risk factors are mumps, testicular microlithiasis and infertility. Of all the testicular neoplasms, 90 to 95% are germ cell tumours while only a small percentage is formed by stromal tumours. Endocrine manifestations are commonly seen in stromal tumours; however these may also be seen in germ cell tumours.

The ovarian neoplasms comprise 25% of all gynaecologic malignancies, with its peak incidence occurring in the sixth decade of life and are the fourth most common cause of cancer deaths among women. Increasing age, nulliparity, family history of ovarian cancer are few of the common risk factors for development of ovarian cancer. The endocrine manifestations are commonly seen in sex cord tumours.

TESTES

Anatomy

The testes are ovoid structures measuring 3 to 5 × 2 to 4 × 3 cm, hung in scrotal sac by spermatic cords. Each of them weighs 12 to 19 gm. These are covered in white fibrous capsule-Tunica albuginea. The substance of each testis is divided into lobules by fibrous septations; each lobule contains numerous seminiferous tubules which join to form tubuli recti→rete testis→efferent ductules →epididymis→vas deferens in spermatic cords.

The arterial supply is through testicular artery, a branch of abdominal aorta; the venous drainage is through testicular veins which drain into IVC on right and left renal vein on left side (Fig. 21.125).

Imaging Modalities

The plain radiographs have no role in imaging of the testicular disorders. Ultrasound is the main diagnostic modality in the initial diagnosis of any testicular disorder; use of Colour Flow Doppler can further aid in establishing the diagnosis of acute conditions such as torsion or discriminating between the various inflammatory disorders. CT scan and MRI have a role in further evaluation of a complex lesion and in staging of neoplasms.

Sonographically, the normal testis has a homogeneously granular appearance. The mediastinum testis is sometimes seen as a linear echogenic band extending craniocaudally within the testis. The septula testis is sometimes seen as linear echogenic or hypoechoic structures. The rete testis may be visualized as a

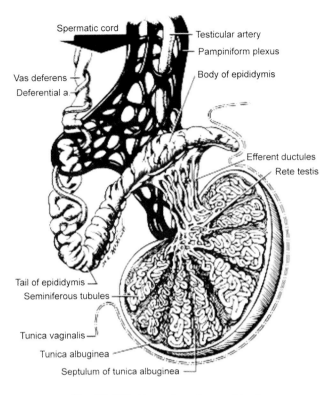

Fig. 21.125: Normal anatomy of testis

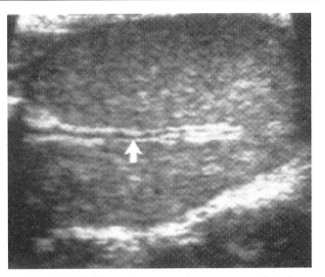

Fig. 21.126: Normal ultrasound appearance of testis (Sagittal section). Arrow points to mediastinum testis

hypoechoic or septate cystic structure adjacent to the head of epididymis (Fig. 21.126).

Imaging Finding

USG remains the diagnostic modality for primary tumour assessment. MRI/CT is used mainly for staging of neoplasms.

Germ Cell Tumours

Seminoma

On USG, these vary from a small nodule to a large mass causing testicular enlargement and appear as uniformly hypoechoic masses without calcification or cystic areas (Fig. 21.127). These tumours may be smoothly margi-nated or ill defined.

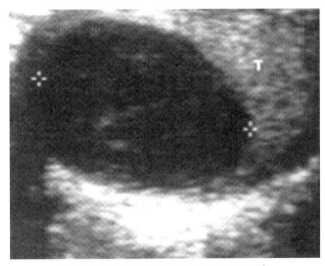

Fig. 21.127: Sagittal ultrasound scan of testis showing seminoma

Embryonal Cell Carcinoma

On USG, these have inhomogeneous appearance (Fig. 21.128). These are poorly marginated and invasion of tunica may occur which leads to distortion in testicular contour. Cystic areas are seen in almost 1/3 of cases and echogenic foci with or without acoustic shadow may also be seen.

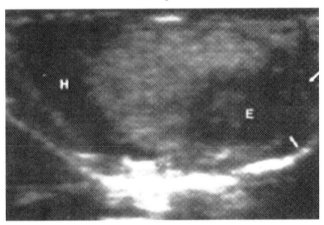

Fig. 21.128: Ultrasound appearance of embryonal cell carcinoma (H–hydrocele, E–embryonal cell carcinoma)

Teratoma

On USG, these appear as well defined masses which are markedly inhomogeneous in echotexture containing cystic as well as solid areas. Dense echogenic foci with acoustic shadow are common because of focal calcification, cartilage, bone or areas of scarring present within the tumour (Figs 21.129A and B).

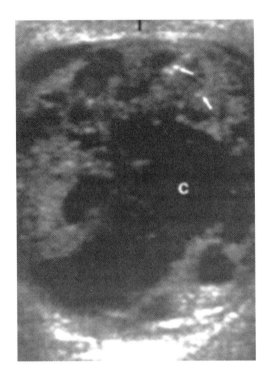

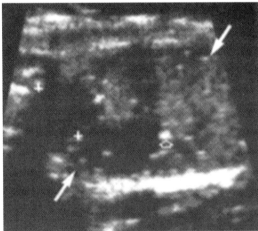

Figs 21.129A and B: (A) Transverse scan of testis with teratoma showing solid and cystic ("C") components and calcific foci (open arrow) (B) Longitudinal scan of testis showing choriocarcinoma with cystic (cursors), calcific foci (arrows) and hyperechoic areas of haemorrhage

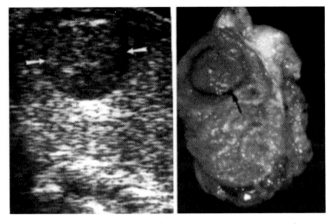

Fig. 21.130: Ultrasound and gross appearance of testicular fibroma

Stromal Tumours

Majority of stromal tumours are Leydig cell tumours and predominantly in third to sixth decades. Patients commonly present with painless testicular enlargement or a palpable mass. About 5% patients may present with gynaecomastia, impotence or loss of libido.

On USG, these are small, solid masses and have a hypoechoic echotexture. However, at times larger lesions may be seen with areas of cystic spaces, haemorrhage and necrosis. Invasion of tunica may be seen as an irregularity in contour in 10 to 15% of cases (Fig. 21.130).

Both USG as well as CT/MRI are used for staging. USS is adequately sensitive in detecting pre- and para-aortic lymphadenopathy; however CT is more accurate for same. CT/MRI also provide better assessment of metastasis in Liver/adrenals. CT/MRI is also useful in assessment of tumours in undescended testis.

OVARIES

Anatomy

The ovaries are ovoid, paired female gonads measuring $3 \times 2 \times 2$ cm. These are intraperitoneal structures connected by suspensory ligament to the lateral pelvic wall, mesovarium to broad ligament and uterus by ovarian ligament—hence have limited mobility and are covered by modified peritoneum. The substance of ovary is divided into cortex which contains developing follicles and medulla which is fibrovascular with ovarian vessels. The arterial supply is through an ovarian artery on each side, a branch of abdominal aorta; the venous drainage is through testicular veins which drain into IVC on right and left renal vein on left side (Fig. 21.131)

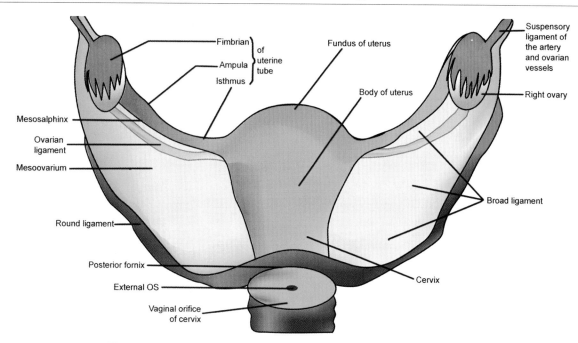

Fimbrian
Ampula
Isthmus
of uterine tube

Fundus of uterus

Body of uterus

Suspensory ligament of the artery and ovarian vessels

Right ovary

Mesosalphinx

Ovarian ligament

Mesoovarium

Round ligament

Posterior fornix

External OS

Vaginal orifice of cervix

Broad ligament

Cervix

Fig. 21.131: Gross anatomy of ovaries and female reproductive system

Imaging Modalities

Like testis, the plain radiographs have little role in imaging of the ovarian disorders. Ultrasound—both trans-abdominal and transvaginal are again the main diagnostic modality in the initial diagnosis of any ovarian disorder. Colour Doppler may have some role in discriminating between benign and malignant masses (still under evaluation). As in testicular disorders, CT scan and MRI have a role in further evaluation of a complex lesion and in staging of neoplasms (Fig. 21.132).

Endocrine Diseases

Imaging Findings

There is no characteristic to differentiate between functional and non-functional tumours. Again, ultrasound is the primary imaging modality; CT and MRI are used mainly for staging. The imaging findings of common functional tumours are described below.

Germ cell tumours Sonographically, cystic teratomas have a variable appearance ranging from completely anechoic to completely hyperechoic. A predominantly cystic mass within an echogenic mural nodule may be seen which is called the 'dermoid plug.' The dermoid plug usually contains hair, teeth or fat and may cast an acoustic shadow. A mixture of matted hair and sebum is highly echoic and has multiple tissue interfaces which may produce illdefined acoustic shadowing obscuring the posterior wall of the lesion—described as

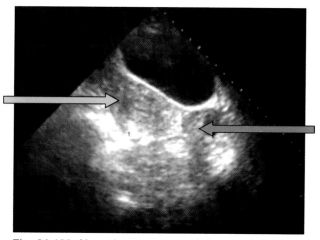

Fig. 21.132: Normal appearance of left ovary (red arrow) and uterus (blue arrow) on ultrasound scans

'tip of the iceberg sign.' Highly echogenic foci with defined acoustic shadowing may be produced by teeth or bone. Multiple linear hyperechogenic interfaces may be seen because of hair fibres which has been referred as 'the dermoid mesh' (Figs 21.133 A to C).

Sertoli-Leydig cell tumours (Androblastoma): On USG, the small tumours appear solid, homogeneous masses whereas the large tumours may have heterogeneous appearance with multiple cysts.

Thecoma and fibromas Both these tumours originate from ovarian stroma and may be difficult to distinguish from each other pathologically and are at times classified

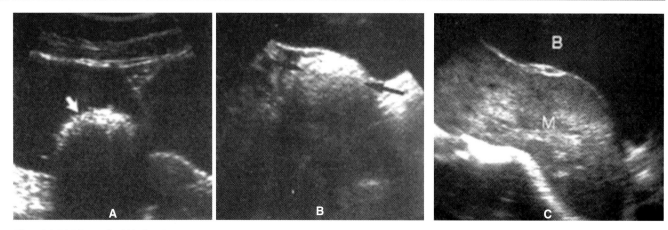

Figs 21.133A to C: (A) Cystic teratoma with echogenic area with posterior acoustic shadowing. (B) 'Tip of the iceberg' sign-cystic teratoma showing highly echogenic mass with poor acoustic shadowing. (C) Dysgerminoma -A solid homogeneous mass (M) posterior to bladder (B)

together as the cofibromas. Tumours with an abundance of thecal cells are classified as thecomas whereas those with abundant fibrous tissue are classified fibromas. Together, these comprise less than 5% of all ovarian neoplasms. These are usually unilateral and benign.

On ultrasound, these are seen as hypoechoic mass with marked posterior attenuation of sound beam (because of homogeneous fibrous tissue) (Figs 21.134A and B).

Granulosa cell tumours This tumour make up 1 to 2% of ovarian neoplasms and has a low malignant potential. These occur in post menopausal women; nearly all are unilateral. These are oestrogenically active ovarian tumour and may manifest as post menopausal bleeding or other signs of oestrogen production.

On USG, the tumours have nonspecific appearances and may appear small, solid, homogeneous masses whereas the large tumours may have heterogeneous appearance with multiple cysts.

CT

CT may be used for primary diagnosis in conditions where satisfactory USS not possible as in obesity, previous surgery or unstable bladder; it also helps in differentiating ovarian from non ovarian pathology. CT is the most commonly performed study for the pre-operative evaluation of a suspected ovarian neoplasms. It is particularly useful in determining the extent of cytoreductive surgery required optimizing subsequent chaemotherapeutic response. The most important role of CT scan is in staging of these neoplasms.

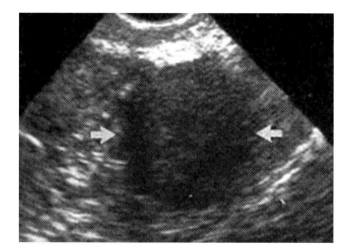

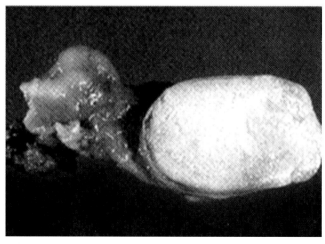

Figs 21.134A and B: Ultrasound and gross appearances of ovarian fibroma

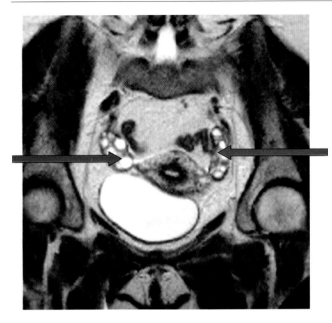

Fig. 21.135: Coronal T2 weighted MR scan of normal female pelvis showing both the ovaries (red arrows)

MRI

MRI of pelvis is increasingly being used in the diagnosis of ovarian disorders because of high soft tissue contrast resolution and multiplanar imaging without any radiation. This has made it the modality of choice for staging.

Several studies have compared MRI to CT and USG for characterizing adnexal masses with mixed results. Both transvaginal US and MRI with IV contrast medium have high sensitivity (97% and 100%) in the identification of solid components within an adnexal mass. MRI,

however, shows higher specificity (98% versus 46%). At present, the relatively high cost of MRI precludes its use as a screening technique and studies suggest that MRI is most appropriately used for characterization of an adnexal lesion in cases where US and clinical examination are indeterminate (Fig. 21.135).

SUMMARY

- Endocrine manifestations are seen rarely in testicular and ovarian neoplasms.
- More common are stromal tumours and are seen in the form of masculinising (Leydig cell tumours) and feminizing features (Theca-granulosa cell tumours in ovaries).
- Imaging modalities cannot differentiate between functional and nonfunctional tumours.
- USG is the primary diagnostic modality for tumour diagnosis and characterization.
- CT/MRI is used for further charcterisation in difficult cases and especially staging of tumour.

FURTHER READING

1. Alex G Pitman, Richard Tello, Nancy Major (Eds): Radiology Care Review, 2002.
2. David A Nyberg. Transvaginal Ultrasound, 1992.
3. David Sutton. Textbook of Radiology and Imaging, 2002.
4. Douglas S Cratz, et al (Eds). Radiology Secrets, 2004.
5. Evan Siegelman (Ed). Body MRI, 2004.
6. Hytton Meire, et al (Eds): Clinical Ultrasound: A Comprehensive Text, 2001.
7. Paul Grech, JG Martin, PG Ell (Eds): Diagnosis of Metabolic Bone Disease, 1985.
8. Ralf Lachman (Ed). Taybi and Lachman's Radiology of Metabolic Syndrome, Metabolic Diseases and Skeletal Dysplasias, 2003.
9. Ralph Weissler, Jack Wittenber, Mukesh G Harisinghani (Eds). Primer of Diagnostic Imaging, 2003.

SECTION

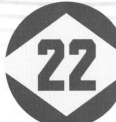

22

MAMMOGRAPHY AND IMAGING

Radiology and Imaging in Breast Lesions

C Mohan, IK Indrajit, Rajul Rastogi

INTRODUCTION

Imaging forms an important investigative tool in evaluation of breast disease. The currently used imaging modalities are mammography, ultrasonography, colour Doppler, magnetic resonance imaging, computed tomography, and scintimammography. These imaging modalities are increasingly applied for a range of different clinical entities on the breast, particularly breast cancer. An early detection of cancer has an excellent prognosis, which allows majority of breast to be preserved and decreases the mortality. Film screen mammography is the only standard imaging modality capable of detecting clinically occult breast cancer with a proven efficacy for the screening of asymptomatic individuals. Improvements over the last decade in the quality of performance and the reporting of mammography studies rank among the most important advances in breast imaging.

Ultrasonography, MRI and CT are useful diagnostic modalities once a lesion has been detected by clinical examination or by mammography. While mammography, sonography have firmly established their place in evaluation and therapy, MRI is increasingly used as a problem-solving tool, availing its inherent advantages in contrast behavioural pharmacokinetics of malignant tumours. Recent developments over the existing mammographic equipment include: full-field digital mammography, computer-assisted detection (CAD), stereotactic mammography-guided biopsy, dose reduction mammographic system, and computed tomography laser mammography.

NORMAL BREAST

The breast parenchyma is composed of glandular and the fatty tissue. Glandular tissue usually comprises of 15 to 20 lobes which are arranged in a pyramidal manner with apex towards the nipple. Each lobe is comprised of a number of lobules which consist of 10 to 100 acini. All lobules and lobes through their interlobular, intralobar and interlobar ducts form mammary ducts, which ultimately converge and open at the nipple.

On mammography, the glandular and ductal tissues are radiodense while adipose tissue that comprises a large portion of breast is radiolucent. In addition to the glandular and ductal components, connective tissue especially extralobular elements also contribute to the breast opacity in mammography. This is responsible for most of the individual variations. Ducts appear as serpiginous structures converging at the nipple. Cooper's ligaments appear as thin opaque septal structures extending from the posterior part of the breast toward the skin and subcutaneous tissues. Vascular structures are seen as thin branching, linear opaque structures that do not converge towards the nipple and can go randomly in any direction.

Postpubertal breast is usually homogeneously dense, with short and thick Cooper's ligaments, endowed with a thin anterior fat plane, and a poorly visible posterior fat plane. With advancing age, glandular parenchyma is replaced by fat which is associated with widening of anterior and posterior fat planes. The breast is more radiolucent and better contrasted in the first half of the menstrual cycle. In the second half, the image becomes denser and connective tissue structures appear thick as a result of diffuse hydration.

Pregnancy and lactation is associated with hypertrophy and increased hydration of glandular and connective tissue structures resulting in a diffuse increase in breast density and a thinned out anterior fat plane. With each pregnancy, breast involution increases and is most marked at the level of medial and inferior quadrants of the breast.

PATHOLOGY OF BREAST DISEASE

Pathological conditions of the breast can involve all the components of the breast parenchyma resulting in different disease entities, as outlined in Table 22.1.

BI-RADS CLASSIFICATION

BI-RADS essentially stands for "Breast Imaging-Reporting and Data System." It is the global standardized lexicon for mammographic descriptions that facilitates a currently acceptable standardized mammographic reporting system. This encourages the generation of a concise mammography report that uses standard terminology to describe features, with clear recommendations understandable both to radiologists, oncologists and other clinicians.

The key analysis in BI-RADS is made on:
a. Mass lesion
b. Calcifications
c. Architectural distortion
d. Associated findings.

BI-RADS ensures that the mammographic evaluation of breast lesions in a given case will be based on the following criteria often seen alone or in combination, with use of descriptors of correct lexicon (Table 22.2).

Mass Lesion

Circumscribed masses are almost always benign with few important exceptions of medullary, colloid, mucinous and intracystic (papillary) carcinoma (circumscribed carcinoma); metastases, lymphoma and sarcoma. The probability of malignancy increases as a lesion becomes more irregular in shape. A spiculated or ill defined margin has a very high probability of being malignant, with few important exceptions of postoperative scar, fat necrosis, haematoma, radial scar, inflammation or abscess, granulomatous mastitis and fibromatosis. Most lesions with spiculated or irregular margins are infiltrative duct carcinoma (75% of all invasive carcinomas) and invasive lobular carcinoma.

TABLE 22.1

Locations	Benign conditions	Malignant conditions
Major duct	Solitary/large duct papilloma Duct ectasia	Papillary carcinoma
Terminal duct	Multiple peripheral papillomas Ductal hyperplasia	Ductal carcinoma *in situ* Invasive ductal not otherwise specified Special types of ductal carcinoma
Lobules	Cysts Fibroadenomas Sclerosing adenosis	Phylloides Lobular neoplasia Invasive lobular carcinoma
Interlobular connective tissue	Pseudoangiomatous stromal hyperplasia	Sarcoma

Classification of breast masses based on site of origin

TABLE 22.2

Shape
- Round
- Oval
- Lobulated
- Irregular

Margins
- Circumscribed
- Microlobulated
- Obscured
- Indistinct
- Spiculated

Density
- High
- Equal
- Low (but not fat containing)
- Fat containing
- Associated microcalcifications
- Calcification

Effect on surrounding tissue
- Architectural distortion
- Halo sign
- Satellite lesions
- Multiple lesions

Mammographic descriptors of breast masses

A low density mass favours a benign process while high density increases the probability of a malignant lesion. Lesions with area of fat density within are benign, for example fat necrosis, hamartoma, galactocele, traumatic oil cyst and lipoma. Halo around a mass favours a benign lesion, with few exceptions as intracystic (papillary) carcinoma and carcinoma arising in a fibroadenoma. In an elderly female, a single well-defined or spiculated lesion carries a high-risk of malignancy but multiple well-circumscribed lesions are usually benign, i.e. cysts and fibroadenoma, with the exception of metastases.

Calcifications

Calcification is a common finding on mammography. In the BI-RADS lexicon, calcifications are divided into categories of typically benign, and high probability of malignancy. The descriptors of calcification includes:

i. *Form:* Round or linear, coarse or fine granular, monomorphic or pleomorphic.
ii. *Size:* Large or small.
iii. *Distribution:* Unilateral or bilateral, diffuse, segmental, focal or multifocal.
iv. *Density:* High or low.
v. Number.

Benign calcifications are usually larger, coarser, often round with smooth margins and easily seen. Typical benign calcifications include skin calcifications with lucent centre, vascular calcification with parallel lines, involuting fibroadenoma with coarse (Fig. 22.1) or "popcorn like" calcification, secretory deposits with large rodlike calcifications, acinar calcification with round configuration (Fig. 22.2), cyst with rim calcifications, cyst sediments with milk of calcium calcifications or punctate well defined less than 0.5 mm calcifications.

Malignant calcifications are characteristically numerous, fine, linear, branching, discontinuous and less than 0.5 mm in width. Their appearance either in a segmental or linear distribution suggests filling of the lumen of a duct involved irregularly by breast cancer. It may be fragmented, irregular, Y-shaped branching, granular or rod-shaped. Microcalcifications are seen in 40 per cent cancers on mammography. Calcification may be seen within a soft tissue mass or may be the only indication of malignancy.

Few other aspects of calcification favouring malignancy include:

i. A "clustered" distribution as suggested by five or more calcifications, each less than or equal to 0.5 mm isolated in 1 cc volume on mammogram.
ii. Irregular pleomorphic or heterogeneous calcifications with varying size and shape but less than 0.5 mm.
iii. Calcifications may be the only sign of malignancy particularly in early noninvasive carcinoma.
iv. Greater the extent of malignant pattern of calcification, the higher is the probability of microinvasion.

Intraductal carcinoma of the comedo type (large cell) are characteristically linear or ductal with irregular size,

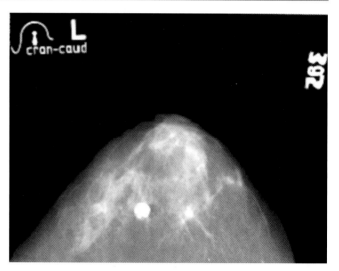

Fig. 22.1: Fibroadenoma. Close-up mammogram shows well defined 20 x 18 mm mass at inferomedial quadrant of left breast with varied calcification within

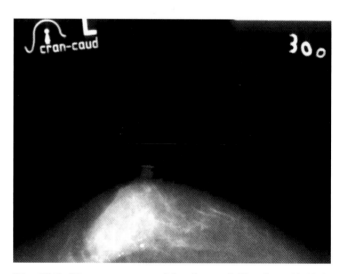

Fig. 22.2: Mammogram and benign calcification. Multiple foci of macrocalcifications with central lucency at all quadrants of right breast. BI-RADS category 2

shape, and density. Cribriform and micropapillary (small cell) intraductal carcinomas are characterised by irregular papillary like extensions with looping arches spokewheel patterns.

Architectural Distortion

It indicates disruption of normal architecture of breast without an obvious mass lesion and can be seen in both benign and malignant diseases. Benign conditions producing architectural distortion include postoperative and radial scar while malignant lesions include invasive lobular carcinoma.

Associated Findings

These include skin retraction, nipple retraction, skin thickening, trabecular thickening and enlarged axillary nodes. They are commonly considered as secondary signs of malignancy.

BI-RADS Assessment Categories

The most important part of a mammography report is the assessment, which describes the category that best represents the mammographic findings, according to the ACR BI-RADS lexicon. These assessment categories, as outlined in Table 22.3, are associated with specific follow-up actions. On the basis of the mammographic features described above, the final impression should assign one of the following categories to the abnormality, to convey the risk assessment to the clinician.

DIAGNOSTIC MAMMOGRAPHY

Introduction

There are two basic types of mammographic examinations: screening mammography and diagnostic mammography. Screening mammography refers to examinations of asymptomatic women to detect clinically occult breast cancers. Used in both, film screen mammography is a special type of soft tissue radiography of breast, aiming at delineation of various structures of breast including pathologies, from surrounding fat. In spite of advances in film screen mammography, the sensitivity ranges from 85 to 95 per cent but its specificity is insufficient for accurate differentiation of many lesions due to significant overlap in the appearance of benign and malignant lesions and detecting subtle soft tissue lesions, especially in the presence of dense glandular tissues.

Basic Technical Requirements

Dedicated mammography equipment capable of producing high quality images with optimum film density, high resolution and low radiation dose is necessary for diagnosing small breast cancers. A good mammographic unit consists of a generator having high output rate to minimise the exposure time, uses low kVp, high mA with minimum possible filtration of X-rays. The films used should have a slow speed, single coating, fine grain, low latitude and high contrast. Orthochromatic films sensitive to green light are preferable.

Optimal mammographic image quality can be achieved by: correct positioning technique, proper exposure, appropriate compression and correct processing technique. Overlying tissues and structures such as shoulder should not come in the X-ray beam. There

TABLE 22.3

Categories	Risk assessment	Status	Differentials
Category 0	Incomplete assessment	Needs additional imaging.	Reserved for the screening situation
Category 1	Normal mammogram	Continue yearly mammography	A negative mammogram
Category 2	Benign finding	This is also a normal mammogram, but with benign findings	Involuting, calcified fibroadenomas Fat containing lesions
Category 3	Probably benign finding	Very high probability of being benign Cases need to be followed at 6 months intervals for a total of 2 years.	Small < 8 mm circumscribed masses Small round clustered microcalcifications Focal asymmetric densities. Multiple rounded densities seen for the first time
Category 4	Suspicious abnormality	May be malignant No characteristics for malignancy but probability of malignancy. Biopsy should be considered.	—
Category 5	Highly suggestive of malignancy	—	Spiculated lesions. Fine, linear, branching microcalcifications with or without secondary signs

(Category 0 is reserved for the screening situation in which additional imaging evaluation is needed. Categories 1 to 5 are final assessments)

Assessment of BI-RADS categories

should be symmetrical images of both breasts. The goal in mammographic positioning is to pull as much breast tissue as possible away from the body so that it can be compressed and imaged.

Breast compression improves the image on mammography by because it:
  i. Decreases the thickness of breast.
 ii. Reduces the scattered radiation with improvement of the contrast.
iii. Reduces motion unsharpness.
 iv. Makes breast thickness homogeneous bringing uniformity in film density.
  v. Discriminates easily compressible cysts and fibro-glandular tissue from the more rigid carcinomas.
 vi. Separates superimposed breast lesions.
vii. Reduces the radiation dose to the breast tissue since a lesser thickness of breast tissue needs to be penetrated.

Standard Film Screen Mammographic Examinations

The standard film screen mammographic examinations consist basically of two views. Mediolateral oblique (MLO) and craniocaudal (CC) views. There are many alternative views, of which spot view and magnification view are considered (Table 22.4).

Mediolateral View

The mediolateral view (MLO view) is the best view to image the breast tissue and the pectoral muscle. A good visualisation of deeper part of breast, axillary tail and inframammary tissue is obtained. The lateral view of the breast has been modified to take advantage of the orientation of the breast tissue in relation to the underlying chest wall and muscle structure. Compression for MLO views is applied from the upper inner quadrant inferolaterally. Relaxation of the pectoral muscle, outward pull of the breast tissue parallel to the underlying muscle fibres, medial mobilisation of the breast and pectoral muscle, and maintaining mobilisation as compression is applied are critical factors in obtaining optimal positioning on MLO views.

Craniocaudal View (CC View)

The cassette is placed under the breast at the level of inframammary fold, and the breast is pulled until the inframammary fold is taut. Compression is then applied and X-ray beam is directed vertically from above. The postero-medial aspect of breast should be included in craniocaudal view as this area is most likely to be

TABLE 22.4

Adequate positioning of common views
1. Mediolateral oblique (MLO) views
• Muscle to level of nipple
• Pectoral muscle convex margin
• Open inframammary fold
• Retroglandular fat laterally
• Pectoral muscle, laterally
2. Craniocaudal (CC) views
• Pectoral muscle (30%--40%)
• Cleavage
• Retroglandular fat laterally
• Posterior nipple line within 1 cm of PNL

Assessing adequate positioning of two commonly used views

excluded in mediolateral projection. A correctly performed CC projection shows the pectoral muscle on the posterior edge of the breast, indicating that the breast has been positioned as far forward as possible. The nipple should be seen in profile including the central part of the retroglandular fat tissue. Adequate positioning is important (Table 22.4).

Spot Compression Views

Spot compression is one of the most commonly used additional study in practice. Primary indications for spot compression views, include the evaluation of densities seen in only one view, potential masses, asymmetry, and possible distortion (Table 22.5). In addition, spot compression images areas and lesions that may have been excluded from routine screening views, like chest wall or axillary tail. Spot compression overcomes blurring related to inadequate compression or underexposed areas.

TABLE 22.5

1. In evaluating questionable areas
• Density
• Possible mass
• Asymmetry
• Distortion
2. To include more tissue
• Posterior
• Axillary tail
3. Technical issues
• Underexposure
• Blurring

Role of spot compression

Magnification Views

Magnification views are useful in evaluating definite masses and microcalcifications detected on screening views (Table 22.6). If there is architectural distortion in isolation or associated with masses, magnification views are helpful in further characterizing the lesion.

TABLE 22.6

1. Mass evaluation
   - Margins
   - Shape
   - Associated calcifications
   - Presence of satellite lesions
2. Microcalcification evaluation
   - Morphology
   - Extent
3. Associated soft tissue abnormality
4. Architectural distortion
   - Associated with mass
   - Associated with calcifications

Role of magnification views

Methods to Improve Accuracy

Mammography is the current gold standard used for detection of breast carcinoma. However, literature reports 10 to 30 per cent of breast cancers are missed at mammography. This lacuna is attributable to a variety of causes like dense parenchyma obscuring a lesion, poor positioning or technique, subtle features of malignancy or slow growth of a lesion. To address this problem measures recommended include avoiding reliance solely on screening views to diagnose an abnormality; adding diagnostic mammography evaluation, reviewing clinical data meticulously, supplementary use of ultrasonography, observing strict adherence to positioning and technical protocols, optimising image quality and comparing current images with all previous studies. In addition, subtle features of breast cancers, looking for other lesions, judging a lesion by its most malignant features are simple and basic analytical tools.

SCREENING MAMMOGRAPHY

Screening mammography for breast cancer fulfils few criteria for ethical, scientific, and financial justification, in that:

i. It detects an important health problem with a high prevalence.
ii. It identifies a recognisable latent or early asymptomatic stage.
iii. It analyses an entity whose natural history is clearly understood.
iv. It can detect lesions prior to onset of signs and symptoms.
v. Facilities are widely available for confirmation of the diagnosis.
vi. Effective treatment is available.
vii. Good evidence is available that early detection and treatment reduce mortality and morbidity significantly.
viii. The expected benefits of early detection and treatment clearly exceeds the risk and cost. Screening mammography complies with other important issues like acceptability, repeatability, validity (accuracy) in terms of sensitivity, specificity, predictive values, is cost effective, can be rapidly performed, and is simple, safe and easy to perform.

Screening mammography has been proven beyond doubt to be of definite use in breast malignancies. The aim behind screening breast cancer is to take advantage of lead-time (the time period by which screening detection precedes usual case detection) to cure the patient/ alter the disease course favourably. Mammography can be used as a screening technique for breast masses but due to its relatively low specificity as compared to USG and MRI, it is not very useful to characterise the lesion. Important indications of screening mammography include:

i. Screening of asymptomatic women
ii. Screening high-risk women, e.g. family history of carcinoma breast
iii. Follow-up of patients after mastectomy of same and
iv. Opposite breast and same breast with transplant, investigation of breast lump
v. Occult primary with secondaries
vi. Benign breast diseases with eczematous skin, nipple discharge and skin thickening.

Since breast is a radiosensitive organ, risk of malignancy increases with exposure of breast to radiation in early age group. The glandular tissue of breast, however, is sensitive to radiation and all efforts should be made to minimise the radiation doses to it. Maximum risk is between 10 to 20 years. Mean dose to the parenchyma should be less than 0.1 c Gy (equivalent to 1 year background radiation). Such low radiation doses have never shown any effect on breast, particularly of women over 40 for whom mammography is especially beneficial. All analyses of radiation carcinogenesis in the breast are based on extrapolation from populations exposed to doses that are at least two orders of magnitude higher than those required for X-ray mammography.

It has also been shown that the breast of women over 40 years (in whom incidence of breast carcinoma is high, are less sensitive to radiation and the risk versus benefit ratio is higher in screenable age group. In women less than 40 years of age any exposure to radiation with screening can lead to mutation and damage of the actively dividing genetic material, leading to increased chances of malignancy.

Current American Cancer Society (ACS) guidelines for early breast cancer detection, recommends mass screening at the interval of two years in women between 40 to 49 years age group. In 2003, the American Cancer Society updated its guidelines for early detection of breast cancer into three groups:

i. Women at average risk: Women in their 20s and 30s should undergo breast self-examination (BSE) or periodic health examination, preferably at least every three years.

ii. Older women: Screening decisions should be individualized by considering the potential benefits and risks of mammography.

iii. Women at increased risk might benefit from additional screening strategies such as earlier initiation of screening, shorter screening intervals, or addition of other screening modalities like USG or MRI.

While there is general agreement that screening mammography reduces mortality from breast cancer in women over 50 years of age, there has been considerable debate over the effectiveness of screening mammography in women who are aged 40 to 49.7 years. Two reports from recent clinical trials also support the use of screening mammography for women in this age group. A 14-year follow-up in the Edinburgh trial has shown a mortality reduction of 21% for women aged 45 to 49 years who were screened with mammography. A 16-year follow-up in the UK Trial of Early Detection of Breast Cancer revealed a 27% decrease in mortality in women who were screened with mammography, and there was no evidence that women who were aged 45 to 46 years at the start of screening received less benefit than older women.

Currently points in favour of screening young women include that:

i. It can detect small, early stage tumour.

ii. Can detect ductal carcinoma *in situ* (DCIS).

iii. Several series have reported no statistically significant difference in size, stage, lymph node status among invasive cancers detected by screening mammography in age groups 40 to 49 as compared to age groups 50 to 64.

However, points against screening of young women are:

i. Dense breast tissue may hide the malignant lesion, and mammogram screening test may be wasteful.

ii. Tumour at these ages, is more aggressive, may have spread by the time screening examination detects it

iii. With a low incidence screening may not be cost effective.

Screening mammography can ensure a statistically significant decrease in mortality (25 to 30%) and assists in the detection of small, node negative tumour, which can be treated with lumpectomy and radiotherapy. False-positive and false-negative results are known risks of the screening mammography programme. False-negative results give false reassurance to the screened woman regarding her disease process. This can be harmful as such women may become negligent towards further screening. The overall sensitivity of screening mammography is 83 to 95 per cent. A 10 per cent reduction in sensitivity is seen for women in age group < 50. This is mainly because of dense breast obscuring the lesions, presence of non-calcified lesions and lobular carcinoma *in situ* (LCIS), poor radiographic technique, missing of the lesions or wrong interpretation by the observer, rapidly growing tumour becoming significant before detection. They can be solved by meticulous technique, double reading of films, use of Computer aided diagnostic systems and decreased interval between screenings. False-positive results unnecessarily increase the workload on a screening programme and make it cost ineffective. Various studies have calculated the false positive results to be in a range of 5 to 50 per cent. Best way to reduce these is to have previous mammograms and results of clinical breast evaluation for comparison.

ULTRASONOGRAPHY BREAST

In the last decade, the use of ultrasonography in the evaluation of patients with breast lesions has been limited to differentiating masses as cystic or solid (Table 22.7). With advances in technology however, the role of ultrasonography has been expanding rapidly, to form an integral part of breast lesion workup. Currently, ultrasonography is used as an adjunct to mammography and in the evaluation of symptomatic patients. Newer technical refinements have enabled use of:

i. Linear array transducers of multiple focal zones at various depths that improves image quality and resolution.

ii. Tissue harmonics that has improved the diagnostic accuracy of breast ultrasonography on cyst versus solid differentiation as well as lesion conspicuity.

TABLE 22.7

Cyst and solid descriptors

- Shape
- Margins
- Echotexture
- Shadowing
- Enhancement
- Microcalcifications
- Duct extension
- Duct branching

Ultrasonography features of breast masses

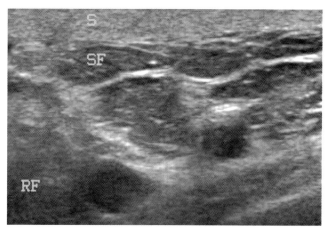

Fig. 22.3: Ultrasonography of normal breast. The skin (S) lies between two bright echogenic lines on the surface of the breast. The subcutaneous fat (SF) is hypoechoic. The fibroglandular tissue (FG) is relatively echogenic. There is also retroglandular fat (RF). The ultrasonographic appearance varies according to the relative proportions of fat and fibroglandular tissue

iii. Easy availability of 7.5 MHz or higher frequency linear array transducer.

Knowledge of normal breast anatomy on ultrasonography is important. The breast constituents imaged are connective tissue, breast parenchyma, and fat. Connective tissue has the highest acoustic impedance, breast parenchyma is intermediate, and fat lowest. Normal skin is less than 2 mm thick and appears as two echogenic lines separated by a hypoechoic band (Fig. 22.3). During real-time scanning, small tubular structures are identified in the thickened skin and subjacent to it; these are thought to be distended lymphatic channels.

Primary indications for breast ultrasonography include the following:
i. Characterization of palpable or clinically occult mammographically detected masses.
ii. Characterization of solid masses.
iii. Evaluation of tissue potentially excluded on routine mammographic views (i.e. superior, medial and axillary tissue).
iv. Evaluation of women with inflammatory symptoms to distinguish mastitis from an abscess.
v. Guidance of interventional procedures.

Abnormalities are analyzed for size, margins, echogenicity, compressibility, posterior acoustic enhancement, shadowing, duct extension, duct branching, orientation, and multiplicity. Breast ultrasonography is used as a complementary examination to mammography in the following situations: evaluation of dense breasts tissue, evaluation of mass in mammography, and guidance of biopsy needle or needle localisation.

Stavros and co-workers have described uniform hyperechogenicity, an ellipsoid shape with a thin echogenic capsule, and fewer than four gentle lobulations as features of solid masses that suggest a benign aetiology. Spiculation, angular margins, anteroposterior dimension exceeding transverse dimension (i.e. taller than wide), marked hypoechogenicity, shadowing, punctate calcifications, duct extension towards nipple), branch pattern away from nipple, and microlobulation are features associated with malignant lesions.

Malignant masses are usually irregular or poorly defined in outline, more hypoechoic, less through transmission with poor definition of posterior wall and distal acoustic shadowing. However, carcinomas can be circumscribed and fibroadenomas may be irregular, to suggest that significant overlap of benign and malignant features can occur at times. Stavros et al have described additional features, which favour malignancy, like spiculations, fine 1 to 2 mm microlobulations, angular margins at junction of the mass and the surrounding tissue. Malignant masses are usually taller than wide because of the fact that benign lesion grows within normal tissue planes whereas malignant growth invades them and grows across the tissue boundaries.

Ductal carcinoma *in situ* accounts for 15 to 20 per cent of all detected breast cancers and 25 to 56 per cent of clinically occult breast cancers detected at mammography. The most common ultrasonography finding in ductal carcinoma *in situ* is microlobulated mass with mild hypoechogenicity, ductal extension, and normal acoustic transmission. Spiculated margins, marked hypoechogenicity, a thick echogenic rim, and posterior acoustic shadowing often suggest the presence of invasion.

Doppler helps to improve benign versus malignant differentiation. Demonstration of vascularity is suspicious for malignancy and infection. Malignant masses commonly show peripheral as well as central or penetrating vessels with disordered morphology of these vessels. In a study of 210 breast masses, Cosgrove *et al* concluded that:

i. Colour Doppler signal in a mass lesion in the breast otherwise thought to be benign, should prompt a biopsy.

ii. Absence of colour in an indeterminate lesion is reassuring. If the breast lesion is extremely hypoechoic on ultrasonography, differentiation of cystic from solid lesion may be difficult. Demonstration of vascularity in such lesion obviously confirms its solid nature.

On spectral analysis, compared to benign lesions the tumour vessels show high PSV (>15 cm/ sec) with high RI (> 0.75). Contrast enhanced power Doppler ultrasonography improves the benign versus malignant differentiation due to improved display of neovascularity (Figs 22.4A and B).

INTERVENTIONAL PROCEDURES

Sonography allows direct real-time guidance of interventional breast procedures that can be done quickly, accurately, safely, and with minimal patient discomfort. The procedures include ultrasonography-guided cyst aspirations, preoperative wire localisations, core biopsies; fine-needle aspiration, percutaneous ductography, and abscess drainage. Ultrasonography guided procedures have few general principles. They are:

i. Generally done freehand.

ii. The needle during procedure is attempted to be seen in its entirety.

iii. Expected trajectory of needle is parallel to chest wall and transducer.

iv. Needles not angled into the breast.

Indications for cyst aspiration include cysts with atypical ultrasonography features (wall irregularity, intracystic mass, internal echoes) and symptomatic cysts. Core needle biopsy are better than fine-needle aspirations, because larger volumes of tissue are obtained that can be processed histologically. Moreover, they are reliable substitutes for excisional biopsies in most patients. The advantages of core biopsies over excisional biopsies include lower cost, less morbidity, and decreased cosmetic deformity as well as the fact that they expedite patient care and increase efficiency in diagnosing breast cancer. The one disadvantage of ultrasonography-guided core biopsies, particularly in women with larger breasts,

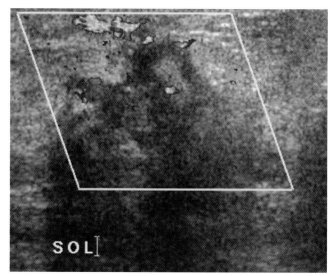

Fig. 22.4A: Radial colour power doppler US image of a primary breast cancer shows central (open arrows) and peripheral (solid arrows) vessels; biopsy proved lesion as an Infiltrating ductal carcinoma

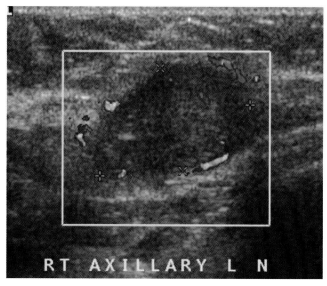

Fig. 22.4B: Radial colour power Doppler US image of a malignant axillary node in a biopsy proven infiltrating ductal carcinoma shows central (open arrows) and peripheral (solid arrows) vessels

is the need to immobilise the lesion, which is done by using the transducer like a compression paddle.

Stereotactic localisation of breast lesions has become a common practice in the diagnosis of breast abnormalities. Carr JJ et al have elaborated on stereotactic localisation which requires a fixed coordinate system. The breast is placed between a compression plate and back breast support to keep the lesion in a fixed position during the procedure.

Problems such as apparent lesion movement, non-visualisation of a lesion, various targeting errors, geometry-related errors (e.g. incorrect X-ray tube positioning, failure to re-reference the biopsy needle, patient motion) are addressed by strategies, that include lesion identification and accurate targeting on both stereo images, application of basic trigonometry for x, y, and z coordinates of the lesion centre, familiarity with geometric configuration of biopsy unit, knowledge of location of reference point and centre of rotation, use of a long-throw core biopsy gun and additional sampling along the z axis, all leading to greater success in stereotactic biopsy sampling.

SCINTIMAMMOGRAPHY AND PET

Scintimammography and PET are imaging techniques wherein breast scanning is performed after the injection of radionuclide-labelled substances, which concentrate in areas of high metabolic activity, including some tumours. ^{99m}Tc Methoxy Isobutyl Isonitrile (MIBI) breast scintigraphy ("scintimammography") has been under investigation for several years. Early reports indicated a high sensitivity (over 90%) and specificity (slightly less than 90%) for breast cancer with this technique.

However, more recent studies have shown a relatively low sensitivity for cancers that are < 1 cm in size (39%) and for lesions that had been identified only on screening mammography (56%). Therefore, the ultimate role of ^{99m}Tc MIBI scintigraphy in breast cancer still needs to be determined. The technique ultimately may be helpful for avoiding unnecessary biopsies of palpable but benign masses that are > 1 cm in size, and which have equivocal mammographic or ultrasonographic features. Another benefit of scintimammography is in differentiating post-surgical and/or post-radiation therapy changes from carcinoma. This is based on an increased uptake of Tc-99m sestamibi at mitochondrial level in carcinoma, due to greater mitochondrial density in breast cancer cells.

Focal radionuclide uptake in breast cancers has also been identified with positron emission tomography (PET) after the injection of fluorine-18 2-deoxy-2-fluoro-D-glucose (FDG), and has been found particularly useful in breast cancer detection in dense breasts and for disease staging. This labelled compound may also accumulate in abnormal axillary nodes. PET scanning requires additional research to determine its sensitivity, specificity, and cost-effectiveness in breast cancer. PET is increasingly used as:

i. An adjunct to standard imaging modalities for staging patients with distant metastasis (Fig. 22.5).

ii. In re-staging patients with locoregional recurrence or metastasis.

iii. As an adjunct to standard imaging modalities for monitoring tumour response to treatment for women with locally advanced and metastatic breast cancer when a change in therapy is anticipated.

It must be remembered that in breast cancer, the status of the axillary nodes is one of the strongest prognostic indicators, and a major factor in determining adjuvant systemic therapy. Sentinel node biopsy (SNB) is a valuable technique in cases of small operable breast cancer. It avoids treatment of the axilla when the nodes were negative for metastasis. Thus patients with negative biopsy with no histologic evidence of metastases, require no further axillary treatment.

^{99m}Tc sulphur colloid and dye like 1% isosulfan blue identifies sentinel nodes in the axilla prior to surgery. Labelled ^{99m}Tc sulphur colloid is injected interstitially by the surgeon near a biopsy-proven breast cancer, with injected material tracking along routes of tumour lymphatic vessels. At subsequent surgery, an axillary sentinel node which drains the primary cancer site, containing the radioactive tracer identified by a radionuclide probe, is removed and evaluated histologically. If the sentinel node is negative for tumour, axillary node dissection and its potential complications may be avoided. However, in practice, a false-negative rate as high as 16.6 per cent on immunohistochemistry is encountered resulting in leaving behind untreated positive non-sentinel nodes in the axilla and a potential risk for axillary recurrence.

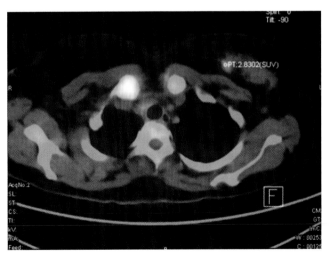

Fig. 22.5: PET/CT in an established case of infiltrating ductal carcinoma , reveals evidence of primary tumour at upper inner quadrant left breast and skeletal metastasis at medial end of right clavicle (*Courtesy:* Department of Nuclear Medicine, AH (R & R), Delhi Cant)

MRI BREAST

A dedicated breast coil is preferable for breast MR imaging. A double coil is preferable, permitting comparison between the two sides. The coils are designed such that the patient is imaged in the prone position, supported by the coil and table, with the breasts pendent in the coil. This position reduces motion artefact from respiratory movement. A variety of MR sequences for contrast-enhanced breast imaging may be used. The morphologic appearance of carcinomas on MRI is similar to that on mammography, except for non-visualisation of microcalcifications. 2D techniques may miss small lesions because of gaps between slices. Echo-planar imaging (EPI) is an ultrafast MRI technique that enables dynamic imaging of multiple levels within the entire breast, in as little as 6 seconds intervals.

The most effective strategy with a high sensitivity for enhancing lesions is a 3D imaging technique using either FLASH (fast low-angle shot), FISP (fast imaging with steady precession), FATS (fast adiabatic trajectory in a steady state), or GRASS (gradient-recalled acquisition in a steady state) sequence, performed before and after injection with Gd-DTPA. These sequences have an advantage of allowing volumetric coverage of the breasts resulting in thin, contiguous slices (1 to 2 mm) that enable detection of extremely small lesions. To differentiate fat from enhancing lesions on gradient echo images, since both display high-signal intensity, fat signals are suppressed by chemical-shift imaging and image subtraction of the pre from the postcontrast images. The optimal dose of Gd-DTPA may range from 0.1 to 0.2 mmol/kg body weight.

The role of contrast-enhanced MRI of the breast at present includes:
  i. Determining the size and extent of known invasive cancers.
  ii. Identifying multi-centric lesions.
  iii. Evaluating the ipsilateral breast of a woman who comes initially to attention with axillary metastases.
  iv. Identifying a recurrent carcinoma in a conservatively treated breast.
  v. Analysis of lesion contrast pharmacokinetics.

The interpretation of breast MRI, standardised by the Lesion Diagnosis Working Group Project is divided into two parts.

The first part is morphologic analysis involving evaluating lesions by morphology, margins, and patterns of enhancement. Morphology yields descriptors like round, oval, lobulated, irregular, or stellate, while margins describes terms like smooth, scalloped, irregular, or spiculated. Smooth and lobulated margins favour benign, while spiculated and irregular margins are associated with malignancy. The second part of the interpretation is the pattern of enhancement, i.e. homogeneous, heterogeneous, rim pattern, enhancing internal separations, or nonenhancing internal separations. Linear enhancement may suggest DCIS.

The second part of the interpretation is kinetic or dynamic analysis of "enhancement intensity versus time curve", with malignant tumours tending to have fast enhancement with fast washout, and with benign lesions tending to have a gradual increase in enhancement.

As a diagnostic modality in breast cancer, MRI of the breast is highly sensitivity (94 to 100%). In addition, in these highly selected patients, MRI demonstrates other unsuspected areas of cancer in approximately one-third of cases. Comparative studies of MRI to mammogram, ultrasonography, and clinical assessment consistently show MRI to have higher accuracy for determining the extent of disease, including the presence of multifocal or multicentric disease. However, the specificity of breast MRI remains low and highly variable (37 to 100%), because of contrast enhancement shown by few benign breast lesions. On proton MR spectroscopy (MRS) high levels of composite choline are likely to be found.

For screening in women at highest risk for breast cancer, as in suspected or known genetic mutations (e.g., BRCA (Breast Cancer Antigen 1 and 2), MRI may be useful as a screening tool. Women with BRCA mutations tend to develop breast cancer at a younger age, when breast density is higher. MRI is useful as a screening modality for breast cancers related to BRCA 1 (as opposed to BRCA 2) mutation since the former is NOT associated with DCIS and its subsequent microcalcifications as well as tends to present with a more benign appearance on mammography, with round/pushing as opposed to irregular margins. However, with BRCA 2 carriers in whom DCIS is more prevalent, mammography, which can detect microcalcifications, is a more valuable screening tool.

RADIOLOGY AND IMAGING IN COMMON BREAST CONDITIONS

Mammographic Findings of Benign Masses

Commonly encountered benign lesions in mammography comprise the following: raised skin lesions, intramammary lymph nodes, and fat containing lesions like lipomas, fat necrosis, oil cysts, galactoceles, hamartomas and haematomas. Besides these, patterns such as central coarse calcification in involuting fibroadenomas, peripheral calcification in involuting fibroadenoma, cysts with calcified walls as in fat necrosis and calcifying large duct papillomas, cysts with precipitated calcium (milk of calcium) are also usually benign.

Benign Proliferative Disorders

These constitute a spectrum of breast conditions from more glandular and/or fibrotic tissue than expected for patient's age and parity to morphologically abnormal tissue. It includes the following:

  i. Adenosis
 ii. Fibroadenoma
iii. Cyst
 iv. Ductal hyperplasia
  v. Papillomatosis/papilloma
 vi. Fibrocystic disease.

These usually coexist and seldom occur in pure forms. Patients with benign breast disease were once considered to be at increased risk for developing malignancy, but it is now established that an entity, atypical epithelial hyperplasia has an increased risk for breast carcinoma, especially those with family history of breast cancer.

Large Duct Papilloma or Intraductal Papilloma

It is the single commonest cause of serous or bloody discharge from the nipple. It occurs due to proliferation of ductal epithelium, projecting into lumen of duct. Papillomas may have a fibrovascular stalk, foci of necrosis, haemorrhage and occasional calcification. A dilated duct may be the only finding on mammography, if papilloma measures only a few millimetres. When the papilloma is of sufficient size, an elongated mass is visualised. Occasionally mulberry-like calcification may be seen in the subareolar region due to multiple papilloma. Ultrasonography may reveal a dilated duct with intraductal solid hypoechoic mass. Colour Doppler may demonstrate the vascular stalk. On MRI, large papilloma has features comparable to fibroadenoma.

Fibroadenoma

Fibroadenoma is the commonest benign tumour of the breast in women of child bearing age and the usual age of presentation is between 30 and 35 years. They are firm, mobile and non-tender masses with variable size; usually less than 3 cm. Multiplicity is reported in about 20% of women. They are the result of overgrowth of the stromal connective tissue within the lobule causing expansion of the lobule and compression of the acini and terminal ducts. The lesions are hormone dependant with cyclical fluctuation in the size of the mass. They undergo involution with advancing age and may develop coarse calcifications. On mammography, the lesions are well-defined, homogeneous round or oval mass with smooth and lobulated margins. The mass density is similar to or slightly more than the normal glandular tissue (Fig. 22.1). The lesion may be partly or completely surrounded by a radiolucent halo. The calcification may be central amorphous or peripheral calcification and sometimes clustered microcalcifications. They are not premalignant lesions, but carcinomas can incidentally arise alongside a fibroadenoma or can develop in epithelium within fibroadenoma.

An ill-defined margin, microcalcification or an increase in size of a fibroadenoma, favours malignancy. A fibroadenoma with a diameter of more than 6 cm is defined as a *giant fibroadenoma* and is usually seen in adolescent and young females. Fibroadenoma occurring in teenagers with faster rate of growth and larger sizes often occupying a major portion of the breast are termed as *juvenile fibroadenoma. Complex fibroadenoma,* a term coined by Dupont and colleagues, describes fibroadenoma that contain cysts greater than 3 mm. On ultrasonography, fibroadenoma appears solid, ovoid, circumscribed, hypoechoic, homogeneous lesions with sharp margins (Fig. 22.6). Posterior acoustic enhancement is seen when the adenoma is highly cellular; posterior acoustic shadowing is seen when the fibrotic component predominates. On Doppler, it is usually avascular but in one-fifth cases minimal to moderate vascularity with low Peak Systolic Velocity and Resistivity Index is noted. On MRI, fibrous fibroadenoma is hypointense on all sequences and shows no enhancement. Cellular adenoma are difficult to differentiate from carcinomatous lesions because of variable appearance and enhancement; hence biopsy is diagnostic.

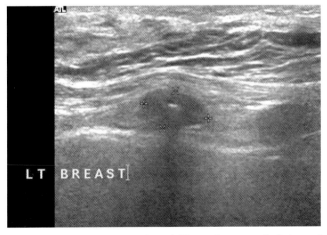

Fig. 22.6: Ultrasonography of fibroadenoma. Left breast Ultrasonography shows a well circumscribed, smooth marginated homogeneous solid mass measuring 1 cm x 1 cm

Fibrocystic Disease

It is a condition characterised by abundance of fibrous tissue and formation of cysts. "Aberrations of normal development and involution" (ANDI) is an emerging nomenclature to describe this entity and is normally diagnosed clinically and pathologically. Mammography reveals dense breasts or multiple predominantly benign cystic masses. US findings are usually normal or show generalised or regional thickening of glandular element, prominent ducts, surrounded by a hypoechoic cuff causing a spongy or mottled appearance. Multiple cysts of varying sizes may be associated.

Implants

Implants are of many types such as:
  i. *Silicone gel* with a 200 to 300 microns outer silicone rubber envelope.
  ii. *Saline implants* with an outer silicone envelope filled with saline.
  iii. *Double-lumen implants* with saline and internal silicone filled implant.

The envelopes of implants vary from smooth silicone, rough surface silicone envelopes and polyurethane covered shells. The silicone gel may migrate across the implant envelope into adjacent patient tissue with the formation of a fibrous capsule around the implant. The complications involving breast implants are varied and are best imaged by MRI. These include:
  i. *Herniation:* Occurs when fibrous capsule becomes disrupted and the intact implant with intact implant envelope herniates into the adjacent tissues.
  ii. *Intracapsular rupture:* Defined as a disruption of the implant envelope, collapsing and falling into the gel (linguine or fallen envelope or collapsed implant shell sign seen on MR imaging) with the implant contents contained by the intact external fibrous capsule).
  iii. *Extracapsular rupture:* Occurs when both the fibrous capsule and implant envelope are disrupted, with free silicone gel extruding into the surrounding tissue; foci of silicone outside the shell (tear drop sign). Rupture or herniation may occur without a history of trauma.
  iv. *Silicone granulomata* may also result from long-standing rupture.
  v. Postoperative complications include haematomas and abscess formation.
  vi. Capsular contraction, that produces a hard implant.

Principles of Imaging in Malignant Conditions of Breast

The four important tasks in breast cancer detection and management while using the currently available modalities are:
  i. Recognition of lesions
  ii. Analysis of lesions
  iii. Interpretation to make a decision
  iv. Disposition by biopsy, follow-up and therapy.

Mammographic Findings that Raise a Suspicion of Malignancy

These comprise of lesion with ill-defined margins, lesion with microlobulated margin, architectural distortion, a distorted parenchymal edge, density increasing over time, clustered microcalcifications and changing calcifications.

Findings that support the possibility of malignancy comprise of asymmetric breast tissue, asymmetric ducts and veins, skin and trabecular thickening, nipple retraction, deviation or inversion, enlarged axillary lymph nodes.

Mammography in Malignant Breast Lesions

The characteristic mammographic features of malignant breast masses are primary signs like mass lesion, microcalcification, architectural distortion, asymmetric density and segmental enlargement of duct. The secondary signs comprise skin changes, nipple/areola, increased vascularity and axillary lymphadenopathy.

Lesion Characterisation in Mammography of Breast Lesions

Since shape and morphology of lesion is an important analytical tool in mammography, attention is to be paid to analyse the same in detail. Broadly, the lesions are either round, oval and macrolobulated or they are irregular, ill-defined and spiculated. Each of these have a range of disease entities either benign or malignant as shown in Table 22.8.

Classification of Breast Cancer

Depending on the site of origin, namely ductal epithelium, lobular epithelium, stromal tissues and metastasis, breast malignancy can be divided into four major histological categories, each further subdivided into various subtypes (Table 22.9).

TABLE 22.8

Round, oval macrolobulated	Irregular, illdefined, spiculated
Benign	**Benign**
Cyst	Fat necrosis-postoperative changes
Fibroadenoma	Radial scar/complex sclerosing lesion
Papilloma	Haematoma (acute)
Sebaceous cyst	Mastitis/abscess
Haematoma	Sclerosing adenosis
Abscess	Fibrosis
Fibrosis	Extra-abdominal desmoid
Pseudoangiomatous stromal hyperplasia	
Phylloides (benign)	
Galactocele	
Sclerosing adenosis	
Malignant	**Malignant**
Invasive ductal carcinoma not otherwise specified (NOS)	Invasive ductal carcinoma not otherwise specified (NOS)
Mucinous	Invasive lobular carcinoma
Medullary	Tubular carcinoma
Papillary	Ductal carcinoma in situ
Metastases	Lymphoma
Lymphoma	Sarcoma
Phylloides (malignant)	
Ductal carcinoma *in situ*	
Invasive lobular carcinoma	

Lesion characterization of breast masses

Furthermore, malignant breast lesions are also divided into the non-invasive and the invasive types.

Ductal Carcinoma in Situ (DCIS)

It is a pre-invasive lesion with histologic progression from atypical hyperplasia to invasive breast cancer. It constitutes 22 to 45 per cent of all breast cancers diagnosed by mammography. It may be multifocal due to discontinuous intraductal growth, in low grade lesions, as opposed to high-grade lesions that are continuous. Nearly 90% of DCIS are diagnosed while they are clinically occult because of mammographic detection of microcalcifications, soft-tissue densities, or both. Mammography shows clusters of pleomorphic, ductally oriented microcalcifications in the majority. A mass with an ill-defined or lobulated margin with or without calcification may also be present. Magnification views are helpful in some cases. 10 to 15% of DCIS have associated invasive carcinoma, found on excision biopsy.

TABLE 22.9

I. Tumours of ductal epithelial origin
   A. Ductal carcinoma in situ (DCIS)
   B. Invasive ductal carcinoma
     • 95 per cent are ductal not otherwise specified (NOS)
     • 5 per cent characterised by specific histological features
     i. Paget's disease (tumour cells involving the nipple)
     ii. Tubular carcinoma (well defined ductal tubular structures)
     iii. Papillary carcinoma (often in a cystically dilated duct)
     iv. Colloid carcinoma (extensive mucin production)
     v. Medullary carcinoma (large reticular cells and lymphoid infiltrate)
     vi. Inflammatory cancer (with early dermal lymphatic invasion)

II. Tumours of lobular origin
   A. Lobular carcinoma *in situ*
   B. Infiltrating lobular carcinoma.
   C. Phylloides tumour

III. Stromal malignancy
   Sarcomas—Fibrosarcoma, angiosarcoma, liposarcoma, osteogenic sarcoma

IV. Metastatic disease of the breast
   A. From primary tumours of melanoma, lung, renal, others
   B. Lymphoma—usually secondary—may be primary rarely

Classification of breast cancers based on histological subtypes

USG shows high specular echoes due to calcification. Associated soft tissue component and architectural distortion may be appreciated as hypoechoic lesions (Fig. 22.7). MRI is inferior to mammography because of its inability to delineate microcalcification. Moreover, only 40 to 50 per cent of DCIS display an enhancement pattern typical of malignancy. Lobular carcinoma *in situ* (LCIS) accounts for 1 to 6% of all carcinomas. The tumour is often multifocal and bilateral. It does not usually show any clinical or mammographic abnormalities. Diagnosis is an incidental finding in biopsy done for other reasons.

Invasive Lesions

Among the invasive breast cancers, invasive ductal carcinoma accounts for nearly 90%, invasive lobular carcinoma for 5.5% and stromal cancers for less than 4% of these lesions.

Invasive ductal carcinoma not otherwise specified (NOS): DCIS may be seen as a component of infiltrating ductal carcinomas. Clinically there may be a palpable mass, focal tenderness, nipple discharge, skin retraction or ulceration. Mammography shows a spiculated,

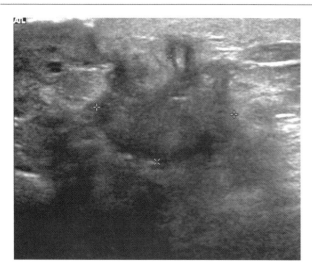

Fig. 22.7: Ultrasonography of carcinoma: A mass (within cursor) has following features suggesting malignancy: ill-defined margins, height equal to or greater than width, and low-level heterogeneous internal echoes

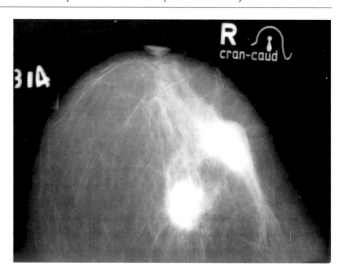

Fig. 22.8: Invasive ductal carcinoma. Close-up mammogram shows a spiculated mass with irregular shape, and clusters of microcalcification is seen at inferomedial quadrant of right breast. The right nipple is retracted. A case of BI-RADS category 5

rounded mass with well-defined or partially defined margins (Fig. 22.8). Architectural distortion may be the only finding. Calcification is seen in 60% tumours. Ultrasonography shows a hypoechoic mass having spiculated or lobulated margin with or without calcification. Distal acoustic shadowing and incomplete posterior wall may be seen.

RECENT ADVANCES

Mammography

The recent advances in mammography breast include introduction of Full-field Digital Mammography, Dose-reduction Mammographic system, Computer-aided Detection for Mammography and Computed Tomography Laser Mammography. Amongst them, the most promising is digital mammography. Full-field digital mammography is similar to standard mammography system, but the system is equipped with a digital receptor and a computer instead of a film cassette. It offers several advantages over traditional film mammography: faster image acquisition, sharper image resolution, shorter examinations, facilitating quicker procedures, easier image storage, easy transmission of images to other physicians, and computer processing of breast images for more accurate detection of breast cancer.

Digital mammography is reported to detect additional cancers, although this may be at the expense of more false-positive results. Digital mammography

may be significantly more sensitive than film mammography in screening women who have dense breasts and women who are younger than 50 years or are premenopausal or perimenopausal. Computer-aided detection for mammography reduces interpretative errors by identifying and marking suspicious features on mammography films that may be associated with breast abnormalities. It enables suspicious regions to be evaluated more closely, with additional diagnostic testing like ultrasonography or biopsy. Computed tomography laser mammography is currently under development. It is a breast imaging system that uses advanced laser technology to produce a near three-dimensional perspective of the breast. In another path of advances, newer machines like microdose system reduce the mammography radiation dosage by 20 per cent.

Breast Ultrasonography

Del Cura JL investigated differences in Doppler features between benign and malignant breast lesions and between malignant lesions with different prognostic factors. Colour flow was more frequently seen in malignant (68%) than in benign (36%) lesions. However, sensitivity, specificity, and positive and negative predictive values for this sign were low (68%, 64%, 58%, and 73%, respectively). The RI and PI values were significantly higher (p < 0.001) in cancers. The authors concluded that flow visualisation on power Doppler sonography indicated a higher possibility of malignancy but is not useful as the main sign for malignancy. However, any lesion with a vessel that has an RI value greater than 0.99 or a PI value greater than 4 within must be considered as probably malignant regardless of any other sonography sign present. Doppler findings were found not useful to predict tumour grade or lymph node involvement.

USG-guided vacuum biopsy is now considered an accurate and well tolerated technique. It is an alternative to surgery for masses less than 15 mm including fibroadenomas and papillomas or in patients with imaging-histologic discordance at core biopsy. In effect, US-guided directional vacuum-assisted large-gauge core needle biopsy acquires larger samples of tissue (compared to automated core biopsy) and potentially avoids under-sampling a lesion which reduces false negative results). This is found useful in certain lesions exhibiting a spectrum of change ranging from atypia to *in situ* cancer or when sampling masses are smaller than 1.5 cm.

Yang et al in a study evaluated benign and malignant breast masses and axillary nodes with echo-enhanced colour power Doppler ultrasonography. The study was based on analysing increased tumour vascularity at Doppler ultrasonography, a characteristic feature of malignancy, by using 10 ml of a 300 mg solution of SHU-508A (Levovist), a galactose-based medium injected at a rate of 2 ml/sec that contains microbubbles, allowing more complete delineation of microvessels anatomy. Microbubble-enhanced colour Doppler US characterises vessel distribution as:

i. Peripheral vessels defined as one or more vessels coursing along the margin of a mass.
ii. Central vessels defined as one or more colour signals within the mass that did not extend to the periphery.
iii. Side-branching vessels defined as one or more colour signals arising from peripheral or central vessels in a branching pattern that were smaller in calibre than the primary vessel.

The study revealed that breast cancers had a greater total number and greater number of peripheral vessels than did benign lesions before and after contrast material administration. Malignant axillary nodes had a greater total number and greater number of peripheral vessels at baseline and after contrast enhancement and a longer enhancement duration (P 5.004) compared with benign nodes. Malignant nodes enhanced more than did corresponding primary breast cancers.

MRI Breast

The recent advances in MRI breast include:
i. Analysis of breast tumour volume in cases of neoadjuvant chemotherapy to predict recurrence-free survival (RFS).
ii. Use of intravenous gadolinium to detect angiogenesis.
iii. Standardisation of MR protocols.
iv. MRI guided biopsy of clinically occult breast lesions detected by MRI but not at mammography/sonography.
v. Fusion of contrast-enhanced breast MR and mammographic imaging data.
vi. MR spectroscopy: Cumulatively, these have pushed MRI as a "problem solving" tool in a significant number of cases.

A recent study using MRI showed that measurement of breast tumour volume can help predict recurrence-free survival (RFS) in patients undergoing neoadjuvant (preoperative) chemotherapy. In the study, 58 breast cancer patients scheduled to undergo neoadjuvant chemotherapy, were suggested to contrast-enhanced MR, before and after one and four cycles of treatment. Initial tumour volume was a strong predictor of recurrence-free survival. Of the women who had tumour volumes of $33~cm^3$ or less on initial MR examination, 93 per cent remained disease-free after two years, compared with 70 per cent of the women with larger tumours. Besides, change in tumour volume with treatment was a valuable predictor of survival. Apparently, patients who had a 50 per cent or greater reduction in MR tumour volume when comparing the first MR examination to the last had a recurrence-free survival rate of 87 per cent after two years, compared with 64 per cent of those with less tumour shrinkage during chemotherapy, irrespective of their initial tumour volumes.

MR enhancement behaviour of breast lesions is emerging as an important advancement by the use of intravenous gadolinium to detect the presence (Figs 22.9 A and B) or absence (Figs 22.10 A to C) of angiogenesis (Table 22.10). On MRI, almost all invasive malignancies enhance with Gd-DTPA. With dynamic MRI, malignancies may enhance at much more rapid initial rates than benign lesions, due to tumour angiogenesis a term implying:
a. Recruitment of large density and concentration of tumour neovessels needed for cancer growth.
b. Neovessels with abnormal basement membranes, resulting in vessel leakiness.

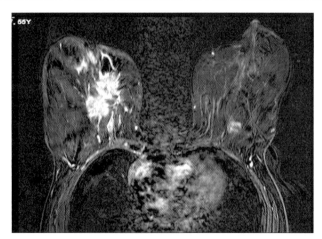

Fig. 22.9A: MRI breast in a woman with breast cancer. Enhanced fat saturated T1-weighted 3D gradient-echo MRI shows two irregularly marginated lesion with intense and heterogeneous enhancement in a proven case of invasive ductal carcinoma. Note the fibroadenoma at left breast

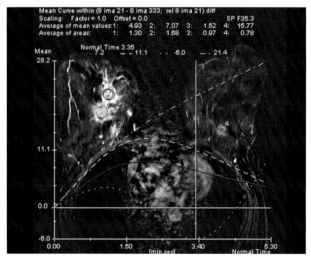

Fig. 22.9B: Dynamic breast MRI time-signal intensity curve of the lesion in the left breast shows a type III curve characterized by 'classic washout curves;' a rapid rise followed by decreased intensity of enhancement, usually indicating malignancy. Lesion underwent excisional biopsy which revealed invasive ductal carcinoma. Note the fibroadenoma at left breast, which shows a type 1 curve, indicating benign pattern

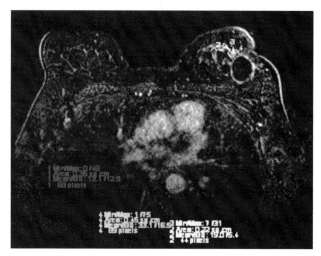

Fig. 22.10A: Follow-up MRI breast of postoperative breast cancer: Enhanced fat-saturated T1-weighted 3D gradient-echo MRI shows large smooth walled lesion in left outer quadrant with rim irregular enhancement. Lesion underwent USG-guided localisation and excisional biopsy. Pathology revealed fibrocystic change without malignancy

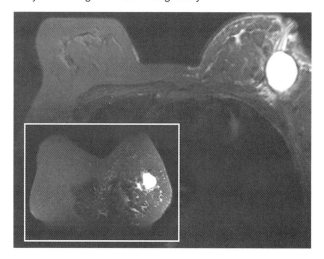

Fig. 22.10B: Follow-up MRI breast of postoperative breast cancer: Enhanced fat-saturated axial T1-weighted 3D gradient-echo MRI shows large smooth walled lesion in left outer quadrant. Inset reveals coronal image. Inset shows coronal view of same. Lesion underwent USG-guided localisation and excisional biopsy. Pathology revealed fibrocystic change without malignancy

Fusion of contrast-enhanced breast MR and mammographic imaging data is a logical evolution, since it combines the advantages of MRI and mammography, thereby overcoming their inherent disadvantages. While the assets of contrast-enhanced MRI are:

i. Providing a three-dimensional (3D) functional information via pharmacokinetic interaction between contrast agent and tumour vascularity.

ii. Its applicability to women of all ages, and

iii. Patients with postoperative scarring, mammography is inherently a modality that offers high-resolution structural information, especially calcification.

The fusion of mammography is complementary, since it brings out microcalcification clusters and fine speculations that are not visible in CE-MRI, alone.

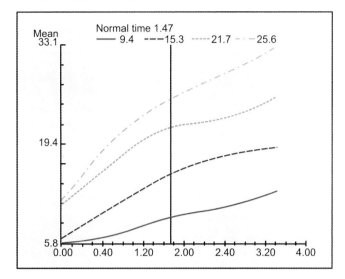

Fig. 22.10C: Dynamic breast MRI time-signal intensity curve of the lesion in the left breast shows a type I curves characterized by a gradual increase in enhancement over time and is supportive of a benign lesion. Lesion underwent USG-guided localization and excisional biopsy. Pathology revealed fibrocystic change without malignancy

MR spectroscopy is useful in patients with suspicious lesions or biopsy-proved cancers. In a recently published study, single-voxel breast MR spectroscopy was performed in patients with suspicious or biopsy-proved malignant lesions measuring 1 cm or larger at MR imaging. A choline peak was present in all cancers and in three of 26 benign lesions, giving MR spectroscopy a sensitivity of 100 per cent and a specificity of 88 per cent. The authors concluded that proton MR spectroscopy was useful in reducing the number of lesions detected at MR imaging that require biopsy.

Another study showed that proton MR spectroscopy was useful for *in vivo* characterization of breast masses when the lesion exceeds 1.5 cm in maximal dimension, but was unable to identify benign breast lesions and phyllodes tumours of benign and borderline malignancy. In the same study, the authors focus their attention on HER2/neu, which is an oncogene that is (a) commonly over expressed in breast cancer, (b) that is associated with poor prognosis due to its role in tumour progression and c) responsible for causing a dramatic increase in levels of choline compounds. The authors suggest that a false-negative spectroscopic result may be related to an absence of HER2/neu over expression in carcinoma of the breast.

SUMMARY

Imaging by mammography has played a significantly beneficial role in detection of breast lesions, particularly

TABLE 22.10

Contrast enhancement in normal and abnormal breasts
- The ideal time for MRI of the breast is approximately between day 5 and 15 of the menstrual cycle, which avoids the luteal phase, where an increase in oestrogen and progesterone leads to oedematous stroma that shows increased enhancement.
- By analysing kinetic or dynamic analysis of contrast enhancement as a function of time, benign and malignant lesions can be differentiated to a certain degree, due to tumour mediated angiogenesis.
- Generally, for tumours to grow more than 2 to 3 mm in size, they have to secrete proangiogenic factors.
- Malignant lesions have microvasculature which undergoes 'tumour mediated angiogenesis' featuring more haphazard distribution, increased capillary permeability and arteriovenous shunting leading to quicker enhancement and quicker washout times.
- Types of contrast enhancement time intensity kinetic curves
    - o Type I curves are characterised by a gradual increase in enhancement over time and is supportive of a benign lesion.
    - o Type II curves are characterised by a rise in enhancement intensity followed by a plateau. Can be benign or malignant lesions.
    - o Type III curves are the 'classic washout curves'; a rapid rise in enhancement followed by a decreased intensity of enhancement, usually indicating malignancy.
- Several invasive cancers, including infiltrating lobular carcinomas, malignant phylloides tumours, tubular carcinoma, colloid and mucinous carcinomas have type I enhancement profiles.
- Several benign lesions like fibrocystic disease, fibroadenomas, sclerosing adenosis, atypical hyperplasia, lobular carcinoma in situ (LCIS), and breast papillomas can occasionally show type III curve.
- DCIS lesions are more commonly missed on MRI, due to they being more dependent on diffusion but less on angiogenesis: Also their main imaging hallmark of microcalcification is usually undetected with MRI.
- Comedocarcinoma variants of DCIS are more likely to enhance than other subtypes, due to increased angiogenesis is therefore required for further growth.
- MRI breast after irradiation therapy shows inflammation associated with radiation that causes enhancement of the tissue. It is therefore recommended to wait at least 9 months, for replacement of inflammation by fibrosis

Caveats in contrast enhanced MRI of normal and abnormal breasts

early breast cancer. Film screen mammography with a low cost, good diagnostic ability and easy availability surpasses all other imaging modalities available for breast imaging, notwithstanding its limitations. At this point in time, mammography equipment and technique have significantly improved since the invention of mammography in the sixties by ongoing advances in digital technology. Ultrasonography and MRI have emerged as useful adjuncts. Keeping with the trends of the past and present. Imaging will continue to occupy a central place in the diagnosis, interventional procedures and follow up of breast lesions, in times ahead.

FURTHER READING

1. American College of Radiology (ACR). Breast imaging reporting and data system (BI-RADS) (3rd edn). Reston, VA: ACR; 1998.
2. Andolina V, Willson KM, Lille SL. Mammographic Imaging—A Practical Guide (2nd edn). New York: Lippincott Williams and Wilkins. 2001.
3. Bauermeister D, Beverly H. Breast Imaging: A Correlative Atlas (1st edn). Thieme Medical Publications, 2002.
4. Berry M, Suri S, Chowdhury V, Mukhopadhyay S. Diagnostic Radiology: Chest and Cardiovascular Imaging (2nd edn). New Delhi: Jaypee Brothers 2003.
5. Cardeñosa G. The Core Curriculum: Breast Imaging (1st edn). New York: Lippincott Willliam & Wilkins, 2003.
6. Cosgrove DO, Kedar RP, Bamber JC, et al. Breast diseases—colour Doppler US in differential diagnosis. Radiology 1993;189:99-104.
7. Harris JR, Lippman ME, Morrow M, Osborne CK. Diseases of the Breast (3rd edn), London: Lippincott Williams & Wilkins 2004.
8. Ikeda DM. Appleton & Lange Review of Mammography. Boston: Elsevier Science Health Science, 2004.
9. Jacobson DR. Rad Tech's Guide to Mammography: Physics, Instrumentation, and Quality Control (Rad Tech's Guide Series) (1st edn). London: Blackwell Publishers 2001.
10. Kopans DB. Anatomy, Histology, Physiology and Pathology in Breast Imaging (2nd edn). New York: Lippincott Williams & Wilkins, 1998.
11. Kopans DB. Atlas of Breast Imaging (1st edn). Philadelphia: Lippincott Williams & Wilkins, 1999.
12. Kuhl CK, Mielcareck P, Klaschik S, Leutner C, Wardelmann E, Gieseke J, Schild HH. Dynamic breast MR imaging: signal intensity time course data useful differential diagnosis enhancing lesions? Radiology 1999;211:101-10.
13. Stavros AT, Rapp CL, Parker SH. Breast Imaging Companion. (1st edn). London: Lippincott Williams & Wilkins, 2003.
14. Stavros AT, Thickmass D, Rapp CL, et al. Solid breast nodules—use of sonography to distinguish between benign and malignant lesions. Radiology 1995;196:123-34.
15. Tabar L, Tot T, Dean PB. Teaching Atlas of Mammography (3rd edn). Berlin: Thieme Medical Publishers; 2001.

Part 5

Section 23
Special Topics in Endocrinology

SECTION

23

SPECIAL TOPICS IN ENDOCRINOLOGY

23.1 Metabolic Syndrome and Vascular Disease

JS Bajaj, Mandeep Bajaj

- Origin and Evolution of Metabolic Syndrome (MS)
- Metabolic Syndrome and Coronary Heart Disease (CHD)
- Diagnostic Criteria: NCEP-ATPIII, WHO, ACE, EGIR Criteria
- Fat Topography and Insulin Resistance in Asian Indians
- National Criteria for MS/ IRS
- Pathophysiology of Insulin Resistance in Asian Indian
- Nutritional Programming in Foetus and Infancy

- Cardiologists' Perspective
- Insulin Resistance, Vascular Biology and
- Cardiovascular Disorders
- Adipocyte Biology, Pathogenesis of MS and Atherosclerosis
- Resistin, Adiponectin
- Summary

ORIGIN AND EVOLUTION OF METABOLIC SYNDROME

The clinical association of coronary heart disease (CHD), diabetes, hypertension, and dyslipidaemia is well-recognised. However, a linkage between a constellation of these disorders and the underlying common feature of insulin resistance, was put in the conceptual framework of syndrome X by Gerald Reaven in 1988. The contour and contents of this syndrome have been better delineated and enlarged in the following years. Likewise, various synonyms have been suggested to reflect its essential features (Table 23.1.1).

TABLE 23.1.1

- Metabolic syndrome
- Dysmetabolic syndrome
- Plurimetabolic syndrome
- Insulin resistance syndrome
- CHO syndrome
  (Carbohydrate intolerance, CHD, hypertension, obesity)
- The Deadly Quartet
- Chronic cardiovascular risk factor syndrome
- Reaven's syndrome
- Syndrome X

Syndromic semantics

In the recently held first-ever World Conference on the Insulin Resistance Syndrome at Los Angeles, California in November, 2003, the term dysmetabolic syndrome, as included in the International Classification of Disease (ICD-9) code 277.7, was the preferred choice. Nevertheless, the term metabolic syndrome (MS) continues to be used by most of the investigators, and shall be used in this review.

Since its original description in 1988, a number of clinical disorders such as nonalcoholic fatty liver disease and polycystic ovary syndrome (PCOS) have been included amongst the constituents of metabolic syndrome. Additional metabolic and endocrinal characteristics, have also been added. Thus visceral adiposity and hypercoagulable state, along with hyperleptinaemia and hypoadiponectinaemia have been added. Increased risk of both diabetes and CHD is linked with insulin resistance possibly through such endocrinal and metabolic alterations. Table 23.1.2 summarises the evolving profile of metabolic syndrome.

TABLE 23.1.2

Original description 1988	Evolving profile 2005
Insulin resistance	Insulin resistance
Glucose intolerance	Glucose intolerance
Hyperinsulinaemia	Hyperinsulinaemia
Hypertriglyceridaemia	Hypertriglyceridaemia
Decreased HDL-cholesterol	Decreased HDL-cholesterol
Hypertension	Hypertension
	Visceral adiposity (Central obesity, truncal obesity)
	High plasminogen activator inhibitor -1
	Non-alcoholic fatty liver disease (NAFLD; hepatic steatosis)
	Polycystic ovaries syndrome (PCOS)
	Hypoadiponectinaemia
	Hyperleptinaemia
	Microalbuminuria
	Hyperuricaemia

Clinical profile of metabolic syndrome

METABOLIC SYNDROME AND CHD

Epidemiologic Evidence

In a cohort of 2,390 subjects in the San Antonio Heart Study, it was observed that a combination of three or more risk factors for CHD (obesity, T2DM, IGT, hypertension, hypertriglyceridaemia, and hyper-cholesterolaemia) in the same cardiac patient was more prevalent than either only a single factor or two factors in combination. Further data analysis convincingly demonstrated a significant increase in the relative risk of constituent disorders with increasing fasting insulin levels at baseline. Basal hyperinsulinaemia reflects the degree of insulin resistance.

The fact that the syndromic synergy becomes operational in early years of life is confirmed in clinical as well as postmortem studies. There is growing evidence that Asian Indians, as an ethnic group, seem to be particularly predisposed to develop central adiposity (high waist: hip ratio) and insulin resistance. More importantly, in Asian-Indians, the risk of T2DM, hypertension and CHD starts to increase rapidly at levels of BMI otherwise considered normal by WHO standards. This is because of the fact that even at lower BMI (~ 23 to 24) Asian-Indians are much more hyperinsulinaemic and insulin resistant, and have increased total body fat as well as visceral fat. Whether there is, in addition, a genetic predisposition to insulin resistance, needs to be further substantiated. In a recent study at the AIIMS, New Delhi, which investigated a group of 38 young healthy non-obese (mean BMI ~22.74), normotensive offspring of hypertensive parents, higher levels of insulin both in the fasting state and during oral GTT were observed in 23 (62%) of the subjects. Furthermore, serum triglycerides were significantly higher, and HDL-cholesterol significantly lower, in this group as compared to BMI-matched, and age-matched controls without family history of hypertension. The findings are suggestive of a genetic basis of insulin resistance. This early phase of hyperinsulinaemia in otherwise normal subjects may be followed by the clinical manifestations of T2DM, hypertension or CHD. In another case-control study of 44 young patients (age <40 years) with CHD, a significantly higher prevalence of obesity, hypertension, IGT, hyperinsulinaemia and dyslipidaemia was observed in this group. These findings support our previous observations regarding hyperinsulinaemia and impaired glucose tolerance in young non-diabetic subjects with CHD. Reaven has recently suggested that

adiposity and physical fitness each accounts for approximately 25% of the variability in insulin sensitivity, with genetic factors responsible for an additional 50% of the variation.

The corroborating confirmatory evidence for the presence of cardiovascular and metabolic abnormalities at a younger age, comes from a postmortem study of atherosclerotic lesions in 204 subjects ranging in age from 2 to 39 years. The arterial lesions were related to antemortem risk factors in a subgroup of 93 subjects in which such data were available. The extent of fatty streaks in the coronary arteries was 8.5 times higher in those with three or four risk factors compared with those in which no such risk factors were present.

Using uniform and standardised diagnostic criteria (see Diagnostic criteria) such as those recommended by the National Cholesterol and Education Programme, Adult Treatment Panel III report (NCEP-ATP III) and more sensitive imaging modalities, a most recent analysis estimated the magnitude of cross-sectional associations between the MS, CHD, and atherosclerosis in 14,502 black and white middle-age patients in the Atherosclerosis Risk in Communities Study (ARIC Study). CHD was ascertained by standardised procedures and subclinical atherosclerosis was determined by measuring carotid intimal medial wall thickness. The overall prevalence of MS was 30%. CHD prevalence was 7.4% among those with MS compared with 3.6% in comparison subjects. Amongst subjects free of CHD and stroke, the average intimal-medial wall thickness of carotid arteries was significantly greater among those with MS (747 vs 704 μm). The study convincingly demonstrates the significant association of MS with the presence of CHD and carotid intimal medial wall thickness, and suggests that identification of subjects with MS may provide opportunities to initiate CHD prevention strategies.

The representative studies cited above across different ethnic groups strongly point out a common underlying pathogenic link of insulin resistance and hyper-insulinaemia. Nevertheless, ethnic differences do exist, both in the pattern of risk factors and in the manifes-tations of the syndrome. For example, in African-Americans with T2DM, circulating levels of HDL-cholesterol tend to be significantly higher, and the triglyceride levels significantly lower, than in the Caucacians. This combination of protective factors is reflected in a reduced risk of CHD in individuals of African origin. In contrast, reverse is the case in the Indian subcontinent where there is higher degree of visceral adiposity disproportionate to the body mass index, along with hypertriglyceridaemia and low HDL-cholesterol concentrations. This may partly explain the increased cardiovascular mortality, both with and without T2DM, in those subjects.

DIAGNOSTIC CRITERIA AND PREVALENCE OF METABOLIC SYNDROME

A reference has already been made to National Cholesterol Education Programme (NCEP) Adult Treatment Panel III (ATP III) criteria. For the diagnosis of MS, any 3 or more of the following must be present:
- Waist circumference > 102 cm in men and > 88 cm in women
- Serum triglycerides ≥ 150 mg/dl (1.69 mmol/L)
- HDL-C <40 mg/dl (1.04 mmol/L) in men, < 50 mg/dl (1.29 mmol/L) in women.
- BP ≥ 130/85 mmHg.
- Fasting serum glucose ≥ 110 mg/dl (6.1 mmol/L).

Applying these criteria to a representative sample of the civilian noninstitutionalised US population recruited into the Third National Health and Nutrition Examination Survey (NHANES), Ford et al analysed data in a population subset of 8,814 men and women aged 20 years or older. The unadjusted and age-adjusted prevalence of MS were 21.8% and 23.7%, respectively. The Mexican Americans had the highest age-adjusted prevalence of 31.9%. The prevalence increased from 6.7% among participants aged 20 through 29 years, to 43.5% and 42.0% for participants aged 60 through 69 years and aged at least 70 years, respectively. Using 2000 census data, Ford et al estimated that about 47 million US residents have the metabolic syndrome.

Using identical criteria, as employed for data analysis of 1988-1994 population sample and cited above, the prevalence rate of MS showed a significant increase in the NHANES 1999 to 2000 sample. The unadjusted prevalence increased to 26.7%. Taking into account the possible variability in measuring waist circumference, an alternate criterion of BMI ≥ 29. 2 kg/m^2 among men and ≥ 24.9 kg/m^2 among women in NHANES 1999 to 2000 was used, and there was a very close agreement in prevalence estimates using these BMI cut-offs instead of waist circumference.

Taking cognizance of the recent recommendation by the American Diabetes Association for lowering fasting glucose cut-off to ≥ 100 mg/dl (5.55 mmols/L) for the diagnosis of impaired fasting glucose (IFG), the NCEP/ATP III criteria for the diagnosis of metabolic syndrome were modified with respect to fasting glucose. This raised the prevalence of MS to 28.0% from 23. 1% (1988-94 data) and from 26.7 to 31.3% (1999 to 2000 dataset). The prevalence estimates of the metabolic syndrome based on the revised criteria (and adjusting for population growth between 1994 to 1999), were accordingly revised to ~64 million US adult citizens in 2000.

While ATP III criteria for the diagnosis of metabolic syndrome have been extensively used by several investigators, alternate criteria have also been proposed by several groups. These include:

WHO Consultation Group

Diabetes, IFG, IGT, or HOMA insulin resistant and ≥ 2 of the following criteria:
- Waist-hip ratio >0.90 cm in men or >0.85 cm in women
- Serum triglycerides ≥150 mg/dl, HDL-C <35 mg/dl in men, or <39 mg/dl in women
- Urinary albumin excretion rate >20 μg/min
- Blood pressure ≥140/90 mmHg.

American College of Endocrinologists (ACE)

Presence of ≥1 of the following factors:
- Diagnosis of CVD, hypertension, PCOS, NAFLD, or acanthosis nigricans
- Family history of type 2 diabetes, hypertension, or CVD
- History of gestational diabetes or glucose intolerance
- Non-caucasian ethnicity with high risk for T2 diabetes or CVD
- Sedentary life style
- Age ≥40 years.
  and ≥2 of the following criteria:
- Triglycerides >150 mg/dl
- HDL-C: Men <40 mg/dl, women <50 mg/dl
- BP >130/85 mmHg
- Fasting glucose 110 to 125 mg/dl or 120 minutes post-glucose challenge 140 to 200 mg/dl (diabetes is excluded from the ACE criteria for diagnosis of insulin resistance syndrome).

European Group for the Study of Insulin Resistance (EGIR)

Fasting hyperinsulinaemia (highest 25%) and ≥2 of the following:

- Fasting plasma glucose ≥6.1 mmol/litre, but nondiabetic (2 hours post-glucose < 11.1 mmol/L)
- BP ≥140/90 mmHg or under treatment for hypertension
- Triglycerides >2 mmol/L or HDL-C <1 mmol/L or treated for dyslipidaemia
- Waist circumference ≥94 cm in men and ≥80 cm in women.

A critical comparative analysis of the criteria proposed by different expert groups convincingly demonstrates a single fact namely, lack of agreement. A major difference between the criteria proposed by the WHO Consultation Group and the others is that the former include definitive diagnosis of type 2 diabetes in the proposed criteria, while all others include only IFG or IGT but specifically exclude persons with type 2 diabetes mellitus. Further, while ATP III criteria emphasise IFG, the ACE criteria recognise the limitations of fasting glucose, and highlight the usefulness of the 2-hour post-glucose challenge blood glucose. Most importantly, ACE criteria take a broader view of syndromes associated with insulin resistance, and accordingly include factors such as PCOS, NAFLD, and acanthosis nigricans, amongst the diagnostic criteria. In contrast, WHO group (consisting of diabetologists rather than endocrinologists) does not take cognisance of such clinical syndromes. Furthermore, while ATP III criteria include waist circumference, the WHO criteria emphasise waist-hip ratio. Finally, urinary albumin excretion rate, as a diagnostic criterion, is included only in the WHO criteria (possibly due to special interest of one of the members of the consultative group).

Dekker presented at the First World Congress on IRS an analysis of the Hoorn study of 2484 persons, initiated in 1989 with persons who were then aged 50 to 75 years. Among both men and women, those with ATP III IRS were more likely to have hypertension, hypertriglyceridaemia, low HDL cholesterol, and higher glucose, higher insulin, and increased waist circumference. Nineteen per cent of men and 26% of women in the study had IRS by the ATP III criteria; 32% and 17%, respectively, had IRS by the WHO criteria; 19% and 26%, respectively, had IRS by the EGIR criteria; and 35% and 33%, respectively, had IRS by the ACE criteria, with 60%

to 80% agreement between the various definitions. Among men, those having IRS according to either the ATP III or ACE criteria had a doubling of risk for CVD, while those with IRS according to the WHO and EGIR had a 1.5-fold increased risk. Among women, the associations were less strong: those with IRS by the ATP III criteria had twice the risk of CVD without increase in fatal CVD; those satisfying the ACE criteria had doubling of nonfatal CVD and a 1.5-fold increase in fatal CVD. The strengths of association were weaker among women for the WHO and EGIR criteria. Using the Hoorn study data, among men, high insulin predicted a 1.5-fold increase in CVD, increased waist circumference predicted a doubling, and hypertension predicted a 2- to 3-fold increase in risk. Among women, high insulin and waist circumference predicted risk of nonfatal CVD, and both low HDL and high triglyceride levels were significant factors predicting both fatal and nonfatal CVD.

Intervention strategies for prevention of CVD must be considered in individuals with a constellation of strong risk factors including obesity, IFG/IGT, hypertension, and dyslipidaemia, especially if there is a strong family history of CVD. The physicians, irrespective of denominational allegiance to cardiology, diabetology or endocrinology, must initiate appropriate interventions for individuals under their care, without complacently awaiting international consensus on diagnostic criteria. Nevertheless, it is obvious that till such a consensus emerges, ATP III recommendations shall continue to be widely used, subject to appropriate modifications warranted by local/regional experiences. It is in this context that the inclusion of 'non-caucasian ethnicity' as one of the ACE criteria warrants detailed consideration as there is evidence indicating that anthropometric measures, such as BMI, WHR, and waist circumference are not comparable across different ethnic groups residing in the US.

FAT TOPOGRAPHY AND INSULIN RESISTANCE IN ASIAN INDIANS

Bajaj and Banerji (2004) have recently reviewed the subject extensively. Epidemiological studies suggest that the distribution of fat, especially central obesity (visceral adiposity) may be an important determinant of insulin resistance, diabetes, and CVD, rather than generalised obesity as indicated by BMI, in Asian Indians. In a study of migrant Indians in the UK, it was observed that for a similar BMI, a four-fold increase in diabetes in migrant Indians was associated with higher waist: hip ratio (WHR) as compared with Europeans living in the UK. Furthermore, for every level of WHR, migrant Indians had higher fasting insulin levels and were more insulin resistant than the Europeans. It has also been shown that Asian Indians have a disproportionately high percentage of body fat relative to BMI and muscle mass, with predominant increase in visceral fat. A reference has already been made to the fact that even with a BMI < 25 m^2/kg, these subjects have significant hyper-insulinaemia and marked insulin resistance. The latter is better correlated with total visceral fat, and not with the subcutaneous adipose tissue volume. Taking cognizance of the need to define appropriate cut-off point for BMI relevant to Indian subcontinent, a recently held WHO Expert Consultation has endorsed a cut-off of 23 kg/m^2 as 'public health action point for Asians.' Our cumulative clinical data, which also include NAFLD and PCOS, show that fasting hypertriglyceridaemia and low HDL-cholesterol are predominant features of dyslipi-daemia, with their levels inversely correlated with each other, and directly correlated with insulin resistance, as ascertained by HOMA and/or by the mathematical model developed by us. Responding to the need of developing diagnostic criteria of local relevance, we propose the revised criteria for national use, and for use in the migrant Indians residing in other countries. In our data analysis, we have considered the presence of insulin resistance (fasting insulin and/or HOMA) as essential criterion. However, as facilities may not be available in all parts of India, we propose the following:

National Criteria for the Diagnosis of MS/IRS

Any 4 or more may be present:
- Waist circumference : >90 cm in men and > 80 cm in women
- Triglyceride/HDL ratio >3
- BP >130/85 mmHg
- Fasting plasma glucose ≥110 mg/dl or
  Fasting plasma glucose ≥100 mg/dl with 2 hr post-glucose challenge plasma glucose ≥140 mg/dl
- Fasting insulin ≧16 μU/ml and/or insulin resistance (HOMA).

Pathophysiology of Insulin Resistance in Asian Indians

It has been suggested that the magnitude of insulin resistance seen even in lean migrant Indians residing in the US may represent a primary metabolic defect (i.e. independent of total body fat) and may account for excessive morbidity and mortality from type 2 diabetes and its cardiovascular complications in this ethnic group. A reference has earlier been made to other factors, including possible genetic predisposition to insulin resistance that may explain pathophysiological basis of insulin resistance in persons in the Indian subcontinent (and possibly in the South-East Asian countries). It is in this context that our original hypothesis of malnutrition-related diabetes wherein foeto-maternal protein-energy deprivation, continuing into neonatal period and early infancy, and leading to endocrinal and metabolic dysfunction, needs a critical reappraisal.

In our clinical and experimental studies initiated nearly thirty years back, and continued for a period of over 10 years, it was convincingly demonstrated that glucose tolerance was impaired in both clinical as well as experimental (sub-human primate model) protein-energy malnutrition. It was also shown that adreno-cortical function was impaired, with high levels of circulating cortisol and abolition of the diurnal rhythm of cortisol. It suggested to us that sustained steroido-genesis and ACTH release was possibly secondary to nutritional and metabolic stress. Subsequent studies showed elevated basal growth hormone levels in the experimental group. More importantly, there was a lack of responsiveness (suppression) of both cortisol and growth hormone following oral or intravenous glucose. The observations provided evidence that abnormalities in hypothalamo-hypophyseal-GH and adrenal regula-tion occur early in response to protein-energy depri-vation. Since both cortisol and growth hormone are known to be contra-insulin hormones with major effects on glucose utilisation and lipolysis, the resultant increase of free fatty acids may enhance triglyceride synthesis in the liver, with an increase in the hepatic as well as intramyocellular lipid. Combined together, these abnor-malities may lead to insulin resistance both in the liver and also in the muscle.

The clinical and experimental observations cited above, find considerable support from the reported data by Bjorntorp and colleagues who noted high prevalence of metabolic syndrome in subjects lacking normal diurnal variation in cortisol levels. Such subjects also showed a blunted cortisol response following food intake, and an impaired suppressibility of plasma cortisol. These investigators have highlighted the striking association between the metabolic syndrome and dysfunction of neuroendocrine axis especially affecting the hypo-thalamopituitary adrenal axis.

Further support for the hypothesis linking mal-nutrition during foetal life and early infancy and insulin resistance has come from several studies in different parts of the world which have confirmed an association between low birth weight (due to maternal malnutrition) and an increase in the prevalence of T2 DM, hypertension and coronary heart disease in adulthood. In a recent review of 48 published studies on the subject of relation-ship between birth weight and glucose/insulin meta-bolism in adult life, it was observed that most studies reported an inverse relationship between birth weight and fasting plasma glucose concentrations (15 of 25 papers), fasting plasma insulin concentrations (20 of 26), plasma glucose concentrations 2 hr after a glucose load (20 of 25), the prevalence of type 2 DM (13 of 16) and measures of insulin resistance (17 of 22). However, the relationship of birth weight with insulin secretion was inconsistent in studies of adults.

Additional evidence was provided in the San Antonio Heart study wherein Valdez (1994) confirmed the relationship between the prevalence of IRS, the birth weight, and the current body weight. It was concluded that in traditionally impoverished and deprived populations that are exposed to affluent environments in a short time span, the transition from low birth weight newborns to obese adults, predominently contributes to T2DM, hypertension and dyslipidaemia.

Nutritional Programming in the Foetus and Early Infancy

The high prevalence of IRS in different parts of the world, and its correlation with low birth-weight and/or body weight in early infancy, coupled with overweight and/or central adiposity in the adults, points to the significant role of nutritional 'programming' in the foetus and early infancy. The concept of nutritional programming empha-sises the import of 'thrifty phenotype', as against the originally proposed 'thrifty genotype' by Neel. Recent work, however, provides a bridging hypothesis, emphasising *in utero* programming of 'mitochondrial genome' as a result of maternal and foetal protein-energy deprivation. This hypothesis provides a molecular basis for the connectivity between low birth weight, insulin resistance, and adult metabolic syndrome. Lee (2001) has proposed that the basis of insulin resistance lies in the quantitative and qualitative changes in the mitochondrial

genome, as a result of maternal malnutrition. Summing up the evidence, Lee argues that 'the mtDNA content would vary, depending upon nutritional status, while nuclear genes would not, making mtDNA more likely as the basis for 'thrifty genome'. Whether maternal malnutrition resulting in quantitative and qualitative changes in mtDNA facilitates the development of insulin resistance and diabetes in those who also have an underlying inherited defect of mitochondrial oxidative phosphorylation, seems to be an attractive hypothesis that merits further exploration.

Metabolic Syndrome: Cardiologists' Perspective

As the primary clinical outcome of metabolic syndrome is in terms of CVD, there is a heightened awareness amongst the cardiologists regarding the definition and diagnosis of metabolic syndrome. The proceedings of NHLBI (National Heart, Lung, and Blood Institute)/ AHA (American Heart Association) conference as approved by the AHA Science Advisory and Coordi-nating Committee, have been recently published (Circulation 2004; 109:433-438). The report highlights abdominal obesity, atherogenic dyslipidaemia, elevated blood pressure, and insulin resistance, alongwith a proinflammatory and a prothrombotic state, as essential characteristics. It further recognises three potential aetiological categories : (i) obesity and disorders of adipose tissue; (ii) insulin resistance; and (iii) a constellation of factors of hepatic, vascular and immunologic origin that mediate specific components of the metabolic syndrome.

For evaluating metabolic syndrome as a risk condi-tion, the participants of the NHLBI/AHA conference were provided detailed analysis of 3,323 Framingham men and women (mean age, 52 years) in 8 years of follow up. In this study, MS alone predicted ~ 25% of all new onset CVD. In the absence of diabetes, MS did not raise 10-year risk for CHD to > 20%. Ten-year risk of CHD in men with MS ranged from 10 to 20%; in women, it did not exceed 10%. Furthermore, it was observed that no advantage was gained in risk assessment by adding the unique risk factors of ATP III defined MS, to the usual Framingham risk factors. Contrary to the lack of advantage for CHD risk assessment, a distinct advantage was discernible when the risk of new-onset diabetes was examined for the Framingham cohort, in both men and women. The presence of MS was highly predictive of new-onset diabetes.

Insulin Resistance, Vascular Biology and Cardiovascular Disorders

It took nearly sixty years following the discovery of insulin to convincingly demonstrate its direct effects on the vasculature in dogs (Liang et al, 1982), and another decade to establish similar vascular effects in humans. Insulin, in concentration at the high physiological range, as observed in the post-parandial phase, produces a nearly two-fold increase in skeletal muscle blood flow in non-obese insulin-sensitive subjects. The vasodilatory effect of insulin occurs within about 30 minutes of administration coinciding temporally with its effects on glucose uptake in the muscle. The mechanism underlying the vasodilatory effect of insulin is through the release of endothelium derived nitric oxide (eNO). Such release of eNO is mediated through signalling pathways involving tyrosine kinase, PI 3-K, and Akt, downstream from the insulin receptor. Thus, the metabolic and vascular actions of insulin share common signalling pathways.

In addition to enhancing blood flow in the skeletal muscle, insulin also augments stroke volume, increases heart rate, as well as cardiac output. Furthermore, insulin causes antinatriuresis, antikaliuresis, and antiuricosuria in healthy human volunteers. Insulin also modulates the response to vasopressor hormones, i.e. norepinephrine, vasopressin, and angiotensin II both at the level of vascular endothelium, as well as at vascular smooth muscle cell independent of the endothelium. Taken together, there is a net effect of insulin on blood pressure. Thus, any imbalance between the vasodilatory effects of insulin and the opposite effects of other vasoconstrictor hormones, may result in elevation of blood pressure and accelerated development of macrovascular disease.

A study of vascular effects of insulin in some of the important clinical components of metabolic syndrome has yielded interesting data. Obesity causes a shift to the left in the vasodilatory response to insulin. The medium effective dose (ED_{50}) for insulin to increase leg blood flow in the obese was approximately four times (~ 160 µU/ml) that in the lean subjects (44 µU/ml). Subjects with T_2DM showed a more pronounced impairment of insulin-mediated vasodilation: only supraphysiologic hyperinsulinaemia (~ 2000 µU/ml) resulted in a 33% increase in blood flow. Similar observations were made when subjects with essential hypertension were studied. It was surmised that the impaired insulin-induced vasodilation as observed in obesity, type 2 diabetes, and hypertension was a result of impaired production of NO.

A sound conceptual framework for the understanding of molecular linkage between insulin resistance, hyperinsulinaemia, and increase risk of cardiovascular diseases or atherosclerosis in metabolic syndrome, has been provided in recent studies. Insulin receptors have been demonstrated on the vascular cells; these receptors are identical with those on the nonvascular cells with respect of structure, affinity, binding kinetics, capacity for tyrosine phosphorylation, and activation of tyrosine kinase. As in other cells, insulin binding with its receptors on vascular cells results in the activation of two separate signal transduction pathways: (i) the phosphatidylinositol (PI 3-kinase pathway; and (ii) the ras-mitogen-activated protein (MAP) kinase pathway. Under physiological concentrations of insulin, the vascular effects are mainly mediated by PI 3-kinase pathway. However, in insulin resistant states with resultant hyperinsulinaemia and persistent elevation of plasma insulin concentrations, MAP-K pathway is continuously activated, leading to proliferation and migration of smooth muscle cells in aorta and large blood vessels, alongwith a marked increase in the synthesis of extracellular matrix proteins in the arterial wall. In addition to these direct effects, insulin may also enhance the mitogenic effect of more potent growth factors, such as platelet-derived growth factor, and insulin-like growth factors.

It has already been mentioned that PI 3-kinase pathways is involved in the release of endothelium derived nitric oxide, and that the vasodilatory effects of insulin are considerably impaired in insulin-resistant states. The role and place of PI 3-kinase and ras-MAP kinase pathways in vascular endothelial cells can now be succinctly conceptualised. At physiological concentrations, insulin-mediated vasodilation is mainly through PI 3-kinase activation, leading to NO production (acute effect) and enhanced gene expression of eNOS (delayed effect). These effects are antiatherogenic. In contrast, insulin-mediated effects through ras-MAP kinase pathway, resulting in vascular smooth muscle cell growth, proliferation and migration, alongwith stimulation of extracellular matrix production, are atherogenic requiring persistently elevated concentrations of insulin as encountered in insulin-resistant states. Thus, accelerated atherosclerosis in metabolic syndrome is due to a combined effect of impaired insulin effects mediated by

PI 3-kinase pathway without the inhibition of insulin effects mediated by ras-MAP kinase pathway. The differential effects of insulin resistance on the PI 3-kinase and MAP kinase-mediated signalling in human muscle, are major determinants of alteration of vascular biology in insulin resistant states such as type 2 diabetes and obesity.

Experimental evidence, generated in recent years, does show that mice with gene disruption of endothelial nitric oxide synthase (eNOS) or neuronal nitric oxide synthase (nNOS) exhibits insulin resistance, hypertension, and dyslipidaemia. Induction of iNOS by endotoxin is associated with impaired insulin-stimulated glucose uptake. In contrast, targeted disruption of iNOS protects against obesity-linked insulin resistance in muscle. Recent clinical studies indicate marked impairment of insulin activation of IRS-1/PI 3-kinase pathway in the muscle of normal-glucose-tolerant insulin-resistant offspring of two diabetic parents. Thus, both the metabolic effects of insulin and its vasodilatory effects are linked together through IRS-1/PI 3-kinase pathway and insulin resistance even at an early stage, when glucose tolerance is normal, results in impairment of both metabolism and vasodilation.

Vascular cell adhesion molecule (VCAM) and intercellular adhesion molecule (ICAM) are established cardiovascular risk markers. It has also been shown that NO modulates leucocyte adhesions to the endothelium by regulating the production/release of ICAM and VCAM by endothelial and vascular smooth muscle cells. In a recent study, NOS activity in skeletal muscle of well controlled type 2 diabetics, who were on diet and/or sulphonylurea therapy, was investigated under basal condition and during a 80 mU/m^2. min euglycaemic clamp. Healthy age-matched, sex matched, BMI matched, and ethnicity matched subjects served as controls. Basal and insulin-stimulated muscle NOS activity was impaired in well controlled type 2 diabetic subjects. The defect in insulin-stimulated NOS activity correlated closely with the severity of insulin resistance as assessed by measurements of insulin-stimulated glucose disposal. In addition, there was a significant increase in plasma ICAM and VCAM concentrations, with an inverse correlation between the increased plasma ICAM and VCAM levels and the reduced muscle NOS activity.

Multiple mechanisms constitute the pathophysiological basis of vascular disorders in metabolic syndrome.

Some of the recent advances in our understanding of endothelial dysfunction secondary to insulin resistance have already been highlighted. In addition, effects of dyslipidaemia, coagulopathy and pro-inflammatory state need elaboration. Small, dense LDLs, and excess triglyceride-rich remnants, which are highly atherogenic, are increased in the insulin-resistant state. There is also an overproduction of very low-density lipoproteins (VLDLs) which can accelerate the atherosclerotic process in several ways, including direct effect on the metabolism and growth of endothelial cells. Low HDLs, an important feature of metabolic syndrome, are unable to reduce the inhibitory effect of LDL on endothelium-mediated vasodilation.

Hypercholesterolaemia increases the expression of endothelial adhesion molecules. More interestingly, recent studies indicate that hypercholesterolaemia decreases NO availability. Administration of NO precursor L-arginine partially restores endothelial dysfunction.

Adipocyte Biology, Pathogenesis of Metabolic Syndrome, and Atherosclerosis

The adipocyte serves as an integrator of endocrine, metabolic and inflammatory signals, imparting considerable survival advantage during human evolution. Thus, the adipocyte functions not only as a mere storage depot for fat, but as an endocrine, paracrine and autocrine organ that releases hormones and peptides in response to specific environmental demands, extracellular stimuli, or changes in metabolic status. These secreted peptides and hormones which include tumour necrosis factor (TNF)-α, leptin, adipsin, resistin, adiponectin (also known as Acrp-30), interleukin 6 (IL-6), plasminogen activator inhibiter 1 (PAI-1), and angiotensinogen amongst others, carry out a variety of diverse functions, and they have been referred to collectively as 'adipokines'. The key to pathophysiological basis of seemingly diverse clinical and metabolic disorders included in the insulin resistance syndrome (IRS), lies in the understanding of the molecular biology of adipokines and the physiology of the adipocyte. The adipokines have been postulated to play an important role in the pathogenesis of insulin resistance, hypertension, disorders of coagulation, dyslipidaemia, atherosclerosis, coronary heart disease, and glucose intolerance abnormalities associated with the insulin resistance syndrome (IRS).

The association between PAI-1, a key inhibitor of fibrinolysis, and atherosclerotic vascular disease is well recognised. The development of thrombosis within the blood vessels depends on the balance between pro-coagulant and thrombolytic factors. Although principally expressed by liver and endothelial cells, PAI-1 is also expressed by human adipocytes; omental adipose tissue explants produce significantly more PAI-1 than the subcutaneous adipose tissue. PAI-1 binds to the active site of both tissue plasminogen activator and urokinase plasminogen activator. Thus increased PAI-1, as seen in metabolic syndrome, leads to decreased fibrinolysis and can predispose to thrombosis. Hyperinsulinaemia, as a result of insulin resistance, further induces accumulation of PAI-1 as shown in experimental euglycaemic-hyper-insulinaemic clamp studies. Angiotensin II, which is also produced by adipocytes, induces PAI-1 and -2 expression in vascular endothelial and smooth muscle cells.

The observation that angiotensinogen, angiotensin converting enzyme (ACE), and type 1 angiotensin receptor genes are widely expressed in human adipose tissue, has sharpened the focus on local renin-angiotensin system (RAS) in the adipocytes, and the interlinkage between obesity and hypertension, the two important clinical constituents of MS. It is of interest to note that angiotensinogen mRNA levels are higher in visceral adipocytes than in the subcutaneous fat cells. The role and place of ACE inhibitors in the management of hyper-tension in patients at high risk of atherosclerotic vascular disease, as a part of metabolic syndrome, needs to be more intensively investigated.

Considerable interest has been recently generated regarding the role of the two most recently discovered adipokines, resistin and adiponectin, which link obesity and insulin resistance, type 2 diabetes mellitus, dyslipidaemia and inflammatory markers of coronary heart disease (CHD).

Resistin is a member of the recently discovered cysteine-rich secretory protein family and is expressed in adipose tissue. The structure of resistin bears close similarity to proteins that are involved in the inflam-matory process. Resistin expression is increased in abdominal compared to thigh adipose tissue. Interestingly, the physiological functions of resistin are also shared by other proinflammatory cytokines, such as IL-6 and TNF-α. These three adipokines not only cause insulin resistance, but may also be causally related to inflammatory process associated with obesity and coronary heart disease. Insulin has been shown to increase resistin protein secretion from human adipocytes *in vitro*, suggesting that increased resistin secretion may provide the connectivity between visceral adiposity, insulin resistance, and hyperinsulinaemia. Administration of pioglitazone in T2DM causes a significant decrease in plasma resistin concentration; the decrease is positively correlated with decrease in hepatic fat content and improvement in hepatic insulin sensitivity. A recent study has shown, for the first time, a significant positive correlation of serum resistin to CRP which remained significant even after adjusting for BMI and type of diabetes, suggesting that proinflammatory properties of resistin may be partially independent of the class (degree) of obesity.

Adiponectin is a recently discovered novel adipose-specific 247-amino acid protein, with high structural homology to TNFα. Adiponectin is considered as an antidiabetogenic and anti-atherogenic adipokine. Plasma levels of adiponectin are reduced in obese rodents and humans as well as in patients with T2DM. It has been suggested that adiponectin might function as an adipostat in regulating energy balance and that its deficiency might contribute to the development of obesity and T2DM.

In addition to its metabolic effects, adiponectin has also been shown to modulate endothelial inflammatory response through TNFα-induced expression of endothelial adhesion molecules. *In vitro* studies in human aortic endothelial cells have shown that human recombinant adiponectin, not only suppresses endo-thelial expression of adhesion molecules but also decreases the proliferation of vascular smooth muscle cells, and reduces lipid accumulation in macrophages, thereby modulating transformation of macrophages to foam cells.

Two clinical studies published recently provide interesting data linking the metabolic and anti-inflammatory roles of adiponectin. In a study of 77 subjects who had diabetes or were at high risk to develop diabetes, there was a significant negative correlation between circulating levels of adiponectin and CRP, PAI-1, and tissue plasminogen activator (tPA). These negative associations remained significant after adjusting for gender and BMI. This study reinforces earlier observation regarding the protective role of adiponectin against inflammation and endothelial dysfunction, and provides evidence of its negative association with tPA, which is known to play a role in impaired fibrinolysis. A similar study in women with prior gestational diabetes mellitus (pGDM) who are known to be at higher risk of developing T2DM and associated cardiovascular complications, showed that plasma adiponectin was significantly lower in pGDM as compared to women with normal glucose tolerance during pregnancy. The differences remained statistically significant even after adjustment for body fat mass. Equally significant were the differences in the levels of PAI-1 and ultrasensitive CRP which were higher in the pGDM group. It was concluded that lower plasma adiponectin concentrations characterise women with previous GDM independently of the prevailing glucose tolerance, insulin sensitivity or the degree of obesity and are associated with subclinical inflammation and atherogenic parameters.

Thus, the role of adiponectin as an integrator of metabolic and inflammatory signals underlying obesity, T2DM, and coronary heart disease has assumed considerable significance, both in terms of its potential as a part of preventive strategies, and also as a prototype molecule for the development of new analogues and related compounds aimed at therapeutic intervention. Further, development of PPAR-γ agonists which increase endogenous adiponectin may be equally promising and rewarding.

Even though recent understanding of the endocrinology of adipocyte has provided a deeper insight into the causes and consequences of insulin resistance and CVD risk, enhanced lipolysis and chronically elevated levels of free fatty acids play a significant role in affecting inhibition of glucose transport and phosphorylation, glycogen synthase and pyruvate dehydrogenase activity, and insulin signalling through the IRS-1, PKC θ, and PI 3-kinase pathways. In a recent study aimed at investigating the molecular mechanism(s) underlying the biochemical basis of insulin resistance due to the effect of elevated FFA on the muscle, a triglyceride emulsion was infused in healthy subjects for 48 hours, followed by muscle biopsy (vastus lateralis muscle), microarray analysis, quantitative real-time PCR, and immunoblots. After lipid infusion, nuclear encoded mitochondrial genes and PGC-1α (peroxisome proliferator activated receptor γ-coactivator-1α) expression were decreased. In contrast, extracellular matrix genes and connective tissue growth factor were significantly over expressed. A marked increase in expression of extracellular matrix-related genes following lipid infusion was of considerable

interest. This pattern charactrerises an inflammatory response leading to extracellular matrix remodelling and fibrosis. Such fibrotic inflammatory responses are mediated by the connective tissue growth factor (CTGF). Furthermore, there is evidence that CTGF mediates fibrotic changes at multiple sites including atheromatous plaques and in the myocardium following ischaemic injury. Such an understanding of pathophysiology may lead to recognition of additional molecular sites for future drug development.

SUMMARY

Insulin resistance is a key feature of a number of clinical disorders, grouped together as metabolic syndrome (MS), with significant cardiovascular manifestations. There is considerable debate regarding the diagnostic criteria and aetiopathogenesis of MS. These have been discussed and the criteria appropriate to Indian population have been suggested.

Genetic basis of insulin resistance is discussed highlighting the possible role of intrauterine malnutrition and nutritional 'programming' of the foetus, as the basis of altered fat topography and insulin resistance particularly in Asian Indians.

Vascular effects of insulin and adipocytokines such as adiponectin have been discussed with emphasis on molecular basis of pathophysiological alterations in vascular biology. In this context, the role of eNOS, including the modulation by NO of the production and release of vascular cell adhesion molecule (VCAM) and intercellular adhesion molecule (ICAM), have been highlighted. Multiple mechanisms, including dyslipidaemia, constitute the pathophysiological basis of vascular disorders in metabolic syndrome.

The emerging epidemics of obesity and type 2 diabetes mellitus are possibly interlinked by the rising prevalence of metabolic syndrome. Though a world-wide phenomenon, genetic factors may play important role in geographical areas such as the Indian subcontinent. Regardless of the diagnostic criteria used, there is general agreement that therapeutic interventions aimed at lifestyle change, with emphasis on normalisation of body weight, constitute primary strategy for the management (including prevention) of metabolic syndrome. Drug treatment to effectively reduce insulin resistance has shown promise for preventing type diabetes, although long-term clinical trials which would convincingly demonstrate reduction of CVD are as yet lacking. In patients in whom lifestyle changes fail to reverse metabolic risk factors, initiating drug treatment of specific abnormalities in these risk factors in accordance with contemporary therapeutic practice, seems worthwhile. The recognition of additional molecular targets is likely to facilitate development of drugs with therapeutic potential.

FURTHER READING

1. Alessi MC, Peiretti F, Morange P, Henry M, Nalbone G, Juhan-Vague I. Production of plasminogen activator inhibitor 1 by human adipose tissue: possible link between visceral fat accumulation and vascular disease. Diabetes 1997;46:860-7.

2. Bajaj M, Suraamornkul S, Piper P, Hardies LJ, Glass L, Cersosimo E, Pratipanawatr T, Miyazaki Y, DeFronzo RA. Decreased plasma adiponectin concentrations are closely related to hepatic fat content and hepatic insulin resistance in pioglitazone-treated type 2 diabetic patients. J Clin Endocrinol Metab 2004;89:200-6.

3. Bajaj JS, Bajaj M. Hepatic fat and insulin resistance: causes and consequences of non-alcoholic fatty liver disease. In Non-alcoholic Fatty Liver Disease. Ranbaxy Science Foundation, 2005 (in Press).

4. Bajaj JS, Bajaj M. Endocrinology of Adipocyte: Molecular Basis of Metabolic Effects. In Gupta SB (Ed): Medicine Update. Mumbai: Association of Physicians of India 2005;15:325-9.

5. Bajaj M, Banerji MA. Type 2 diabetes in South Asians: a pathophysiologic focus on the Asian-Indian epidemic. Current Diabetes Reports 2004;4:213-8.

6. Bajaj JS, Subba Rao G, Subba Rao J, Khardori R. A mathematical model for insulin kinetics and its application to protein-deficient (Malnutrition-related) diabetes mellitus. J Theor Biol 126:491-503.

7. Bajaj JS. Diabetes mellitus; the third dimention. In Mngola E (Ed): Diabetes 1982. Amsterdam: Excerpta Medica 1983;11-7.

8. Bajaj JS. Lilly Lecture. Diabetes mellitus: a global perspective. In Larkins RG, Zimmet PZ, Chisholm DJ (Eds): Diabetes 1988. Amsterdam: Excerpta Medica; 1989:7-16.

9. Bajaj M, DeFronzo RA. Metabolic and molecular basis of insulin resistance. J Nucl Cardiol 2003;10:311-23.

10. Bajaj M, Suraamornkul S, Hardies LJ, Pratipanawatr T, DeFronzo RA. Plasma resistin concentration, hepatic fat content, and hepatic and peripheral insulin resistance in pioglitazone-treated type II diabetic patients. Int J Obes Relat Metab Disord 2004;28:783-9.

11. Balkau B, Charles MA, for the European Group for the Study of Insulin Resistance (EGIR). Comment on the provisional report from the WHO consultation. Diabetic Medicine 1999;16:442-3.

12. Barker DJP, Hales CN, Fall CHD, Osmond C, Phipps K, Clark PMS. Type-2 (non-insulin-dependent) diabetes mellitus, hypertension and hyperlipidaemia (syndrome X): relation to reduced foetal growth. Diabetologia 1993;36:62-7.

13. Baron AD, Brechtel G. Insulin differentially regulates systemic and skeletal muscle vascular resistance. Am J Physiol 1993;265:E61-E67.

14. Berenson GS, Srinivasan SR, Bao W, Newman WP, Tracy RE, Wattigney WA. Association between multiple cardiovascular risk factors and atherosclerosis in children and young adults. N Engl J Med 1998;338:1650-6.

15. Bjorntorp P. Obesity and diabetes mellitus. In Daniel Porte, Jr , Robert S Sherwin (Eds): Diabetes Mellitus. Appleton and Lange, Stanford, Connecticut 1997;5:553-64.

16. Bloomgarden ZT. Highlights from the first World Congress on the insulin resistance syndrome. Medscape Diabetes and Endocrinology 2004;1-6.

17. Chandalia M, Abate N, Garg A, Stray-Gundersen J, Grundy SM. Relationship between generalized and upper body obesity to insulin resistance in Asian Indian men. J Clin Endocrinal Metab 1999;84:2329-35.

18. Dekker J. The Hoorn study. Presented at the First Annual World Congress on the insulin resistance syndrome. November 20-22, 2003; Los Angeles, California.

19. Dusserre E, Moulin P, Vidal H. Differences in mRNA expression of the proteins secreted by the adipocytes in human subcutaneous and visceral adipose tissues. Biochim Biophys Acta 2000;1500:88-96.

20. Einhorn D, Reaven GM, Cobin RH, et al. American College of Endocrinology position statement on the insulin resistance syndrome. Endocr Pract 2003;9:237-52.

21. Engeli S, Gorzelniak K, Kreutz R, Runkel N, Distler A, Sharma AM. Co-expression of renin-angiotensin system genes in human adipose tissue. J Hypertens 1999;17:555-60.

22. Feener EP, Northrup JM, Aiello LP, King GL. Angiotensin induces plasminogen activator inhibitor-1 and -2 expression in vascular endothelial and smooth muscle cells. J Clin Invest 1995;95:1353-62.

23. Ford ES, Giles WH, Mokdad AH. Increasing prevalence of the metabolic syndrome among US. Adults Diabetes Care 2004; 27:2444-9.

24. Genuth S, Alberti KG, Bennett P, et al. Follow-up report on the diagnosis of diabetes mellitus. The Expert Committee on the diagnosis and classification of diabetes mellitus. Diabetes Care 2003;26:3160-7.

25. Howard BV. Insulin resistance and lipid metabolism. Am J Cardiol 1999;84:28J-32J.

26. Kashyap SR, Roman LJ, Lamont J, Masters BSS, Bajaj M, Suraamornkul S, Belfort R, Berria R, Kellogg L, Liu Y, DeFronzo RA. Insulin resistance is associated with impaired nitric oxide synthase (NOS). J Clin Endo and Metab 2005;90:1100-5.

27. King GL, Davidheiser S, Banskoto N, Oliver FJ, Inoguchi T. Insulin receptors and actions on vascular cells. In Smith U, Bruun Ne, Hedner T, Hokfelt B (Eds): Hypertension as an Insulin-Resistant Disorder. Genetic Factors and Cellular Mechanisms. Elsevier Science Publishers, Amsterdam. 1991;183-97.

28. Laakso M, Edelman SV, Brechtel G, Baron AD. Decreased effect of insulin to stimulate skeletal muscle blood flow in obese men. J Clin Invest 1990;85:1844-52.

29. Laakso M, et al. Impaired insulin-mediated skeletal muscle blood flow in patients with NIDDM. Diabetes 1992;41:1076-83.

30. Lacoste L, Lam JY, Hung J, Letchacovski G, Solymoss CB, Waters D. Hyperlipidemia and coronary disease. Correction of the

increased thrombogenic potential with cholesterol reduction. Circulation 1995;92:3172-7.

31. Lee HK. Method of proof and evidences for the concept that mitochondrial genome is a thrifty genome. Diabetes Res Clin Pract 2001;54(Suppl. 2):S57-S63.

32. Lithell HO, Mckeigue PM, Berglund L, Mohsen R, Lithell U-B, Leon DA. Relation of size at birth to non-insulin dependent diabetes and insulin concentrations in men aged 50-60 years. Br Med J 1996;312:406-10.

33. McNeill AM, Rosamond WD, Girman CJ, Heiss G, Golden SH, Duncan BB, East HE, Ballantyne C. Prevalence of coronary heart disease and carotid arterial thickening in patients with the metabolic syndrome (The ARIC Study). The Am J Card 2004;94:1249-54.

34. McKeigue PM, Shah B, Marmott MG. Relationship of central obesity and insulin resistance with high diabetes prevalence and cardiovascular risk in South Asians. Lancet 1991;337:382-6.

35. Misra A, Cherukupalli R, Reddy KS, Mohan A, Bajaj JS. Hyperinsulinaemia and dyslipidemia in non-obese, normo-tensive offspring of hypertensive parents in Northern India. Blood Pressure 1999;8:1-5.

36. Misra A, Reddy RB, Reddy KS, Mohan A, Bajaj JS. Clustering of impaired glucose tolerance, hyperinsulinemia and dyslipidaemia in young North Indian patients with coronary heart disease : a preliminary case-control study. Ind Heart J 1999;51:275-80.

37. McTernan CL, McTernan PG, Harte AL, Levick PL, Barnett AH, Kumar S. Resistin, central obesity, and type 2 diabetes. Lancet 2002; 359: 46-7.

38. McTernan PG, Fisher FM, Valsamakis G, Chetty R, Harte A, McTernan CL, Clark PM, Smith SA, Barnett AH, Kumar S. Resistin and type 2 diabetes : regulation of resistin expression by insulin and rosiglitazone and the effects of recombinant resistin on lipid and glucose metabolism in human differentiated adipocytes. J Clin Endocrinol Metab 2003;88:6098-106.

39. Muscelli E, Natali A, Bianchi S, et al. Effect of insulin on renal sodium and uric acid handling in essential hypertension. Am J Hypertens 1996;9:746-52.

40. Nakai K, Itoh C, Kawazoe K, Miura Y, Sotoyanagi H, Hotta K, Itoh T, Kamata J, Hiramori K. Concentration of soluble vascular cell adhesion molecule-1 (VCAM-1) correlated with expression of VCAM-1 mRNA in the human atherosclerotic aorta. Coronary Art Dis 1995;6:497-502.

41. National Institutes of Health. Third Report of the National Cholesterol Education Program Expert Panel on Detection, Evaluation, and Treatment of High Blood Cholesterol in Adults (Adult Treatment Panel III). Bethesda, Md: National Institutes of Health; 2001. NIH Publication 01-3670.

42. Naruse K, King GL. Effects of diabetes on endothelial function. In Johnstone MT, Veves A (Eds): Diabetes and Cardiovascular Disease. Human Press: Totowa, New Jersey 2001;45-64.

43. Newsome CA, Shiell AW, Fall CHD, Phillips DIW, Shier R, Law CM. Is birth weight related to later glucose and insulin meta-bolism?—a systematic review. Diabetic Medicine 2003;20:339-48.

44. Neel JV. Diabetes mellitus: a thrifty genotype rendered detrimental by 'progress'. Am J Hum Genet 1962;14:353-62.

45. Phillips DIW, Barker DJP, Hales CN, Hirst S, Osmond C. Thinness at birth and insulin resistance in adult life. Diabetologia 1994; 37:150-4.

46. Reaven GM. Banting Lecture 1988: role of insulin resistance in human disease. Diabetes 1988;37:1595-1607.

47. Reaven G. The insulin resistance syndrome : past, present, and future. Presented at the First Annual World Congress on the Insulin Resistance Syndrome; November 20-22, 2003; Los Angeles, California.

48. Reaven GM, Chen YD, Jeppesen J, Maheux P, Krauss RM. Insulin resistance and hyperinsulinemia in individuals with small, dense low density lipoprotein particles. J Clin Invest 1993;92:141-6.

49. Schneider DJ, Nordt TK, Sobel BE. Attenuated fibrinolysis and accelerated atherogenesis in type 2 diabetic patients. Diabetes 1993; 42:1-7.

50. Shapiro L, Scherer PE. The crystal structure of a complement-1q family protein suggests an evolutionary link to tumour necrosis factor. Curr Biol 1998;12:335-8.

51. Shetty GK, Economides PA, Horton ES, Mantzoros CS, Veves A. Circulating adiponectin and resistin levels in relation to metabolic factors, inflammatory markers, and vascular reactivity in diabetic patients and subjects at risk for diabetes. Diabetes Care 2004; 27:2450-7.

52. Valdez R, Athens MA, Thompson GH, Bradshaw BS, Stern MP. Birthweight and adult health outcomes in a biethnic population in the USA. Diabetologia 1994;37:624-31.

53. Vogel RA. Cholesterol lowering and endothelial function. Am J Med 1999;107:479-87.

54. Weyer C, Funahashi T, Tanaka S, Hotta K, Matsuzawa Y, Pratley RE, Tataranni PA. Hypoadiponectinemia in obesity and type 2 diabetes: close association with insulin resistance and hyperinsulinemia. J Clin Endocrinol Metab 2001;86:1930-5.

55. Winzer C, Wagner O, Festa A, Schneider B, Roden M, Todesca DB, Pacini G, Funahashi T, Willer AK. Plasma adiponectin, insulin sensitivity, and subclinical inflammation in women with prior gestational diabetes mellitus. Diabetes Care 2004;27:1721-7.

56. WHO Expert Consultation. Appropriate body-mass index for Asian populations and its implications for policy and intervention strategies. Lancet 2004;363:157-63.

57. Yusuf S, Sleight P, Pogue J, Bosch J, Davies R, Dagenais G. Effects of an angiotensin-converting-enzyme inhibitor, ramipril, on cardiovascular events in high-risk patients. The Heart Outcomes Prevention Evaluation Study Investigators. N Engl J Med 2000;342:145-53.

23.2 Hormone Resistance Syndromes

AK Das

- Introduction
- Insulin Resistance

- Resistance to Thyroid Hormones
- Resistance to Androgens
- Adrenal Steroids Resistance Syndromes

INTRODUCTION

Ever since the concept of hormone resistance was introduced by Fuller Albright, information on them has grown rapidly along with the advances made in biochemistry and molecular biology. Among hormone resistance syndromes following 3 are seen commonly in medical practice:

1. Resistance to insulin
2. Resistance to thyroid hormones
3. Resistance to androgens.

Less common are adrenocortical and growth hormone resistance syndromes.

INSULIN RESISTANCE (IR)

Definition: IR is defined as the impaired ability of plasma insulin at usual concentrations to effectively promote: peripheral glucose removal, contain hepatic glucose and inhibit VLDL secretion from the liver.

By 2020, there would be an estimated 250 million diabetics, most of them type 2 diabetes (T2DM)—with insulin resistance playing major role. One in 3 or 4 US adults have insulin resistance syndrome, and 90% of diabetics are insulin resistant. The insulin resistance in Asians and Indians is extremely common.

IRS is responsible for about 60% of deaths in the diabetic population and about 6% in the non-diabetic population.

Molecular Mechanisms

Insulin Sensitivity

Insulin sensitivity is influenced by heredity. Heritability (proportion of variance in a trait attributable to additive effects of genes) of various clinical entities are as follows: insulin resistance 47 to 66%; fasting insulin 35%; 2 hour post-OGTT 13%.

Insulin-receptor Gene Mutation

Insulin receptor gene mutations (usually recessive) impair insulin receptor biosynthesis, affect post-translational modification of receptor molecule, impair insulin binding to its receptor. It also retards the activation of receptor tyrosine kinase or can cause accelerated receptor degradation.

Cellular Mechanism

Cellular mechanisms of insulin resistance studied by nuclear magnetic resonance (NMR) spectroscopy-isotopes ^{1}H,^{13}C, ^{31}P, showed that muscle glucose uptake (peripheral glucose disposal which accounts for all the nonoxidative metabolism) was 50% lower in diabetics than in insulin resistant offspring of diabetic patients. A primary glucose transport defect especially in GLUT-4 and a hexokinase II defect—were studied using NMR-spectroscopy; intracellular glucose and glucose-6-phosphate increased proportionally if it was due to a transporter defect rather than a disproportionate increase of intracellular glucose if it primarily was due to hexokinase enzyme defect. Glucose transport is rate limiting step in muscle glycogenosis by GLUT-4. Skeletal muscle takes up 70 to 80% insulin stimulated glucose *in vivo*; GLUT-4 is reduced in obesity and T2DM especially in fat but preserved in skeletal muscle. Insulin augments GLUT-4 translocation to sarcolemma in human muscle from the microsomes while in insulin resistance, more of GLUT-4 are in the microsomes than in plasma membrane.

Mutation in Insulin Receptor

Insulin receptor mutations are rare. The clinically important ones are:

1. Leprechaunism
2. Type A insulin resistance
3. Acanthosis nigricans.

However, these do not play any important role in the pathophysiology in typical T2DM or obesity. PPAR with its two isoforms and a rare naturally occurring mutation causes obesity without significant insulin resistance.

Decreased Expression of Insulin Receptor

Decreased expression of insulin receptor and tyrosine kinase activity is seen in diabetics and obese individuals which improves with weight loss. Possibly down regulation of insulin receptor expression and tyrosine kinase activity occur secondary to obesity and hyperinsulinaemia. IRS levels are reduced to 54% of those in nonobese skeletal muscle. In less obese diabetics, IRS1 is decreased in adipocytes but not in skeletal muscle. Hyperinsulinaemia may also contribute by causing internalisation of receptor and secondary insulin resistance.

Autophosphorylation

Insulin receptor autophosphorylation occurs on tyrosine residues; activated insulin receptors then phosphorylate insulin receptor substrates. Receptor autophosphorylation takes place after activation of one of the beta subunit of the receptor which occurs after insulin binding. Activation of insulin receptor phosphorylates IRS which are nine in number IRS 1,2,3,4 [which are more specific], Gab 1, Shc, p62 dok, and all of these bind only transiently and dissociate from the activated insulin receptor substrate (IRS)1, and its polymorphisms that are common in type 2 diabetics has a prevalence of 5.8 and 10.7% in normal and diabetic Caucasians respectively. Other polymorphisms in IRS2, IRS 3, IRS 4 are not associated with diabetes mellitus.

PI 3-Kinase

PI 3-kinase, a lipid kinase that relays ligand signals by protein-protein interactions without any intrinsic enzymatic activity (and hence an adaptor protein) which is responsible for binding to IRS and its inhibition abolishes insulin stimulated uptake and GLUT-4 translocation to the sarcolemma membrane. PI 3-kinase activity is reduced in both obesity and T2DM. Fatty acids also affect glucose transport by alterations in trafficking, budding, fusion and alteration in the activity of GLUT-4. Fatty acid metabolites activate phosphorylation of serine/threonine substrates—which causes decreased activation of PI kinase and decreased activation of glucose transport which contrasts the earlier theories that increased acetyl CoA from free fatty acids caused increased levels of citrate which inhibits the phosphofructokinase enzyme leading on to accumulation of intracellular glucose-6-phosphate.

Polycystic Ovary Syndrome (PCOS)

PCOS have 7 times chance of developing IR along with anovulation and androgenism described as diabetes of "bearded women" in 1921. There is a significant decrease in glucose uptake due to reduction in GLUT-4 transporters (irrespective of obesity, girth ratios, glucose intolerance and decreased PI 3-kinase in skeletal muscles.

Genetics of IRS

The role played by genes is shown in Tables 23.2.1 and 23.2.2. Counter regulatory hormones like norepinephrine, epinephrine, cortisol, glucagon and growth hormone antagonise action of insulin especially immediately after hypoglycaemic states. TNFα which is secreted by adipose cells along with macrophages have a positive correlation with BMI, decreasing with weight reduction. They increase serine phosphorylation of IRS 1 which inhibits insulin receptor kinase activity.

Leptin expressed in the hypothalamic arcuate nuclei regulates feeding behaviour and reduces food intake while increasing energy expenditure and leptin level correlates with fasting insulin levels and hence is a marker of insulin resistance syndrome.

Role of Resistin

Diet induced hepatic insulin resistance was shown to be due to resistin levels which are secreted by adipocytes. Rat models show that insulin resistance with increasing resistin levels was reversed by antisense oligonucleotide to resistin.

TNFα

TNFα is over-expressed in obese and insulin resistant states. Many macrophage specific genes were up-regulated in obese mice associated with increase in macrophage numbers and TNFα is a potent activator of macrophages and the obesity induced macropage accumulation correlates with insulin resistance; macrophage accumulation is direct response to abnormal fat metabolism (restricted to white adipose tissue) in these mice. Thiazolidenediones can attenuate macrophage activation *in vitro* mediated by PPAR γ in macrophages; the molecular signals which can activate macrophage accretion in these adipocytes include decreased adiponectin (which decreases adhesion of macrophages to endothelial cells) and increased leptin (promotes cholesteryl ester synthesis), and C3a (chemotaxin of macrophages). Inflammation in macrophages produce TNFα, IL1, IL6 and that causes insulin resistance in adipocytes thereby increasing lipolysis and rising levels of free fatty acids (FFA) which cause insulin resistance.

Peripheral Glucose Uptake

Seventy per cent of peripheral glucose uptake is by skeletal muscle; fat tissue with 95% of triglyceride mass does hardly any work in the way of glucose disposal.

TABLE 23.2.1

Insulin receptor pathway defects	Fat cell defects-lipid homeostasis pathway	Hypothalamic level defects, Leptin-POMC-MC$_4$R pathway	Miscellaneous
Mutation in the insulin receptor. Type A syndrome	Congenital generalised lipodystrophy (mutations in 11q13, BSCL2, AGPAT2 gene on 9q34)	POMC mutations	Proteases-CALP10
		MC4R mutations	Impaired processing of pro-hormones, prohormone convertase deficiency (PC1)
		MC3R mutations	Oestrogen receptor mutations
Leprechaunism	Dunnigan's syndrome (lamin mutations)	Leptin mutations	
Rabson-Mendenhall syndrome	Kobberling's syndrome (mutation in the PPAR-γ gene)	Leptin receptor gene mutation, ghrelin polymorphisms, neuropeptide Y5 receptor polymorphisms, cocaine- and amphet-amine-regulated transcript polymorphisms, cholecystokinin A receptor polymorphisms	
Polymorphism in plasma cell membrane glycoprotein -1 (PC-1)	Allelic variation in PPAR-γ influence body fat mass by effects on adipocyte; polymor-phisms of PPARα gene can lead to higher triglyceride and insulin levels; polymorphism of the lipo-protein lipase gene was both linked and associated with insulin resistance; polymorphism of UCP1, UCP2, UCP3 genes; polymorphism of β2- and β3-adrenergic receptors	Single-gene defects leading to disruption of hypothalamic pathways of energy regulation	
		Prader-Willi syndrome (15q11.2-q12, uniparental maternal disomy), Alström syndrome (ALMS1 gene mutants in the hypothalamus might lead to hyperphagia followed by obesity and insulin resistance), Bardet-Biedl syndrome, Cohen syndrome, Beckwick-Weidemann syndrome, Biemond syndrome II, choroideremia with deafness	

Genetics in insulin resistance syndrome

TABLE 23.2.2

Acquired IR pathway defects	Acquired fat cell defects	Acquired miscellaneous
Type B immune-mediated insulin resistance	Lipodystrophy associated with HIV protease inhibitors; acquired generalised lipodystrophy-Lawrence syndrome is caused by antibodies against adipocyte-membrane antigens	Excess counterregulatory hormones; glucocorticoids, catecholamines, PTH, GH, placental lactogen in case of stress, infection, pregnancy, starvation, uraemia, cirrhosis, ketoacidosis, ageing, inactivity
	Barraquer-Simons' syndrome (partial acquired cephalothoracic lipodystrophy) have accelerated complement activation and a serum IgG, called C3 nephritic factor, that is thought to cause lysis of adipose tissue expressing adipsin	

Acquired mechanisms—insulin counterregulatory hormones

Obesity, impaired insulin secretion and action along with increased endogenous glucose output are the major metabolic aberrations in diabetes mellitus; prospective studies show that obesity and insulin resistance predict the development of diabetes in many populations, there was a progressive worsening of insulin action with decreased glucose uptake (non-oxidative disposal). Insulin secretion was also reduced at an early stage of development of diabetes; endogenous glucose output which was found to be a comparatively late event was in part due to declining sensitivity of liver to insulin.

Mechanism of Insulin Resistance in the Elderly

Mechanism of insulin resistance in the elderly are not entirely clear. Because of the inability to attain glucose disposal rates comparable to the non-elderly with highest achievable insulin effect (with adequate monocyte and adipocyte receptors), a post-receptor defect is being hypothesised; decreased daily dietary chromium intake in elderly subjects with low normal chromium stores (which is associated with insulin resistance) can also be considered as possible mechanisms along with decreasing physical robustness and decreasing aerobic activity.

HYPERTENSION

Only 50 per cent of hypertensives are insulin resistant. Putative mechanisms include failure of vasodilation (that can occur due to insulin which stimulates the secretion of nitric oxide), volume overload that is caused by sodium and water retention (due to hyperinsulinaemia) causing volume dependent hypertension and chronic overactivity of the sympathetic nervous system.

Insulin resistance, hyperinsulinemia can cause a precoagulable state due to increased levels of fibrinogen, factor VII and plasminogen activator inhibitor 1 which are all independent risk factors for coronary artery disease.

Insulin resistance causes hydrolysis of triglycerides in adipose cells, increased release of free fatty acids along with decreased uptake of free fatty acids which flood the liver and leads to increase in secretion of VLDL by the liver. In plasma, VLDL transfers triglycerides to both HDL and LDL while in turn, cholesteryl esters are transferred to VLDL. Thus, VLDL is able to deliver more cholesterol per particle to reach the vessel wall and also increases post-prandial hyperglycaemia.

Hyperinsulinism and insulin resistance-mediated organ-specific symptoms and pathologies are enumerated in Table 23.2.3A.

TABLE 23.2.3A

Skin Hyperkeratotic AN, skin tags Striae Hirsutism Frontal alopecia	*Gastrointestinal* Hepatic steatosis, NASH, pancreatitis, cholecystitis, colon cancer
Adipose tissue Obesity, increased intra-abdominal fat Fat infiltrations of muscle, liver, pancreas	*Gonads* Virilisation or hirsutism, menstrual irregularity, persistent acne, scalp hair loss, hyperhidrosis, infertility or precocious pubarche in childhood
Cardiovascular Increased arterial wall thickness Endothelial dysfunction Early atherosclerosis CHD, stroke Hypertension	*Adrenal* Premature adrenarche, increased cortisol production and excretion, increased adrenal androgens and DHEA, normal catecholamines
Kidney Focal segmental glomerulosclerosis	*GH axis* Pseudoacromegaly, accelerated linear growth and bone age, decreased GH secretion, low IGFBP-1
Immune system Impaired cellular mediated immunity Asthma, eczema, Increased cancer risk, e.g. breast	*Inflammation* Increased levels of CRP, raised erythrocyte sedimentation rates and increased TNFα levels, increased autoimmune thyroiditis
Psychological Depression, poor self-esteem, ? cognitive defects	*Neurological* Stroke Pseudotumour cerebri
Respiratory Obesity hypoventilation syndrome Sleep apnoea, ventilation/perfusion mismatches	*Musculoskeletal* Coxa vara, slipped capital epiphysis, degenerative arthritis, Blount's disease, gout, muscle cramps

Organ specific symptoms in IRS

Clinical Features

Fasting levels of insulin >15 μU/ml or post OGTT > 150 μU/ml suggest hyperinsulinaemia. Table 23.2.3B gives the main clinical manifestation of insulin resistance syndrome as seen in adult and paediatric clinical practices.

Treatment

It should be started early and aggressively especially in childhood before decompensation occurs. Treatment includes multiple components among which behaviour

TABLE 23.2.3B

Adult IRS	Paediatric IRS
Striae white	Positive family history of DM
Centrally biased obesity	obesity, hypertension,CHD/stroke
Hirsutism, ovarian hyperan- drogenism and infertility	H/O gestational DM
Dyslipidaemia ($\uparrow$ TG, $\downarrow$ HDL)	SGA (mostly) or LGA (less often)
Premature atherosclerosis	Asthma or allergic rhinitis
Hypertension	Premature pubarche
Hyperuricaemia/gout	Red (new) and white (old) striae,
Allergies/asthma	from adrenarche onward
Fatty liver (NASH)	Decreasing resting expenditure
Chronic pancreatitis	Low resting fat to carbohydrate
Focal glomerulosclerosis	oxidation rates
Glucose intolerance	Acanthosis nigricans
Type 2 diabetes	Tall stature/pseudoacromegaly
Increased cancer risk	Hirsutism/PCOS with adolescence
Increased Alzheimer's disease	Adipomastia/gynecomastia
	Acute pancreatitis
	Premature atherosclerosis
	Hypertension/glomerulonephritis
	Type 2 DM

Main clinical manifestations of IRS as seen in adult and paediatric population

modification(family-based in case of paediatric patients) especially in regard to a definite exercise programme which increases peripheral glucose utilisation by the skeletal muscle, increases HDL levels and decreases insulin resistance.

Metformin is the drug of choice with its gastro-intestinal side effects also playing a small part, for it increases insulin sensitivity by insulin receptor binding even in mutant receptors, downregulates TNFα and is useful in pregnant women too. PPAR γ agonists such as thiazolidendiones are not useful in reducing weight, nevertheless very useful in insulin resistance syndrome since it decreases adipose tissue inflammation by diminishing cytokines release along with fatty acid release and thus improves insulin sensitivity. Fibrates and statins are indicated along with dietary restriction of carbohydrate when risk of pancreatitis and acute coronary events are high. Aspirin in low doses can be started when patients turn thirty. Surgery can be used to reduce carbohydrate intake, reduce weight or treat complications such as sleep apnoea.

THYROID HORMONE RESISTANCE

Recognition of target organ resistance to thyroid hormone was first studied in 1967. Resistance to thyroid hormones may be of two types—related to TSH or related to T_3/T_4.

TSH receptor related mutations form the first while mutations in the thyroid hormone receptor beta form the other group (Fig. 23.2.1).

TSH Resistance

TSH resistance is again classified as being either partial or complete; the former presents with euthyroidism, high levels of TSH, normal FT_3/FT_4 while the latter has hypothyroidism, high levels of TSH and normal levels of FT_3 and FT_4.

T_3/T_4 RESISTANCE

Resistance to thyroid hormone (RTH) is due to a thyroid hormone receptor (beta isoform) mutation that leads to interference of wild type by the mutant thyroid receptor decreasing sensitivity to T_3 mediated inhibition of TSH production. This is also called dominant negative inhibition of the mutant receptor because it interferes with the activation of positive response elements and repression of negative response elements of the normal receptor in a heterozygous state.

Types of Thyroid Hormone Resistance

RTH is of two types (Fig. 23.2.1): Generalized RTH, where the response of T_3 to both periphery and pituitary is inhibited; pituitary RTH, in which there is normal response of peripheral tissues but the pituitary is unable to sense and suppress high T_3 levels and hence there is T_3 toxicity and are linked to mutations in the beta isoform of the thyroid receptor. Generalised RTH present with symptoms of hypothyroidism while the pituitary present with thyrotoxicity; mutations in the β locus cause them to express mutant thyroid receptors which when expressed, interfere with the inactivating positive

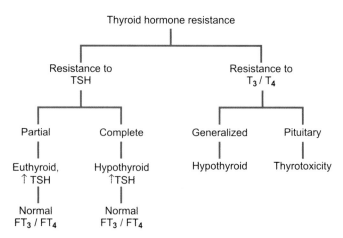

Fig. 23.2.1: Two types of thyroid hormone resistance

response elements or repressing negative response elements, also called the dominant negative activity of the mutant receptor. RTH without the classical defect (mutant receptor) in the beta isoform has been postulated to be due to a cofactor defect, the clinical features being similar.

The prevalence of RTH is 1 in 50000 live births and the inheritance is autosomal dominant. Hearing impairment is common along with attention deficit, hyperactivity disorder and low IQ- severe sensorineural deafness is a typical trait of homozygous deletion of the TR β gene.

Treatment

They need to be distinguished from Graves' disease so as not to inappropriately treat them and reduce T_3/T_4 levels. There is no effective treatment—hormone replacements are indicated for ablated glands due to mis-diagnosis that has lead to poor thyroid reserve. Beta-blockers such as atenolol are useful for treating symptoms such as tremors and tachycardia (especially in peripheral RTH) when used in conjunction with anxiolytics. Neonatal TSH screening programmes in the west have enabled to treat infants much earlier when they present with seizures, failure to thrive and raised levels of TSH in the presence of a family history.

ANDROGEN RESISTANCE

Androgen resistance is a X-linked disorder and are mostly due to mutations in the ligand binding domains (60%), DNA binding domains (20%) of the androgen receptor and due to interruptions in the reading frame of the androgen receptor gene, especially in the critical DNA binding domain that is localized to the COOH terminal. Clinical spectrum includes abnormalities ranging from complete testicular feminization syndrome, incomplete testicular feminization syndrome, Reifenstein syndrome, infertile male to undervirilised fertile males. The continuum of clinical syndromes are due to various levels of responsiveness of the androgen receptor to androgens and involves both nuclear receptors and cell signalling systems. Role of coregulators in human resistance syndromes has been observed in mouse models. Mutations are partly common due to the fact that abnormalities are noted at birth and are likely to be evaluated early.

CORTISOL RESISTANCE

Cortisol resistance is a rare syndrome due to defective glucocorticoid receptor, with a spectrum of presentations ranging from being asymptomatic to being hypertensive

TABLE 23.2.4

Hormone specific manifestations	Hormone studies
(a) *Glucocorticoid* Asymptomatic, hypertension, hypokalaemic alkalosis, chronic fatigue; a women: hyperandrogenism, children: virilization	Hypercortisolism, DOC↑, adrenal androgens↑, diurnal rhythm+ response to metyrapone + Response to ACTH, CRH: cortisol↑, adrenal androgens↑; dexamethasone resistance
(b) *Mineralocorticoid* Hypotension, salt loss, hyperkalaemic acidosis (hypoaldosteronism)	Aldosterone, PRA↑ Fludrocortisone resistance
(c) *Androgens* Males: hypomasculinization, females: masculinization	LH, FSH, Te↑
(d) *Oestrogens* Tall stature, osteoporosis delayed bone age	LH, FSH↑
(e) *Progesterone* Infertility	Normal LH, FSH, E2, P4 abnormal endometrial maturation

Steroid hormones resistance syndromes

with hypokalaemic alkalosis in its severest form with occasional adrenal insufficiency. Most patients have raised cortisol in serum and corresponding excretion in urine without features of Cushing's syndrome. Though dexamethasone resistance was observed, some subjects responded to low dose dexamethasone suppression (Table 23.2.4).

GROWTH HORMONE RESISTANCE

Growth hormone resistance is autosomal recessive as studied in offspring of consanguineous marriages. GH resistance can be of two types: primary GH resistance or insensitivity (otherwise called the classical Laron syndrome) and secondary GH resistance or insensitivity due to acquired disorders. Primary GH resistance can be due to receptor or post-receptor defects or due to defects in synthesis of IGF-1 (Tables 23.2.5 and 23.2.6). Most receptor defects are due to mutations in the extracellular domain with some reports of transmembrane and intracytoplasmic domain mutations. Overnight fasting levels of GH are high and they respond normally to both hypoglycaemia and glucose infusion.

TABLE 23.2.5

1. Primary GH resistance (insensitivity) syndrome = classical Laron syndrome (hereditary conditions)
   a. GH receptor defects (quantitative and qualitative)
   b. Abnormalities of hGH signal transduction (postreceptor defects)
   c. Primary defects of synthesis and action of IGF-I
2. Secondary GH resistance (insensitivity) diseases (acquired conditions; sometimes transitory)
   a. Circulating antibodies to hGH that inhibit GH action (hGH gene deletion patients treated with hGH)
   b. Antibodies to the hGH receptor
   c. hGH insensitivity caused by malnutrition
   d. hGH insensitivity caused by liver disease
   e. GH insensitivity caused by uncontrolled diabetes mellitus
   f. Other conditions

Classification of hGH resistance (Insensitivity)

TABLE 23.2.6

- Dwarfism (height = <4-10 SD score)
- Marked obesity
- Delayed puberty
- Late closure of bony epiphyses
- Thin bones
- Small gonads but full sexual development and reproductive potential
- Thin skin; early wrinkling
- High-pitched voice
- Reduced lean body mass
- Reduced muscular strength
- Reduced bone density (osteopenia)
- Variable psychological performance (from normal to marked retardation)

Signs and symptoms of primary IGF-I deprivation during puberty and adulthood

SUMMARY

Insulin resistance appears to be the commonest among hormone resistance syndromes and has wide ramifications affecting various body systems and organs. Other common hormone resistance conditions are where resistance is due to thyroid hormones, androgens, growth hormone and adrenocortical steroids. A brief account is given mentioning their clinical significance.

FURTHER READING

1. Beck-Peccoz P, Persani L. Syndromes of hormone resistance in thyroid field. Revue de l'ACOMEN, 1999;5:298-9.
2. Chrousos GP. A new 'New' syndrome in the new world. Is multiple post receptor steroid hormone resistance due to a coregulator defect? J Clin Endocrinol Metab1999;84:12.
3. Chrousos GP, Vingerhoeds A, Brandon D, Eil C, Pugeat M, deVroede M, Loriaux DL, Mortimer B. Primary cortisol resistance in man—a glucocorticoid receptor mediated disease. J Clin Invest 1982;69:1261-9.
4. Ferrannini E, Natali A, Bell P, Cavallo-perin P, Lalic N. Mingrone G on behalf of the European group for the study of insulin resistance. J Clin Invest1997;100:166-73.
5. Fink RI, Kolterman OG, Griffin J, Olefsky JM. Mechanisms of insulin resistance in aging. J Clin Invest 1983;71:1523-5.
6. Ginsberg HN. Insulin resistance and cardiovascular disease. J Clin Invest 2000;106:453-8.
7. Hughes IA. Minireview: sex differentiation. Endocrinology 2001;142:3281-7.
8. Hu H, Barnes GT, Yang Q, Tan G, Yang D, Chou CJ, Sole J, Nichols A, Ross JS, Tartaglia LA, Chen H. Chronic inflammation in fat plays a crucial role in the development of obesity related insulin resistance. J Clin Invest 2003;112:1821-30.
9. Jameson JL. Editorial: Thyroid hormone resistance: pathophysiology at the molecular level. J Clin Endocrinol Metab 1992;74:708-11.
10. Lamberts SWJ, Koper JW, Beimond P, den Holder FH, de Jong FH. Cortisol receptor resistance : the variability of its clinical presentation and response to treatment. J Clin Endocrinol Metab 1992;74:313-21.
11. Laron Z. Extensive personal experience. Laron syndrome (Primary growth hormone resistance or insensitivity): the personal experience 1958-2003. J Clin Endocrinol Metab 2004;89:1031-44.
12. McPhaul MJ. Molecular defects of the androgen receptor. Recent Prog Horm Res 2002;57:181-94.
13. Muse ED, Obici S, Bhanot S, Monia BP, Mckay RA, Rajala MW, Scherer PE, Rosetti L. Role of resistin in diet induced hepatic insulin resistance. J Clin Invest 2004;114:232-9.
14. Nagaya T, Eberhardt NL, Jameson JL. Thyroid hormone resistance: correlation of dominant negativity and location of mutations. J Clin Endocrinol Metab 1993;77:1982-90.
15. Pohlenz J, Weiss RE, Macchia PE, Pannain S, Lau IT, Ho H, Refetoff S. Five new families with resistance to thyroid hormone not caused by mutations in the thyroid hormone receptor beta gene J Clin Endocrinol Metab 1999;84:3919-28.
16. Sakurai A, Takeda K, Ain K, Ceccarelli P, Nakai A, Seino S, Bell GI, Refetoff S, Degroot LJ. Generalised resistance to thyroid hormone associated with a mutation in the ligand binding domain of the human thyroid hormone receptor β. Proc Natl Acad Sci USA, 1989; 86: 8977-81.
17. Schulman GI. Cellular mechanisms of insulin resistance. J Clin Invest 2000;106:171-6.
18. Stern MP. Strategies and prospects for finding insulin resistance genes. J Clin Invest 2000;106:323-7.
19. Ten S, Maclaren N. Insulin resistance syndrome in children. J Clin Endocrinol Metab 2004;89:2525-39.
20. Venkatesan AM, Dunaif A, Corbould A. Insulin resistance in polycystic ovary disease : progresses and paradoxes. Recent Prog Horm Res 2001;56:295-308.
21. Virkamaki A, Ueki K, Kahn CR Protein-protein interaction signaling and the molecular mechanism of insulin resistance. J Clin Invest 1999;103: 931-43.
22. Wan W, Farboud B, Privalsky ML. Pituitary resistance to thyroid hormone (RTH) syndrome is associated with T3 receptor mutants that selectively impair β2 isoform function. Mol Endocrinol 2005;1-39.
23. Weiss RE, Refetoff S (Editorial). Treatment of resistance to thyroid hormone-primum non nocere. J Clin Endocrinol Metabol 84:401-4.
24. Weyer C, Bogardus C, Mott DM, Prattley RE. The natural history of insulin secretory dysfunction and insulin resistance in the pathogenesis of type 2 diabetes mellitus. J Clin Invest 1999;104:787-94.

23.3 Immunologic Syndromes Affecting Multiple Endocrine Organs

Narendra Kotwal

INTRODUCTION

When immune dysfunction affects two or more endocrine glands and other nonendocrine immune disorders are present, the polyglandular autoimmune (PGA) syndromes should be considered. The PGA syndromes are classified as two main types:

Type I syndrome starts in childhood and is characterized by mucocutaneous candidiasis, hypothyroidism, and adrenal insufficiency.

Type II, or *Schmidt syndrome*, comprises of adrenal insufficiency, thyroiditis, and type I diabetes mellitus. However, the type II syndrome is heterogenous and may consist of autoimmune thyroid disease along with a variety of other autoimmune endocrine disorders.

AUTOIMMUNE POLYGLANDULAR SYNDROME TYPE I

The spectrum of its manifestations is broad. The most frequent disease components—chronic mucocutaneous candidiasis (MC), hypoparathyroidism (HP), and adrenocortical insufficiency (AI)—frequently appear in childhood and often in the order listed; however, none of them is constant. Many other disease components occur, and keratoconjunctivitis, hepatitis, flashing erythema with fever, or even diarrhoea may dominate the early clinical picture. The disease may become clinically recognizable only in adulthood. The prevalence of most disease components increases with age; hence, only age-specific prevalence figures have full meaning.

Immune Defect

Oral candidiasis usually is the first manifestation. It is chronic in most cases but, in some, it is recurrent, being evident only during impaired general condition (e.g. febrile illness). Its peak incidence is during first two years of life, but susceptibility is variable, and the disease may appear only in adulthood. In the mild cases, there is intermittent angular cheilosis. Severe forms include acute inflammation of the oral mucosa, hyperplastic chronic MC with thick white coating of the tongue, and atrophic disease with scant coatings and a scarred thin mucosa with leucoplakia-like areas. This chronic condition is carcinogenic. Candidal oesophagitis is also common and may appear in the absence of oral candidiasis. It causes substernal pain and odynophagia and may lead to stricture with dysphagia. Perianal candidal eczema is common. Intestinal mucosal candidiasis may cause abdominal pain, meteorism and diarrhoea. The infection may spread to the skin of the hands, face and the nails. Many post-pubertal female patients often suffer from candidal vulvovaginitis.

Humoral immunity against *Candida* develops normally. Generalised candidiasis has only been reported in a patient on immunosuppressive medication. Serious lung disease may occur. Splenic atrophy may add a secondary immunodeficiency, especially susceptibility to pneumococcal sepsis. Splenic atrophy may be common. It appears to be due to a progressive autoimmune-mediated destruction or vascular insult.

Endocrinopathies

Hyperparathyroidism (HP)

The peak incidence of HP is at the age of 2 to 11 years. Early in its development, only the reserve secretory capacity of parathyroid glands may be lost, and hypocalcaemia occurs only during periods of hypo-calcaemic stress (e.g. fasting, exceptionally low Ca intake or high phosphate intake, therapy with loop diuretics). Several patients suffer for years, before a clear manifestation, from vague tetany, which in some patents appears as clumsiness. In addition to frank tetany, grandmal seizures may occur. Hypomagnesemia is common and may complicate the condition with painful muscular cramps.

Adrenocortical disorders: The peak incidence of AI is at 4 to 12 years. Deficiency of cortisol and aldosterone may appear several years apart. In one patient, clear salt craving and hyponatraemia subsided with in a year, with no further adrenal problem over the next 26 years, despite persistent autoantibodies against three adrenocortical enzymes.

Hypogonadism (HG): It manifests as primary gonadal failure. Half the affected female patients have primary amenorrhoea, many of them with spontaneous partial pubertal development.

Diabetes mellitus (DM): It affects 18% of the series, 4.5- to 9-fold more than in other large series. This parallels the prevalence of type I DM in the general population. Antibodies to glutamic acid decarboxylase (GADab) are present in high titres in many nondiabetic patients. Both fasting plasma C-peptide concentration and the first phase insulin response to intravenous glucose were lower in nondiabetic patients for the GADab-positive than the GADab-negative group, which suggests subclinical insulitis in the GADab-positive patients, although some of them appear never to develop clinical DM.

Thyroid disease: Hypothyroidism is relatively uncommon and hyperthyroidism is rare. Hashimoto's thyroiditis may occur at a frequency equal to hypothyroidism.

Gastrointestinal Disorder

Pernicious anaemia (autoimmune gastritis) is the most common gastrointestinal problem with the peak incidence at the age of 10 to 20 years. Intestinal dysfunction such as periodic or chronic diarrhoea, usually with steatorrhoea, and severe obstipation, often alternating with diarrhoea, are common. In most cases, the diarrhoea is secondary to HP and results from hypocalcaemia, as it does sometimes in HP of other aetiologies. Most patients, however, never have diarrhoea, despite equally severe hypocalcaemia; some patients develop HP only years after diarrhoea, or not at all.

The diarrhoea may become very severe through a vicious cycle with hypocalcaemia; diarrhoea impairs absorption of calcium and the calciferol drugs, worsening the diarhoea and making the hypocalcemia difficult to control by oral medication. Hypocalcaemia impairs the secretion of cholecystokinin by the duodenal mucosa in response to a meal, leading to failure of the physiologic stimulus for normal gallbladder contraction and pancreatic enzyme secretion. Autoimmune hepatitis may, on occasion, be the first manifestation. Although autoimmune hepatitis is chronic and almost asymptomatic in most cases, it may lead to cirrhosis, or be fulminant and lethal.

Ocular Diseases

Keratoconjunctivitis is independent of HP; several patients develop HP years after keratoconjunctivitis.

Skin Diseases

Alopecia is the first or part of the initial manifestation in 4% of the patients. Appearing as patchy loss of hair, it may become universal. Vitiligo is of variable extent. In a few patients, initial spots fade, but in most cases they grow larger.

Ectodermal Dystrophies

The pathomechanism of ectodermal dystrophies is unknown. The most frequent abnormality is enamel hypoplasia of permanent teeth, which affects three-fourths of the patients. Pitted nail dystrophy is present in half of the patients. Calcium salt deposits exist in the tympanic membrane in a third of the patients, with no history of middle ear disease. They are obvious on standard otoscopic examination.

Variation in the Clinical Picture and its Determinants

The clinical picture varies widely in many aspects. In one of the series, total number of components in individual patients was 2 to 10 and the number of endocrine components was 1 to 5. Some patients lead a normal life taking a few tablets daily, whereas others suffer from visible or incapacitating components. The patient's fear of developing new components may remain stressful.

The triad of MC, HP, and AI was present in 50% of the patients at the age of 20 years, 55% at age 30, and 40% at age 40. Some of the rare components may dominate the picture with none of the triad present.

Patients with AI as the first component other than MC developed fewer components than the others. Iranian Jewish patients appear different from other patients in having no keratopathy and lower prevalence of MC and AI (four and five of 24 patients, respectively). Italian patients differ from Finnish patients by having less keratoconjunctivitis (12% vs 21%) and DM (2% vs 1%). There is evidence for dependence of the clinical picture on the type of AIRE (autoimmune regulator) mutation only with regard to the prevalence of MC and, perhaps AI. Class II major histocompatibility complex appear to be involved, in that HLA-DRB1* 3 is positively associated with AI, and HLA-DRB1 15-DQB1 *1602 is negatively associated with type I DM. These two associations are clear in other kinds of autoimmune AI and DM.

AUTOIMMUNE POLYGLANDULAR SYNDROME II (APS II)

APS II is defined by the coexistence of autoimmune adrenocortical insufficiency (AAI), or serologic evidence of adrenalitis with either autoimmune thyroid disease (AITD), or type I diabetes mellitus (TIDM). Adrenal failure or autoantibodies plus autoimmune thyroiditis is termed Schmidt syndrome. Adrenal failure or auto-antibodies plus AITD and TIDM constitute Carpenter syndrome. AITD encompasses a spectrum of thyroid disorders, including atrophic thyroiditis, euthyroid thyroid-auto-antibody-positive goitre, and Graves' disease. The presence of AITD without adrenal disease but associated with either TIDM, pernicious anaemia, vitiligo, or alopecia has been referred to as APS III. Alternatively, and most commonly investigators refer to this latter associations by name exclusive to the APS nomenclature. For example, instead of APS III, coexistent AITD and autoimmune pernicious anaemia are termed thyrogastric autoimmunity.

Clinical Aspects (Table 23.3.1)

APS II

Unlike APS I, APS II usually has its onset in adulthood, particularly in the third or fourth decade, although it may occur at any age. APS II is atleast three times more common in females than males. In approximately 50% of APS II cases, adrenocortical failure is the initial endocrine abnormality. Several of the disease components may be present at diagnosis, and thus the clinician should be alerted to the possibility of a second major endocrine disorder once one component of the syndrome is diagnosed. When a patient presents with Addison's disease, TIDM and AITD are found to coexist, in about one-fifth and two-thirds of the time respectively. Therefore, the diagnosis of both TIDM and AITD should be vigorously sought when Addison's disease is first

TABLE 23.3.1

Clinical profile	APS I	APS II
Comparative frequency	Less common	More common
Onset	Infancy/early childhood	Late childhood, adulthood
Heredity	Autosomal recessive	Polygenic
Gender	Males = females	Female predominance
Genetics	AIRE gene; no HLA association	HLA associate: DR/DQ
Hypoparathyroidism	77 to 89%	None
Mucocutaneous candidiasis	73 to 100%	None
Ectodermal dysplasia	77%	None
Addison's disease	60 to 86%	70 to 100%
Type I diabetes	4 to 18%	41 to 52%
Autoimmune thyroid disease	8 to 10%	70%
Pernicious anaemia	12 to 15%	2 to 25%
Gonadal failure		
• Females	30 to 60%	3.5 to 10%
• Males	7 to 17%	5%
Vitiligo	4 to 13%	4 to 5%
Alopecia	27%	2%
Autoimmune hepatitis	10 to 15%	Rare
Malabsorption	10 to 18%	Rare

Clinical profile: APS I and APS II

diagnosed. Coexistent AITD is more common in females. AITD occurs in 80 to 90% of females with APS II. AITD is the single most common component of APS II that occurs as an isolated condition.

Ovarian failure, seen as either primary or secondary amenorrhoea, is present in approximately 10% of women with APS II under 40 years of age. Among females with biopsy-proven lymphocytic oophoritis, adrenocortical failure or subclinical AAI is often present. Progression to gonadal failure is very rare among males with Addison's disease, even in the presence of high-risk steroidal cell autoantibodies. Pituitary involvement is occasionally seen in APS II. Hypophysitis and empty sella syndrome have been described leading to isolated failure of secretion of GH, ACTH, TSH, FSH, or LH. Several nonendocrinological conditions have been reported in association with APS II. These include ulcerative colitis, primary biliary cirrhosis, sarcoidosis, achalasia, myositis, and neuropathy.

AITD (Autoimmune Thyroid Disease) without Addison's

In isolation, AITD has an increased incidence during the teen years, with a peak appearing in the fifth and sixth decades. Hashimoto's disease (chronic lymphocytic thyroiditis) is the most common form of AITD, although Graves' disease and postpartum thyroiditis are not uncommon. Pancreatic islet autoimmunity or overt TIDM coexists in 3 to 8% of cases. About 1% of patients with isolated AITD display serological evidence of adrenal autoimmunity. Polyglandular involvement is thus infrequent in patients with AITD.

AITD, or a family history of AITD, however, is common in patients with pernicious anaemia, vitiligo, alopecia, myasthenia gravis, and Sjogren syndrome, and the diagnosis of AITD should be sought in all such patients. Although a higher percentage of patients with APS I and APS II have vitiligo, most patients with vitiligo and another autoimmune disease have APS II, since APS I is far less common than APS II.

Type I Diabetes (TIDM) without Addison's Disease

A gender discrepancy is not present in patients with isolated TIDM; however, a female dominance occurs in APS II patients. This difference is almost certainly related to the coexistence of AITD. AITD (often asymptomatic), detected by the presence of circulating thyroid microsomal (thyroid peroxidase) or thyroglobin autoantibodies, is present in about 20% of the patients with

TIDM, with females significantly outnumbering males. Likewise, a female disproportion is found in patients with TIDM and gastric parietal cell autoimmunity, again reflecting the likely coexistence of AITD.

Gastric parietal cell autoantibodies (PCA) occur in approximately 10% of females and 5% of males with TIDM. Progression to overt pernicious anaemia rarely occurs in young patients. The disease typically affects women usually after the fifth decade. Atrophic gastritis may lead to megaloblastic anaemia due to the absence of intrinsic factor, and thus an inability to absorb vitamin B_{12}. Iron deficiency anaemia has also been reported in adolescents and adults. It results from decreased acid production (e.g. hypochlorhydria or achlorhydria), which leads to poor iron absorption. AAI (autoimmune adrenal insufficiency) is much less frequent among patients with TIDM, with serological evidence reported in 0.4 to 2.7% of cases. Coeliac disease occurs in 2 to 3% of the patients with TIDM and should be suspected in patients with unexplained diarrhoea, weight loss, a failure to gain weight, or failure to thrive. Transglutaminase or endomysial autoantibodies are used to screen for coeliac disease.

Screening Recommendations

A high index of suspicion for additional autoimmune disorders in patients who have autoimmune polyendocrine syndrome type I or autoimmune polyendocrine syndrome type II, and their relatives, is essential. Patients should be advised of the symptoms of the disorders for which they are at high risk: hypoglycaemia (especially when they are receiving insulin therapy), fatigue, and hyperpigmentation (in some cases) for Addison's disease; polyuria, polyphagia, polydipsia, and nausea and vomiting with ketoacidosis for diabetes; coordination difficulties for pernicious anaemia; and anaemia, osteopenia, abdominal pain, and diarrhoea for coeliac disease.

The constellation of disorders of autoimmune polyendocrine syndrome type I relates to immunodeficiency and chronic candidiasis as well as the frequent development of additional autoimmune disorders. It is important for follow-up to include aggressive treatment of candidiasis if needed, antibiotic prophylaxis if asplenism develops (e.g. if asplenism is detected by screening for Howell-Jolly bodies), tests for early detection of hepatitis (e.g. by screening for elevated serum levels of liver enzymes), and assessment for additional endocrine disorders with autoantibody and hormone testing.

Patients with autoimmune polyendocrine syndrome type II and their first-degree relatives (and patients with "isolated" type 1A diabetes and Addison's disease) should be periodically monitored for the development of hypothyroidism. The presence of autoantibodies against thyroid peroxidase usually precedes overt hypothyroidism. Given the high prevalence of thyroid disease due to autoimmunity thyrotrophin with a sensitive assay should be able to detect both hypothyroidism and hyperthyroidism. We also recommend screening for autoantibodies against 21-hydroxylase and transglutaminase. Currently, there is not enough information to define optimal intervals for testing, but anecdotal data indicate that autoantibodies can develop at any age, and therefore it is recommended to screen patients for autoantibodies even if their initial autoantibody tests are negative. Annual measurement of the corticotrophin level and the level of cortisol both before and after cosyntropin stimulation (at 8 AM) in those with autoantibodies against 21-hydroxylase seems prudent to detect adrenal damage before a hypotensive crisis

The majority of persons identified in programmes screening for autoantibodies associated with coeliac disease, even those who have high levels of transglutaminase autoantibodies, are "asymptomatic." Recent studies suggest that many of them may be at risk for osteoporosis and may have detectable changes in growth and nutrition, as well as anaemia. Intestinal T-cell lymphomas develop in a subgroup of patients with symptomatic coeliac disease. The level of transglutaminase autoantibodies often fluctuates in asymptomatic patients, and it is advisable to obtain a small-bowel biopsy specimen when the levels are high. Islet autoantibody determination in first-degree relatives of patients with autoimmune polyendocrine syndrome type II is best reserved for research settings, although appropriate rapid diagnosis and therapy for new-onset diabetes are important, especially in young children.

Therapy

At present, the treatment of the polyendocrine autoimmune syndromes is dictated by the individual disorders. Knowledge of the syndromes allows early therapy of component disorders. An important clinical caveat is that in patients with suspected concomitant Addison's disease and hypothyroidism, thyroid replacement should not precede the necessary glucocorticoid replacement, since thyroid replacement may precipitate the hypotension and adrenal crisis due to the action of thyroxine in increasing hepatic corticosteroid metabolism. Long-term goals are therapies that address the underlying autoimmunity associated with these disorders and, in particular, preventive therapies. Although prediction of type 1A diabetes is now possible, the preventive therapies studied to date have not altered disease progression. For coeliac disease, removal of gliadin from the diet is an effective treatment. Autoimmunity can be an important barrier to transplantation however with the current immunosuppressive regimens, allogenic pancreatic transplantation is possible and the results of islet transplantation have improved dramatically. Currently, for the clinician and family, recognition of the syndromes and early detection of the component disorders can contribute to the prevention of illness and, in some cases, death.

SUMMARY

The most basic pathogenic lesion of the polyendocrine autoimmune syndromes is an inherited tendency to target self-molecules immunologically. The disease associations and the inheritance pattern make it possible to detect additional components of these syndromes in patients before the appearance of serious manifestations and to make the diagnosis in some first-degree relatives with unrecognized disease. Detection and diagnosis can now be facilitated by autoantibody assays with good sensitivity and specificity.

FURTHER READING

1. Ahonen P. Autoimmune polyendocrinopathy-candidosis-ectodermal dystrophy (APECED): autosomal recessive inheritance. Clin Genet 1985;27:535-42.
2. Eisenbarth GS, Wilson PW, Ward F, et al. The polyglandular failure syndrome: disease inheritance, HLA-type and immune function. Ann Intern Med 1979;91:528-33.
3. Gambelunghe G, Falorni A, Ghaderi M, et al. Microsatellite polymorphism of the MHC class I chain-related (MIC-A and MIC-B) genes marks the risk for autoimmune Addison's disease. J Clin Endocrinol Metab 1999;84:3701-7.
4. Schatz WA, Winter WE. Autoimmune polyendocrine syndrome type II. Endocrinol Metab Clin North Am 2002;31:339-52.
5. Vaidya B, Imrie H, Geatch DR, et al. Association analysis of the cytotoxic T lymphocyte antigen-4 (CTLA-4) and autoimmune regulator-1 (AIRE-1) genes in sporadic autoimmune Addison's disease. J Clin Endocrinol Metab 2000;85:688-91.

23.4 Thyroid Associated Ophthalmopathy

Madhu Bhadauria, Devender Paul Vats

INTRODUCTION

Thyroid associated ophthalmopathy refers to a variety of ophthalmic signs and symptoms typically associated with autoimmune thyroid disease. Affected patients may have clinical hyperthyroidism or, more rarely, even hypothyroidism. Sometimes, the patient never manifests thyroid dysfunction, or the type of thyroid function may evolve and change over a period of time. Thyroid ophthalmopathy includes orbital soft tissue changes and their effects on other ocular tissues like optic neuropathy, venous congestion, oedema and corneal changes like exposure keratopathy and dry eyes. Thyroid ophthalmopathy is clinically evident in about 50% of cases and only 3 to 5% of them require intensive treatment modalities like immune-modulation or surgery.

HISTORICAL BACKGROUND

The association of hyperthyroidism, goitre and exophthalmos has been attributed to the work of Celeb Hillier Parry, Robert James Graves and Carl von Basedow. Parry observed first case of thyroid enlargement and protrusion of eyes, which was reported in 1825. Graves published a complete and detailed description of thyroid disease and exophthalmos in 1835. Basedow presented four cases of exophthalmos goitre and palpitations. In 12th century Persian writing of Sayyid Ismail Al-Jurjani described a relationship between goitre and exophthalmos.

EPIDEMIOLOGY

The incidence of Graves' disease in general population ranges from 0.4 to 2% with male to female ratio being 1:4. Hyperthyroidism and ophthalmopathy usually present during fourth and fifth decades of life. In one large series the age range was 15 to 86 years with median of 52 years. Neonatal or congenital Graves' disease is a rare disorder found in infants born to mothers who have been hyperthyroid during pregnancy. Less frequently it may appear in acquired form in children and young adults. Thyroid ophthalmopathy is the most common orbital disorder; and is the commonest cause of unilateral or bilateral proptosis. Cigarette smoking has been found to be associated with increased risk of Graves' disease. Patients treated with ^{131}I have been found to be at an increased risk for developing or worsening of ophthalmopathy.

Exact nature of ophthalmopathy and its association with thyroid disease is controversial as it may be present in any thyroid state; however most patients with hypothyroidism are treated patients of hyperthyroidism and most euthyroid patients develop hyperthyroidism subsequently. It is less often encountered in patients of Hashimoto's disease (2%) and rarely found in thyroid cancer and thyroid inflammations. Ophthalmopathy does not occur in patients of toxic multinodular goitre, toxic adenoma and diffuse multinodular goitre. It also does not occur in situations of inappropriate thyroid stimulation like tumours, molar pregnancy and hypothalamic pituitary abnormalities.

AETIOPATHOGENESIS

Since the time of initial reporting of Thyroid Associated Ophthalmopathy, there has been increasing evidence that it is an autoimmune disorder but even after decades of research the pathogenic event that triggers the process is unknown. A large number of immunological alterations are seen in thyroid associated ophthalmopathy, which have led to its acceptance as an autoimmune disease. In particular there is evidence that eye muscle tissue may be the key target in the autoimmune process. Orbital connective tissue especially orbital fibroblasts may also be target cells. Therefore there can be two types of ophthalmopathies. One type of disease involves extraocular muscles, and other involves orbital and other soft tissues. These two processes can occur in isolation or can coexist.

This disease process involves sensitization of T cells to retroocular antigens and presence of circulating antibodies to extraocular muscles in serum. Cross-reacting autoantibodies to thyroid gland and extraocular muscles and cytotoxic antibodies to myoblasts have also been isolated in some patients. It is currently believed that autoantibodies directed at the thyroid gland may be capable of binding to orbital tissues. The prime candidates for mediating this process are thyroid-stimulating hormone receptor antibodies (TRab) that bind to TSH receptors in the thyroid gland and then stimulate thyroid hormone synthesis, resulting in hyperthyroidism. It has recently been demonstrated that a subset of TSH receptor autoantibodies can bind to orbital fat and, perhaps, extraocular muscles, and may lead to stimulation of the orbital adipocytes with resultant proliferation and secretion of substances such as glycosaminoglycans. This process leads to a cascading effect and has been found to be responsible for the clinical manifestations encountered.

The presence and binding capability of thyroglobulin to orbital tissues has been confirmed in patients with thyroid-associated ophthalmopathy. It has been suggested that orbital thyroglobulin may bind to glycosaminoglycans, but whether this binding mediates further orbital processes is unknown. Autoimmune thyroid disease is associated with the presence of a variety of autoantibodies directed against thyroid peroxidase, and thyroglobulin. IgA alpha-fodrin autoantibodies are found in less than 1% of normal blood donors and in 22% of patients with thyroid associated ophthalmopathy. It is speculated that alpha-fodrin is an autoantigen in thyroid associated ophthalmopathy and that it may be important in mediating the orbital process. The role of immunogenic abnormalities or specific HLA antigens associations is unclear. Several associations have been reported with Graves' disease, including HLA B-8, HLA Bw 35, HLA-Cw3 and HLA-DR 3.

A striking association between cigarette smoking and Graves' ophthalmopathy has been observed. Smokers have larger thyroid and higher thyroglobulin levels than non-smokers. Smoking causes thyroid damage and orbital hypoxia. Free radicals contained in tobacco smoke lead to orbital fibroblast proliferation. The levels of interleukin-1 receptor antagonists are lowered so the effect of interleukin-1 on orbital inflammatory process is enhanced.

PATHOLOGICAL CHANGES IN ORBITAL TISSUES

Enlargement and inflammation of the extraocular muscles and orbital fat are characteristic of thyroid associated ophthalmopathy. In advanced disease extraocular muscles on gross examination appear enlarged, firm, rubbery and dark red. Histological findings evolve with severity and stage of disease. In early stages only interstitial oedema and inflammatory cells are seen involving the muscle belly and sparing tendons. Immunohistochemical studies have revealed that 80% of the inflammatory cells are B lymphocytes and 20% T lymphocytes. The earliest inflammation occurs in the area of endomysial connective tissue. Endomysial fibroblasts respond with production of glycosamino-glycans specifically hyaluronic acid. In the later stages fibrosis and fatty degeneration dominate the histological picture, functionally leading to restrictive myopathy. Orbital fibroblasts that are located in orbital connective tissue have also been found to be capable of forming new collagen and glycosaminoglycans. Orbital fat inflammation and hypertrophy has never been demonstrated histologically but imaging studies have shown hypertrophy of orbital fat with minimal muscle involvement. Lachrymal gland may show mild to moderate involvement in inflammatory process but not severe enough to cause fibrosis or degeneration. Optic neuropathy in thyroid associated ophthalmopathy has been found to be due to mechanical compression of the optic nerve rather than inflammation of the optic nerve itself. Tendons of muscles and meninges of the optic nerve do not get inflamed but spill over inflammation may involve them in contiguous pathology.

NATURAL HISTORY

Usually eye signs appear a few months after the onset of hyperthyroidism but occasionally may appear months to years before or after the onset of hyperthyroidism. Eventually up to 50% patients of hyperthyroidism develop ophthalmopathy but only 10% of them show severe visual dysfunction. Thyroid associated ophthalmopathy is a self-limiting disorder and stabilises in 12 to 36 months spontaneously. Periorbital oedema and other inflammation signs improve but mobility and proptosis only stabilise.

Classification

The American Thyroid Association has recommended Werner's Classification (mnemonics NOSPECS) which is based on signs and symptoms (Table 23.4.1). This classification is neither used in routine practice nor in

TABLE 23.4.1

Class	Grade	Suggestions for grading
0		No signs or symptoms
I		Only signs
II		Soft tissue involvement with symptoms and signs
	0	absent
	a	minimal
	b	moderate
	c	marked
III		Proptosis
	0	absent
	a	3 to 4 mm increase over upper normal
	b	5 to 7 mm increase
	c	above 8 mm increase
IV		Extraocular muscle involvement
	0	Absent
	a	limitation motion in extremes of gaze
	b	evident restriction of motion
	c	fixation of globe
V		Corneal involvement
	0	absent
	a	stippling of cornea
	b	ulceration
	c	clouding, necrosis, perforation
VI		Sight loss caused by optic nerve involvement
	0	absent
	a	disc pallor or choking or visual field defect Vision 20/20 to 20/60
	b	vision 20/70 to 20/200
	c	vision 20/200 to blindness

Werner' classification of thyroid associated ophthalmopathy (Mnemonics NOSPECS from the first alphabet of the six classes)

TABLE 23.4.2

Ballet's	Palsy of one or more extraocular muscles
Boston's	Uneven jerky motion of the upper lid on inferior movement
Cowen'	Jerky pupil constriction to consensual light
Dalrymple's	Lid retraction
Enroth's	Oedema of lower lid
Gifford's	Difficulty in everting upper lid
Goldzieher's	Deep injection of conjunctiva especially temporally
Griffith's	Lower lid lag on upward gaze
Jellinek's	Abnormal pigmentation of the upper lid
Joffroy's	Absence of forehead wrinkling on upward gaze
Means'	Increase superior scleral show on upward gaze
Mobius'	Deficient convergence
Payne-Trousseau's	Dislocation of globe
Pochin's	Reduced amplitude on blinking
Rosenbach's	Tremors of closed lids
Saintons	Frontalis contraction after cessation of levator activity
Stellwag's	Infrequent blinking
Suker's	Poor fixation
Vigouroux's	Puffiness of lids
Von Graef's	Upper lid lag on downgaze
Wilder's	Jerking of eyes on movement from abduction to adduction

List of eye signs and their eponyms

assessing the outcome of treatment. Since all the patients do not progress through all the stages, this classification does not have much prognostic or therapeutic significance.

Clinical Features

Clinical presentation of thyroid associated ophthalmopathy is variable and is associated with hyperthyroid state in most of the cases and it may precede, develop with or follow the onset of hyperthyroidism. Up to 25% of the patients seek appointment for their ocular symptoms before the diagnosis of thyroid disease (Table 23.4.2). Patients suspected to be suffering from thyroid associated ophthalmopathy should have a thorough history, a general physical examination, careful ophthalmic evaluation and thyroid function tests. History of medications received for thyroid disease is important as the modalities of treatment causing improvement in thyroid disease do not concurrently cause improvement in thyroid associated ophthalmopathy. Treatment with radioactive iodine may exacerbate symptoms and signs of ophthalmopathy. Relationship between thyroidectomy and thyroid associated ophthalmopathy remains inconclusive. Family history of thyroid disease is found positive in 30% patients. Diabetics are known to have more severe form of thyroid associated ophthalmopathy and myasthenia gravis may be found as an associated disease.

Amongst the personal factors, smoking increases the incidence by two folds and also increases severity and progression of the disease. Psychosomatic factors can trigger or aggravate the ophthalmopathy.

Clinical picture evolves essentially due to either one or the combination of the ocular tissues involved. The basic groups of tissues are as follows:
a. Lids
b. Orbital fat
c. Extraocular muscles
d. Optic nerve

SYMPTOMS

Symptoms can be mild to very severe with a waxing and waning course. Early and mild symptoms consist of foreign body sensation, photophobia and watering due to dry eye state.

Specific symptoms include eyelid retraction, unilateral or bilateral proptosis, redness, chemosis and diplopia that is initially transient in up gaze. Convergence insufficiency leading to diplopia for reading is greatest in the mornings. Later complaints include squint due to fibrosis of rectus muscles and decreased visual acuity due to corneal or optic nerve involvement. Greying of vision or loss of vision are indicators of optic neuropathy.

CLINICAL SIGNS

Comprehensive evaluation requires both functional tests and objective measurements.

Lid Retraction

Lid retraction is seen in 37 to 92% patients of thyroid associated ophthalmopathy. In normal position superior limbus is taken as anatomical marker and upper lid covers 2 mm of superior limbus. In lid retraction upper eye lid is observed above its normal resting level in a patient who is relaxed and looking straight ahead (Fig. 23.4.1). Thyroid associated ophthalmopathy is the commonest cause of upper lid retraction (Dalrymple's sign). Temporal flare is the advanced stage when more sclera is seen laterally. In early stages it is caused by sympathomimetic response. In later stages lid retraction is seen due to enlargement, fibrosis and adhesions of levator muscle with other orbital tissues. Proptosis accentuates appearance of lid retraction. Lower eyelid retraction can occur in a similar manner (Figs 23.4.2A and B).

Lid Lag

Additional lid retraction that is seen in downward gaze is called lid lag and is also known as Graefe's sign (Fig. 23.4.3).

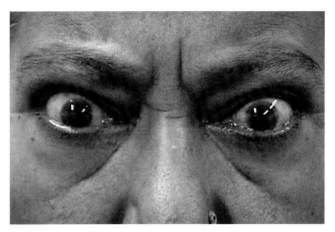
Fig. 23.4.1: Upper lid retraction

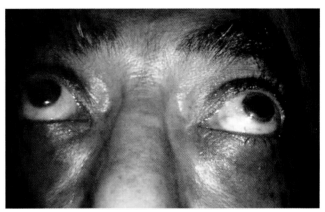
Fig. 23.4.2A: Restriction of lower lid elevation due to inferior rectus fibrosis

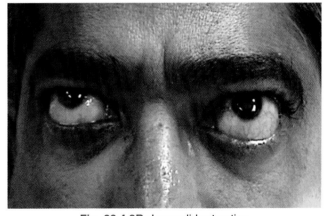
Fig. 23.4.2B: Lower lid retraction

Proptosis

Proptosis occurs in 60% (34 to 94%) of the patients with thyroid eye disease and conversely Thyroid Associated Ophthalmopathy is also the commonest cause of proptosis. It can be unilateral or bilateral. It may also be symmetric or asymmetric. Proptosis is caused by

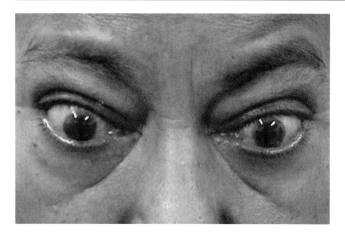

Fig. 23.4.3: Lid lag, conjunctival chemosis

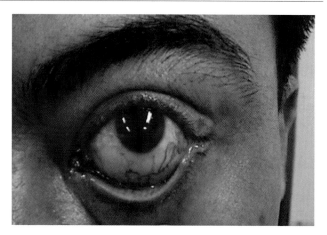

Fig. 23.4.4: Cork screw vessels at muscle insertion

increased soft tissue mass due to enlargement of extra-ocular muscles, increase in volume of fat due to deposition of products of antigen antibody reaction and venous stasis. Increase in orbital volume is an accommodative phenomenon and protects against compressive optic neuropathy. The patients who have more proptosis develop lesser optic neuropathy.

Inflammation and Congestion

Congestion is seen over the insertion of the horizontal recti muscles. Conjunctiva in palpebral aperture shows chemosis along with skin puffiness and mild erythema, which gives an allergic appearance (Fig. 23.4.4).

Periorbital Oedema

Forward displacement of normal orbital fat due to increasing orbital soft tissue mass gives rise to periorbital oedema. Another confounding factor to this is venous congestion. Oedema is seen maximum after a night's sleep as head remains in dependent position (Fig. 23.4.5).

Ocular Dysmotility

Ocular dysmotility occurs due to impaired relaxation, hence, restriction of movement is seen in the direction opposite to the action of the muscle. Patients are symptomatic due to diplopia. The order of frequency in which muscles get involved are inferior rectus, media rectus, superior rectus and lateral rectus. Quantitative assessment of extraocular muscles limitation is the best way to assess and follow progression of the disease and to follow potential for visual loss.

Methods to assess ocular dysmotility are:
i.   Range of movement in six cardinal positions of gaze.

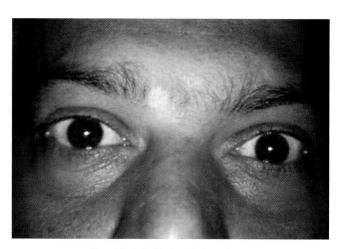

Fig. 23.4.5: Periorbital oedema

ii. Diplopia charting in five gazes: up, down, right, left, and central.
iii. Force duction test.
iv. Prism cover test.
v.   Lancaster R and G test.
vi. Range of fusion.

All these tests may be repeated after tensilon test in case myasthenia is suspected.

In the later stages patient develops squint due to muscle fibrosis and shortening. Inferior and medial recti are the most commonly involved muscles that give rise to characteristic 'down and in' position of the globe.

Corneal Disorders

The combination of lid retraction and proptosis leads to corneal exposure, which is the most frequently described anterior segment abnormality. Infrequent blinking, increased palpebral fissure width and involvement of

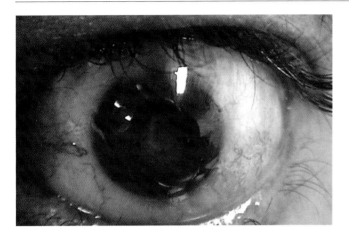

Fig. 23.4.6: Corneal opacity, uveitis, complicated cataract

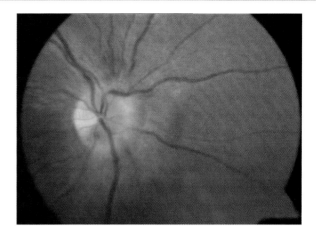

Fig. 23.4.7: Disc oedema due to optic neuropathy

lachrymal gland in immune process lead to dry eye state with increased tear osmolarity. Patients with corneal exposure typically complain of irritation, foreign body sensation, photophobia, and watering. Slit lamp examination reveals conjunctival congestion and punctate keratopathy that appears inferiorly (Fig. 23.4.6). This is especially more prominent on Rose Bengal staining. Nocturnal lagophthalmos is a particular problem and patient should be observed during sleep.

Most of the changes in vision in this group are related to refractive errors induced by malposition of the upper lid and to the effects of corneal exposure or dry eye conditions. Inadequate treatment of corneal exposure leads to corneal ulceration and perforation and severely compromised vision. Damage to the ocular surface directly correlates to the extent of ophthalmopathy. Corneal exposure secondary to more malignant exophthalmos is usually also accompanied by optic nerve compromise.

Glaucoma

Associated glaucoma could be primary open-angle glaucoma, ocular hypertension, secondary open-angle glaucoma, normal tension glaucoma and angle-closure glaucoma. Intraocular pressure should not only be measured in primary gaze but up and down gaze also. Pseudo-increase in intraocular pressure may be due to restrictive myopathy and altered scleral rigidity. Visual field defects may be varied or fluctuating and do not confirm and correlate to the optic disc status. Visual field loss may also be due to compressive neuropathy and vascular insufficiency.

Optic Neuropathy

It is caused by enlargement of extraocular muscles and compression at orbit apex. Incidence ranges between 5 and 8.6%. Patients complain of diminished vision. Pupils show afferent pupillary defect. Fundus examination may show normal optic disc, papilloedema or optic atrophy (Fig. 23.4.7). Colour vision usually gets affected. Visual fields show field defects depending upon the degree of severity. Central scotoma and inferior altitudinal scotoma are characteristic. However, an enlarged blind spot, para-central scotomas, nerve fibre bundle defects and generalised constriction of visual fields may also be seen. Contrast sensitivity in uncomplicated ophthalmopathy without optic neuropathy shows abnormally elevated threshold in medium-high special frequencies. Loss of contrast sensitivity in low frequency signifies onset of optic neuropathy as optic neuropathy causes loss of all the frequencies.

INVESTIGATIONS

A patient of thyroid associated ophthalmopathy is investigated for assessment of thyroid status, extraocular muscle volume and function, functions of optic nerve and measurement of proptosis.

Thyroid Function Tests

The patients of thyroid associated ophthalmopathy should have baseline investigations and periodic monitoring. The measurement of thyroid function include TSH, total and free serum triiodothyronine (T_3), total and free serum thyroxin (T_4) and thyroid antibodies.

Investigations for Extraocular Muscles (EOM)

Examination of range of EOM in all the directions of gaze is documented clinically and by Hess charting to quantify the range of movement, progression and/or regression. Diplopia charting also gives useful information regarding muscle dysfunction. For volume change in EOM, various imaging modalities are available.

Imaging

Imaging modalities in thyroid associated ophthalmopathy mainly involve ultrasound, CT and MRI. MRI is still very expensive and does not add much information over CT findings and hence is used sparingly in specific situations.

Role of Imaging: To Confirm

1. The diagnosis and see the degree of muscles involvement.
2. Bilateral disease when clinically it is appreciated on one side only.
3. Compressive optic neuropathy and its pre- and postoperative status when contemplating orbital decompression.
4. Thyroid associated ophthalmopathy in the absence of clinical/laboratory evidence of thyroid disorder.

Ultrasonography

Ultrasound is performed with 'A scan' in amplitude mode and 'B-scan' in brightness mode. B scan is performed with probe frequency of 10 MHz or more. The normal extraocular muscles are medium to high reflective on A scan and less echo dense than surrounding orbital soft tissue on B scan. B scan is useful for documenting gross size and contour of the muscle where as A scan is useful in differentiating different causes of muscle enlargement. Muscle thickening in thyroid associated ophthalmopathy has a very characteristic appearance. In most cases the insertion is spared while mid and the posterior portion of the muscle belly are involved. Internal reflectivity of the muscle is medium to high and quite regular. This appearance results from large interfaces between muscle fibres and surrounding oedema. Other associated findings include swelling of the orbital fat and lid tissues, thickening of the periorbital tissue and enlargement of lachrymal gland. Fluctuation in the size of extraocular muscles is noted on follow-up examination.

Advantage of USG Ultrasound is a highly useful available office test and is preferred by clinicians due to low cost, no ionising radiation and ease of availability. However, it has a limited role in inexperienced hands and in imaging of orbital apex.

Normal extraocular muscle values are:

Superior rectus/levator palpabrae superioris	—	3.9 to 6.8 mm
Lateral rectus	—	2.2 to 3.8 mm
Inferior rectus	—	1.6 to 3.6 mm
Medial rectus	—	2.3 to 4.7 mm

These normal values may not truly reflect all age and population groups.

Computed Tomography

Computed tomography is done for assessing extraocular muscle enlargement and crowding at orbit apex. For orbital imaging 3 to 4 mm axial and coronal scans are taken as superior and inferior recti are cut tangentially on axial scans hence subtle enlargement may be missed in absence of coronal scans.

Findings Increased extraocular muscle size with tendon sparing is characteristic of thyroid associated ophthalmopathy. Involvement is mostly bilateral. Occasionally muscle tendons may get involved. In chronic cases, muscles may show fatty densities within. Increase in EOM muscle volume correlates well with the degree of severity of optic neuropathy. Increased orbital fat may be the only finding. Increase in fat on CT scan may also be due to obesity or Cushing's disease. Mottled density seen on scan in retrobulbar fat is due to lymphocyte infiltration. Sometimes, remodelling of bony walls may be seen due to orbital fat displacing orbital structures. Lachrymal gland enlargement may be seen occasionally. Superior ophthalmic vein may be prominent.

MRI

MRI is superior to CT due to its inherent soft tissue contrast, better resolution and multipurpose capability. Under normal circumstances, there is no added advantage over CT but has a role to play in cases of optic neuropathy and planning of radiotherapy. Extraocular muscles with elevated T2 time are indicative of increased water content, which occurs in acute inflammatory stage and they are more responsive to radiotherapy than EOM that have a normal T2 time.

Optic Nerve Function

Investigations for Optic Nerve Function

Patients suspected of optic nerve involvement are subjected to contrast sensitivity testing, colour vision testing, computerised automatic visual field examination and visual evoked potentials to assess early signs of compression. Compression is assessed the best by MRI as the tissues at the apex of orbit are not well differentiated on ultrasound and CT.

Proptosis

Proptosis can be seen clinically and can be measured by Hertle's exophthalmometer, specifically for measuring the variation in proptosis. It is preferable to use it without orbital rim contact. Fixation adaptor in regular Hertle's exophthalmometer rests on forehead and nasion. It is useful in patients following lateral orbitotomy for orbital decompression. For the purpose of diagnosis, an absolute value of more than 21 mm or a difference of more than 2 mm between the two eyes is taken as exophthalmos.

MANAGEMENT

Thyroid associated ophthalmopathy has been divided into two broad phases depending upon the immunological activity of the disease process.

Phase one is the phase of acute inflammation and congestion, which is self-limiting and lasts for 6 to 36 months. It is mainly characterized by activity of lymphocytes and fibroblasts and responds to treatment by steroids, immunosuppressive and radiotherapy.

Phase two is chronic stable permanent phase characterized by fibrosis and hypertrophy of extraocular muscles fat and lachrymal grand. Effective treatment for this phase is mainly surgical.

Short-term Goals

In acute phase, treatment is directed at conserving useful vision and decreasing the symptoms by medical treatment.

Long-term Goals

Restoration of anatomic and functional integrity of eye ball and orbit to minimize the physical, psychological and economic impact of the disease. Restorative surgery should be performed only after disease has been quiescent for at least six months. Management of concomitant hyperthyroidism may alleviate some

transient ocular signs like lid retraction caused by sympathetic over activity.

General Management

Medical Treatment

Being a self-limiting disease, all cases do not require treatment for thyroid associated ophthalmopathy. Indications for medical treatment are:
• Optic neuropathy
• Severe exposure keratopathy
• Malignant exophthalmos
• Continued disease progression despite radiation or surgical therapy.

Medical therapy is applicable only in acute or inflammatory phase and two types of treatments have been found useful.
i. Anti-inflammatory and immunosuppressive medication.
ii. Orbital irradiation.

Corticosteroids may be used alone or in combination with immunosuppressive drugs, radiation or surgery. Mechanism of action is by suppressing lymphocytes and fibroblasts. Oral prednisolone is given 60 to 100 mg daily for several days and then tapered off slowly over weeks. Thyroid associated ophthalmopathy with chronic orbital changes does not respond to treatment by steroids. Periocular steroids can be given in some cases to reduce soft tissue symptoms of thyroid associated ophthalmopathy if systemic steroids are contraindicated and other modes of therapy are ineffective. Disadvantage is inherent risk of infection and its lower efficacy. IV methyl prednisolone is indicated in acutely severe or malignant exophthalmos.

The role of steroids in ophthalmopathy, that is not vision threatening is controversial and should not be given in absence of optic neuropathy. Cyclosporine is second preferred drug after steroids for immunosuppressive therapy. It has been found to be effective in 22% of cases. Lower doses of cyclosporine in combination with steroids are especially useful in reducing the dose of steroids and side effects. Plasmapheresis is used to remove humoral factors in autoimmune process and is then followed by a short course of immunosuppressive therapy to achieve optimum effect.

Radiotherapy (RT)

Exact mechanism of action of radiotherapy is not known. Probable mechanisms of action are specific immunosuppression of lymphocytes and nonspecific immuno-suppression of fibroblasts. Active orbital inflammation and congestion are decreased significantly following a course of RT. Optic neuropathy improves in 65 to 85% of cases but only a minimal improvement is seen in proptosis. Strabismus shows little change and chronic orbital fat changes show no improvement.

Indications for radiotherapy (RT)
• Optic neuropathy when steroids and/or surgery are contraindicated.
• Preoperatively to reduce inflammation and fibrosis.

Effects of radiotherapy: Effects start showing 1 to 8 weeks following treatment. Radiotherapy reduces orbital inflammation and decreases congestion just like steroids but effects are less dramatic and more prolonged. In 65 to 85% of cases of optic neuropathy improvement is seen and more so in cases which are more severely affected. Visual improvement has been found to be the most marked clinical improvement. Radiotherapy should be used early, as it has no effect in later stages.

Method of radiotherapy treatment: CT scan dosimeter mapping is done. The radiation field is concentrated in posterior orbit from lateral orbital rim to the border of sella-turcica. Each orbit is irradiated separately. Lens and retina are shielded. Cobalt 60 unit delivers a well collimated photon beam with a total dose of 2000 cGy in 10 fractions.

Management of Specific Symptoms and Signs

Management of Surface Symptoms

Mild ocular irritation, foreign body sensation and watering is treated by tear substitution and lubricants. In addition,use of sun glasses and frequent conscious closure of lids may help relieve the dry eye symptoms. Temporarily nocturnal lagophthalmos may be treated by generous application of ointment along with taping of the lids at bed time.

Management of Glaucoma

Glaucoma is managed by a nonaggressive approach. Treatment is started with treating the primary cause. Associated compressive neuropathy should be treated first. Treatment is started by instituting antiglaucoma therapy and surgery is reserved for nonresolving and refractory glaucoma with documented progression. Prior to glaucoma surgery the eye should be quiet and maximally decompressed with no lid retraction. The choice of surgery is a standard trabeculectomy with mitomycin as these patients have increased sub-conjunctival fibrosis. As the orbital and intraocular pressure is high, pre-placed sutures and tight suturing of the flap is preferred during surgery.

Tarsorrhaphy

Tarsorrhaphy is indicated for temporary correction of mild to moderate exposure keratopathy, chemosis with conjunctival prolapse and sterile corneal ulcers. Tarsorrhaphy is done under local infiltrative anaesthesia. A 5/0 nylon suture is used to weave through the lid margins from one end to the other with the ends taped or tied. This technique offers easy reversibility and temporary loosening to examine underlying cornea and prevents any damage to the lid margin.

Management of Periorbital Swelling

Periorbital swelling can be reduced by head elevation in bed along with diuretics and low salt diet. The effect of oral prednisolone is transient and due to its role being controversial steroid therapy is not justified. Orbital decompression when performed produces dramatic results. Surgery is indicated when disease process goes into chronic phase and oedema becomes less tense. Lid laxity and herniation of fat appears as result of chronic prolonged oedema. Surgical excision of fat lobules, careful dissection and release of scars and blepharoplasty are performed as and when required. Levator dehiscence repair is undertaken if needed. Conservative excision of skin, especially the lower lid is done in selected cases.

Management of Diplopia

Diplopia remains variable in early phase and is worse in the morning. Prisms can manage mild diplopia. Up to 8 prism dioptres, prisms can be directly mounted on the spectacles equally divided in both eyes. From 8 to 30 dioptres Fresnel's prisms are used. Prisms are mounted on spectacles for near and distant vision separately. Temporary occlusion of alternate eyes can also be done to avoid diplopia.

Stable diplopia Diplopia is considered stable when no change is noticed in last 6 months on prism bar cover test. Small deviations are treated by permanent grounding of prisms on glasses. Large deviation need to be corrected by surgery. As muscle paresis is extremely uncommon, resections are not performed. Maximum recession of the involved muscles yields best results as it relieves restrictive force. To minimize secondary deviation from contralateral muscle postoperatively bilateral variable recession may also be considered.

Adjustable sutures may facilitate early postoperative alignment. However, they are not often used due to the unpredictability, difficulty, possibility of slipped muscle and late postoperative muscle imbalance. Most patients require more than one muscle surgery. Most of the patients are left with residual diplopia for either distance or near gaze for which prisms are to be prescribed. Eyelid malposition occurs as a result of rectus muscle surgery, slipped muscles and under correction.

Management of Proptosis

 i. Prednisolone may reduce proptosis by 1 to 2 mm but such minimal effect does not justify its use due to associated systemic side effects.
 ii. Radiation therapy and immune suppression have not proved beneficial in reducing proptosis.
 iii. Surgery is the only modality that reduces proptosis and is performed only when the ophthalmopathy becomes quiescent.

Orbital decompression-orbitotomy: Aim is to create enlargement of confining space by partially removing bony walls and periostium. This causes prolapse of posterior orbital soft tissues into adjacent spaces thus relieving pressure on the optic nerve and reduction in proptosis. There are various approaches. Two wall approach is antral-ethmoidal decompression. Three wall decompression including lateral wall and four-wall decompression including the roof of the orbit into anterior cranial fossa. Multi-speciality approach has been found to be the beneficial way to obtain optimal results and minimize complications.

Indications of orbitotomy
 i. Moderate to severe proptosis.
 ii. Globe luxation.
 iii. Severe lagophthalmos with exposure keratopathy.
 iv. Disfiguration from the bug eye appearance.
 v. Visual loss from optic neuropathy.

Management of Lid Retraction

Mild to moderate lid retraction is treated by medical treatment.

Guanethidine sulphate used as 2 to 5% eyedrops produces ptosis of 1 to 1.5 mm. Drops can be used from alternate day to thrice a day. Effect is easily reversible. Side effects of these drops are superficial punctuate keratitis, miosis and conjunctival vessel dilatation. Other similar drugs like bethanidine and thymoxamine may be used.

Botulinium toxin A has been in use for chronic fibrotic lid retraction. An injection of 2.5 to 5 units is given into the subcutaneous plane in superior subtarsal border just lateral to the centre of the upper lid. The effect lasts for 8 to 32 weeks. Surgery for lid retraction is performed as last of all rehabilitative surgeries on the thyroid patient. Therefore, it is important to be familiar with the relationship of eyelid retraction, temporal progression and need for eyelid retraction repair. As in strabismus surgery, eyelid position must be documented stable for at least 6 months.

Indications for surgery for lid retraction
 i. Severe upper lid retraction with lagophthalmos and resultant exposure keratopathy.
 ii. Cosmetically disfiguring eyelid retraction.
 iii. Eye lid retraction with symptomatic dermatochalasis of upper or lower lid.
 iv. Residual exposure keratopathy/lagophthalmos following upper lid retraction repair.

SUMMARY

Thyroid associated ophthalmopathy presents itself from minor symptom of grittiness to severe vision threatening optic neuropathy due to compression and exposure keratopathy due to proptosis. Complete ophthalmic evaluation is important (Table 23.4.3). Often these patients suffer from residual disabling squint, diplopia and disfiguring proptosis. All the patients can be helped to a variable degree by use of symptomatic medication, immunosuppression (steroids, antimetabolites), radiotherapy and surgery. Surgery in acute phase is useful in saving damage to optic nerve and cornea, and in late fibrotic phase in correction of squint, lid retraction and proptosis. Thyroid associated ophthalmopathy is a self-limiting disease and subsides in 12 to 36 months. The clinical course cannot be altered substantially in most of the cases but treatment helps in prevention of complications and is usually used for a few months only. The sequence and timing of treatment require mature clinical judgement for optimization. In 95% of patients only symptomatic treatment with lubricants suffices. All other patients are managed on individual merits of the case. However, all those who need definitive treatment need all the caution, care and titration of all available treatment

TABLE 23.4.3

History

Symptoms

1. **Nonspecific:** Watering, redness, photophobia, foreign body sensation

2. **Specific:** Lid retraction, lid lag, proptosis, redness, diplopia, squint, decreased visual acuity or loss of vision

H/o Thyroid disease: Weight loss/gain, appetite increased/decreased, intolerance heat/cold, sleep (insomnia/hypersomnia), treatment h/o thyroid disease, drugs, radioactive iodine, thyroidectomy

Family h/o thyroid disease

Personal history
Smoking
Psychosomatic factor

Systemic disease
Diabetes, myasthenia

Examination

Lid retraction, oedema including nocturnal lid lag

| Periorbital oedema | Proptosis-measurements |
| | Hertle's exophthalmometry |

Ocular motility	**Visual acuity Distance and near**
Ocular movements, convergence	Contrast sensitivity
Cover test—prism cover test	Colour vision—Ishihara's
Force duction test	Farnsworth Munsel's 100 hue test
Diplopia charting	**Pupillary reactions:** RAPD (Relative afferent pupillary defect)

Range of fusion

Slit lamp examination: Corneal examination, opacities and irregularities

Rose bengal and fluorescein staining (as and when needed).

Congestion on the insertion of horizontal recti, Tear film—Schirmer's test, Tear film breakup time

Anterior chamber: Shallow/normal   **Gonioscopy**

Tension—Primary position   Looking up   Looking down (differential tonometery)

Fundus examination

Optic-disc: Normal, disc oedema, optic atrophy, cup/disc ratio

Visual fields: Central, full fields.

Investigations: Thyroid function tests, ultrasonography, computed tomography, magnetic resonance imaging

Comprehensive ophthalmological work-up

modalities. All the patients of thyroid associated ophthalmopathy cannot be brought back to premorbid state but most of them can be rehabilitated visually and functionally. Management of severe thyroid associated ophthalmopathy should not be done by endocrinologist or ophthalmologist alone. Treatment should be a team approach by skilled ophthalmologists in this subspeciality in close collaboration with endocrinologists to prevent permanent visual loss.

FURTHER READING

1. Albert Daniel M, Jakobiec Frederick A. Principles and Practice of Ophthalmology. Philadelphia (Pennsylvania): WB Saunders and Co., 2000;(4)3082-8.

2. Bartalena L, Marcocci C, Gorman CA, Wiersinga WM, Pinchera A. Orbital radiotherapy for Graves' ophthalmopathy: useful or useless? Safe or dangerous? J Endocrinol Invest 2003;26:5-16.

3. Cockerham KP, Kennedell JS. Thyroid associated orbitopathy, in focal points (AAO) vol XV Number Q, 1997.

4. Coday MP, Netland PA, Dallow RL. Principles and Practice of Ophthalmology. Philadelphia (Pennsylvania): WB Saunders and Co., 2000;(5)4742-59.

5. Hatton MP, Rubin PA. The pathophysiology of thyroid-associated ophthalmopathy. Ophthalmol Clin North Am 2002;(1):113-9.

6. Jack Rootman. Graves' Orbitopathy in Diseases of the Orbit. Philadelphia: Lippincott Co.,1998;241-80.

7. Kalmann R, Mourits MP. Prevalence and management of elevated intraocular pressure in patients with Graves' orbitopathy. Br J Ophthalmol 1998;82:754-7.

8. Kenneth D, Burman MD. Graves' Ophthalmopathy; Highlights of the 74th Annual Meeting of the American Thyroid Association; October 10-13, 2002; Los Angeles, California.

9. Traisk F, Tallstedt L. Thyroid associated ophthalmopathy: botulinum toxin A in the treatment of upper eyelid retraction—a pilot study. Acta Ophthalmol Scand 2001;79(6):585-8.

10. Tucker SM, Tucker N A, Linberg JV. Thyroid eye disease. Duane's Clinical Ophthalmology, volume 2. Philadelphia, 1999;Chapter 36.

11. Vander Meulen JC. Ocular Plastic Surgery. Mosby, Wolfe, 1996.

12. Vaseghi M, Tarin TT, Levin PS, Terris DJ. Minimally invasive orbital decompression for Graves' ophthalmopathy. Ann Otol Rhinol Laryngol 2003;112:57-62.

13. Yokoyama N, Nagataki S, Uetani M, Ashizawa K, Eguchi K. Role of magnetic resonance imaging in the assessment of disease activity in thyroid-associated ophthalmopathy. Thyroid 2002;12(3):223-7.

14. Zimmermann-Belsing T, Feldt-Rasmussen U, Fledelius H. Ultrasound measurement of the horizontal external eye muscles in patients with thyroid disease. Is orbital involvement associated with thyroid autoantibodies? Eur J Ophthalmol 2002;12(5):351-8.

23.5 Pulmonary Manifestations of Endocrine Disorders

BNBM Prasad

INTRODUCTION

Endocrine disorders affect respiratory system at various levels including respiratory centre, respiratory pump, airways, lung and pulmonary vasculature.

Respiratory dysfunction associated with endocrine disorders may be mild to life-threatening. Proper management of endocrine disorders demands prompt recognition of various manifestations including respiratory involvement, understanding their pathogenesis and institution of appropriate therapy. This chapter outlines the various pulmonary manifestations of various endocrine disorders.

DIABETES MELLITUS

In diabetes mellitus, lung is considered as a target organ. The pathological finding of pulmonary microangiopathy seen in diabetes mellitus, is characterized by thickening of alveolar epithelial and pulmonary capillary basement membrane. Acute or chronic complications of diabetes mellitus affect respiratory system in numerous ways. Both hypoglycaemic and hyperglycaemic coma predispose to aspiration pneumonia. Respiratory insufficiency can occur due to development of dyselectrolaemia and hypophosphataemia while treating hyperglycaemic coma.

Infections

Diabetes mellitus is an independent risk factor for development of lower respiratory infections and also for higher mortality. The increased risk of infection is related to hyperglycaemia, altered immune cell functions (impaired phagocytic, chemotactic, and bactericidal activity of white blood cells), impaired cytokine production, pulmonary microangiopathy and effects of non-enzymatic glycation on alveolar membrane and pulmonary basal lamina.

Pneumonias

Bacterial pneumonias caused by both gram-positive and gram-negative organisms are common. Usual pathogens of bacterial pneumonia include *Escherichia coli*, *Klebsiella pneumonia*, and *Staphylococcus aureus*. Pneumonia in diabetes mellitus is usually severe with tendency for suppuration and abscess formation (Figs 23.5.1 to 23.5.3). Aggressive antibiotic therapy with proper diabetic control is vital for better outcome. In diabetes mellitus, infections caused by *Legionella*, *Streptococcus pneumoniae* and influenza virus may be associated with high morbidity and mortality. Gastroparesis and laryngeal dysfunction complicating diabetes, predispose to aspiration pneumonia.

Mucormycosis

There is also increased incidence of nonbacterial infections such as fungal infections and tuberculosis. Diabetics particularly those with complications and poor control are prone to mucormycosis that usually presents with rhinocerebral infections. Pulmonary mucormycosis in diabetes mellitus is associated with major airway involvement, vascular invasion and high mortality and the disease mimics invasive aspergillosis. Endobronchial mucormycosis presents with hoarseness of voice, dyspnoea, mediastinal widening and haemoptysis. Massive haemoptysis can also occur due to necrotising lung infections and pulmonary infarction due to vascular invasion by mucor species. Treatment consists of control of diabetes, systemic antifungal therapy, surgical

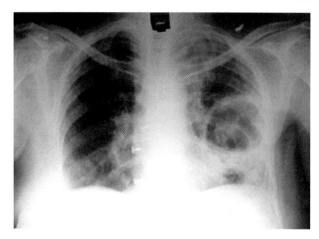

Fig. 23.5.1: Chest X-ray PA view showing a large lung abscess

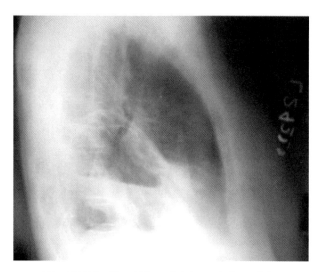

Fig. 23.5.2: Chest X-ray left lateral view of the same patient

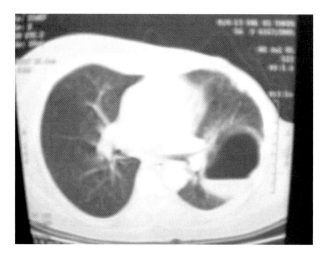

Fig. 23.5.3: CECT chest depicting pulmonary cavity with a fluid level (left lower lobe)

resection if disease is localised and supportive measures. Fatality is due to fungal sepsis, respiratory failure and massive haemoptysis.

Pulmonary zygomycosis with spectrum of acute, subacute and chronic necrotising pneumonia can also occur in diabetes mellitus.

Pulmonary Tuberculosis

The incidence of pulmonary tuberculosis is 2 to 5 times higher among diabetics. Those with tuberculosis have a higher prevalence of diabetes and infection- related stress and malnutrition might play a role in the pathogenesis. The spectrum of pulmonary tuberculosis in diabetes described includes lower lobe involvement rather than classical involvement of posterior-apical segments of upper lobes, infiltrates in any lobe, multilobar involve-ment, cavitory disease and pleural effusion. There is no significant increase in relapse rate of tuberculosis among diabetics so long as glycaemic control is satisfactory when compared with those without diabetes and the treatment of tuberculosis is similar to non-diabetics. There is no major dissimilarity of disease pattern as well as treatment outcome amongst different types of diabetes.

Some of the antituberculous drugs have endocrine and metabolic effects. Rifampicin, a potent inducer of cytochrome P-450 hepatic microsomal enzymes, enhances steroid hormone metabolism. In those with damaged adrenals with subacute adrenal insufficiency, rifampicin administration is associated with develop-ment of an acute adrenal crisis usually within 2 weeks after starting therapy. This can be prevented in esta-blished cases of adrenal insufficiency with tuberculosis by increasing the dose of glucocorticoids. There is no need to alter the dose of mineralocorticoids in such cases since the effect of rifampicin on mineralocorticoids metabolism is less pronounced.

Rifampicin decreases the levels of both $25(OH)D_3$ and $1, 25(OH)_2 D_3$ by enhancing the catabolism of vitamin D to inactive compounds. Consequently parathormone levels are increased significantly and this can result in hypocalcaemia and even osteomalacia in those with low vitamin D reserves. Isoniazid also affects vitamin D metabolism by inhibiting 1 alpha hydroxylase activity and by reducing synthesis of calcitriol. When isoniazid is given in combination with rifampicin there is not only a substantial decrease in levels of both $25(OH) D_3$ and $1,25(OH)_2D_3$ but also an increase in levels of parathormone. This predisposes to development of hypocalcaemia and osteomalcia in those with marginal vitamin D stores. Although rifampicin increases extrathyroidal metabolism of thyroid hormones, it has no clinical significance. Rifampicin also increases the insulin requirements in type 1 diabetes mellitus by augmenting glucose absorption from the intestine.

Para-aminosalicylic acid (PAS) and ethionamide inhibit synthesis of thyroid hormones and cause goitre and hypothyroidism. PAS can induce hypoglycaemia.

Pulmonary Dysfunctions

Various respiratory dysfunctions related to severity of diabetes mellitus can occur. However, these dysfunctions are not severe enough to cause significant respiratory embarrassment in vast majority of patients. Causes of pulmonary dysfunctions in diabetes are attributed to alterations of lung connective tissue due to nonenzymatic glycation, pulmonary microangiopathy, diabetic autonomic neuropathy, and diaphragmatic dysfunction. Pulmonary dysfunctions observed in diabetes mellitus include decrease in lung volumes, diminished total lung capacity and vital capacity, reduced pulmonary elastic recoil, impaired pulmonary diffusion and impaired bronchial responsiveness with increased threshold for cough response.

Sleep Apnoea

It is common in diabetes mellitus particularly in those with autonomic neuropathy. Central sleep apnoea and periodic breathing are often observed. Sleep is disrupted particularly in those with painful neuropathy and periodic leg movements during sleep is more common. In diabetes mellitus ventilatory response to hypoxia may be impaired with preserved hypercapnic ventilatory response. Type 2 respiratory failure can occur in diabetes mellitus due to central hypoventilation and respiratory muscle weakness/myopathy consequent to diabetic microangiopathy of muscles. Increased levels of insulin and impaired glucose tolerance have been observed in those with sleep apnoea independent of obesity and these changes are considered to be secondary to increased sympathetic activity. Nasal continuous positive airway pressure (CPAP) ventilation may improve insulin sensitivity.

Miscellaneous

Diabetic ketoacidosis can be complicated by pulmonary oedema due to altered pulmonary capillary permeability, fluid overload and pulmonary microangiopathy. Pleural effusions are common among diabetics particularly in those with left ventricular dysfunction and the exact mechanism of such effusions remains unclear. Diabetic ketoacidosis may be associated with pneumomediastinum due to acidosis induced hyperpnoea and severe vomiting. Mucus plugging of major airways has been observed in diabetic ketoacidosis and is contributed by altered vagal tone, autonomic neuropathy and altered mentation. Foetal pulmonary immaturity can occur if maternal blood glucose remains high in diabetic mothers.

THYROID DISORDERS

In thyroid disorders, the respiratory system can be affected by both thyroid enlargement and dysfunction.

Goitre

Both extra- and intrathoracic goitres cause extrinsic compression of surrounding structures. In intrathoracic goitre, a greater portion of thyroid mass lies below thoracic inlet. In 80% of cases of intrathoracic goitre, the thyroid mass arises from isthmus or inferior pole of thyroid gland and presents as anterior mediastinal mass lying anterior to trachea. In rest of the cases, thyroid mass arises from posterior aspect of thyroid gland and it lies in posterior mediastinum behind and usually right of trachea. Intrathoracic goitre may remain asymptomatic and is discovered incidentally in chest radiograph. Airway compression occurs in 31 to 33% cases and manifests with dyspnoea, stridor and irritative cough. Cough can be distressing and usually subsides after the removal of goitre. Dyspnoea can be life threatening, acute or chronic. Life-threatening/acute dyspnoea is rare and occurs in a setting of intragoitre haemorrhage and in thyroid malignancy. Dyspnoea and dysphagia due to tracheoesophageal compression are common in thyroiditis. Compression of recurrent laryngeal nerve is observed in less than 1% of cases of benign goitres and it results in vocal cord palsy and stridor. Superior vena caval syndrome is not uncommon and has been reported among 4 out of 32 cases of retrosternal goitres in one study. Compression of thoracic duct and bracheocephalic vessels cause chylothorax. Goitre lying anterior to trachea is seen on chest skiagram as sharply defined lobulated or smooth homogeneous density in the anterior mediastinum often displacing trachea posteriorly and laterally. Radioisotope studies with ^{131}I thyroid scan are diagnostic. Flow volume loop is useful in assessing the degree of airway obstruction. In those cases of goitre with compression or displacement of trachea, surgery in the form of thyroidectomy is the treatment of choice. Tracheal stenting to maintain patency or radioactive iodine ablation can be done in those where surgery cannot be done. Life-threatening tracheal obstruction requires tracheostomy or bronchoscopically guided stent placement in trachea. Pulmonary metastasis in thyroid cancer can be single or multiple pulmonary nodules and occurs in 5 to 20% of cases.

Thyrotoxicosis

It is associated with dyspnoea (thyrotoxic dyspnoea), proximal myopathy, pulmonary functional abnormalities and worsening of bronchial asthma.

Thyrotoxic Dyspnoea

Thyrotoxic dyspnoea occurs at rest and is due to increased metabolism, respiratory myopathy, altered lung mechanics, and cardiac dysfunction. Excessive circulating thyroid hormones enhance central respiratory drive through enhanced adrenergic stimulation since beta blockade restores normal ventilatory drive in patients with thyrotoxicosis. There is increase in respiratory rate and oxygen consumption. Dyspnoea in thyrotoxicosis may be secondary to cardiac involvement such as cardiomyopathy with congestive cardiac failure, pleural effusion and pulmonary oedema. Occasionally, hyperthyroidism may have benign, often mild and asymptomatic thymic hyperplasia. Rarely thymic hyperplasia may present with anterior mediastinal mass and cause dyspnoea by extrinsic compression of trachea.

Proximal Myopathy

Proximal myopathy with significant decrease in inspiratory and expiratory maximal pressures and exercise intolerance due to muscle dysfunction are seen in significant number of cases with thyrotoxicosis. The respiratory muscle strength is related to severity of thyrotoxicosis with marked decrease in muscle strength in severe cases. Treatment of thyrotoxicosis reverses respiratory muscle dysfunction.

Pulmonary Functional Abnormalities

Pulmonary functional abnormalities in the form of decrease in vital capacity and lung compliance with normal diffusion capacity for carbon monoxide and increased work of breathing are observed.

Bronchial Asthma

Worsening of coexistent bronchial asthma has been observed in hyperthyroidism possibly due to increased bronchial reactivity consequent to reduced beta adrenergic responsiveness and down regulation of beta receptors. Treatment of hyperthyroidism helps control asthma in such cases. Bronchodilator therapy may not benefit much since bronchodilators accelerate metabolic rate. Beta blockade to treat hyperthyroidism may worsen asthma. Similarly, thyroxine treatment of hypothyroidism in asthmatics may worsen asthma.

Miscellaneous Effects

Iodinated glycerol, a mucolytic agent for treating chronic obstructive pulmonary disease (COPD) can induce thyrotoxicosis in those with subclinical hyperthyroid state. Potassium iodide used in the past as an expectorant, can aggravate asthma by inducing thyrotoxicosis. Aspiration pneumonia due to bulbar palsy, a known complication of thyrotoxicosis can occur. Granulocytopenia due to administration of thiourea to thyrotoxicosis can lead to pulmonary infections.

Hypothyroidism

Hypothyroidism affects respiratory system in several ways:

Hypoventilation

Hypoactivity of respiratory centre with depressed hypoxic and hypercarbic ventilatory drive is seen in 10% of patients with myxoedema. Reduction of hypoxic ventilatory response is more marked than the reduction in hypercapnoic ventilatory response. Thyroid hormone replacement in these cases promptly restores normal hypoxic response though there is delay for restoration of normal hypercapnoeic drive. 30 to 40% of hypothyroid cases have myopathy that manifests with respiratory muscle weakness with diminished maximal inspiratory as well as expiratory pressures and maximum voluntary ventilation with improvement on restoration of euthyroid state. Hypothyroid neuropathy particularly phrenic neuropathy with diaphragmatic muscle weakness presents with dyspnoea. Hypoventilation may be responsible for coma in one-third of patients with myxoedema coma, a condition common in elderly obese females with hypothyroidism.

Sleep Apnoea

It is observed in patients with hypothyroidism and associated obesity may be one of the confounding factors (Figs 23.5.4 and 23.5.5). 50% of hypothyroid cases have episodes of partial or complete upper airway obstruction during sleep as compared to 29% euthyroid control cases. Myxoedema coma that is rare now is probably due to severe sleep apnoea and hypercapnoeic respiratory failure. The causes of sleep-related breathing disorders in hypothyroidism include mucopolysaccharide and protein infiltrations in the upper airways and tongue, upper airway muscle dysfunction and reduced central drive to upper airway muscles. Sleepiness is a common

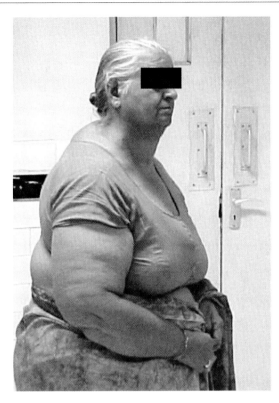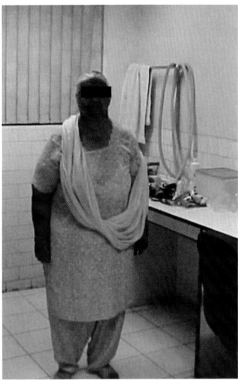

Fig. 23.5.4: Physical profile of a hypothyroid patient with obesity

symptom in hypothyroid state. Central sleep apnoea occurs in hypothyroidism due to abnormalities in ventilatory control with blunted hypoxic ventilatory response and is corrected by thyroid hormone replacement therapy which also resolves obstructive sleep apnoea. Besides sleep apnoea, primary central effects of hypothyroid state may be a cause for sleepiness. Sleep studies in hypothyroid cases reveal marked reduction in slow wave sleep.

Pleural Effusions

Pleural effusions either unilateral or bilateral can occur in hypothyroidism. The exact incidence of pleural effusion is not known. Up to 25% of cases have radiographic evidence of pleural effusions. Usually myxoedematous pleural effusions have concomitant pericardial effusion and, many have congestive cardiac failure and ascites. Hypothyroid related effusions are mild, detected on roentgenographic examination, transudates or exudates, generally non-inflammatory and resolve with therapy for hypothyroidism. Pleural effusion associated with pericardial effusion is a transudate. The pathogenesis of pleural effusion is controversial but increased pulmonary or pleural capillary permeability may play a role.

Miscellaneous

Hypothyroidism can result in alterations in pulmonary function tests and if associated with obesity the impairment is pronounced. Mild impairment of diffusion capacity for carbon monoxide with decrease in oxygen saturation and small increase in alveolar-arterial oxygen difference occur in hypothyroidism and these pulmonary functional abnormalitis may be due to ventilation perfusion mismatch. Hypothyroidism is associated with shift of oxygen dissociation curve to left, thereby worsening tissue supply of oxygen. Decrease in vital capacity in the absence of heart failure is noted in myxoedema and is most likely due to muscle weakness or myopathy. Adequate thyroid hormone therapy restores pulmonary functional abnormalities. In asthmatics, development of hypothyroidism results in reduced bronchospasm and improvement of asthma symptoms.

In hypothyroidism, roentegenographic abnormalities in the form of soft, patchy and nodular pulmonary infiltrates with resolution of lesions following thyroid hormone replacement have been reported. The exact cause of these infiltrates is not known and is attributed to atelectasis due to decrease in surfactant production. Thyroid hormone plays a vital role in growth and

Sleep Apnoea Report

WIFE OF H/CAPT RA SHARMA, 78

Date of Recording 8/25/05 (7 hours and 19 minutes, starting at 10:27:34 PM)

Apnea analysis   **AHI = 79.0**

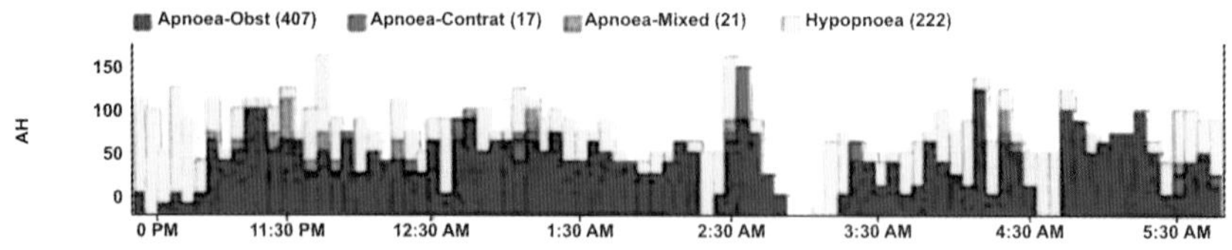

■ Apnoea-Obst (407)   ■ Apnoea-Contrat (17)   ■ Apnoea-Mixed (21) | Hypopnoea (222)

Respiration	Number	AHI	Mean	(±STD)	Shortest	Longest
Apnoea	445	61	20 s	(±11.5 s)	10 s	83 s
Obstructive	407	58	20 s	(±11.5 s)	10 s	83 s
Central	17	2	14 s	(±3.3 s)	10 s	20 s
Mixed	21	3	25 s	(±14.5 s)	12 s	66 s
Hypopnoea	222	30	25 s	(±15.6 s)	10 s	116 s
Total	578	79	21 s	(±12.6 s)	10 s	116 s

Oxygen saturation analysis   **ODI = 67.8**

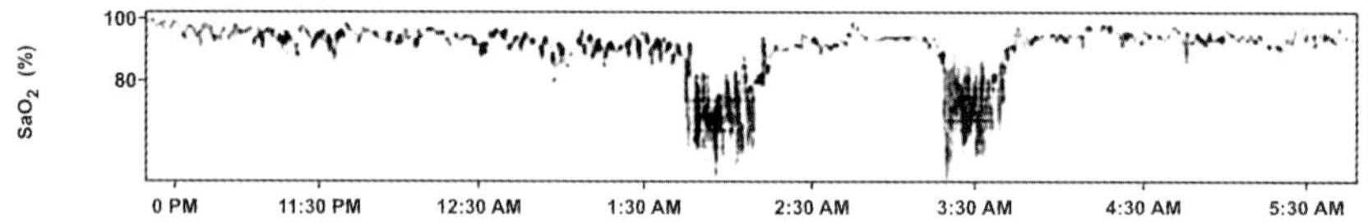

Desaturation	Number	Cumulative Number	ODI	Cumulative ODI
Total	496	496	68	68
2%	104	496	14	68
3%	103	392	14	54
4%-9%	237	289	32	39
10%-20%	27	52	4	7
>20%	25	25	3	3

Saturation	Mean	Base	(±STD)	Min	Max
	92	94	2	56	98

Fig. 23.5.5: Polysomnogram (PSG) of above patient showing severe obstructive sleep apnoea (OSA)

Comments: Overnight sleep study/polysomnography (PSG) is used to document sleep apneas in patients who have fragmentation of sleep with day time hypersomnolence. Sleep apnoea implies cessation of airflow at nose and mouth during sleep lasting more than 10 seconds. In central apnoea there is transient abolition of central respiratory drive. In obstructive sleep apnoea airflow ceases due to complete occlusion of upper airways at oropharyngeal level despite continued activation of inspiratory muscles. PSG in sleep apnoea syndrome reveals more than 5 episodes of apnoea per hour (apnoea index of 5 or more) with oxygen desaturation. PSG done in above patient shows severe OSA as evidenced by apnoea/ hypopnoea index of 79 (578 apnoeas/ hypopnoeas, 407 obstructive apnoeas, 496 oxygen desaturation events during 7 hours and 19 minutes of sleep) and oxygen desaturation index (desaturation events per hour of sleep) of 67.8 with minimal oxygen saturation of 56%. Such cases can develop sudden and catastrophic cardiovascular events during sleep

development of lung and maturation of lung surfactant system. Thyroid hormone levels in premature infants with respiratory distress syndrome are decreased and this may be related to decreased thyroxine binding to proteins. Pulmonary haemosiderosis has been reported in cases of thyrotoxicosis and autoimmune hypothyroidism.

Riedel's Thyroiditis

In this rare condition there is extensive and dense fibrosis of thyroid gland often extending to strap muscles and adjacent structures in the neck. Respiratory manifestation include airway obstruction due to extrinsic compression, both upper lobe fibrosis and lymphocytic interstitial pneumonia.

PARATHYROID DISORDERS

Parathyroid disorders affect respiratory system indirectly. Both hypoparathyroid and hyperparathyroid states are associated with muscle weakness, which can result in mild restrictive ventilatory defect. Parathyroid tumours may be located within thorax and are visible as anterior mediastinal masses on chest radiography. They are usually small and encapsulated. Mediastinal parathyroid can be identified in about 11% of cases who undergo surgical exploration for hypercalcaemia. It is observed that serum calcium levels are higher in those with mediastinal parathyroid tissue than in those with hyperactive parathyroid glands in neck. Ectopic parathyroid glands in thorax can be detected more accurately by sestamibi scintigraphy. Computerised tomography (CT), magnetic resonance imaging (MRI) and single photon emission tomography (SPECT) can find out the exact location of the gland in the thorax. Most of the ectopic intrathoracic parathyroid tumours are functioning and present with hypercalcaemia. Rarely, hypercalcaemic crisis with pulmonary oedema can occur. More often hypercalcaemic state is associated with metastatic calcification or calcinosis of the visceral organs. In the lungs, diffuse metastatic calcification are seen often in secondary hyperthyroidism of end-stage renal disease. Rarely it can occur in primary hyperparthyroidism. Metastatic calcification occurs when calcium-phosphorus double product increases above 70 mg^2/dl. In pulmonary metastatic calcification, the calcific nodules are distributed in the alveolar septa (with predilection for apical portions of the lungs possibly due to alkaline pH in these areas) and are associated with septal thickening and fibrosis. Bronchial and pulmonary arterial walls may also have foci of metastatic calcification.

Most of the patients with metastatic pulmonary calcification remain asymptomatic with normal lung functions. However, those with heavy calcification may have dyspnoea and dry cough. Metastatic calcifications in lungs are better visualised by CT thorax than by plain chest skiagram. Radionucleotide bone scans show increase uptake in the lungs and other affected organs. Parathyroidectomy or treatment with new vitamin D analogue can reverse organ calcium deposition.

Parathyroid cancer can present with respiratory symptoms either by laryngeal nerve involvement or by nodular pulmonary metastasis. Occasionally enlarged mediastinal parathyroid cysts may manifest with tracheal compression with stridor and/ or vocal cord impairment and hoarseness. Parathyroid surgery can cause airway obstruction by laryngeal spasm due to hypocalcaemia, compression of airways by haematoma and by vocal cord palsy due to recurrent laryngeal nerve injury.

ACROMEGALY

Acromegaly is characterised by additional bony growth and soft tissue proliferation in adults due to growth hormone excess. Patients have macroglossia, oropharyngeal airway narrowing, vocal cord restriction, and pneumomegaly. Pneumomegaly/large lungs defined by a vital capacity of more than 120% of predicted value is found in about 34% patients. Lung size is increased due to increase in alveoli and hypertrophy and over distension of individual alveoli. Lung volumes, total lung capacity, vital capacity, lung compliance and diffusion capacity are increased.

Sleep Apnoea

In acromegaly sleep disordered breathing is extremely common with reported occurrence of 39 to 91%. Both central and obstructive sleep apnoeas occur in acromegaly. Obstructive sleep apnoea occurs due to narrowed upper airways and is contributed by craniofacial changes and soft tissue proliferation of hypopharynx. There is osseous enlargement, swelling and hyperplasia of oropharyngeal soft tissues and macroglossia with subsequent collapse of upper airways during sleep. Flow volume loop exhibits variable extrathoracic obstruction in 30 to 50% of patients and intubations may be difficult in such cases. Thickening of laryngeal mucosa can cause stridor and progressive dyspnoea in some cases of acromegaly. In some cases somatostatin analogue-octreotide or pituitary ablation helps reduce obstructive sleep apnoea.

High prevalence of central sleep apnoeas due to abnormalities in central respiratory control has been observed in acromegaly with figures ranging from 34 to 66%. The precise cause of this is not known but has been attributed to alterations in central somatostatin pathways disinhibiting respiratory control, or due to effect of growth hormone on respiratory centre either directly or through metabolic alteration. Though there is defective respiratory control due to action of excessive growth hormone on respiratory centres, the hypercapnoeic response remains normal. Sleep apnoea may not resolve after cure of acromegaly. Sleep apnoea in acromegaly as well as acromegaly *per se* can contribute for the increased risk of hypertension in patients with acromegaly. Somnolence is one of the clinical features of acromegaly and is due to associated sleep apnoea besides direct effect of growth hormone in promoting sleep and effect of cranial radiotherapy used to treat acromegaly.

ADRENAL DISEASES

Respiratory system is involved indirectly in adrenal disorders. They include:

Mediastinal Lipomatosis

Abnormal deposition of fat occurs in anterior mediastinum (mediastinal lipomatosis) and in both pleuropericardial angles in cases of Cushing's syndrome and in those on long-term corticosteroid therapy. Chest skiagram in those with mediastinal lipomatosis shows widening of the upper mediastinum extending from thoracic inlet to both hila. CT thorax confirms diagnosis by demonstrating lipid density in the mediastinum.

Muscle Weakness

Electrolyte imbalance notably hyperkalaemia in adrenal insufficiency may present with muscle weakness. Cushing's syndrome may be associated with osteoporosis, wedge fractures of vertebrae and kyphosis with restrictive chest wall. Cushing's syndrome may be initial manifestation of bronchial carcinoids that may be occult on chest skiagram. CT thorax helps locate the disease in such cases.

Infections

Those with endogenous Cushing's syndrome due to various causes including small cell lung cancer, bronchial carcinoid, islet cell tumour of pancreas and adrenal neoplasia are prone to infections.

The hazard for infections particularly mucocutaneous fungal infections and opportunistic pulmonary infections are much more in those with ectopic tumours and adrenal neoplasia than pituitary Cushing's disease since they are associated with much higher cortisol levels. Those who are on long-term corticosteroid therapy are also prone to number of unusual and opportunistic infections. Most common pulmonary infections seen in such conditions associated with hypercortisolism are caused by *Cryptococcus, Aspergillus, Nocardia, Pneumocystis,* and *Mycobacterium tuberculosis. Pneumocystis carinii* pneumonia tends to occur in those with high morning cotisol levels. It is important to correct hypercortisolism while treating infections for better outcome. Asthmatics on high doses of aerosolized corticosteroid therapy are at increased risk of developing oropharyngeal candidiasis and also suppression of adrenal function.

MISCELLANEOUS

Adrenal insufficiency due to tuberculosis is common in India and other developing countries. Infants with adrenalin insufficiency are more prone for bronchopulmonary dysplasia.

Oedema due to catecholamine-induced cardiomyopathy can occur in phaeochromocytoma. Sudden surge of catecholamines from phaeochromocytoma can cause pulmonary oedema similar to neurogenic pulmonary oedema and manifests with severe respiratory distress. Rarely, haemoptysis due to paroxysms of hypertension seen in phaeochromocytoma can occur.

Paragangliomas

Paragangliomas are the tumours of extra-adrenal paraganglion system. Their common varieties include carotid body chemodectoma, glomus jugulare tumours and globus tympanicum tumours. Mediastinal paragangliomas are slow growing, locally invasive and indolent tumours with a high local recurrence. They are usually found in posterior mediastinum and above the aortic arch near subclavian arteries. They may be asymptomatic or present with hoarseness, cough, dysphagia and chest pain. Distant metastasis can occur. Extra-adrenal paraganglioma in association with pulmonary chondromata, multicenteric epitheloid leiomyosarcoma also known as "Carney triad" has clinical features of haemetemesis, anaemia, and hypertension with multiple pulmonary nodules and mediastinal widening on chest skiagram. Pulmonary lesions are usually uncalcified and cause no symptoms. Adrenal carcinoma with pulmonary metastasis is extremely rare.

REPRODUCTIVE SYSTEM DISORDERS

Respiratory manifestations are rare. Ovarian carcinoma may be associated with malignant pleural effusions. Benign ovarian tumour may present with Meig's syndrome that is characterized by unilateral (usually right sided) or bilateral pleural effusions and ascites. Pulmonary metastases occur with granulosa cell tumours, Sertoli-Leydig cell tumour and choriocarcinoma. In endometriosis, ectopic endometrial tissue deposits in pleura can occur usually on right side, which may complicate with pneumothorax during menstruation.

SUMMARY

Various endocrine conditions can affect respiratory system. Among them diabetes and hypothyroidism are common. In diabetes mellitus respiratory infections are common and they account for significant morbidity and mortality. Diabetics are particularly prone to develop tuberculosis and mucormycosis. In diabetes mellitus pulmonary tuberculosis may present with multilobar infiltrates, lower lobe lesions, cavitory lesions and pleural effusion. Pulmonary mucormycosis is characterized by propensity to invade vascular structures and airways and is associated with high mortality. In diabetes mellitus, lung is considered as a target organ with pulmonary microangiopathy. Various pulmonary dysfunctions related to severity of diabetes including reduced elastic recoil, impaired pulmonary diffusion and reduced lung volumes can occur. Diabetic autonomic neuropathy is associated with increased threshold for cough response, impaired ventilatory response to hypoxia, sleep-related disordered breathing, respiratory muscle weakness and hypoventilation. Diabetic ketoacidosis may be complicated by pulmonary oedema, hypokalaemic hypoventilation, pneumomediastinum, mucus plugging of airways and aspiration pneumonias. In acromegaly, pneumomegaly and sleep apnoea syndromes are common. Thyroid disorders affect respiratory systems in many ways. Goitres both intra- and extrathoracic cause extrinsic compression of airways. Intrathoracic goitre manifests as a mediastinal mass and may be complicated by dyspnoea, chronic cough, dysphagia, recurrent laryngeal nerve palsy, chylothorax and superior vena caval obstruction. Thyroiditis is associated with higher incidence of tracheoesophageal compression. Life threatening tracheal obstruction due to intrathoracic goitre occurs due to haemorrhage within the gland and malignancy. Thyrotoxicosis may manifest with dyspnoea at rest (thyrotoxic dyspnoea), respiratory muscle weakness and decreased lung compliance. In hypothyroidism decreased central ventilatory drive, obstructive sleep apnoea, hypoventilation, pleuro-pericardial effusions and shift of oxygen dissociation curve with tissue hypoxia are frequent which usually resolve with restoration of euthyroid state. In bronchial asthma with thyroid disorder, asthma control worsens in hyperthyroid state and improves in hypothyroid state due to alterations in the airway reactivity. Riedel's thyroiditis causes compressive symptoms due to dense fibrosis of thyroid and surrounding structures. Mediastinal parathyroid tumours are generally small and encapsulated and rarely present as anterior mediastinal mass. Hypercalcaemia is a feature of mediastinal parathyroid tumours and is associated with metastatic calcification. Cushing's syndrome and long-term corticosteroid therapy can result in mediastinal lipomatosis. Long-term corticosteroid therapy predisposes to opportunistic infections such as tuberculosis, *Pneumocystis carinii* pneumonia and cryptococcosis. Aerosolized corticosteroid therapy for asthma in mega doses is associated with oral candidiasis and suppression of adrenal functions. Phaeochromocytoma can cause both cardiogenic and non-cardiogenic pulmonary oedema. Mediastinal paraganglioma are indolent and locally invasive tumours. Diseases of reproductive system rarely manifest with respiratory involvement and ovarian tumours may present with pleural effusions.

FURTHER READING

1. Bacakoglu F, Basoglu OK, Cok G, et al. Pulmonary tuberculosis in patients with diabetes mellitus. Respiration 2001;68:595-600.
2. Brussel T, Matthay MA, Chernow B. Pulmonary manifestations of endocrine and metabolic disorders. Clin in Chest Med 1989;10:646-53.
3. Cooper BG, Taylor R, Alberti KG, et al. Lung function in patients with diabetes mellitus. Respir Med 1990;84:235-9.
4. Grunstein RR, Ho KY, Sullivan CE. Acromegaly and sleep apnoea. Ann Intern Med 1991;115:527-32.
5. Hansen IA, Prakash UBS, Colby TV. Pulmonary complications in diabetes mellitus. Mayo Clin Proc 1989;64:791-9.
6. Kim SJ, et al. Incidence of pulmonary tuberculosis among diabetics. Tubercle Lung Dis 1995;76:529-33.
7. Lamy AL, Fradet GJ, Luoma A, et al. Anterior and middle mediastinum paraganglioma: complete resection is the treatment of choice. Ann Thorac Surg 1994;57:249-52.
8. McElvancy GN, Wilcox PG, Fairbarn MS, et al. Respiratory muscle weakness and dyspnoea in thyrotoxic patients. Am Rev Respir Dis 1990;141:1221-7.
9. Prakash UBS, King, Jr. TE. Endocrine and metabolic diseases. In Crapo JD, Glassroth J, Karlinsky J, King, Jr. TE (Eds): Baum's Textbook of Pulmonary Diseases (7th edn). Philadelphia: Lippincott Williams and Wilkins 2004;1237-53.
10. Prasad GA, Sharma SK, Mohan A, et al. Adrenocortical reserve as morphology in tuberculosis. Indian J Chest Dis Allied Sci 2000;42:83-93.
11. Rajagopal KR, Abbrecht PH, Derderian SS, et al. Obstructive sleep apnoea in hypothyroidism. Ann Intern Med 1984;101:491-4.
12. Zimmerman L. Pulmonary complications of endocrine disease In Murray JF, Nadel JA, Mason RJ, Boushey HA (Eds): Textbook of Respiratory Medicine (3rd edn). WB Saunders Company, 2000;2309-15.

23.6 Skin and Endocrines

SK Sayal

INTRODUCTION

Skin, the largest organ of the body, is heterogeneous in composition having both cellular and non-cellular components, each cell having unique metabolic pattern. A wide variety of biochemical reactions occur in skin, some of which are governed by hormones. Consequently, endocrinal disorders exert profound effects on the skin, some of which can offer vital diagnostic clues to the alert and observant clinician.

EMBRYONIC DEVELOPMENT OF SKIN

All constituents of skin are derived from either ectoderm or mesoderm. The epidermis, epidermal appendages, namely hair follicles, sebaceous glands, apocrine glands, eccrine glands and nail units are ectodermal in origin. Melanocyctes, nerves and specialized sensory receptors originate from neuroectoderm. Other elements of skin, i.e. connective tissue, blood vessels, lymph vessels, muscles and subcutaneous fat originate from mesoderm.

Development of skin starts in 3 weeks old embryo with single layer of flattened epithelial cells. All layers of epidermis are developed by 6 months. Epidermal appendages start developing by 3 months and are complete by 7 months. Development of dermis from mesenchymal cells starts by 3 months and is complete by 8 months. By third trimester characteristics arterial and venous plexuses develop. Subcutaneous tissue develops by second trimester from the lobules of mesenchymal cells surrounding blood vessels. Finalization of structure and complete adult skin pattern is established by third trimester and continues in postnatal life.

The events of development of skin are basically genetically programmed. However, these may be partly governed by hormonal influences. Thyroid hormones play a pivotal role in the embryonic development of skin and maintenance of normal functions in adult also. They are necessary for initiation as well as maintenance of hair growth and for normal secretion of sebum. Sebaceous glands also require androgens for their development.

STRUCTURE AND FUNCTIONS OF SKIN

Skin is composed of 3 distinct components. From above downwards they are epidermis, dermis and subcutaneous tissue. Epidermis is cellular structure. Keratinocytes are the predominant cells which are arranged in different layers, i.e. basal layer, spinous layer, granular layer and cornified layer. Other cells of epidermis are melanocytes (in basal layer), Langerhans' cells (in spinous layer), and Merkel's cells (in basal layer). Dermis consists mostly of connective tissue composed of collagen fibres, elastic fibres and ground substance, all derived from fibroblasts. Within dermis are epidermal appendages, i.e. hair follicles, sebaceous glands, apocrine sweat glands, eccrine sweat glands, errector pilorum muscles, blood vessels, lymph vessels, nerves and specialized nerve endings. Beneath dermis lies the subcutaneous tissue, which consists of lobules of adipocytes.

Through these structures, skin performs several important functions:
- Protective functions from external physical, chemical and biological insults (keratinocytes).
- Barrier function to loss of fluid, electrolytes, etc. (keratinocytes).
- Pigment production and photoprotection (melanocytes).
- Immunological functions (Langerhans' cells).
- Sensory perceptions (cutaneous nerves, free nerve endings and specialized receptors).

The author is grateful to Professor (Brigadier) JS Saini VSM for allowing him to print some of his patients' photographs

- Temperature regulation (cutaneous vasculature, eccrine sweat glands).
- Regulation of fluid and electrolytes (sweat glands).
- Seceretory and excretory functions (sweat glands).
- Synthesis of vitamin D (keratinocytes).
- Synthesis and storage of fat (adipocytes).
- Psychosexual functions (texture of skin, hair and nails).

EFFECTS OF ENDOCRINE HORMONES ON SKIN FUNCTIONS

Endocrine glands secrete a variety of hormones, which may have direct influence on the development of different structures of skin and their functions. These influences are either positive (stimulate) or negative (inhibit). Hormones can also have effects on skin indirectly as a result of generalized derangement in endocrinal disorders. Table 23.6.1 summarizes the effects of endocrine hormones on skin.

Thyroid Hormones

- Thyroid hormones have distinctive influence on the embryonic development of skin as well as on the maintenance of functions of adult skin.
- Increase epidermal mitotic activity and protein synthesis.
- Necessary for initiation and maintenance of hair growth and sebaceous secretion.
- Retard accumulation of mucin in dermis.
- Effects on heat production and altered cardiovascular dynamics.

Glucocorticoids

- Decrease dermal fibroblast activity thereby decrease mass of dermal connective tissue.

- Regulate diurnal variation in mitotic activity of epidermis.
- Stimulate hair growth and follicular keratosis.
- Cause altered distribution of subcutaneous fat.

Androgens

- Trophic actions on skin particularly sexual zones.
- Increase mitotic activity of epidermis.
- Stimulate growth and activity of sebaceous glands.
- Effects on hair growth (small amounts cause growth of pubic and axillary hair, moderate amount cause growth of facial, trunk and extremity hair whereas excessive amount in genetically predisposed cause loss of scalp hair).

Oestrogen

- Induce keratinization of vaginal mucosa.
- Suppress sebaceous gland activity.
- Stimulate melanocyte activity.

Pituitary Hormones

- Regulate activity of other endocrinal glands.
- MSH and ACTH stimulate melanocyte activity.

Parathyroid Hormone

- Regulates the flux of calcium between extra- and intracellular compartments in responsive tissues (kidney and bone).
- May affect collagen synthesis in dermal fibroblasts.
- Abnormalities in calcium and phosphate metabolism can produce skin changes.

CUTANEOUS MANIFESTATIONS OF ENDOCRINE DISORDERS

Endocrinal disorders result from imbalance in the feed back loops maintaining endocrine homeostasis.

TABLE 23.6.1

Hormones	Keratinocyte proliferation	Melanocyte activity	Hair growth	Sebaceous secretion	Fibroblast activity	Mucin deposition	Vascular dynamics	Lipo-genesis
Thyroid	+		+	+			+	
Corticosteroid	–		+		–			+
Androgen	+		+/–	+				
Oestrogen	+	+	–	–			+	+
Growth hormone	+	+			+			
MSH		+						
ACTH		+						
Insulin							+	+

Hormonal effects on various components of skin

+ Stimulate/increase
– Inhibit/decrease

Derby Hospitals NHS Foundation Trust
Library and Knowledge Service

Endocrine dysregulation of skin functions produces manifestations in skin and in some instances, the initial and most prominent features of endocrine disorders are related to alterations in skin. Cutaneous manifestations of some common endocrinal disorders are described in Tables 23.6.2 to 23.6.7.

TABLE 23.6.2

	Thyroid hormone excess (Graves' disease, subacute thyroiditis)	Thyroid hormone deficiency (hypothyroidism)
Physical skin changes	• Peripheral vasodilatation. Increased blood flow Skin warm, moist, smooth. Increased sweating	• Vasoconstriction. Reduced core body temperature skin cold, dry xerotic. Decreased sweating (Figs 23.6.1 to 23.6.3)
	• Persistent flush of the face.	• Pale skin (deposition of mucin).
	• Redness of the elbow and palmar erythema.	• Yellowish hue in palms, soles, nasolabial folds (accumulation of carotene in stratum corneum) (Figs 23.6.5).
Hair	• Scalp hair fine and soft, diffuse alopecia, alopecia areata.	• Hair coarse and brittle, hair growth slow in scalp, beard and sexual areas. Patchy alopecia. Diffuse thinning of scalp hair. Loss of outer third of eyebrows and diminished body hair.
Sebaceous glands	• Less oily secretion.	• Sebum secretion decreased.
Nails	• Onycholysis (Plummer`s nails).	• Brittle and slow growing.
Specific	• Pretibial myxoedema—localized thickened, oedematous plaques on legs.	• Myxoedema—entire skin puffy with boggy non-pitting oedema due to deposition of mucin in dermis (Fig. 23.6.4).
		• Characteristic facial changes: Nose broadened, lips thickened, tongue enlarged, smooth (Figs 23.6.6 and 26.6.7).
Miscellaneous	• Generalised pruritus.	
	• Chronic urticaria.	• Poor skin healing.

Cutaneous manifestations of thyroid dysfunctional states

TABLE 23.6.3

	Excess Hypercortisolism (Cushing's syndrome, Cushing's disease, Non-pituitary neoplasia, exogenous glucocorticoids)	Deficiency Addison's disease (Primary adrenal failure, secondary adrenal failure)
Physical skin changes	• Fat deposition in certain areas (clavicle and back-buffalo hump); abdomen, cheeks-(moon facies), loss of subcutaneous fat of extremities, truncal obesity	—
Texture	• Thin, atrophic, friable	—
	• Striae	
Sebaceous gland	• Acne	—
Vascular	• Telangiectasia, petechiae, ecchymoses (Vascular fragility)	
	• Purplish mottling of lower extremities cutis marmarota (decreased vascular tone)	
Pigmentary	• Hyperpigmentation in Cushing's disease.	
	• Acanthosis nigricans.	• Hyperpigmentation—diffuse but especially involving sun exposed areas, areas of trauma, naturally pigmented areas, sexual areas, etc. (Figs 23.6.8 and 23.6.9)
Hair	• Hypertrichosis	• Loss of body hair—diffuse; mostly in axillae.
Infections	• Increased proneness for bacterial, fungal, candidal infections.	• Mucocutaneous candidiasis

Cutaneous manifestations of adrenocortical disorders

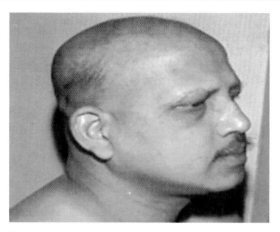

Fig. 23.6.1: Polyglandular syndrome with alopecia

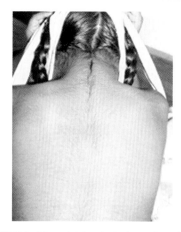

Fig. 23.6.4: Hypertrichosis in hypothyroidism

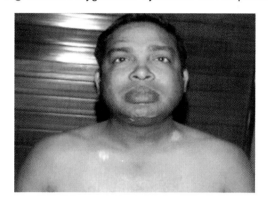

Fig. 23.6.2: Hypothyroidism with vitiligo

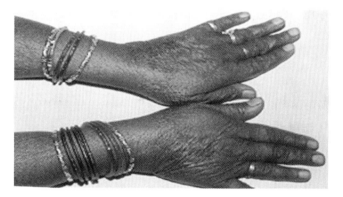

Fig. 23.6.5: Xerosis in hypothyroidism

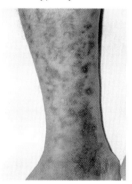

Fig. 23.6.3: Vasculitis in hypothyroidism

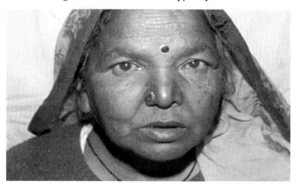

Fig. 23.6.6: hypothyroid facies
(Broad nose, madarosis, thick lip, puffy face)

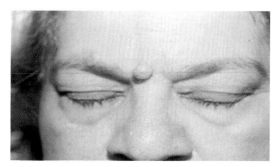

Fig. 23.6.7: Xanthelasma in hypothyroidism

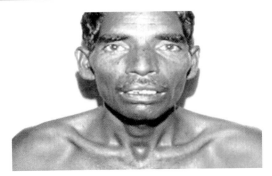

Fig. 23.6.8: Hyperpigmentation in Addison's disease

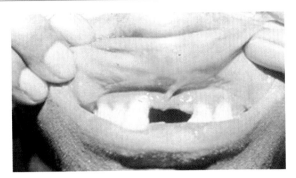

Fig. 23.6.9: Gingival pigmentation in Addison's disease

TABLE 23.6.4

	Excess	Deficiency
ANDROGENS		
Females	• Virilization • Hirsutism • Alopecia (diffuse) • Acne • Increased oiliness • Male pattern baldness in genetically predisposed	• Decreased oiliness • Improvement in acne a. Onset before puberty Eunuchoidism absent/decreased beard, axillary, pubic hair. Small penis
Males	• No other detectable changes	b. Onset after puberty Little change in facial, truncal, pubic or axillary hair, decreased oiliness vasomotor phenomenon
OESTROGEN	• Precocious puberty (in preadolescent girls)	
Females	• Hyperpigmentation • Decreased oiliness of skin • Vascular changes—erythema, telangiectasia • Spider angioma	• Early onset menopause • Atrophy of genitalia • Atrophy of breast • Vasomotor instability
Males	• Gynaecomastia • Testicular atrophy • Features of androgen deficiency	• No detectable cutaneous change

Cutaneous manifestations of sex hormones abnormalities

TABLE 23.6.5

	Excess growth hormone	Deficiency panhypopituitarism
Texture	• Generalized thickening of skin with doughy feel, furrowing and increased folds (due to epidermal and dermal hyperplasia) especially over face and extremities.	• Pallor, yellow tinge • Increased sensitivity to sunlight
Hair	• Hypertrichosis—chest, extremities, pubes and axillae • Hyperpigmentation in 44% cases.	• Early loss of body hair • Less pigmentation of traumatized skin
Pigmentary	• Lower lip enlarged, macroglossia. • Nose—hypertrophic (Fig. 23.6.10).	• Face expressionless
Miscellaneous	• Pads of digits fleshy, fingers blunted, heel pad thickened • Nails thickened and hard • Excessive eccrine and apocrine sweating • Oily skin	• Fine wrinkling around eyes and mouth

Cutaneous changes in acromegaly and hypopituitarism

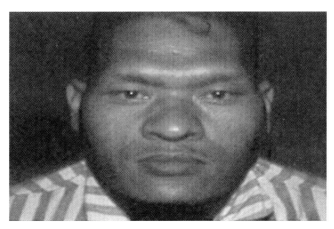

Fig. 23.6.10: Acromegaly facies

TABLE 23.6.6

	Parathyroid excess	Parathyroid deficiency
	Not associated with cutaneous manifestations except, rarely, pruritus and deposition of calcium	
Physical skin changes	—	Dry, scaly and puffy
Hair	—	Coarse and sparse
Nails	—	Opaque and brittle
Infections	—	Chronic mucocutaneuous candidiasis
Miscellaneous	—	Eczematous dermatitis maculopapular eruptions

Cutaneous changes in parathyroid disorders

HAIR AND ENDOCRINE HORMONES

Hormones may cause increase as well as decrease in growth of hair by affecting hair growth cycle and pattern of distribution of hair. There is interchange between vellus hair (soft, fine, lightly pigmented) and terminal hair (coarse, longer, pigmented). From the point of view of effects of hormones, hair can be grouped as nonsexual, ambosexual and male sexual types. The effects of hormones on hair has been summarised in Table 23.6.8

Though growth hormone basically determines growth of non-sexual hair, it plays synergistic role for androgenicity and secondary sexual hair. Deficiency of growth hormone results in loss of hair from scalp as well as pubic and axillary regions. Hair are thus under dual control of androgen and growth hormone.

TABLE 23.6.7

Metabolic disturbances
- Pruritus—Localized or generalized
- Xanthoma
- Carotenaemia

Infections
- Bacterial—Pyodermas, especially due to *Staphylococcus aureus*
- Fungal—Dermatophytosis, candidiasis, mucormycosis

Vascular manifestations
- Pretibial pigmented patches (diabetic dermopathy)
- Rubeosis
- Atherosclerosis—Ischaemic skin ulceration, digital gangrene

Neurologic lesions
- Neurotrophic ulcer (Figs 23.6.11 and 23.6.12)
- Charcot's joints
- Amyotrophy

Lipodystrophic conditions
- Progressive lipodystrophy (cephalothoracic type
- Lawerence-Seip disease
- Lipodystrophy secondary to insulin injections

Skin lesions due to diseases associated with diabetes
- Acromegaly
- Haemochromatosis
- Porphyria cutanea tarda
- Cushing's syndrome
- Werner's syndrome
- Mauriac's disease

Unexplained associations
- Kyrles's disease
- Reactive perforating collagenosis
- Asymptomatic parotid gland enlargement
- Kaposi's sarcoma
- Granuloma annulare
- Necrobiosis lipoidica
- Bullous diabeticorum
- Scleroedema adultorum
- Vitiligo
- Alopecia areata
- Acanthosis nigricans
- Dupuytren's contracture
- Peyronie's disease

Drug reactions
- Insulin preparations—Local wheal, urticaria
- Oral hypoglycemic compounds—Allergic and photosensitive skin eruptions

Cutaneous lesions associated with diabetes mellitus

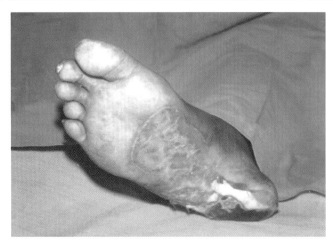

Fig. 23.6.11: Diabetic foot

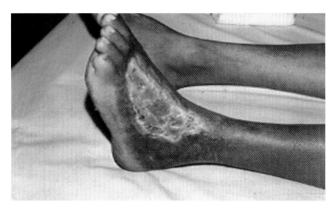

Fig. 23.6.12: Peripheral vascular disease in diabetes mellitus with ischaemic cutaneous ulceration left foot

The individual variation is genetically determined and not solely governed by androgen levels. Regional differences in hair growth are dependent upon the capability of target site to convert testosterone to dihydro-

testosterone (DHT). The final outcome of hormonal events on the hair follicles are determined by:
a. 5-alpha reductase activity, which converts testosterone to more active dihdrotestosterone.
b. Sex hormone binding globulin (SHBG). More the level of SHBG, less is the availability of free androgen and vice versa.
c. The presence of receptors at the target site.

Other hormones that affect the growth of hair are oestrogen and thyroid hormones. Oestrogen prolongs the growing stage (anagen) of hair. Postpartum reduction in oestrogen level cause shedding of hair (Telogen effulvium). Low level of thyroid hormones leads to thinning and sparsening of hair. High level may also have similar effects.

Hirsutism

Hirsutism is a response of hair follicle to androgenic stimulation and therefore an indication of hyper-androgenism. Hirsutism can be defined as male pattern of hair growth in a female. It has profound cosmetic and psychological implications. However, hirsutism is more often a relative term in vogue depending upon the social and acceptable hair growth pattern in females in a particular race, geographical region. It can occur alone or as a component of virilization. Table 23.6.9 enumerates the common causes of hirsutism and usual investigational results seen.

Approach to a Case of Hirsutism

An approach to a case of hirsutism is outlined in Table 23.6.10. History taking and clinical examinations are important. Detailed endocrinal investigations are required in cases in whom onset is in childhood, or is sudden in nature, has a rapid course or is associated with virilization or menstrual irregularity.

TABLE 23.6.8

Types of hair	Hair regions	Pre-pubertal	Post-pubertal	Hormones	Source
Nonsexual	Eyebrows, eye lashes	Terminal	Terminal		
	Forearms, legs	Vellus	Terminal	Growth	Pituitary
	Lower part of scalp	Terminal	Terminal	hormone	
Ambosexual	Axillary and lower pubic triangle	Vellus	Terminal	Androgens in low concentration	Adrenals and ovaries (Females)
	Temporal and vertical regions of scalp	Terminal	Vellus		Adrenals (Male)
Male sexual	Beard, moustache, trunk (sternal) upper pubic triangle	Vellus	Terminal	Androgens in high concentration	Testes
	Temporal and vertical regions of scalp	Terminal	Vellus		

Hormonal classification of hair pattern

TABLE 23.6.9

Causes	Clinical features	Investigations
Idiopathic	Often familial clustering. Mediterranean or Asian background	Normal
Polycystic ovary syndrome/tumour	Obesity, oligomenorrhoea or secondary amenorrhoea, infertilty	• LH : FSH ratio > 2.5 : 1 • Minor elevation of androgen • Mild hyperprolactinaemia • Normal 17 oxosteroid excretion • Enlarged sclerocystic ovary
Congenital adrenal hyperplasia (95% 21 hyroxylase deficiency)	Pigmented Jewish background, history of salt wasting in childhood, ambiguous genitalia, adrenal crisis when stressed	• Increased androgen levels which suppress with dexamethasone • Abnormal rise in 17 OH progesterone with ACTH
Androgen secreting tumours of ovary or adrenal cortex	Rapid onset, virlization (Husky voice, coarse skin, increased muscle mass, breast atrophy, clitoromegaly) male/female pattern alopecia, acne vulgaris/acanthosis nigricans	• High androgen levels which do not suppress with dexamethasone or oestrogen • Low LH, FSH • 17 oxosteroid excretion increased.
Cushing's syndrome	Moon facies, buffalo hump, truncal obesity thin limbs, facial plethora, purple striae, poor wound healing	• Normal or mild elevation of adrenal androgen • Loss of normal circadian rhythm for cortisol • Blood sugar may be high
Exogenous androgen administration (Androgens, anabolic steroids, oral contraceptives, glucocorticoids, minoxidil, phenytoin, diazoxide, psorlen, etc.)	Athletes, virilization	• Low LH, FSH • Increased urinary pregnanetriol • Androgen detection depends on which steroid is being taken

Causes of hirsutism and related investigations

Male Pattern Alopecia (Androgenetic Alopecia)

This term was coined by Orentreich in 1960. It refers to common type of male baldness having frontotemporal recession and vertical thinning and loss of hair in genetically predisposed individuals under the influence of androgens. Although varied pattern are seen, but in males bitemporal recession and loss of hair from the vertex, the so called Hamilton pattern is the commonest. Occipital and parietal regions are spared. Women have relative sparing of frontal hairline and have more diffuse loss. Also known as Ludwig pattern. In both sexes, genetically predisposed hair follicles undergo changes involving shortening of anagen phase of hair cycle with consequent increase in the proportion of telogen hair, a phenomenon called as 'miniaturization,' the resultant structural changes from terminal hair to finer hair and ultimately vellus hair.

These changes in the predisposed hair follicles take place with the conversion of testosterone to dihydrotestosterone by type II isoenzyme of 5 alpha reductase, the same isoenzyme which is also present in liver, prostrate, epididymis and seminal vesicles. Finasteride, an inhibitor of type-II isoenzyme is used for androgenetic alopecia.

Treatment

Male pattern alopecia in males is considered essentially a physiologic event. Although all adult women have alopecia, though of lesser degree, after menopause when oestrogen levels have declined and thus more androgenic environment prevails, women having profound androgenetic alopecia should be clinically assessed. History of amenorrhoea or oligomenorrhoea may indicate polycystic ovary disease, and galactorrhoea indicates increased prolactin levels. If features of cutaneous virilism like hirsutism are present, investigating for prolactin, LH, FSH and testosterone level is essential.

Effect of Hormones on Melanocytes

Marked regional variation is seen in the sensitivity of Melanocytes to specific hormones. The hormone induced and endocrine related changes in pigmentation might be summarized as under (Table 23.6.11).

TABLE 23.6.10

History	Onset:	Precocious	• Congenital adrenal hyperplasia
		Pubertal, post pubertal	
	Course:		• Ovarian causes
		Slow	• Polycystic ovary
		Rapid	• Tumour
	Family history:		
	Drug intake (glucocorticoids, anabolic steroid, oral contraceptives, etc.)		• Could be in all groups
			• Could be drug induced
	Menstrual history:		
	Oligomenorrhoea, amenorrhoea, infertility		• Polycystic ovary
	Acne vulgaris,		
	Male/female pattern alopecia		
	Acanthosis nigricans		• Hyperandrogenism
Clinical associations	Virilisation (Husky voice, coarse skin, increased muscle mass, clitoromegaly)		• Hyperandrogenism
	Moon facies, buffalo hump, truncal obesity, striae.		• Cushing's syndrome
	Imaging:		
	(Ultrasound, CT scan, MRI)		• For ovarian/adrenal/pituitary tumour/cyst
Investigations (Depending on merit of the case and in consultation with gynaecologist and endocrinologist	Hormone assay		
	a. LH and FSH		• Polycystic ovary
	LH:FSH>2.5		• Androgen secreting tumour
	Low LH and ↑FSH		• Exogenous androgens
	b. Androgen estimation (Testosterone, DHEAS)		
	Mild increase		• Polycystic ovary
	Considerable increase		• Androgen secreting tumour
	c. Cortisol:		
	Loss of circardian rhythm		• Cushing's syndrome
	d. Dexamethasone suppression test		
	Androgen secretion suppressed		• Congenital adrenal hyperplasia
	Androgen secretion not suppressed		• Androgen secreting tumour
	Cortisol level not suppressed		• Cushing's syndrome tumour
	e. Other hormones assay		For more detailed work up

Approach to a case of hirsutism

TABLE 23.6.11

Increased pigmentation		Decreased pigmentation	
Generalised	*Localised*	*Generalised*	*Localised*
Adrenal	Pregnancy and anovulatory drugs	Panhypopituitarism	Vitiligo associated with thyroid diseases, Addison's disease
Ectopic ACTH and MSH, and MSH producing neoplasms	Acanthosis nigricans associated with endocrinopathies	—	—
Thyrotoxicosis	Neurofibromatosis and phaeochromocytoma	—	—

Endocrine related changes in pigmentation

Oestrogen and progesterone augment pigmentary changes at specific sites in pregnancy, resulting in hyperpigmentation of nipples areola, linear nigra and melasma. The latter is accentuated by ultraviolet rays.

Acanthosis Nigricans

Hyerpigmented soft velvety excrescences usually seen in obese individuals, also seen in endocrinal disorders like diabetes mellitus, lipodystrophic diabetes, adrenal insufficiency, hyperpituitarism and Cushing's disease.

Chloasma (Syn. Melasma)

It is another common condition seen in women of reproductive age and may be regarded as physiological changes of pregnancy. In some cases it is associated with the use of oral contraceptives. Occasionally, it is also seen in males. An endocrine mechanism is postulated but its nature is unknown. It manifests as hyperpigmented macules on cheeks, nose, forehead, chin and other areas It becomes more apparent following sun exposure.

Hypopigmentation

Hypopituitarism is associated with generalized hypopigmentation, pallor and failure to tan because of deficient stimulus in form of ACTH and MSH for melanocytes.

Localised Depigmentation

It, in form of vitiligo, is associated with thyroid disorders, Addison's disease and diabetes. Myxoedema, thyroiditis and thyrotoxicosis are the commonest thyroid problems to be associated with it. In Addison's disease it may be superimposed upon hyperpigmentation. Vitiligo may even precede these disorders.

Sebaceous Glands and Acne

Sebaceous glands and hair follicles are predominantly the target for sex hormones, though other hormones also have influence on these glands.

Effect of Sex Hormones

Androgens

Sebaceous glands on face, upper back and chest are dependent upon androgenic stimulus for their development as well as the activity. Androgens cause acne not only by increase in the size of sebaceous glands but also due to increase in mitotic activity and cellular turnover, and thus increased sebum production, as these are holocrine glands. Glands are rudimentary before puberty. Under the influence of androgen these enlarge and sebaceous production increases multifold. In males it is mainly the androgen of testicular origin and partly from adrenals, whereas in females ovaries and adrenal both contribute to androgen production and causation of Acne. Adrenal androgen affects sebum production also by getting converted to testosterone.

Acne bearing skin produces 2 to 20 times more dihydrotestosterone (DHT) than normal skin. Regional differences in acne are thus dependent upon the capability of sebaceous glands to convert testosterone to DHT. It is dihydrotestosterone, the more active metabolite of testosterone, which is the stimulus for sebaceous activity. The reaction is carried out by 5 alpha reductase, isoenzyme type I, which is present in the sebaceous glands and also in epidermal and follicular keratinocytes. Isoenzyme type II of same enzyme is present in selective hair follicles on scalp and also in prostrate, epididymis and seminal vesicles. Therefore, the antiandrogen which inhibit isoenzyme type II have action on sex organs and scalp hair but no effect on acne. Steroid antiandrogen like cyproterone acetate, progesterone and 17 methyl nortestosterone inhibit sebaceous activity by lowering level of androgen and also reducing cellular division in sebaceous glands.

Oestrogen

Conversely oestrogen inhibits sebum production by decreasing cellular turnover time, as well as size of the glands.

Progesterone

It is a competitive inhibitor of 5 alpha reductase and therefore might reduce sebaceous activity, but paradoxically it has also been found to increase sebum production and cause acne when given to elderly women.

Non-sex Hormones and Acne

Adrenocortical hormones—ACTH causes hypertrophy of sebaceous glands in prepubertal males and postpubertal females. Exogenous corticosteroids, anabolic steroids, gonadotrophin and contraceptive pills cause acne mainly over shoulders and upper arm and much less on face. Such acne is monomorphic and lacks comedones.

Pituitary hormones act on sebaceous glands directly as well as through other endocrinal glands. Growth hormone has direct stimulant effect on sebaceous glands, whereas ACTH has effect through adrenal androgen. Thyrotrophic hormone acts through thyroid gland.

Endocrinal disorders which affect sebum production may be due to:
a. Adrenal tumours, Cushing's disease and adrenogenital syndrome causing excess androgen production and therefore increased sebum and acne.
b. Ovarian disease, e.g. tumour or polycystic disease of ovary.
c. Acromegaly (see Fig. 23.6.11)

Isotretinoin, a vitamin A derivative is nonhormonal substance having antiacne activity. It reduces sebum production by decreasing size of sebaceous gland, decreasing 5 alpha reductase activity and its anti-inflammatory effect.

The various influences of hormones in causation of acne are operative under physiological conditions also and are apparent at adolescence, when there is insurgence of sex hormones. Individuals who develop acne at unusual age, or have continuation of acne till fourth decade, when sebaceous activity is expected to be low, may have acneform eruptions or endocrine acne. The term endocrine acne should be reserved only when patient has other features of endocrinal disease like Cushing's disease, adrenogenital syndrome and polycystic ovarian disease. Hormonal assay and investigation for underlying likely cause are warranted only in such cases.

Effects of Hormones on Dermis

Corticosteroid hormones accelerate the catabolism of collagen and thereby reduce collagen synthesis by fibroblasts. Therefore, in Cushing's syndrome, skin becomes relatively transparent, gives a plethoric look and causes atrophic striae to look purple. Lack of support to vasculature, because of decreased collagen causes easy bruisability and ecchymosis, poor wound healing is attributed to diminished fibroblastic activity.

Growth hormone increases fibroblastic proliferation and increased laying down of collagen. Thyroid and sex hormones affect the metabolism of dermal glycosamino-glycan. Therefore, there is accumulation of glycosamine specially hyaluronic acid in the dermal ground substance. Hyaluronic acid being hydrophilic gives rise to doughy non pitting swelling of skin in hypothyroidism. Pretibial myxoedema is due to localized collection of mucin in the anterolateral aspect of legs, generally in Graves' disease under the influence of TSI. These appear as waxy plaques with prominent hair follicles giving the "peau d'orange' appearance. Localized hypertrichosis may be seen. Sex hormones also affect glycosaminoglycan metabolism.

In hyperthyroidism there is hyperdynamic circulation and therefore increase in cutaneous flow resulting in increased sweating. Oestrogen levels may be increased in pregnancy, in patient on oestrogen therapy or due to reduced degradation in hepatic disorders, which accounts for palmar erythema and spider angiomas in these patients.

Multiple factors operate to cause various alterations in vasculature in diabetes mellitus. The clinical manifestation are governed by the size of vessels involved, peripheral large vessel insufficiency resulting from concominant arteriosclerosis results in hair loss, shiny skin and cold distal parts of extremities, specially legs causing leg ulcers and propensity to gangrene, microagiopathy associated with diabetes further accentuates the damage. Microangiopathy is in form of basement membrane thickening and intimal proliferation resulting in endarteritis obliteration. Necrobiosis lipodica diabeticorum, diabetic bullae and pigmented spots over legs are also attributed to vascular changes.

Necrobiosis Lipodica Diabeticorum

The earliest lesions are sharply elevated papules, which do not disappear under diascopy. These develop into round or oval sclerotic plaques having glazed surface, the centre becomes depressed and attains yellowish hue in which telangiectasia may be seen. The classical lesions are well defined hard, depressed, waxy, yellowish atrophic patches on the skin. More than half of the patients have diabetes mellitus or abnormal glucose tolerance test but it is only a small proportion of diabetics (0.3%) who have these lesions. Female to male ratio is 3:1.

Histopathologically, there are necrobiotic foci of collagen looking pale, homogeneous and without nuclei, elastic fibres being absent. A palisading granuloma consisting of Langhans' giant cells, monocytes and lymphocytes is seen in vicinity of degenerating collagen, predominantly in perivascular region.

SUMMARY

Skin is an organ with heterogeneous cellular and non-cellular components. It comprises of rapidly proliferating keratinizing epidermal cells and hair follicles, sebum producing sebaceous glands, pigment producing melanocytes, dermal connective tissue responsible for production of fibrous tissue and ground substance, lipid synthesizing and storing subcutaneous tissue. Each cellular component has its own distinctive metabolic pattern and therefore skin is capable of performing a wide variety of biochemical activities.

Endocrine glands secrete a variety of hormones, many of them are associated with embryonic development, growth and maintenance of cutaneous structures and influence their functions and regulate cutaneous homeostasis. Hormones themselves get metabolised in the skin to become activated. The clinical features of effects of hormones range from physiological changes to the manifestations of hyper- or hyposecretion. The changes may be alteration in texture, sebum production, sweating, dermal changes or other effects. Depending upon the level of melanocyte stimulating hormone (MSH) and adrenocorticotrophic hormone (ACTH), there can be hyperpigmentation or hypopigmentation, either diffuse or at specific sites.

Sebaceous glands have receptors for androgens, which determine the severity of acne by increasing the size of sebaceous gland as well as sebum production. It requires conversion of testosterone to dihydro-testosterone (DHT) by 5 alpha reductase which is present at the target sites. Other factors also operate simultaneously.

Hair at various sites and at different periods of life, under physiological conditions respond to androgens to give the characteristics pattern of their distribution in pre- and postpubertal stage and differences in males and females. The common male pattern baldness is determined largely genetically under the influence of dihydrotestosterone (DHT) on selective hair follicles on scalp. Females also develop androgenetic alopecia but of more diffuse nature. However, when associated with features of endocrinal dysfunction, it warrants investigations. Hirsutism in the same way should be analyzed cautiously, whether in the realms of physiological limits or beyond it, keeping in mind the racial and geographical variations. Alterations in hair can also be caused by thyroid hormones, which also influence texture of skin, sweating, vascular response and deposition of mucin (ground substance) in dermis. Corticosteroids reduce collagen synthesis by suppressing fibroblastic activity and also cause redistribution of subcutaneous fat leading to a variety of manifestations.

In this subsection an updated, comprehensive analysis of mechanism of actions of endocrine hormones on skin and their correlations with cutaneous manifestations of hormones excess and deficiency have been discussed so as to harmonize the diagnostic approach.

FURTHER READING

1. Fenigold KR, Elias PM. Endocrine-skin interactions. J Am Acad Dermatol 1987;17:21-40.
2. FreinkelR K, Freinkel N. Dermatological manifestations of Endocrine disorders. In Fitzpatrick TB, Eisen AZ, Wolff K, Freedberg K, Austen KF (Eds): Dermatology in General Medicine. New York: Mc Graw Hill 1986;2063-81.
3. Glass RH. Hirsutism. In Speeroff L, Kase N G (Eds): Clinical Gynaecologic Endocrinology and Infertility.Baltimore.Williams and Wilkins 1999;746-8.
4. Grando SA. Physiology of Endocrine Skin Interrelations. J Am Acad Dermatol 1993;981-92.
5. Jakubovic HR, Ackerman AB. Development, morphology and physiology of skin. In Moschella SL, Hurley HJ (Eds): Dermatology. Philadelphia: WB Saunders 1985;1-74.
6. Parker SH. Skin and hormones. In Textbook of Endocrinology. Philadelphia: WB Saundars 1991;1080-96.
7. Paus R, Cotsarelis G. Hair disorders. In Thiers BH, Lang PG (Eds):Yearbook of Dermatology and Dermatologic Surgery Mosby 1999;194-6.
8. Rittmaster RS, Loriaux DL. Hirsutism. Ann Intern Med 1987;106:221-47.
9. Siddappa K, Ravindra K. The skin in systemic disease. In Walia RG, Valia AR (Eds): IADVL Textbook of Dermatology. Bhalani 2001;1048-53.
10. Weismann K, Graham RM. Systemic diseases and skin. In Champion RH, Burton JL, Burns DA, Breathnach (Eds): Rook, Wilkinson, Ebling Textbook of Dermatology. Blackwell Science1998;2703-77.

23.7 Endocrine Manifestations of Systemic Disease

KM Suryanarayan, Narendra Kotwal, SP Kalra

INTRODUCTION

Hormones are produced by various endocrine glands and their overproduction or deficiency affect most body systems to a greater or lesser extent. However, many hormone secretions occur as a result of ectopic hormone production, various systemic diseases and are not due to the intrinsic disease of endocrine glands. The endocrine responses may be adaptive in nature to the stress induced by these illnesses or manifestation of biological changes precipitated by the nonendocrine disorders. Medical, surgical and psychiatric disorders often have repercussion on the endocrine system. The endocrine manifestations of systemic disease in this chapter, will be broadly outlined under the following groups.

- Paraneoplastic endocrine syndromes
- Euthyroid sick syndrome
- Endocrine abnormalities in chronic renal failure
- Endocrine abnormalities in sarcoidosis
- Endocrine abnormalities in leprosy
- Endocrine abnormalities in malnutrition
- Endocrine abnormalities in fluorosis.

PARANEOPLASTIC ENDOCRINE SYNDROMES

Paraneoplastic endocrine syndromes are caused by factors produced by cancer cells that often act at a distance from both the primary cancer site and its metastases. Mostly the tumours are derived from neuroendocrine or neural crest tissue such as small cell lung cancer, carcinoid tumours. The genetic mechanisms involved are not clear. Oncogenes may activate other cellular genes, including genes that encode hormones, which are normally silent. Alternatively, demethylation of normally methylated inactive genes may permit expression in rapidly dividing cells. The three major classes of hormones are steroids, monoamines and peptides. Malignant tumours rarely produce steroid

hormones. Lymphomas produce 1, 25-dihydroxy vitamin D from circulating 1-hydroxy vitamin D and it results in hypercalcaemia. Epinephrine and norepinephrine, which are monoamines are not ectopically secreted by malignant cells. Ectopic peptide hormone production results in most of the paraneoplastic endocrine syndromes. A peptide hormone is generally encoded by mRNA that is translated into a larger prohormone molecule, which undergoes a number of post-translational modifications. Tumour cells may produce proteins that are immunoreactive but biologically less active than the normal hormones. The severity of paraneoplastic endocrine syndrome often parallels the clinical course of the cancer. Hormones even though produced by tumour cells, are not very good tumour markers (Table 23.7.1).

Baylin and Mendelsohn have established validation criteria for ectopic hormone production that include:

a. Clinical or biochemical evidence of abnormal endocrine function in a patient with a tumour.
b. Cessation of endocrine abnormality after ablation of tumour.
c. Presence of an arteriovenous gradient across the tumour vascular bed.
d. Demonstration of hormone in tumour tissue and documentation of hormone synthesis by tumour cells in culture of extraction of appropriate mRNA from the tumour.

Hypercalcaemia of Malignancy

Hypercalcaemia of malignancy is the most common paraneoplastic syndrome. It is responsible for approximately 40% of all hypercalcaemia and is usually caused by increased bone resorption by skeletal metastases or the production of PTHrP. PTHrP is composed of 139 to 173 amino acids and produces most of the biologic effects

TABLE 23.7.1

Syndrome	Proteins	Tumours typically associated with syndrome
Hypercalcaemia of malignancy	Parathyroid hormone-related peptide (PTHrP), Parathyroid hormone (PTH)	Non-small cell lung cancer Breast cancer Renal cell carcinoma Head and neck cancer Bladder cancer
Syndrome of inappropriate antidiuretic hormone scretion (SIADH)	Arginine vasopressin (AVP) Atrial natriuretic peptide	Small cell lung cancer Head and neck cancer Non-small cell lung cancer
Cushing's syndrome	Adrenocorticotrophic hormone (ACTH) Corticotrophin-releasing hormone (CRH)	Small cell lung cancer Carcinoid tumours
Acromegaly	Growth hormone-releasing hormone (GHRH), growth hormone (GH)	Carcinoid tumours Small cell lung cancer Pancreatic islet cell tumours
Gynaecomastia	Human chorionic gonadotrophin (hCG)	Testicular tumour Lung cancer Carcinoid tumours of the lung and gastrointestinal tract
Non-islet cell tumour	Insulin-like growth factor-2 (IGF-2)	Sarcomas

Common paraneoplastic endocrine syndromes

of PTH by acting on PTH receptor in the bone and kidney. The various actions that result in hypercalcaemia include increased bone resorption, decreased bone formation, increased renal tubular reabsorption of calcium, increased phosphaturia, and also from increased levels of urinary cyclic AMP. Ectopic production of PTH is very rare. Hypercalcaemia in lymphomas can occur due to production of metabolically active 1,25 dihydroxy vitamin D [1, 25(OH)$_2$ D]. Breast and lung cancers are among the most common PTHrP producing tumours. Certain cytokines, notably IL-1 and growth factors, notably TGF-β, can also produce hypercalcaemia by stimulating osteoclastic bone resorption. All patients with underlying cancer and hypercalcaemia should be initially evaluated to rule out other causes of hypercalcaemia including hyperparathyroidism. A normal PTH level in the absence of bone metastases supports the diagnosis of PTHrP related hypercalcaemia. The median survival in cancer patients with hypercalcaemia of malignancy is only a few months and treatment should be directed to ameliorate the acute metabolic effects of hypercalcaemia.

Syndrome of Inappropriate Antidiuretic Hormone Secretion (SIADH)

A primary defect in arginine vasopression (AVP) secretion or action can result in osmotically inappropriate

antidiuresis. SIADH is characterized by hyponatraemia secondary to increased total body water as a result of impaired renal free water excretion. There is failure to suppress AVP secretion even when the plasma osmolality falls below the normal osmotic threshold for stimulating AVP secretion. Ectopic production of AVP by lung cancer or other neoplasm results from unregulated expression of AVP-NPII gene. The ectopic release of AVP in acute infections and strokes results in SIADH. The underlying mechanism which disrupts autoregulation is not known. Clinical criteria for diagnosis of SIADH include:

a. The patient must have true hypoosmolality with a urine osmolality that is greater than maximally dilute (i.e. > 100 mOsm/kg H$_2$O).
b. Elevated urine Na$^+$ excretion), i.e. 30 mmol/L).

Approximately 10 to 20% of patients who fulfil the criteria for SIADH do not have measurably elevated plasma AVP levels. When the hyponatraemia develops gradually it may not produce any symptoms. However when it develops acutely, features of acute water intoxication in the form of headache, vomiting, seizures and altered sensorium can occur. Restriction of fluid intake to less than the sum of insensible losses and urine output is important in the management of patients of SIADH.

Ectopic Pro-opiomelanocortin or ACTH Syndrome

Ectopic ACTH syndrome is a unique disorder of pro-opiomelanocortin (POMC) gene expression in non endocrine tumours. They constitute a small but significant percentage of patients presenting with clinical hypercortisolism.

Tumours associated with the ectopic ACTH syndrome are:
- Small cell lung cancer
- Non-small cell lung cancer
- Pancreatic tumours (including carcinoids)
- Thymic tumours (including carcinoids)
- Lung carcinoids
- Medullary carcinoma of thyroid
- Phaeochromocytoma and related tumours
- Rare carcinoma of prostate, breast, ovary, gall-bladder, colon.

The clinical presentation depends on the nature of underlying tumour. Indolent tumours, such as benign bronchial carcinoids that produce ACTH, present with clinical features that are typical of Cushing's syndrome and may be biochemically similar to patients with Cushing's disease. Cases occurring in the setting of highly malignant tumours such as small cell carcinoma of bronchus exhibit high circulating ACTH levels and cortisol secretion rates. As a result, the duration of symptoms from onset to presentation is short, patients are pigmented, and metabolic manifestations of glucocorticoid excess are often rapid and progressive. Weight loss, myopathy and glucose intolerance are prominent features. The diagnosis is established by the demonstration of ACTH dependent Cushing's syndrome with elevated cortisol and ACTH levels, absence of suppression of cortisol on high dose dexamethasone suppression test. Imaging studies will facilitate localization of the lesion. Management depends on the nature of underlying tumour.

Non-islet Cell Tumour and Hypoglycaemia

In patents with non-islet cell tumours of pancreas such as sarcomas, mesotheliomas and hepatomas, production of insulin like growth factor-2 (IGF-2) is responsible for hypoglycaemia. The IGF-2 may act as autocrine growth factor for the tumour. Hypoglycaemia results from the metabolic actions of IGF-2, which are similar to that of insulin and with classical symptoms occurring particularly in the fasting state. Diagnosis is mostly made on clinical grounds, as plasma IGF-2 levels are typically not elevated. However, the levels of IGF binding proteins may be elevated. In those patients where successful resection of tumour is not possible, conservative therapy with frequent oral feeds and intravenous glucose infusion will be helpful to overcome the hypoglycaemic symptoms.

Gynaecomastia

Gynaecomastia can be a manifestation of paraneoplastic syndrome. Altered ratio of oestrogen to testosterone leads to proliferation of breast tissue and gynaecomastia. Ectopic production of hCG is the commonest cause and leads to increased oestrogen production by Leydig cells in testes. Alternatively aromatase enzymatic activity in a tumour such as hepatoma or germ cell tumour with choriocarcinoma elements can result in conversion of circulating androgens to oestrogens. Evaluation includes examination of testes, serum hCG measurement and to detect any underlying malignancy. The therapy of gynaecomastia is directed towards the underlying cancer.

Ectopic Acromegaly

Growth hormone releasing hormone (GHRH) stimulates the secretion of growth hormone (GH) in adenohypophysis which in turn increases production of insulin like growth factor (IGF-1) in peripheral tissues. Ectopic production of GHRH is the predominant cause of ectopic acromegaly and very rarely ectopic production of GH by tumours may be the cause. Ectopic acromegaly is rare disease and clinical features develop over several years. Carcinoid tumours of the bronchus, pancreatic islet tumours and small cell lung cancer can be associated with ectopic acromegaly. Diagnosis is established in a patient of cancer with acromegaly by nonsuppressed serum GH levels to glucose, as well as by demonstrating elevated serum GHRH and IGF-1 levels. Management consists of surgical resection of underlying tumour or radiotherapy. Long-acting somatostatin analogue (octreotide) reduces pituitary GH secretion and can be used to relieve symptoms.

EUTHYROID SICK SYNDROME

The global pattern of changes in thyroid physiology that occur during illness in the absence of underlying thyroid disease is known as euthyroid sick syndrome, non-thyroid illness or the low T_3 syndrome. Similar physiological changes occur during fasting but to a lesser extent. The fall in T_3 may provide a mechanism for limiting catabolism during starvation or severe illness. The changes in thyroid function are a continuum, with the abnormalities becoming progressively more severe in accordance with the patient's clinical condition and changes can be arbitrarily divided into three stages. These alterations reverse after recovery from illness, confirming the absence of underlying thyroid disease. The major cause of these hormonal changes is attributed to the release of cytokines.

Stage 1. In patients with mild illness, generally there is a reduction of upto 50 percent in circulating T_3, a modest increase in serum rT_3, but no change in serum free T_4, total T_4 or TSH. T_4 conversion to T_3 via peripheral deiodination is impaired, leading to increased rT_3. Despite this effect, decreased clearance rather than increased production is the basis for increased rT_3.

Stage 2. The clearance of T4 is significantly reduced but pulsatile TSH secretion persists, leading to a modest increase in free T4. This is generally accompanied by further decrease in serum T_3 and increase in rT_3.

Stage 3. These changes occur in addition to loss of pulsatile secretion of TSH and a fall in T4 and T3 levels. The T4 level may be initially normal but is eventually reduced. Serum rT_3 levels are elevated earlier, but return to normal later if T_4 levels fall. Total serum T_3 may be almost undetectable. Mortality is high at this stage of disease.

In addition to central changes to TSH regulation and the abnormalities in peripheral hormone metabolism, changes in circulating binding proteins and reduction in TBG affinity can occur. Therapeutic agents, such as dopamine, dobutamine and glucocorticoids which act on the central thyroid axis and suppress TSH may complicate the abnormality. The level of TSH, which is reduced during acute illness may increase above normal range during recovery and persist till T_3 and T_4 levels return to normal. The picture can meet the biochemical criteria for primary hypothyroidism. However, follow-up generally reveals normalization within one or two months. Despite the severity of these abnormalities, most controlled studies have failed to show any benefit of T_3 or T_4 supplementation in these critically-ill patients. It is documented that there is significant inverse relationship between severity of reduction in serum T_4 concentration in non-thyroidal illness and mortality rates.

ENDOCRINE ABNORMALITIES IN CHRONIC RENAL FAILURE

Endocrine abnormalities are common and develop early in chronic renal failure with moderate renal insufficiency but become more manifest as renal failure progresses. The pathophysiologic mechanisms for these abnormalities may include.

- Decreased synthesis of hormones, endogenous and exogenous to the kidney.
- Reduced metabolic clearance of hormones by renal and extra-renal mechanisms.
- Alteration in homeostatic signalling mechanisms.
- Altered hormone binding.
- Altered tissue responsiveness to hormones.

Erythropoietin Deficiency

Erythropoietin is a hormone endogenously synthesised by the kidney and foetal liver. It is derived mostly from interstitial cells in the renal cortex and stimulates erythroid precursors in bone marrow to sustain normal erythropoiesis. Regulation of erythropoietin secretion is by tissue oxygen sensing mechanisms that may be mediated by intracellular redox conditions and also by haemproteins. As kidney failure progresses, erythropoietin production typically decreases. Impaired erythropoietin production is the major factor in the anaemia of chronic renal failure. Occasionally, patients of chronic renal failure due to cystic diseases of kidneys may not have severe anaemia due to preservation of normal erythropoietin secretion. Recombinant human erythropoietin (EPO) has been extensively used in the treatment of anaemia of chronic renal failure.

Vitamin D and PTH Metabolism

The kidney is the major site of conversion of vitamin D to its active metabolites. Vitamin D derived from diet or; synthesized in the skin undergoes initial hydroxylation in liver to form 25 hydroxy vitamin D [25(OH)D] by hepatic mitochondrial and microsomal enzymes and subsequently to 1,25 dihydroxy vitamin D [1,25(OH$_2$) D] in the kidney. 1,25 dihydroxy vitamin D binding protein is delivered to various target organs. The active form of vitamin D acts directly on the parathyroid gland to suppress PTH secretion and enhance intestinal absorption of calcium and phosphate reabsorption and promote resorption of these ions from bone. In addition, 1,25 (OH$_2$) D probably opposes the phosphaturic actions of PTH in the renal tubule by augmenting rather than diminishing, phosphate reabsorption. Loss of nephron mass with advancing renal disease, leads to impairment of vitamin D hydroxylation. Phosphate retention also impairs vitamin D hydroxylation. The levels of 1,25(OH$_2$) D are diminished in circulation and the receptors that mediate its action in parathyroid glands are also diminished. The plasma PTH levels increase due to diminished inhibitory influences. The net result of these changes in chronic renal failure is hypocalcaemia and hyperparathyroidism. Phosphate retention occurs when

GFR falls below 25 ml/min. Resistance of bone to the calcaemic effect of PTH and reduced PTH degradation, by kidneys in uraemia also contributes to hyperparathyroidism, combination of hypocalcaemia; phosphate retention and hyperparathyroidism are the principal determinants of bone changes in renal osteodystrophy. Dialysis, dietary adjustments, therapy with vitamin D and phosphate binders is important tools in the management of this disorder.

Fertility and Sexual Dysfunction

Sexual problems such as decreased libido and infertility in males and females, erectile dysfunction in males and menstrual disorders in females affect many CRF patients. Abnormalities involving prolactin, gonadotrophin and gonadal steroids occur early in chronic renal failure, worsen as renal function deteriorates and get corrected on successful kidney transplantation. Hyperprolactinaemia due to increased production, is a common feature and does not respond to suppressive of stimulatory manoeuvres. A lack of midcycle LH and oestradiol peaks, absent progestational changes in endometrium denotes anovulatory cycles resulting in infertility in females Amenorrhoea is a common feature and does not respond to suppressive or stimulatory manoeuvres. The changes are attributed to hypothalamo-pituitary dysfunction. In males, reduction in testosterone levels occurs from blocking factor to LH at receptor level in Leydig cells. Low testosterone levels and decreased metabolic clearance of LH result in elevated LH levels. Impaired spermatogenesis leads to infertility in males.

ENDOCRINE ABNORMALITIES IN SARCOIDOSIS

Hypercalcaemia has been described in many granulomatous disorders and sarcoidosis in particular. Sarcoidosis is a chronic, multisystem, noncaseating epitheloid granulomatous disorder of unknown cause. Although lung is the most frequently affected organ, involvement of the skin, eye, liver and lymph nodes is also common. Diabetes insipidus can occur due to involvement of hypothalamic-pituitary axis. Rarely anterior pituitary, adrenals and reproductive organs can be involved resulting in hormone deficiencies.

Hypercalcaemia can rarely be a manifestation of sarcoidosis. Overproduction of the enzyme 25-hydroxylase D1-hyroxylase in macrophages increases conversion of 25 hydroxy vitamin D[25(OH)D] to its active form 1,25 dihydroxy vitamin D[1,25(OH$_2$)D] resulting in hypercalcaemia. Recent observations reveal that PTHrP produced by these macrophages can also produce hypercalcaemia. Glucocorticoids are the drug of choice in sarcoidosis and overall prognosis is good.

ENDOCRINE ABNORMALITIES IN LEPROSY

Testicular involvement in leprosy results in infertility and undervirilization. Testicular atrophy occurs in 10 to 20% of men with lepromatous leprosy as the result of invasion of the tissue by the bacilli. The result is a decreased plasma testosterone level and elevated plasma LH and FSH levels. Obstructive azoospermia due to obstruction of the ejaculatory system can also occur.

ENDOCRINE ABNORMALITIES IN MALNUTRITION

Malnutrition can have varied effects on various endocrine disorders. Iodine deficiency or excess results in varied thyroid dysfunction. Euthyroid or hypothyroid goitre may occur in iodine deficiency, depending on iodine levels and homeostasis. Antithyroid agents also occur naturally in foods. These are widely distributed in the family Cruciferae or Brassicaceae, particularly in the genus Brassica, including cabbages, turnips, kale, kohlrabi, rutabaga, mustard, and various plants that are not eaten by humans but that serve as animal fodder. It is likely that some thiocyanate is present in such plants (particularly cabbage). Cassava meal, a dietary staple in many regions of the world, contains linamarin, a cyanogenic glycoside, the metabolism of which leads to the formation of thiocyanate. Ingestion of cassava can accentuate goitre formation in areas of endemic iodine deficiency. Except for thiocyanate, dietary goitrogens influence thyroid iodine metabolism in the same manner as do the thionamides, which they resemble chemically; their role in the induction of disease in humans is uncertain. Water-borne, sulphur-containing goitrogens of mineral origin are believed to contribute to the development of endemic goitre in certain areas of Columbia. A number of synthetic chemical pollutants have been implicated in causing goitrous hypothyroidism, including polychlorinated biphenyls and resorcinol derivatives.

Malnutrition is associated with delayed puberty or failure to progress through the stages of puberty. It is necessary to distinguish the effects of malnutrition, which can lead to functional hypogonadotrophic hypogonadism, from the primary effects of the disease. In general, weight loss of any cause to less than 80% of ideal weight for height can lead to gonadotrophin deficiency and low serum leptin levels; weight regain usually restores hypothalamic-pituitary gonadal function over a variable period.

Inadequate caloric and protein intake is the most common cause of growth failure. Marasmus refers to cases with an overall deficiency of calories, including protein malnutrition. Subcutaneous fat is minimal, and protein wasting is marked. Kwashiorkor refers to inadequate protein intake, although it may also be characterized by some caloric undernutrition. In both conditions, multiple deficiencies of vitamins and minerals are apparent. Frequently, the two conditions overlap. Decreased weight growth generally precedes the failure of linear growth by a very short time in the neonatal period and by several years at older ages. Stunting of growth in early life has life-long consequences, resulting in diminished height growth.

Both acute and chronic malnutrition affects the GH-IGF system. The impaired growth is usually associated with elevated basal and stimulated serum GH levels, but in generalised malnutrition (marasmus) GH levels may be normal or low. In both conditions, serum IGF-I levels are reduced. Malnutrition may consequently be considered a form of Growth hormone insensitivity (GHI), with serum IGF-I levels reduced despite normal or elevated GH levels. GHBP levels, as a reflection of GHR content, are decreased. GHI may be an adaptive response, whereby protein is spared by the lipolytic and anti-insulin actions of GH. Reduced serum IGF-I levels would serve to shift calories from anabolic to survival requirements. These adaptive mechanisms are accompanied by changes in serum IGFBPs to further limit IGF action during periods of malnutrition.

ENDOCRINE ABNORMALITIES IN FLUOROSIS

Excess fluoride ingestion causes fluorosis, a painful condition associated with extraosseous calcification and brittle bones. High doses of fluoride can stimulate osteoblasts. However bone that is formed may be abnormal and the effect on fracture rates is unclear. Secondary hyperparathyroidism may occur due to decreased resorption of calcium from bones. Calcium and Vit D supplementation helps to ameliorate bone pains and altered calcium kinetics.

SUMMARY

Systemic disorders and general ailments affect many endocrine glands and reflect adversely on their hormonal values. As such the disturbed hormonal levels must be interpreted intelligently before initiating any hormonal therapy. The chapter covers some of the commonly seen systemic conditions which produce widely known and well documented endocrine manifestations.

FURTHER READING

1. Baylin SB, et al. Ectopic (inappropriate) hormone production by tumours. Mechanisms involved and the biological and clinical implications. Endocr Rev 1990;1:45-77.
2. Braunstein GD. Gynaecomastia. N Engl J Med 1993;328:490.
3. Chopra IJ. Euthyroid sick syndrome: is it a misnomer? J Clin Endocrinal metab 1997; 82: 329.
4. Ezzat S. Acromegaly. Endocrine Metab Clin North Am 1997;26:703.
5. Leonard J, et al. Hypercalcaemia in malignant and inflammatory diseases. Endocrine Metab Clin North Am 2002;31:141.
6. Sachdev YR. A clinical study of endocrine profile in protein-energy mulnutrition. Final report AFMRC project. 1239/81 of 1984.
7. Sachdev YR. Alterations in hypothalamic-anterior pituitary target gland axis in chronic renal failure MJAFI 1991;47:96-102.
8. Wajchenberg BL, et al. Ectopic adrenocorticotropic hormone syndrome. Endocr Rev 1994;15:752-87.

23.8 Syndromes of Ectopic Hormone Secretion

HB Singh, BN Kapur

INTRODUCTION

Tumours can produce signs and symptoms at sites distant from the primary or metastatic site and these signs and symptoms form what are called paraneoplastic syndromes. These syndromes are due to:
a. Tumour producing biologically active substances.
b. Depletion of an essential substance.
c. Host response to the tumour.

Biologically active substances secreted by the tumour range from hormones, to growth factors and cytokines to antibodies. This chapter will deal with paraneoplastic syndromes due to ectopic production of hormones.

HISTORY

In 1928, Brown first described the syndrome of ectopic secretion of corticotrophin (ACTH), 4 years before Cushing's description of the syndrome. In 1941, Albright recorded hypocalcaemia in renal cancers and suggested that tumours can secrete hormones. Hyponatraemia due to syndrome of inappropriate secretion of antidiuretic hormone (SIADH) seems to have been first described by Winkler and Crankshaw in 1938. In 1957, Schwartz demonstrated the presence of a substance with bio-assayable ADH activity in tumour tissue in bronchogenic carcinoma. In 1967, Bartter and Schwartz conceived of the syndrome of inappropriate ADH secretion and laid down the criteria for diagnosis but it was only in 1969 that Liddle coined the term ectopic hormone syndrome for such clinical situations.

The term ectopic does not mean that the hormone is secreted by tissues that normally do not do so. On the contrary, most of the secreted hormones are usually present in small amounts in the normal tissues (e.g.

vasopressin and ACTH in neuroendocrine cells that form small cell lung carcinoma (SCLC); parathyroid hormone related peptide (PTHrP) in squamous cells). It is the quantity produced that is out of place ("ectopic").

AETIOPATHOLOGY

There are a number of hypotheses regarding the aetiology of such syndromes as none offers a complete explanation. The simplest explanation for the secretion of hormones by tumour cells is the *"derepression"* hypothesis. It is known that every cell has the capacity to perform any task but once specialized, these genes are repressed. The derepression hypothesis assumes that control over the repressed genes are lost. However, loss of control should be random but as hormone secretion is specific to some tumours, this is an unlikely explanation.

Another hypothesis is the *"dedifferentiation"* hypothesis, whereby tumour cells transform retrogradely to their more primitive state and produce foetal proteins. While some tumours do produce foetal proteins (carcinoembryonic antigen or CEA, alfa-fetoprotein or AFP), there is no evidence of generalized pattern of expression of primitive genes.

The third *"dysdifferentiation"* hypothesis suggests that clonal expansion of a normally rare population of committed cells could lead to secretion of a hormone, or this could also be due to clonal expansion of a primitive cell type not normally present in mature epithelium.

Some tumours derive a growth advantage by secreting hormones, such as small cell lung carcinona (SCLC) that are stimulated by hormones such as GRP and beta-endorphins. Insulin like growth factor (IGF) II is another growth factor for some tumours.

COMMON CHARACTERISTICS

Features common to ectopic hormone syndromes include:
a. Association with advanced malignancy.
b. Loss of suppressibility by feedback mechanism due to autonomous nature.
c. Lack of use of such hormones as tumour markers.
d. Secretion of related or incompletely processed peptides to produce the syndrome.

DIAGNOSIS

Syndrome of ectopic hormone secretion should be suspected in two clinical situations:
a. Person of known malignancy where some signs and symptoms are not explained by the presence of either primary tumour or its metastases.
b. Person with an endocrine syndrome where the symptomatology/work-up shows ambiguous results.

Certain criteria have been drawn up to help in the diagnosis.

Clinical Criteria

a. Hormone excess associated with a neoplasm.
b. Inappropriately high plasma/urine levels.
c. Nonsuppressible hormone levels.
d. Other causal mechanisms excluded.
e. Reversible by resection of tumour.

Research Criteria

a. Detectable in tumour tissue (hormone or mRNA).
b. Detectable in culture of tumour tissue.
c. Arteriovenous gradient present across the tumour.

The strongest evidence of hormone secretion by a tumour, either the demonstration of an arteriovenous gradient of the hormone across the tumour, or reversal of the syndrome on resection of the tumour are infrequent occurrences and not often essential for the diagnosis.

COMMON ECTOPIC HORMONE SYNDROMES

1. Humoral hypercalcaemia of malignancy
2. Syndrome of inappropriate ADH (SIADH) secretion
3. Ectopic ACTH syndrome
4. Hypoglycaemia
5. Hypocalcaemia
6. Acromegaly.

Other syndromes are uncommon and are enlisted in Table 23.8.1.

TABLE 23.8.1

Conditions	Examples
1. Hypocalcaemia	Bone metastases due to breast cancer
2. Acromegaly	Carcinoids
3. Gynaecomastia	Germ cell tumours
4. Precocious puberty	Germ cell tumours
5. Oncogenous osteomalacia	Mesenchymal tumours
6. Erythrocytosis	Renal and hepatocellular carcinoma
7. Verner-Morrison syndrome	Neuroendocrine tumours
8. Glucagonoma syndrome	Neuroendocrine tumours

Less common ectopic hormone syndrome

Humoral Hypercalcaemia of Malignancy

Up to 40% of patients with cancer have hypercalcaemia at some point in their clinical course, making hypercalcaemia the most common paraneoplastic syndrome. Malignant tumours are the commonest cause of hypercalcaemia in hospitalized patients.

Lung cancer (squamous and large cell), breast cancer and multiple myeloma account for more than 50% of all cases. Other causes are given in Table 23.8.2.

TABLE 23.8.2

Malignancy	Frequency (%)
Lung (squamous and large cell)	35
Breast	25
Haematological (myeloma)	14
Head and neck	6
Renal	3
Prostate	3
Unknown primary	7
Others	7

Hypercalcaemia of malignancy

Humoral hypercalcaemia of malignancy is caused by the production of parathyroid hormone-related protein (PTHrP) by the tumour. This protein has homology with parathyroid hormone and similar functional activity, but they are structurally different. PTHrP increases bone resorption, renal resorption of calcium and phosphate excretion. It is associated most commonly with squamous cell carcinoma of the lung and has been purified from a cultured lung cancer cell line. Other mechanisms of hypercalcaemia associated with malignancy include direct bony metastases, hormonally mediated local activation of osteoclasts by cancers that have invaded bone, and rare production of steroid hormones (e.g. 1,25-dihydroxyvitamin D) by tumours.

Clinical features of hypercalcaemia include fatigue, lethargy, mental status change, weakness, abdominal pain, constipation, nausea, vomiting, anorexia, and polyuria. Laboratory features of hypercalcaemia with hypophosphataemia is consistent with the diagnosis of primary hyperparathyroidism except that the serum level of PTH is less than 20 pg/ml. Vitamin D level is also suppressed (exception: lymphomas). Electrocardiographic abnormalities occur, including prolongation of the PR interval, widening of the QRS interval, and shortening of the QT intervals, followed by bradycardia and finally heart block.

Patients with humoral hypercalcaemia have elevated levels of PTHrP by assay. This elevation is not detected by conventional assays for parathyroid hormone. Other causes of hypercalcaemia should be ruled out, including primary hyperparathyroidism; medications, such as thiazides and lithium; hyperthyroidism; sarcoidosis; and osseous metastases.

Prognosis of such patients is poor with a median survival of 4 to 8 weeks. However, breast cancer and multiple myeloma patient will survive longer (up to years with a good quality of life) and aggressive measures are indicated in these cases.

All cases of hypercalcaemia should be treated regardless of symptoms, if the serum calcium level is above 14 mg/dl (3.5 mmol/L) (the upper limit of normal being 10.5 mg/dl (2.6 mmol/L). Therapies include vigorous intravenous hydration with normal saline and the administration of diuretics once the intravascular volume has been repleted. Loop diuretics are the diuretics of choice because they promote calciuresis and avoid volume overload. Bisphosphonates, particularly pamidronate and more recently zoledronate are effective hypocalcemic agents but their effect is delayed. Dose of pamidronate is 90 mg infusion over 4 hours and of zoledronate is 4 mg over 15 minutes, in calcium free solutions. These agents function mainly by inhibiting osteoclastic bone resorption.

For immediate effect, other than hydration and frusemide, calcitonin is effective (2 to 8 U/kg IM or SC 6 or 12 hrly) but is infrequently available. Gallium nitrate is another effective therapy. Gallium also functions through the inhibition of osteoclastic bone resorption. It can worsen renal function by the formation of renal tubular plugs and is contraindicated in the presence of severe renal impairment. Close monitoring of renal function and the avoidance of other nephrotoxins are recommended in patients receiving the drug. Other treatment options include the use of plicamycin.

Humoral hypercalcaemia of malignancy develops in patients with advanced, aggressive cancer and is associated with an increased frequency of metastases and poor prognosis. As such, the clinician must consider the appropriatness of reversing the hypercalcaemia in malignancies other than those of breast and myeloma.

Half of lymphoma patients with hypercalcaemia have raised calcitriol levels due to unregulated extrarenal production of this hormone. As in sarcoidosis, this hypercalcaemia is responsive to steroids.

Rare causes of hypercalcaemia of malignancy include secretion of parathyroid hormone by the tumour, usually of neuroendocrine origin, and due to local osteolysis by various cytokines that can activate osteoclasts, such as TNF and IL-6.

Syndrome of Inappropriate ADH (SIADH)

SIADH is the second most common endocrine complication in cancer patients and hyponatraemia is a frequent finding in patients with lung cancer. It was originally described by Winkler and Crankshaw in 1938, and more fully by Bartter and Schwartz in 1957 who also laid down the criteria for it, viz:

a. Hyponatraemia with corresponding hypo-osmolality of the serum and extracellular fluid.
b. Continued renal excretion of sodium.
c. Absence of clinical evidence of fluid volume depletion (i.e. normal skin turgor and blood pressure).
d. Osmolality of the urine greater than appropriate for the concomitant osmolality of the plasma, i.e. urine less than maximally dilute.
e. Normal renal function.
f. Normal adrenal function.

It is more commonly a sign of small cell lung carcinoma (SCLC), where it is usually caused by the ectopic secretion of arginine vasopressin. Although most small cell lung cancer tissues stain positive for this hormone, only about 7 to 11% of individuals with SCLC actually develop SIADH. Up to 50% of small cell lung carcinomas have elevated levels of ADH, but fewer than 10% have clinically apparent disease.

Atrial natriuretic peptide also is produced ectopically in some patients. The contribution of this ectopic production to hyponatraemia is unclear.

The cardinal features of SIADH are water intoxication and hyponatraemia. Hyponatraemia rarely causes symptoms unless the serum sodium falls below 125 mmol/L. Symptoms are related to the rate of sodium decline more than the absolute value. Clinical features include mental status changes, confusion, lethargy, and seizures. Although the hyponatraemia is usually severe, only few patients are symptomatic at the time of diagnosis. The lack of symptoms at diagnosis is related to the prolonged period of time during tumour growth, in which the syndrome develops (i.e. slow rate of sodium decline).

SIADH is diagnosed by finding an inappropriately increased urinary sodium (> 20 mEq/L) and osmolarity in the setting of low serum sodium and reduced serum osmolarity. The ADH level is elevated. Other causes of SIADH (e.g. medications) and hyponatraemia (e.g. renal, adrenal, thyroid dysfunction) should be excluded.

Therapy should begin with treatment of the underlying tumour. SCLC is a chemosensitive tumour and chemotherapy leads to resolution of SIADH in most cases. Additional management of the hyponatraemia may be necessary while awaiting a response to chemotherapy or when the tumour is resistant to therapy. This management involves fluid restriction (800 ml to 1.0 L per day) and medications, such as demeclocycline, lithium carbonate, and phenytoin. These agents act by interfering with the effect of ADH at the collecting duct. Demeclocycline (600 to 1200 mg/day in divided doses) is the drug of choice because of the side effects of the other agents. Fludrocortisone (0.1 to 0.3 mg per day) is another option but side effects include fluid overload and CCF.

Administration of oral salt does not always help in such patients—this is thought to be due to rapid excretion of salt in urine, due to suppressed plasma aldosterone due to expanded plasma volume.

In severe, symptomatic hyponatraemia (< 120 mEq/L), hypertonic saline (3 or 5%) and/or a combination of saline and frusemide administration may be necessary. Rapid correction of hyponatraemia should be avoided because it may lead to central pontine myelinolysis. Recommended correction is a rate of 0.5 mmol/L/hour till serum sodium level reaches 120 to 125 mmol/L.

The prognosis of patients with small cell carcinoma and SIADH is similar to those without SIADH. Dilutional hyponatremia recurs in up to 70% of cases when the tumour relapses.

Ectopic ACTH Syndrome

Twenty per cent to 30% of Cushing's syndrome cases are caused by the ectopic production of adrenocorticotrophic hormone (ACTH). Lung cancer is the cause of this ectopic production approximately 50% of the time. Small cell carcinoma accounts for most cases, but carcinoid tumours and non-small cell carcinomas also have been responsible. Although up to 50% of patients with lung carcinoma may have elevated levels of ACTH by assay, case series report a prevalence of clinically significant disease of only 2 to 10% of individuals with small cell carcinoma and 0.4 to 2% of patients with lung cancer overall.

Normal human lung produces small amounts of the parent compound pro-opiomelanocortin (POMC). POMC is cleaved to pro-ACTH, ACTH, β-lipotropin, N-terminal peptide of POMC, and β-endorphin. Although the exact cause of ectopic Cushing's syndrome is not known yet, it is believed that the increase in POMC levels seen in the setting of malignancy is the result of overexpression of the gene responsible for its production.

In contrast to the female predominance of Cushing's disease, ectopic Cushing's syndrome occurs with equal frequency in men and women. The clinical manifestations of ectopic Cushing's syndrome are less prominent than with Cushing's disease because of the shorter time period that the individual is exposed to excessive ACTH because the underlying cancer is aggressive in nature. The classic symptoms are often absent and the entire syndrome rarely is observed. Peripheral oedema, proximal myopathy, and moon facies most commonly are reported, with weight loss being more common than weight gain. Hypertension is common. Biochemical abnormalities also differ. Hypokalaemia and alkalosis are seen in nearly all cases, and hyperglycaemia is present in most.

Carcinoid secreting ACTH is more likely to present with classical Cushingoid features such as moon facies, centripetal obesity, polydipsia and polyuria. Hyperpigmentation and hirsutism are also common.

The differential diagnosis of Cushing's syndrome includes Cushing's disease, adrenal dysfunction, ectopic Cushing's syndrome and corticotrophin releasing hormone (CRH) overproduction.

Tumours that produce ACTH include SCLC (45%), carcinoids (thymic/bronchial/others) (30%), islet cell tumours (10%), phaeochromocytoma (2%) and ovarian adenocarcinomas (rare).

The diagnosis of ectopic Cushing's syndrome is made by first finding an excess of cortisol and then determining whether this is ACTH dependent. An elevated 24-hour urinary free cortisol level and an elevated plasma cortisol level confirm the first level; and an elevated plasma ACTH that does not decrease after administering a high-dose dexamethasone suppression test (2 mg every 6 hours for a total of 8 dosages) are essential steps in the diagnosis.

Imaging studies (e.g. Chest X-ray, CT scanning, MR imaging, and radioactive isotope studies like somatostatin receptor scintigraphy) are then used to locate the source of ectopic production if not previously known. Inferior petrosal vein sampling, with or without corticotrophin releasing hormone (CRH) or metyrapone stimulation, is occasionally necessary to assist in the diagnosis.

The primary therapy of ectopic Cushing's syndrome is treatment of the underlying tumour, which is mainly by surgery. Adjuvant radiation to the tumour bed is given in some centres, while the role of chemotherapy is debatable, except in metastatic disease. If patients experience significant clinical effects from the hypercortisolism, cortisol production blockers (steroid synthesis inhibitors, "medical adrenalectomy"), such as aminoglutethimide (250 mg thrice daily, mitotane, metyrapone (250 to 500 mg thrice daily), and ketoconazole (200 to 400 mg twice daily), or suppressors of ACTH production, such as the somatostatin analogue octreotide have shown some efficacy. Bilateral adrenalectomy may be an effective therapy for the patient with refractory disease.

The presence of clinically apparent ectopic Cushing's syndrome (but not simply elevated ACTH levels) in the setting of small cell carcinoma has been associated with a reduction in responsiveness to chemotherapy, an increase in the rate of chemotherapy-related toxicity, an increase in the rate of severe opportunistic infection after the initiation of treatment, and decreased survival.

Cushing's syndrome due to secretion of corticotrophin releasing hormone (CRH) is rare.

Hypoglycaemia

Insulinomas produce hypoglycaemia but this is not an ectopic production. Hypoglycaemia due to non-islet cell tumours cause fasting hypoglycaemia and are true paraneoplastic syndromes. Fibrosarcomas, rhabdomyosarcomas, leiomyosarcomas, mesotheliomas and haemangiopericytomas account for 50% of cases while hepatocellular carcinomas, carcinoids and adrenocortical carcinomas account for another 25%. Infrequent causes include leukaemia and lymphomas.

Tumours cause hypoglycaemia by a variety of methods including production of insulin-like growth factors, hypermetabolism of glucose, liver damage, production of substances stimulating ectopic insulin release, insulin receptor proliferation and rarely, ectopic insulin production. However, the commonest mechanism is the production of insulin-like growth factors, IGF I and II (somatomedins), especially IGF II.

Standard treatment is the resection of the tumour; even partial debulking is sometimes effective. In case this is not possible or effective, medical methods include therapy with growth hormone, glucagon, steroids or somatostatin.

Hypocalcaemia

Hypocalcaemia is actually more common than hypercalcaemia in patients with lytic bone metastasis, but is usually asymptomatic. Bone metastasis due to cancer of breast, prostate and lung are common causes; rare causes include tumours that secrete calcitonin (such as medullary carcinoma of thyroid). Those with features of neuromuscular irritability (positive Chvostek's or Trousseau' sign) or frank tetany may need calcium infusions.

Acromegaly

Acromegaly due to non-pituitary tumours is rare (< 1%) and most are due to ectopic secretion of growth hormone releasing hormone (GHRH) secretion and not due to GH. Associated diabetes mellitus, amenorrhoea and galactorrhoea are common, as are other paraneoplastic syndromes like Cushing's syndrome, primary hyperparathyroidism and Zollinger-Ellison syndrome. Carcinoids are the commonest tumours causing acromegaly.

Hypothalamic tumours, including hamartomas, choristomas, gliomas and gangliocitomas are the usual causes of GHRH secretion. Immunoreactive GHRH is present in several tumours, including carcinoid tumours, pancreatic cell tumours, small-cell lung cancers, adrenal adenomas, and phaeochromocytomas which have been reported to secrete GHRH. Acromegaly in these patients however, is uncommon.

Standard treatment is surgery. Octreotide is the choice in unresectable cases.

MISCELLANEOUS HORMONES

Human chorionic gonadotrophin (hCG) can be produced by trophoblastic and germ cell tumours and can cause gynaecomastia and isosexual puberty. hCG producing tumours include lung, hepatocellular, adrenocortical and renal cancers.

Erythropoeitin produced ectopically has been implicated in erythrocytosis associated with renal carcinomas (1 to 4%), hepatocellular cancers (5 to 10%) and cerebellar haemangioblastomas. However, this relation is not consistent.

Calcitonin is usually produced by the C cells of the thyroid and is a normal product in medullary carcinomas of thyroid. Ectopic production of calcitonin is seen in SCLC, and in some other cancers and cause hypocalcaemia rarely.

Vasoactive Intestinal Peptide (VIP) is produced in pancreatic islet cells and also by other neuroendocrine tumours and cause pancreatic cholera (also called Verner-Morrison syndrome or WDHA - watery diarrhoea, hypokalaemia, achlorhydria). Somatostatin and its analogues are effective in these tumours.

Rare syndromes are produced by the ectopic production of somatostatin, glucagons, GRP, endothelin, human placental lactogen (hPL), prolactin, TSH, etc. The latter is occasionally associated with gestational trophoblastic disease and produce hyperthyroidism. Ectopic luteinising hormone (LH) secretion has been associated with anovulation.

Oncogenic osteomalacia is a rare condition usually associated with benign mesenchymal tumours. Raised levels of fibroblast growth factor-23 (FGF-23) is associated with renal loss of phosphates, leading to a condition resembling X-linked hypophosphataemic rickets with osteomalacia. The condition dramatically responds to the removal of the tumour; if however, the tumour is not resectable or cannot be found, calcitriol and oral phosphates are the treatment of choice.

SUMMARY

Ectopic hormone syndromes are a fascinating but infrequent cause of endocrine syndromes. A high clinical index of suspicion and active search is needed to diagnose these cases. They are frequently missed as they occur in advanced cases of malignancies that are potentially incurable. However, the exceptions to this rule must be remembered (e.g. hypercalcaemia in breast cancer and multiple myeloma) and early diagnosis and aggressive management could result in good quality of life for years in this subgroup.

FURTHER READING

1. Arnaldi G, Angeli A, Atkinson AB, et al. Diagnosis and complications of Cushing's syndrome: a consensus statement. J Clin Endocrinol Metab 2003;88:5593-5602.
2. Berensen JR. Treatment of hypercalcaemia of malignancy with bisphosphonates. Semin Oncol 2002;(6 Suppl 21)12-8.
3. Beuschlein F, Hammer GD. Ectopic pro-opiomelanocortin syndrome. Endocrinol Metab Clin North Am 2002;31:191-234.
4. Body JJ. Hypercalcemia of malignancy. Semin Nephrol 2004;24:48-54.
5. Bollanti L, Riondino G, Strollo F. Endocrine paraneoplastic syndromes with special reference to the elderly. Endocrine 2001;14(2):151-7.
6. Carpenter TO. Oncogenic osteomalacia—a complex dance of factors. N Engl J Med 2003;348:1705-8.
7. De Herder WW, Lamberts SWJ. Tumor localization-the ectopic ACTH syndrome.J Clin Endocrinol Metab 1999;84:1184-5.
8. Doga M, Bonadonna S, Burattin A, Giustina A. Ectopic secretion of growth hormone-releasing hormone (GHRH) in neuro-endocrine tumours: relevant clinical aspects. Ann Oncol 2001;12 Suppl 2:S89-94.
9. Hirshberg B, Conn PM, Uwaifo GI, et al. Ectopic luteinizing hormone secretion and anovulation. N Engl J Med 2003;23: 348:312-7.
10. Isidori AM, Kaltsas GA, et al. Discriminatory value of the low-dose dexamethasone suppression test in establishing the diagnosis and differential diagnosis of Cushing's syndrome. J Clin Endocrinol Metab 2003;88:5299-306.
11. Janicic N, Verbalis JG. Evaluation and management of hypo-osmolality in hospitalised patients. Endocrinol Metab Clin North Am 2003;32:459-81, vii.
12. Mazzone PJ, Arroliga AC. Endocrine paraneoplastic syndromes in lung cancer. Curr Opin Pulm Med 2003;9:313-20.
13. Newell-Price J. Proopiomelanocortin gene expression and DNA methylation: implications for Cushing's syndrome and beyond. J Endocrinol 2003;177:365-72.
14. Newell-Price J, Trainer P, Besser M, Grossman A. The diagnosis and differential diagnosis of Cushing's syndrome and pseudo-Cushing's States. Endocrine Reviews 1998;19:647-72.
15. Reimondo G, Paccotti P, Minetto M, et al. The corticotrophin-releasing hormone test is the most reliable noninvasive method to differentiate pituitary from ectopic ACTH secretion in Cushing's syndrome. Clin Endocrinol (Oxf). 2003;58:718-24.
16. Terzolo M, Reimondo G, Ali A, Bovio S, et al. Ectopic ACTH syndrome: molecular bases and clinical heterogeneity. Ann Oncol 2001;12 (Suppl 2):S83-7.
17. Tomassetti P, Migliori M, Lalli S, et al. Epidemiology, clinical features and diagnosis of gastroenteropancreatic endocrine tumours. Ann Oncol 2001;12 (Suppl 2):S95-9.
18. Wong LL, Verbalis JG. Systemic diseases associated with disorders of water homeostasis. Endocrinol Metab Clin North Am 2002; 31:121-40.

23.9 Hormones and Cancer

Ajit Venniyoor, BN Kapur

INTRODUCTION

The development of four major cancers-breast, endo-metrial, ovarian, and prostate—are affected by hormones in the body. There are many hormonal agents used in the treatment of patients with cancer. The primary use of these agents is in hormonally responsive cancers such as breast, prostate, or endometrial carcinomas. Other indications for some hormonal therapy include paraneoplastic syndromes, such as carcinoid syndrome, or symptoms caused by cancer, including anorexia.

BREAST CANCER

Therapy of breast cancer is a multimodality discipline. It depends on stage and hormone positivity. It involves a combination of chemotherapy, surgery, radiotherapy and hormonal therapy. The sequence being dictated by the stage of the tumour. Simultaneous exhibition of hor-mones and chemotherapy is not recommended.

Hormones have been used before surgery (neo-adjuvant setting), after surgery (adjuvant setting) or metastatic setting.

There are two major types of breast cancer. In hormone-dependent breast cancer, the tumour cells have Oestrogen receptors (ER positive tumours) and need Oestrogen to grow. In hormone-independent breast cancer, the cells lack oestrogen receptors (ER negative tumours) and oestrogen is not required for tumour growth.

Oestrogen (Table 23.9.1)

The connection between breast cancer and oestrogen has been recognized for more than a century. It was demons-trated that bilateral oophorectomy resulted in the cure of breast cancer in premenopausal women. Oestrogens promote the development of mammary cancer by both direct and indirect proliferative effects on cultured

TABLE 23.9.1

Risk factors	Low risks	High risks
Menarche age	> 14 years	<12 years
Age at birth of first child	< 20 years	$\geq$ 20 years
Breast-feeding	> 16 months	0 month
Parity	> 5	0
Menopause age	<45 years	>55 years
Serum oestradiol	Lowest quartile	Highest quartile
Bone density	Lowest quartile	Highest quartile
Oestrogen therapy	Never	Current
Oral contraceptives	Never	Ant point of time
Breast density on mammogram	0	>75
Postmenopausal BMI	<30	>30

Hormonal indicator of breast cancer risk factors

human breast-cancer cells. The risk of breast cancer could be determined by the cumulative exposure of breast tissue to oestrogen. Indirect evidence of this sequence includes the increased risk of breast cancer associated with early menarche, late first full-term pregnancy, and late menopause as well as the reduced risk associated with early menopause. The predictive value of these factors for risk of breast cancer is increased by combi-nation of these factors. Tumour-initiating effects may occur, through the activation of oncogenes and through the production of growth factors, e.g. transforming growth factor and epidermal growth factor. Mutation of key genes involved in cell proliferation, DNA repair, or Apoptosis must accumulate to produce cancer. It is likely that mutagenic and mitogenic effects of oestradiol act in concert to initiate and promote the development of breast cancer.

Oestrogen Source (Fig 23.9.1)

The source of oestrogen varies with the menopausal status of the woman.

In premenopausal women, the ovaries are the predominant source of serum oestrogen, and only a small proportion of serum oestrogen comes from peripheral organs. In contrast, the little oestrogen that is produced in postmenopausal women comes predominantly from aromatization of adrenal and ovarian androgens in extragonadal tissues such as the liver, muscle, and fat tissues. Breast can synthesize oestradiol through aromatization of androgen to oestrogen or cleavage of oestrone sulphate.

Oestrogen Synthesis (Fig 23.9.2)

P-450 enzymes are involved in oestrogen biosynthesis. Polymorphisms of the P-450 aromatase gene are associated with an increased risk of breast cancer. It has also been seen that the promoters of P-450 change from PI.4 to PII and PI.3, which are more active and can result in increased synthesis of P-450 aromatase mRNA.

Oestrogen Receptor

Oestrogens diffuse passively through cell and nuclear membranes. In specific cells and tissues containing oestrogen receptors, oestrogen then binds to the receptor, and this ligand-receptor complex binds to and activates specific sequences in the regulatory region of genes responsive to oestrogen, known as oestrogen-response elements. These genes in turn regulate cell growth and differentiation. Though oestrogen-receptor levels are low in normal breast tissue, they vary from woman to woman, and high levels have been directly correlated with an increased risk of breast cancer.

Catabolism of Oestrogens (Fig 23.9.2)

Oestrogens are catabolized mainly by two different hydroxylation reactions. 2-hydroxylation and 16-hydroxylation control the proportions of carcinogenic and anticarcinogenic metabolites formed. Thus, women who metabolize a larger proportion of endogenous oestrogen through the 16α-hydroxylation pathways may have a higher risk of breast cancer than women who metabolize more oestrogen through the 2-hydroxylation pathway.

Antioestrogens in Breast Cancer

Oestrogen deprivation remains a key therapeutic approach in breast cancer. Selective oestrogen-receptor modulators (SERMs) exemplified by tamoxifen and aromatase inhibitors are two different classes of

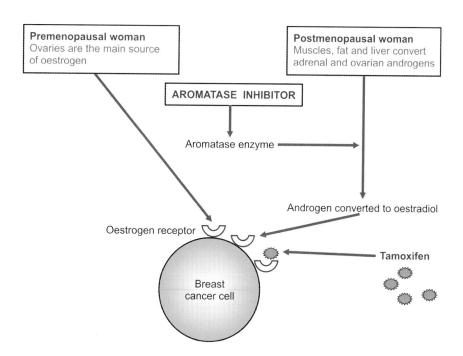

Fig. 23.9.1: Oestrogen source in premenopausal and postmenopausal woman

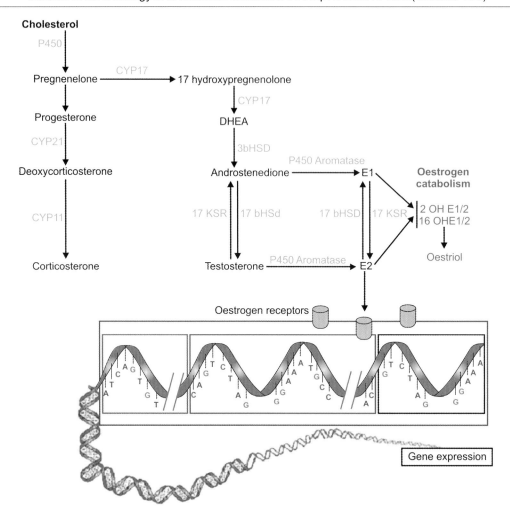

Fig. 23.9.2: Oestrogen synthesis and catabolism

compound used in treatment of breast cancer. Tamoxifen inhibits the growth of breast tumours by competitive antagonism of oestrogen at its receptor site however, and it also has partial oestrogen-agonist effects. These partial agonist effects are beneficial, by preventing bone demineralization and detrimental, since they are associated with increased risks of uterine cancer. In contrast, aromatase inhibitors markedly suppress plasma oestrogen levels in postmenopausal women by inhibiting or inactivating aromatase, the enzyme responsible for the synthesis of oestrogens from androgenic substrates. Unlike tamoxifen, aromatase inhibitors have no partial agonist activity.

Aromatase Inhibitors (Fig. 23.9.3, Table 23.9.2)

Aromatase is present, at lower levels, in several nonglandular tissues, including subcutaneous fat, liver, muscle, brain, normal breast, and breast-cancer tissue.

Residual oestrogen production after menopause is solely from nonglandular sources, in particular from subcutaneous fat.

Investigation of aromatase inhibition in breast cancer before menopause has been minimal, as it leads to an increase in gonadotrophin secretion because of reduced feedback of oestrogen to the hypothalamus and pituitary, and in some animal models lead to an increase in the weight of the ovaries. The data in the current review, however, pertain solely to postmenopausal women.

Aminoglutethimide, the first aromatase inhibitor, was initially developed in 1978. Side effects, including drowsiness and rash, limited its use and stimulated the development of numerous new inhibitors. They are described as first, second, and third generation inhibitors according to the chronologic order of their clinical development. They are further classified as type 1 or type 2 inhibitors according to their mechanism of action.

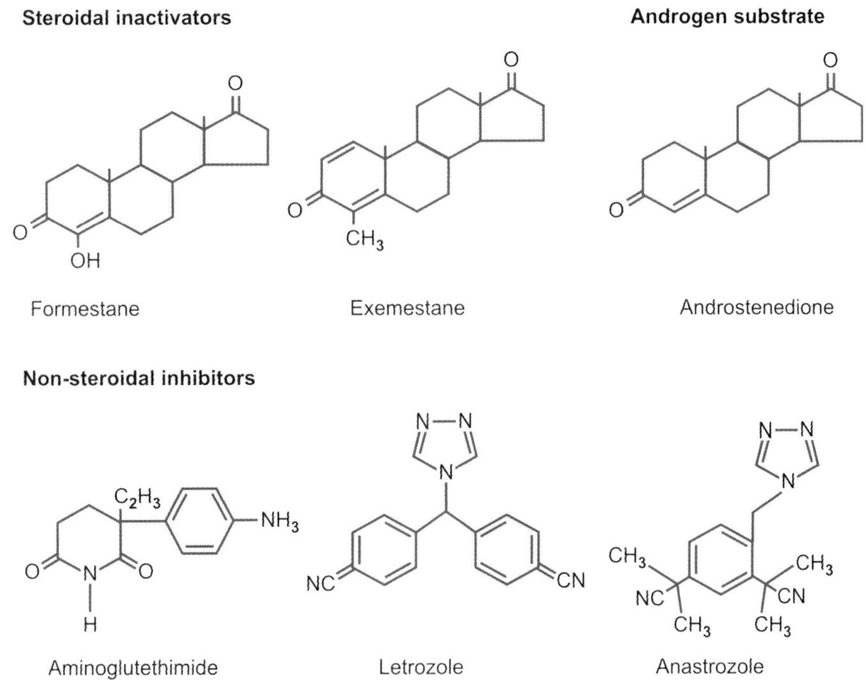

Steroidal inactivators **Androgen substrate**

Formestane   Exemestane   Androstenedione

Non-steroidal inhibitors

Aminoglutethimide   Letrozole   Anastrozole

Fig 23.9.3: Aromatase inhibitors pharmacology

Type 1 inhibitors are steroidal analogues of androstenedione and bind irreversibly, therefore, they are now commonly known as enzyme inactivators. Type 2 inhibitors are nonsteroidal and bind reversibly to the haem group of the enzyme by way of a basic nitrogen atom; anastrozole and letrozole, both third-generation inhibitors, bind at their triazole groups (Table 23.9.2).

In metastatic breast disease, letrozole is clearly superior to tamoxifen as first-line therapy. For

TABLE 23.9.2

Generation	Type 1	Type 2
First	None	Aminoglutethimide
Second	Formestane	Fadrazole
Third	Exemestane (25 mg OD) (used after 2 to 3 years of tamoxifen)	Anastrozole (1 mg OD) • Alternative to tamoxifen Letrozole (2.5 mg OD) • Neoadjuvant setting • Metastatic disease • Sequential after 5 years of tamoxifen

Classification of aromatase inhibitors

anastrozole, the data on superiority are contradictory, but the drug is convincingly at least as good as tamoxifen. The data on the use of letrozole for neoadjuvant therapy are preliminary but are promising as alternative to mastectomy for older patients with large, oestrogen-receptor-positive cancers. Trials of adjuvant therapy with the third-generation aromatase inhibitors are on going. The first analysis of Arimidex and Tamoxifen Alone or in Combination [ATAC] trial conducted at a median follow-up of 33 months, showed a small but statistically significant reduction in the rate of relapse with anastrozole as compared with tamoxifen: 89 per cent of the patients assigned to anastrozole were relapse-free at 3 years, as compared with 87 per cent of those assigned to tamoxifen (relative risk reduction, 17 per cent; P = 0.013). The results of the ATAC trial with regard to the chemoprevention of contralateral invasive breast cancer (in 30 [1.0%] of those receiving tamoxifen vs. 9 [0.3%]) of those receiving anastrozole. This suggests that anastrozole might reduce the early incidence of breast cancer to an even greater extent and thus have more potential in chemoprevention than tamoxifen. The commonest of these effects were hot flashes, vaginal dryness, musculoskeletal pain, and headache. In contrast to findings with tamoxifen, there is no evidence to suggest an increased risk of uterine carcinoma with aromatase inhibitors or venous thromboembolism. The risk of important long-term skeletal problems, including osteoporosis, may increase with the use of aromatase inhibitors.

In the Intergroup Exemestane Study (IES) exemestane therapy after two to three years of tamoxifen therapy significantly improved disease-free survival as compared with the standard five years of tamoxifen treatment. MA-17 trial shows that use of letrozole 5 years after tamoxifen significantly prolongs disease free survival.

The use of aromatase inhibitors in premenopausal women with breast cancer who have normal ovarian function is contraindicated due to reasons alluded before. Thus aromatase inhibitors have improved disease free survival in postmenopausal hormone positive breast cancer patients used as alternative to tamoxifen (Anastrozole in ATAC trial), after 5 years of tamoxifen (trial) and after 2 to 3 years of tamoxifen (Exemestane in IES study).

Cancer results from excessive hormonal stimulation of an organ where growth is under endocrine control. The cumulating action of hormones results in progressing from normal growth to hyperplasia to cancer. Indirect evidence of this sequence includes the increased risk of breast cancer associated with female

sex, early menarche, late first full-term pregnancy, and late menopause as well as the reduced risk associated with early menopause. The effect of obesity varies with menopausal status of the patient. Premenopausal obese woman are likely to have more anovulatory cycles and thereby lower levels of oestrogen. On the other hand postmenopausal woman have a lower levels of oestrogen binding globulin and therefore greater levels of oestrogen. Diet is also known to influence the incidence of breast cancer with lower incidence being reported in places consuming soya and flaxseed. This is attributed to phytoestrogen which are present in plant which are similar to oestrogens with both agonist and antagonist property. The role of oral contraceptives is difficult to dissect as they cause anovulation which is protective against cancer and on the other hand it may stimulate mitotic activity in breast tissues with reports for increased risk in BRCA 1 and BRCA 2 mutation. However the incidence of mortality is more than offset by reduced cardiac deaths.

SERMs (Tamoxifen, Raloxifene)
(Table 23.9.3, Fig 23.9.4)

On binding an agonist or an antagonist, the oestrogen receptor (the α or β isoform) undergoes a conformational

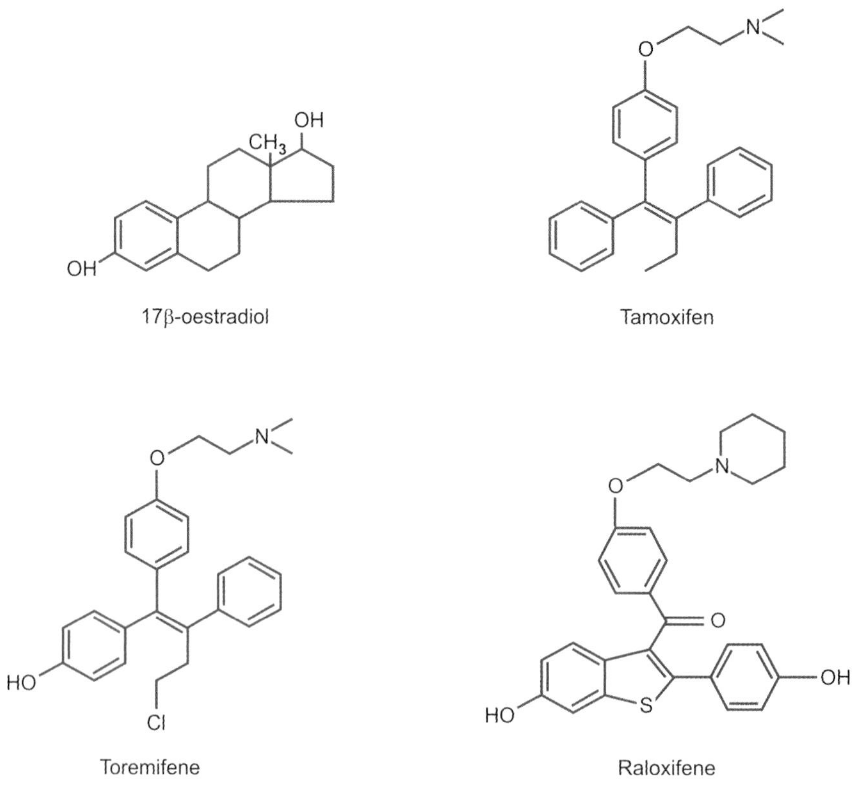

Fig. 23.9.4: Chemical structure of SERMs and oestrogens

TABLE 23.9.3

Action	Oestrogens	Tamoxifen	Raloxifene	Torimefene
Endometrial cancer	↑↑	↑	→	??
Breast cancer	↑↑↑	↓↓	↓↓	↓↓
Bone loss	↓↓	↓↓	↓↓	→
Hot flashes	↓↓↓	↑	↑	↑
Venous thrombosis	↑	↑	↑	??
Favourable lipid profile	↑	↑	↑	↑

Comparative action of different SERMs

change that permits its spontaneous dimerisation and facilitates the subsequent interaction of the dimer with oestrogen response elements (EREs) located within target genes. It has been determined that oestrogen facilitates the interaction of the oestrogen receptor with coactivators. An antagonist-activated oestrogen receptor, on the other hand, interacts preferentially with a corepressor protein.

Unlike antioestrogens, which are uniformly antagonists, the SERMs exert selective agonist or antagonist effects on various oestrogen target tissues. The SERMs are chemically diverse compounds that lack the steroid structure of oestrogens.

The binding of different SERMs to the receptor permits it to adopt conformational states distinct from that induced by classic agonists or antagonists. The weight of available evidence suggests that the structure of some SERM-oestrogen-receptor complexes favours corepressor recruitment and that of others favours some affinity for known coactivators. Some SERMs may also facilitate the interaction of the oestrogen receptor with yet-to-be-identified coactivators with which it would not normally couple. The implication of this model is that SERM activity will be influenced by the relative levels of expression of the cofactors (corepressors and co-activators) in target cells.

Most of the unique pharmacology of SERMs can be explained by three interactive mechanisms: differential oestrogen-receptor expression in a given target tissue, differential oestrogen-receptor conformation on ligand binding, and differential expression and binding to the oestrogen receptor of coregulator proteins.

Different SERMs have different effect on different tissues.

Bone: Tamoxifen has been reported both to increase and to decrease the risk of hip fracture. The use of tamoxifen in premenopausal women is that it acts as a bone antagonist that results in bone loss in this age group. Raloxifene decreased markers of bone turnover by 30 to 40 per cent after one year and increased bone density at several scanning sites by 2 to 3 per cent after three years

Breast: The proportional reduction in recurrence was 47 per cent after 5 years of treatment with tamoxifen and the proportional reduction in mortality was 26 per cent after 10 years. The absolute improvements in 10-year survival were 10.9 per cent in node-positive and 5.6 per cent in node-negative breast cancer.

Uterus: Unlike raloxifene, tamoxifen is associated with a 2.5-fold increase in endometrial carcinoma; so vaginal bleeding in women receiving tamoxifen should be promptly investigated.

Cardiovascular system: SERM therapy induces a beneficial serum lipid profile; tamoxifen, toremifene, and raloxifene also decrease LDL cholesterol but, unlike oestrogen, do not increase triglycerides. Toremifene, unlike other SERMs, increases HDL cholesterol. Raloxifene decreases cardiovascular events by 40 per cent. Tamoxifen, and raloxifene therapy are associated with increases by a factor of 1.5 to 3 in venous thromboembolic disease, although the absolute risk is small.

Therapy of breast cancer today involves local therapy in form of surgery and radiotherapy. For addressing micrometastatic disease, chemotherapy followed by tamoxifen in premenopausal woman and aromatase inhibitors in postmenopausal woman is recommended today. This contrasts with a year ago when tamoxifen was the standard of care for all woman with breast cancer.

PROSTATE CANCER

Dietary factors (evidence suggest that total energy intake is a risk factor for prostate cancer and diet rich in soyabean products and fish, might be protective against prostate cancer), lifestyle-related factors, and androgens have long been recognised as contributors to the risk of prostate cancer.

State-of-the-art treatment in prostate cancer provides prolonged disease-free survival for many patients with localised disease but is rarely curative in patients with locally extensive tumour. Surgery is usually reserved for patients in good health who are under the age of 70 and who elect surgical intervention. Candidates for definitive radiation therapy must have a confirmed pathological diagnosis of cancer that is clinically confined to the prostate and/or surrounding tissues (stages I, II, and III). Asymptomatic patients of advanced age or with concomitant illness may warrant consideration of careful observation without immediate active treatment, especially those patients with low-grade and early-stage tumours. Hormonal treatment is the mainstay of therapy for distant metastatic (stage D2) prostate cancer. Cure is rarely, if ever, possible, but striking subjective or objective responses to treatment occur in the majority of patients. The role of adjuvant hormonal therapy in patients with locally advanced disease has been analysed in a meta-analysis. The metaanalysis found a difference in 5-year overall survival in favour of radiation therapy plus continued androgen suppression compared to radiation therapy alone (hazard ratio = 0.631, 95% CI = 0.479-0.831). Hormone therapy has also been used in neoadjuvant androgen deprivation therapy (ADT) with radical prostatectomy in localized prostate cancer (Table 23.9.4).

Androgen-dependent and Androgen-independent Clones

The dependence of the growth of prostate cancer on androgens is well documented. DHT binds to androgen receptor and serves as a major regulator of prostate cancer growth. Androgen ablation triggers a cascade of biologic events that ends in irreversible damage to the DNA of androgen-sensitive prostate-cancer cells. Such treatment, traditionally reserved for men with metastatic disease, results in major objective and subjective benefits in most patients. However, in approximately 50 per cent of patients, disease progression occurs 12 to 18 months after the initiation of treatment, and as a result, survival

rates have not increased over the past five decades. Androgen ablation controls the tumour only temporarily because prostate cancer consists of androgen-dependent and androgen-independent clones. Tumour progression after androgen ablation is due to the proliferation of androgen-independent cells. At present, there is no conclusive evidence that androgen-deprivation therapy improves survival.

Hormonal Therapy

Hormonal therapy is the mainstay of treatment for men with disseminated prostate cancer. Though unequivocal evidence of a survival benefit is lacking, about 85 per cent of patients have an objective response. A change in the serum PSA concentration is a good indicator of a response. Several different hormonal approaches can benefit men in various stages of prostate cancer. These approaches include bilateral orchidectomy, oestrogen therapy, LHRH agonists, antiandrogens, ketoconazole, and aminoglutethimide.

Orchidectomy

Orchidectomy, a minor, outpatient operation that can be performed under local anaesthesia, is a time-honoured method of reducing serum testosterone concentrations. Benefits of bilateral orchiectomy include ease of the procedure, compliance, its immediacy in lowering testosterone levels, and low cost. Disadvantages include psychologic effects, loss of libido, impotence, hot flashes, and osteoporosis.

TABLE 23.9.4

Hormonal manipulation	Dose	Advantage	Disadvantage
Orchidectomy		• Compliance • Immediacy in lowering testosterone levels • Low cost	• Psychologic effects • Loss of libido • Impotence • Hot flashes • Osteoporosis
Diethylstilboestrol	3 mg/day		• Thrombosis • Impotence • Gynaecomastia
LHRH agonists Leuprolide, goserelin, buserelin	3.75/ 7.5/22.5 3.6 mg	Reversible loss of androgens	• Impotence • Hot flashes • Loss of libido
Antiandrogen Flutamide Bicalutamide	250 mg tid 50 mg od		• Diarrhoea • Breast tenderness • Nausea • Nonfatal liver toxic effects
Ketoconazole	1200 mg		• Impotence • Pruritus • Nail changes • Adrenal insufficiency

Hormones in prostate cancer

Oestrogen

Oestrogen therapy is as effective as orchidectomy, and there is no benefit from combining the two treatments. Diethylstilboestrol in daily doses of 3 mg or more causes cardiovascular toxicity; a daily dose of 1 mg is effective without excessive toxic effects but does not reliably reduce serum testosterone concentrations to the range associated with castration.

Gonadotrophin-releasing Hormone Agonists (Leuprolide, Goserelin, and Buserelin)

Gonadotrophin-releasing hormone agonists: Gonadotropin-releasing hormone (GnRH) analogues result in a medical orchidectomy in men and are used as a means of providing androgen ablation for metastatic prostate cancer. Testosterone secretion rises and then declines, resulting in very low serum testosterone concentrations after two to three weeks. The initial rise in serum testosterone concentrations may stimulate tumour growth; therefore, patients who have spinal cord compression, pathological fracture, or urinary obstruction from tumor growth should receive antiandrogen therapy during the testosterone surge. Treatment with gonadotrophin-releasing hormone agonists is as effective as treatment with diethylstilboestrol or orchidectomy and offers the psychological advantage of avoiding castration; a disadvantage is its high cost.

Nonsteroidal Antiandrogens (Bicalutamide, Flutamide)

Flutamide is a nonsteroidal antiandrogen agent that acts by blocking the binding of testosterone (and dihydrotestosterone) to its intracellular receptors. Flutamide also blocks the inhibitory effect of testosterone on gonadotrophin secretion, and therefore serum luteinizing hormone and testosterone concentrations increase, so that many patients remain potent.

GnRH Antagonists

These compounds also suppress FSH, and represent the latest class of agents introduced for hormonal treatment, but phase III studies with survival data are not yet available.

Other Hormonal Agents

Progestins, such as megestrol acetate, act primarily by inhibiting the release of luteinizing hormone; they also block androgen receptors. With all progestins, an escape phenomenon occurs in which serum testosterone concentrations gradually rise after 6 to 12 months of treatment. Escape can be prevented by adding a low dose of oestrogen (0.1 mg of diethylstilboestrol daily), which by itself is insufficient to suppress testosterone secretion, but which, by synergizing with the progestin, maintains testosterone suppression

Finasteride is a 5-alpha-reductase inhibitor that is only marginally effective in the treatment of prostate cancer.

Maximal Androgen Ablation

The most controversial issue concerning hormonal therapy for prostate cancer is maximal androgen ablation—that is, combined therapy to reduce the effects of both gonadal and adrenal androgens, such as the use of a gonadotrophin-releasing hormone agonist plus flutamide. Combined therapy may confer at most a six-month overall survival benefit; however, for patients with early metastatic disease, survival may be increased by as long as 20 months. Maximal androgen ablation as an option in patients with metastatic disease has a modest beneficial effect.

Optimal Anti-androgen Therapy

LHRH agonist (medical castration) and bilateral orchidectomy (surgical castration) are equally effective. Combined androgen blockage (medical or surgical castration combined with an anti-androgen) provides limited benefit over castration alone. Serial use of anti-androgen and LHRH agonist have not been adequately studied but empirically used. Anti-androgen therapy should precede LHRH agonist and be continued in combination for one month for patients with overt metastases who are at risk of developing symptoms associated with the flare in testosterone with initial LHRH analogue alone.

Treatment of Patients with Disease Refractory to Hormonal Therapy

Secondary Hormonal Therapy

The results of secondary hormonal therapy with high-dose oestrogen, an antiandrogen, or an inhibitor of androgen synthesis are poor. Though subjective responses occur in 10 to 20 per cent of patients, they last only about six months. Cancers that have recurred after hormonal therapy but are still responsive to androgenic stimulation, lifelong androgen suppression should be maintained. The one exception is patients who have been treated with flutamide. In these patients, flutamide should be discontinued. Objective responses lasting about six months have been reported after discontinuation of flutamide in patients with hormone-refractory disease.

Intermittent Hormonal Therapy

The scientific basis for intermittent hormonal therapy is that hormonally dependent clones of prostate cancer cells may potentially prevent the growth of hormonally independent cells through the elaboration of growth inhibitory factors. Alternatively, the reintroduction of androgen after androgen withdrawal may result in the generation of differentiated tumour cells. It might be advantageous, therefore, to allow the reintroduction of androgen after androgen withdrawal to delay the emergence of an androgen-independent phenotype.

Androgen deprivation therapy also can cause osteoporosis. A small nonblinded study with short follow-up suggests that the bisphosphonate, pamidronate can prevent bone loss in men receiving a gonadotrophin-releasing hormone agonist for prostate cancer.

ENDOMETRIAL CARCINOMA
Excessive Oestrogen

Excessive oestrogen is associated with most of the risk factors that have been linked to endometrial carcinoma. Excessive oestrogen produces continued stimulation of the endometrium, which can result in endometrial hyperplasia.

Risk Factor

Obesity is a risk factor for endometrial carcinoma. The development of cancer in obese women is believed to be mediated by endogenous oestrogen, through the conversion of androstenedione to oestrone by aromatase in adipose tissue can result in endometrial hyperplasia.

Twenty-five per cent of women with endometrial cancer are premenopausal, and 5 per cent are less than 40 years of age. The majority of young women with endometrial carcinoma are obese or have high levels of unopposed endogenous oestrogen because they have chronic anovulation, such as those with polycystic ovary disease.

Although serum oestrogen and progesterone concentrations increase during pregnancy, progesterone is the predominant hormone of pregnancy. Pregnancy confers protection from endometrial carcinoma by interrupting the continued stimulation of the endometrium by oestrogen. Nulliparity is thus a risk factor for endometrial carcinoma.

Tamoxifen is a synthetic antioestrogen (oestrogen antagonist) that is used in the treatment of breast cancer. In addition, tamoxifen has been shown to have oestrogenic (agonist) effects on the endometrium and to increase the risk of endometrial carcinoma. Progesterone confers protection from endometrial cancer. Cigarette smoking decreases the risk of endometrial carcinoma by inactivating oestrogen through hydroxylation at the 2-alpha position.

Oestrogen and Progesterone Receptors

The most extensively studied biologic markers in endometrial carcinoma are oestrogen and progesterone receptors. It has been shown that high levels of oestrogen and progesterone receptors directly correlate with better tumour differentiation, less myometrial invasion, and a lower incidence of nodal metastases and that they independently predict better survival.

Certain characteristics including well-differentiated tumours, a long disease-free interval, and positivity for oestrogen and progesterone receptors identify a subgroup of women who are most likely to respond to hormonal therapy. There is no apparent difference in activity among the numerous progestational agents that have been used.

Drugs in Adjuvant and Recurrent, Metastatic Setting

The results of treatment with tamoxifen are generally inferior to those obtained with progestogens. It remains to be seen whether tamoxifen in sequential combination with progestogens (to modulate receptors) will have an advantage over progestogen therapy alone. Other hormonal manipulations are increasingly under study. These include not only combinations of tamoxifen and MPA, but also other selective oestrogen receptor modulators such as raloxifene, luteinizing hormone-releasing hormone (LHRH) agonists and antagonists, aromatase inhibitors, and miscellaneous other drugs. The presence of oestrogen and progesterone receptors in tumours has been shown to correlate with well-differentiated cancers and with response to progestogens. Sequentially alternating tamoxifen and MPA or megestrol acetate regimens are based on the concept of up-regulation of progesterone receptors by the antioestrogen.

COLONIC CANCER
Oestrogen Hormones

Clinical and experimental evidences have been reported showing that oestrogen hormones may be involved in malignant colorectal tumours. The sex differences in site-specific incidence, the increased incidence of colonic cancer in women with breast cancer, the protective effect of increasing parity and the reduced risk among women taking postmenopausal hormones, are all elements suggesting that sex hormones may play a role. Studies suggest that oestrogens and their receptors play an important role in the growth and progression of colorectal tumours, by interacting with other molecules required for cell proliferation like growth factors and polyamines.

In the only WHI randomized trial, the use of oestrogen plus progestin was associated with a statistically significant decrease in the incidence of colorectal cancer among postmenopausal women.

Possible mechanisms of the effect of postmenopausal hormone therapy on the risk of colorectal cancer include the influence of oestrogen on bile acids, changes mediated by oestrogen receptors on intestinal epithelium, and alteration of insulin and insulin-like growth factor.

GI Peptides

Some GI peptides, including gastrin and gastrin-releasing peptide (GRP) (mammalian bombesin), appear to be involved in the growth of neoplasms of the colon. Certain growth factors such as insulin-like growth factor (IGF)-I, IGF-II and epidermal growth factor and their receptors that regulate cell proliferation are also implicated in the development and progression of colonic cancer.

OVARIAN CANCER

Ovarian carcinoma continues to be the leading cause of death due to gynaecologic malignancies and the vast majority of it is derived from the ovarian surface epithelium (OSE) and its cystic derivatives. Epidemiological evidence strongly suggests that steroid hormones, primarily oestrogens and progesterone, are implicated in ovarian carcinogenesis. Ovarian tissue is sensitive to gonadotrophins. Gonadotrophins receptors are present in the epithelium and stroma of the ovary. Data from epidemiological study clearly shows, that development of tumour is correlated with morphological and biochemical processes taking place in the gonad.

New convincing data have indicated that oestrogens favour neoplastic transformation of the OSE. Specifically, oestrogens, particularly those present in ovulatory follicles, are both genotoxic and mitogenic to OSE cells.

Progesterone

Epidemiological evidence suggests that elevated levels of the pregnancy hormone progesterone might play a role in the reduced risk of women to develop ovarian cancer. *In vitro* studies have supported this hypothesis by demonstrating negative effects of this hormone on the growth and proliferation of cultured ovarian carcinoma cells.

Androgens

Numerous studies indicate that the steroid hormones have been implicated in the aetiology and/or progression of epithelial ovarian cancer and support a role for androgens. The supporting evidence includes the observation that:
a. Androgen receptor (AR) is present in primate ovaries at almost all stages of the menstrual cycle and involve folliculogenesis and ovulation.
b. High androgen serum levels show high risk of ovarian cancer and ovarian cancer occurring after menopause when the balance of ovarian steroid production shifts from oestrogens to androgens.
c. Ovarian cancer tissue shows a 90% AR positive rate and is associated with favourable outcomes.
d. Androgens promote or inhibit ovarian cancer cell growth.
e. Chemotherapy decreases androgen production from cancer cells.

Cytotoxic Luteinizing Hormone-releasing Hormone

Binding sites for LHRH (now known in genome and microarray databases as GNRH1), were found on about 80% of human ovarian cancers.

SUMMARY

The breast, ovarian, endometrial and prostate cancers are hormone dependent. In hormone-dependent breast cancer, the tumour cells have oestrogen receptors and progesterone receptors (ER and PR positive tumours) and need oestrogen and progesterone for its growth. This tumour responds to anti-oestrogen and progesterone therapy.

Hormonal therapy is the mainstay of treatment for disseminated prostate cancer. Different hormonal approaches benefit in various stages of prostate cancer. These approaches include oestrogen therapy, LHRH agonists, antiandrogens, ketoconazole, and aminoglutethimide.

Excessive oestrogen is linked to endometrial carcinoma. The results of treatment with tamoxifen are generally inferior to those obtained with progestogens. Other hormonal manipulations are increasingly under study. These include not only combinations of tamoxifen and megestrol acetate, but also other selective oestrogen receptor modulators such as raloxifene, luteinizing hormone-releasing hormone (LHRH) agonists and antagonists and aromatase inhibitors.

Epidemiological evidence strongly suggests that steroid hormones, primarily oestrogens and progesterone, are implicated in ovarian carcinogenesis. Ovarian tissue is sensitive to gonadotrophins. Gonadotrophins receptors are present in the epithelium and stroma of the ovary. It has been seen that androgens promote or inhibit ovarian cancer cell growth and chemotherapy decreases androgen production from cancer cells and thus helps in reduction of tumour loads.

FURTHER READING

1. Arnett-Mansfield RL, deFazio A, Mote PA, Clarke CL. Subnuclear distribution of progesterone receptors A and B in normal and malignant endometrium. J Clin Endocrinol Metab 2004;89:1429-42.

2. Arnett-Mansfield RL, deFazio A, Wain GV, Jaworski RC, Byth K, Mote PA, Clarke CL. Relative expression of progesterone receptors A and B in endometrioid cancers of the endometrium. Cancer Res 2001;61:4576-82.

3. Baum M, Budzar AU, Cuzick J, et al. Anastrozole alone or in combination with tamoxifen versus tamoxifen alone for adjuvant treatment of postmenopausal women with early breast cancer: first results of the ATAC randomised trial. Lancet 2002;359:2131-9. [Erratum, Lancet 2002; 360:1520.

4. Berrino F, Muti P, Micheli A, et al. Serum sex hormone levels after menopause and subsequent breast cancer. J Natl Cancer Inst 1996;88:291-6.

5. Early Breast Cancer Trialists' Collaborative Group. Tamoxifen for early breast cancer: an overview of the randomised trials. Lancet 1998;351:1451-67.

6. Eisenberger MA, Walsh PC. Early Androgen deprivation for prostate cancer? N Engl J Med 1999;341:1837-8.

7. Forrest ARW. Aromatase Inhibitors in Breast Cancer. N Engl J Med 2003;349:1090.

8. Goss PE, Ingle JN, Martino S, et al. A randomized trial of letrozole in postmenopausal women after five years of tamoxifen therapy for early-stage breast cancer. N Engl J Med 2003;349:1793-802.

9. Goss PE, Strasser K. Aromatase inhibitors in the treatment and prevention of breast cancer. J Clin Oncol 2001;19:881-94.

10. Gruber CJ, Tschugguel W, Schneeberger C, Huber JC. Production and actions of estrogens. N Engl J Med 2002;346:340-52.

11. Hellerstedt BA, Pienta KJ. The current state of hormonal therapy for prostate cancer. CA Cancer J Clin 2002;52:154-79.

12. Hulka BS. Epidemiologic analysis of breast and gynecologic cancers. Prog Clin Biol Res 1997;396:17-29.

13. Hsing AW, Reichardt JK, Stanczyk FZ. Hormones and prostate cancer: current perspectives and future directions. Prostate 2002;1;52(3): 213-35.

14. McDonnell DP. The molecular pharmacology of SERMs. Trends Endocrinol Metab 1999;10:301-11.

15. Piccart-Gebhart MJ. New Stars in the sky of treatment for early breast cancer. N Engl J Med 2004;350:1140-2.

16. Rowan TC, Jean WW. Estrogen plus progestin and colorectal cancer in postmenopausal women. J Natl Cancer Inst 2004;350(10):991-1004.

17. Taplin ME, Ho SM. The Endocrinology of prostate cancer. J Clin Endocrinol Metab 2001;86:3467-77.

18. Toniolo PG, Levitz M, Zeleniuch-Jacquotte A, et al. A prospective study of endogenous estrogens and breast cancer in post-menopausal women. J Natl Cancer Inst 1995; 87:190-7.

23.10 Effect of Ageing on Endocrine System

Y Sachdev

INTRODUCTION

The human physiology undergoes a variable change with ageing. The change affects all body systems; the brunt, though, is borne by the immune and endocrine systems. The protein synthesis, defence mechanism, physical activity, stamina, muscle strength and bone densitometry—all show a reduction. Clinically, an elderly person is relatively frail, has general muscle weakness, poor hand grip, impaired mobility and poor balance. Some of these functions can be improved upon by physical training programmes while the others are due to the ageing process and continue showing age-related downward alterations.

Out of endocrine system, the maximum deterioration is seen in the pancreas and hypothalamic-anterior pituitary axes.

Pancreas

Changes in pancreatic insulin receptor and post-receptor events are two critical components of ageing. The insulin secretion in response to various stimuli is diminished showing delayed and blunted response (Figs 23.10.1A to D). The efficacy of secreted insulin is reduced due to insulin resistance and insensitivity of the peripheral tissues. Meagre dietary intake, diminished physical activity, lean muscle mass and increased abdominal fat

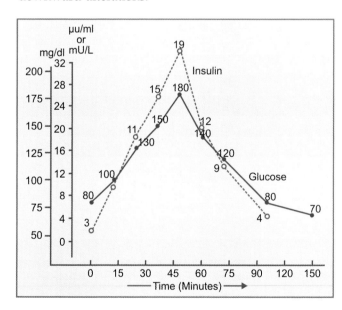

Fig. 23.10.1A: Plasma glucose and insulin values during OGTT in a young healthy man of 25 years

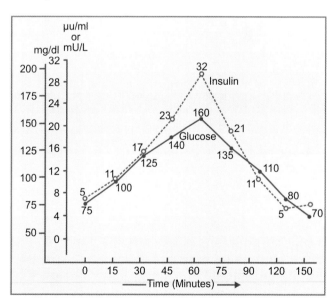

Fig. 23.10.1B: Plasma glucose and IRI values during OGTT in a normal 22-year-old man

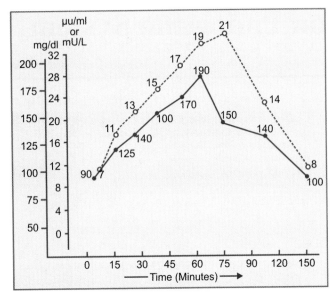

Fig. 23.10.1C: Plasma glucose and insulin values during OGTT in a healthy normal 75-year-old man

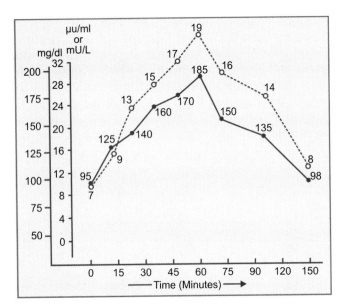

Fig. 23.10.1D: Plasma glucose and IRI values during OGTT in a healthy old man of 70 years

are some of the main contributory factors associated with insulin resistance. The prevalence of impaired glucose tolerance and frank diabetes mellitus increases with advancing age. It is reported to be 50 to 80% above the age 80 years and 40 to 55% between 65 and 74 age group. Risk of macrovascular complications increase with age.

Thyroid

Many (5%) of the elderly aged 60 years and above, who stay in iodine-deficiency goitrous areas have multi-

nodular goitre while those who stay in non-endemic areas where a small goitre is commonly seen in younger population register decrease in thyroid size. Such changes are usually observed above the age of 60 years. Resting metabolic rate (RMR) decreases with age. T_4 secretary rate shows a gradual decrease with age. FT_4 value, however, is not significantly different than in young adults. There is reduction in peripheral conversion of T_4 to T_3 with consequent elevation in rT_3 values. Elderly over the age of 70 years demonstrate a marginal reduction in TSH and FT_3. TSH response to TRH test may be delayed and abnormal showing higher 60 minutes value compared to that at 20 minutes.

Hypothalamic-Anterior Pituitary-Gonadal Axis

The pituitary gland decreases in size with age. The GnRH oscillations and pulses decrease with age. In males there is gradual decline in Leydig cell mass and their response to gonadotrophin is reduced and blunted (Fig. 23.10.2). Total and free testosterone values are diminished resulting in diminished libido and sexual performance. These changes have been labelled as 'andropause.' With testosterone (Te) therapy in elderly patients with low Te value, muscle power and physical activity may increase. The objective of Te treatment is to bring the Te level to the age related normal value and not to the adult level. Caution has to be exercised as there is a risk of prostate malignancy. Oral testosterone undecanoate (20 to 40 mg/day) is not favoured and recommended in elderly men due to unreliable absorption and hepatotoxicity, especially if transdermal device is available. Transdermal delivery is best in the form of 'testoderm' or 'androderm'. It is to be appreciated that Te therapy is recommended only if there is deficiency of Te and not otherwise. When androgen replacement therapy (ART) is initiated, basal

Age (yr)	Plasma Te Values		
	Basal	Peak at 24 hr. after 1st hCG inj.	Peak at 48 hr. after 2nd hCG inj.
21 to 30	564 ± 224	786 ± 156	894 ± 135
31 to 40	484 ± 236	810 ± 164	886 ± 126
41 to 50	498 ± 210	874 ± 172	912 ± 153
51 to 60	448 ± 192	672 ± 165	716 ± 136
61 to 70	367 ± 128	562 ± 95	610 ± 115
Above 70	312 ± 124	----	----

Fig. 23.10.2: Showing progressive age-related decrease in plasma Te response (mg/dl) to injection hCG (Sachdev Y 1984)

and periodic check on PSA, Te (FTe), LFT, haemogram and lipid profile is obligatory. Prostrate and breast carcinoma are absolute contraindications.

Hypothalamic-Anterior Pituitary-adrenocortical Axis

The age related change in adrenocortical secretion is labelled as 'adrenopause.' There is reduction in dehydro-epiandrosterone (DHEA) and dehydroepiandrosterone sulphate (DHEA-S). ACTH and cortisol values, however, remain unchanged. The ACTH and cortisol secretary circadian rhythms diminish.

Growth Hormone and Insulin Like Growth Factor 1 (IGF 1)

GH and IGF-1 undergo a gradual decline with age. The mean pulse amplitude of GH decreases though the pulse frequency is not much affected: the GH secretary bursts are very few, infrequent and short lived. GH secretion declines by approximately 14% per decade so that it is approximately 15% of the puberty level by 45 to 55 years. Serum IGF-1 level is lower in elderly individuals by 20 to 80% compared to healthy young individuals. GHRH and ghrelin secretion decreases with ageing. These changes lead to decline in functional capacity in the elderly and has been labelled as 'somatopause'.

Serum concentration of IGF-1 can be restored by GH therapy (0.15 to 0.3 mg/day (maximum 1.2 mg a day) for 4 to 6 months). By this treatment lean body mass increases and bone density improves. IGF-1 values must be kept in mid-normal range for age and sex. However, if the therapy is continued for a longer time, the positive effect on the bone mineral density is lost. The therapy is also liable to result in adverse effects like carpal tunnel syndrome, gynaecomastia, hyperglycaemia and fluid retention. There appears to be no significant effect on muscle strength and functional capacity. GHRH injections have been observed to have positive effect on GH secretion indicating that perhaps it is a hypothalamic problem. GH-releasing peptides (GHRPs) also increase GH secretion and could be an alternative therapy in somatopause. Presently there is insufficient evidence to recommend this or any other therapy to rejuvenate healthy elderly individuals unless, of course, the hormonal deficiency is proven by minimum of two dynamic tests.

Treatment of Endocrine Ageing

a. It must be appreciated that ageing results not by hormonal alterations alone. The process is far more complex and intricate. All the same, appropriate hormone replacement in andropause and in somatopause may help delay or prevent some problems of ageing.
b. Testosterone therapy in elderly reduces body fat mass and increases lean mass without much effect on the muscle power. If it is decided to use testosterone aim should be bring its value to an age matched normal range.
c. In adrenopause while DHEA and DHEA-S deficiency is observed, DHEA replacement (50 mg daily) has given limited benefits especially in women. DHEA being a precursor of both oestrogens and androgen, its judicious use is expected to result in an increased overall well-being feeling, libido, sex interest and bone density. However, the safety of long-term use of this hormone is not known and more research is needed.
d. For somatopause, the role of GH replacement is well documented with pros and cons. Long-term safety of GH and IGF-1 therapy in elderly is a matter of concern in view of increased risk of prostate, colon and breast cancer and other side effects. GHRP and GHRH analogues may prove a better alternative in time to come.

CLIMACTERIC AND MENOPAUSE

Introduction

Life span for a woman at the time of Roman Empire was 28 years. At the time of discovery of America it was expected to be 30 years and even in Victorian era it was only 45 years. In the 17th century only 28% of American women lived to experience menopause and only 5% survived upto the age of 75 years. Presently nearly 95% women in India and other developing countries expect to reach menopause and over 50% reach the age of 75 years. Thus a large majority of Indian women spend more than one-third of their life in menopause. Menopause is an age-related ovarian and reproductive senescence which is marked by reduction in ovarian steroid secretion and altered target responses.

Physiology of Menstrual Cycle

The menstrual cycle is characterized by repetitive changes in hypothalamic-pituitary-ovarian hormone secretion that regulate the development and release of a mature ovum and coordinate the preparation of the reproductive tract for fertilization and implantation. If pregnancy does not ensure, each cycle culminates in menstrual bleeding which signals the beginning of the next menstrual cycle.

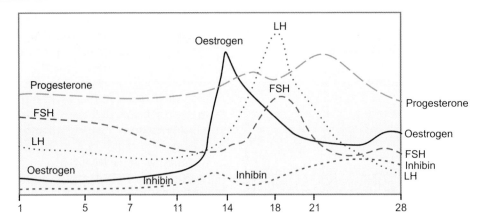

Fig. 23.10.3: LH, FSH, progesterone and oestrogen during normal menstrual cycle

During menses a slight but physiologically significant rise in serum follicle-stimulating hormone (FSH) occurs which acts on the small antral follicles, stimulates their growth and ability to synthesize oestradiol. It takes approximately 14 days for a 5 mm follicle to reach pre-ovulatory size of over 20 mm in diameter. The number of follicle in the cohort of developing follicles is gradually reduced throughout the follicular phase of the cycle while a dominant follicle destined to be the ovulatory follicle is selected by the day 7 of the cycle. Although the number of growing follicles is reduced, the capacity of the dominant follicle to secrete oestradiol increases accounting for gradual elevation of serum oestradiol level during the follicular phase. After serum oestradiol levels reach approximately 150 pg/ml and remain there for about 36 hours, LH and FSH surge is triggered (Fig. 23.10.3). This gonadotrophin (Gn) surge induces ovulation and subsequently promotes the transformation of the ovulatory follicle into a corpus luteum.

The corpus luteum becomes functional and secretes large amount of progesterone within 2 days of the (Gn) surge. Oestradiol is also secreted from the corpus luteum but at nearly half the rate of the preovulatory follicle. If the ovulated oocyte is not fertilized, the corpus luteum degenerates within 14 days. Both progesterone and oeatradiol levels fall, the uterine endometrium is not maintained and menses ensures.

Physiology of Climacteric and Menopause

As a woman reaches menopause, her menses become irregular with prolonged intervals and ultimately stop altogether. Menopause is generally seen between 40 to 55 years (average 46.2 years in Indian women in 1982; in 2002 it was 49.4 years) and is accompanied by a complete loss of oocytes. The climacteric or perimenopause is a critical transitional period which encompasses the change from ovulatory cycles to cessation of menses and is marked by irregularity of menstrual bleeding, prolonged cycle intervals, elevated FSH value, decreased inhibin level, normal LH level and slightly elevated oestradiol level. These changes in hormone value reflect a declining ovarian follicular reserve and is best detected between 2 to 3 day of menstrual cycle. During climacteric, serum oestradiol value is somewhat higher than seen in younger woman and is due to increased follicular response to elevated FSH. The decline in inhibin production by the follicle, allowing elevated FSH level reflects diminishing follicular reserve and competence. Inhibin starts declining after 30 years of age and its reduction is significant after 40 years.

The climacteric or perimenipausal women are liable to conceive due to occasional ovulation and functional corpus luteum. It is, therefore, advisable to use contraception unless the menses cease completely or FSH value measured at two separate occasions is higher than 40 IU/L.

The postmenopausal human ovary contains very few primordial follicles, and these follicles are rarely, if ever, stimulated to develop into ovulatory follicles. The ovarian cysts, however, are seen quite often upto 10 year after menopause. The loss of follicular structures and the resulting absence of ovulation and luteal formation account for the 50% decrease in the weight of the post-menopausal ovary compared with ovaries of younger normal cycling women. The capacity of postmenopausal ovary to synthesize and secrete oestradiol 17-β is dramatically reduced to as low as 20 μg per day. This results in an abrupt fall in serum oestradiol levels from peak values of 150 pg per ml to 13 to 15 pg per ml. The pattern of steroids genesis also shifts and oestrone and not oestradiol becomes the dominant oestrogen synthesized by the postmenopausal ovary.

The major cell types within the postmenopausal ovary are corticostromal and hilar cells. the corticostromal cells appear to be derived from the theca of atretic follicles and possess various enzymes involved with the synthesis of steroids and ultrastructural characteristics of steroidogenecally active 'luteinized' cells. The 'luteinized' stromal cells are observed in 35 to 40% ovaries of the women aged 56 to 76 years. LH and FSH binding sites have been localized within these cells suggesting that circulating Gn still influence the steroidogenesis. Similarly, hilar region of the postmenopausal ovary contains not only connective tissue and the blood vessels but also steroidogenically active hilar cells. The amount of steroid hormones that a postmenopausal ovary contributes to the circulation is relatively small—30% of the serum androgen and virtually none of oestradiol.

As the steroid secretion is severely attenuated after menopause, the LH and FSH levels rise in both plasma and urine. Characteristically, the plasma oestradiol is below 20 pg per ml and LH and FSH value increase 5- and 15-fold respectively.

Reproductive Tract Changes in Menopause

The following changes are due to lack of oestrogens. Urogenital tract suffers the maximum:

The Labia Majora and Minora

They are less prominent and the vulval skin becomes only a few cells thick. Subcutaneous fat is lost and atrophic changes extend to the perineum and anus. There is loss of pubic hair.

Vagina

Oestrogen deficiency allows the vaginal wall to become thin, dry and atrophic, with loss of rugae and decreased vascularity. Vaginal cytology demonstrate fall in karyopyknotic index as its cells show a predominance of small basal and parabasal cells with large deeply staining nuclei. Vaginal distensibility is diminished and there is loss of glycogen.

Cervix

It shrinks and becomes almost flush with the vaginal wall. The crypts and ducts atrophy and the cervical canal decreases in size.

Uterus

It diminishes in size and loses weight which may be as much as 50%. The endometrium becomes athophic with fever glands.

Urethra

Lower urathral and vaginal mucosa have a same origin, it shows atrophy, becomes thin and its vascularity decreases.

Hormonal Changes in Menopause

LH, FSH levels increase, oestradiol value falls markedly. Oestrone level is maintained. Testosterone value increases.

Symptomatology

The symptoms are variable and depend on the amount and rate of oestrogen depletion; the inherited and acquired ability to withstand the natural ageing process, and the psychological impact of the changes in life.

The symptoms may be divided into vasomotor, emotional, sexual and musculoskeletal symptoms.

Vasomotor symptoms The most frequent are the hot flushes (or flashes) and night sweats. The exact cause of hot flushes is unknown. The hot sweats that occur at night produce insomnia, palpitation, tension and even migraineous headache.

Emotional symptoms These may manifest as diminished energy, reduced drive, decreased power of concentration, depression, poor work performance, irritability, aggression, nervous exhaustion, mood fluctuation, tension and introversion.

Sexual symptoms Dyspareunia, decreased libido, diminished sexual interest and pleasure are the main sexual symptoms. Some women may complain of constant irritation and vaginal itching due to atrophic vaginitis. As the bladder, urethra and genital tract have a common embryological origin, the trigone and periurathral vascular tissue gets atrophic causing urinary urgency, frequency and incontinence.

Musculoskeletal symptoms Due to increased laxity of ligaments and reduced muscle strength, the backache, pain in the shoulders, elbows or small joints are common complaints.

Treatment

- Reassurance and self confidence building advice is helpful in symptomatic menopausal women.
- In some, standard doses of beta blockers are effective in controlling hot flashes and related symptoms, while others are benefited by vitamin E.
- Local use of lubricant vaginal creams will help in control of dry vaginitis.

- Hormonal replacement therapy (oestrogen and progesterone), given orally or transdermal, has been in use over 20 years based on data available from observation studies. However, since 1998, large number of randomized control trials have negated many previous observations and presently it is no longer recommended for all women. One of the largest trials, Women's Health Initiative (WHI) covering 16,000 postmenopausal women for an average of 5.2 years proved that HRT women were 26% more likely to develop breast cancer. In another study, heart and Estrogen/progesterone replacement study (HEPS), 4 years combination therapy was associated with 27% increase in breast cancer risk. The incidence of cholecystitis, venous thrombo-embolism, CHD and stroke are also higher in HRT women.

On the positive side HRT removes the majority of distressing symptoms, creates a feeling of well being, improves the bone densitometry and is associated with lower incidence of colorectal cancer. HRT is contra-indicated in those with deep vein thrombosis, active liver disease, unexplained vaginal bleeding and history of endometrial malignancy.

Therefore the present guidelines for HRT are to administer it for a period of 6 to 12 months in recent menopausal women to control their distressing symptoms. If on stoppage of HRT, their symptoms recur, the HRT may be given for a longer time. It may also be given for a longer period in those women who undergo premature menopause where it could be continued till the age of normal menopause. It is not advised to improve bone density or for cardio-protection as for the first condition better drugs are available and for the second no concrete evidence is available. Addition of progestogens to oestrogen interferes with the replenishment of nuclear oestrogen receptors, increases the activity of 17β-oestradiol dehydrogenase which converts it to less potent oestrone thus reducing the risk of endometrial cancer.

The recommended doses are given in Table 23.10.1. To protect the bone density, drugs like:

a. Selective oestrogen receptor modulators (SERMs) are helpful. Both tamoxifene and reloxifene (60 mg/day) have anti-osteoporotic effect and their use is being encouraged to improve upon bone density. Other agents which are being tried are iodotoxifene and droloxofene.

b. Drugs like bisphosphonates (alendronate 10 mg daily or 70 mg weekly) and risedronate (5 mg daily or 35 mg weekly), vit D_3 and calcium supplements are

TABLE 23.10.1

1. Bone protecting oestrogen	
• Conjugated equine oestrogen	0.625 daily
• Oestrogen sulphate	1.5 mg daily
• Oestradiol 17-β	
• Oral	1 to 2 mg daily
• Transdermal	0.05 mg daily
• Implant	50 mg × 6 monthly
2. Oral progesterone for endometrial protection	
• Norgestrel	0.15 mg × 12 days
• Noresthisterone	1 mg × 12 days
• Medroxyprogesterone acetate	10 mg × 12 days
• Micronized progesterone	200 mg × 12 days

Hormone replacement regimens

also useful to the bones. Long acting bisphosphontes (pamidronate 30 to 60 mg IV infusion 3 to 6 months or zolendronate 4 mg IV annually) may also be used.

SUMMARY

Endocrine glands undergo a progressive age-related change in their functional performance and response to various stimuli. The main effect of ageing process is seen on the carbohydrate tolerance, thyroid and hypo-thalamic-anterior pituitary-gonadal axis.

The subsection describes, in brief, various clinically significant changes which take place in some of the endocrine glands and their management.

FURTHER READING

Andropause

1. Basaria S, Dobs AS. Hypogonadism and androgen replacement therapy in elderly men. Am J Med 2002;110:563-72.
2. Bhasin S, Bremnner WJ. Emerging issues in androgen replacement therapy. J Clin Endocrinol Metab 1997; 82:3-8.
3. Juul A, Skakkeback NE. Androgen and ageing male. Human Reprod Update. 2002;8:423-33.
4. Snyder PJ, Peachey H, Berlin JA, et al. Effects of testosterone replacement in hypogonadal men. J Clin Endocrinol Metab 2000; 85:2670-7.
5. Wang C, Sweerdloff RS, Iranmanesh A, et al. Transdermal testosterone improves sexual function, mood, muscle strength, and body composition parameters in hypogonadal men. J Clin Endocrinol Metab 2000; 85:2839-53.
6. Wespes E. Schulmann CC. Male andropause: myth, reality and treatment. Int J Import Res. 2002; 14(suppl 1): 593-8.
7. Morales A, Lunenfeld. The standard guidelines and recommendations of the International Society for the study of ageing male (ISS AM). Investigations, treatment and monitoring

of late onset hypogonadism in males. The Ageing Male. 2002;5: 74-85.

Adrenopause

1. Baulies E E. Studies on dehydroepiandrosterone (DHEA) and its sulphate during ageing. CR Acad Seji III, 1995; 378:7-11.
2. Kalmijn S, Launer L J, Stolk RP, et al. A prospective study on cortisol, dehydroepiandrosterone sulphate and cognitive function in the elderly. J Clin Endocrinol Metab 1998;83,3487-92.
3. Moraes AJ, Nolan JJ, Nelson JC, et al. Effects of replacement dose of dehydroepiandrosterone in men and women of advancing age. J Clin Endicrinol Metab 1994;78:1360-7.

Somatopause

1. Consensus guidelines for the diagnosis and treatment of adults with growth hormone deficiency. Summary statement of the growth hormone research society. Workshop on adult growth hormone deficiency. J Clim Endocrinot Metal 1998;83:379-81.
2. Carroll PV, Christ ER, Bengtsoon BA, et al. Growth hormone deficiency in adulthood and the effects of GH replacement. A review. J Clin Endocrinol Metab 1998;83:382-95.

Menopause

1. Clemett D, Spancer C. Raloxifene: a review of its use in post-menopausal osteoporosis. Drugs 2000; 60: 379-411.
2. Diez J. Skeletal effects of selective oestrogen receptor madulators (SERMs). Human Reprod Update 2000; 6:255-8.
3. Postmenopausal estrogen/progesterone interventions (PEPI) trial. Effects of estrogen or estrogen/progesterone regimes on heart disease risk factors in postmenopausal women. JAMA 1995; 273: 199-208.

Part
6

SECTION

24

GLUCOSE METABOLISM AND HYPOGLYCAEMIA

24.1 Pancreas and Insulin

Y Sachdev

ANATOMY, PHYSIOLOGY AND EMBRYOLOGY OF PANCREAS

Anatomy

The pancreas is a flat elongated racemose gland measuring 12 to 15 cm in length with approximately 80 G weight. Its anatomical divisions are a head (30% of the gland), a neck, a body and a tail (70% of the gland) (Fig. 24.1.1). The head is lodged within the curve of the duodenum. Sometimes, a portion of the pancreatic head is actually embedded within the duodenal wall. The boundary between the head and the neck is marked anteriorly by the groove for the gastroduodenal artery. The neck has the superior mesenteric vessels as its posterior relation. Behind the neck, near its upper border, the superior mesenteric vein joins the splenic vein to form the portal vein. The tail is narrow and is contained, along with the splenic vessels, within the two layers of the lieno-renal ligament. The anterior surface of the neck and body is covered by peritoneum. The posterior surface is in contact with the aorta, the left adrenal gland, left kidney and its vessels.

The arteries of the pancreas are derived from the splenic and pancreatico-duodenal arteries. Its venous drainage is in the portal, splenic and superior mesenteric veins. The name pancreas is derived from the Greek *pan* (all) and *kreas* (flesh).

Physiology

A normal adult human pancreas gland weighs 50 to 150 G, of which only approximately 1 G is the islet tissue.

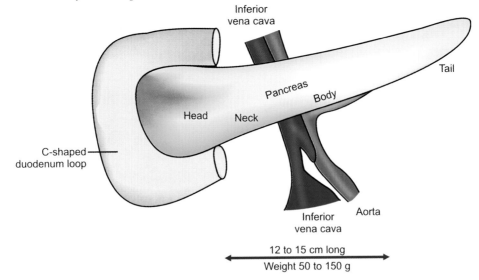

Fig. 24.1.1: The human pancreas

It possesses between a quarter and one and three quarter million islets of Langerhans (average about one million) which are scattered throughout the pancreas. The tail contains proportionately higher number of islets than the body and head. Individual islets vary from 75 to 175 microns in diameter and from a few dozen to several thousand of cells. Paul Langerhans (1869) was the first who recognized the islets as dense clusters of clear cells embedded in the exocrine pancreas. They were named after Langerhans 24 years later by Laguess. The major cell types in the islets are alpha (α), beta (β), delta (δ) and pancreatic polypeptide (PP) cells. α cells are further subdivided into α_1 and α_2 cells. The β cells account for nearly 70 to 80% of the total cells. α_1 cells secrete gastrin and α_2 cells glucagon, β insulin, δ somatostatin and PP cells secrete pancreatic polypeptide respectively. Some other pancreatic islet cells products are pancreastatin, chromostatin and amyloid polypeptide.

Embryology

Embryologically, the islets are derived from the specialized buds of epithelial cords from which arise the pancreatic ducts and acinar cells. These endocrine cells separate around the third month of gestation:
a. α cells appear around 9 weeks
b. δ cells at 10 weeks
c. β cells at 11 weeks while
d. PP cells appear the last.

Though the islets constitute only about or less than 2% of the total pancreatic mass, they receive nearly 20% of the total pancreatic blood flow. Islets are also rich in innervation from the coeliac plexus, parasympathetic, cholinergic, sympathetic adrenergic and various polypeptidergic nerves. These polypeptidergic nerves contain peptides such as VIP which stimulates release of all islet hormones, and neuropeptide Y (NPY) which inhibits insulin secretion. The overall role of these neuropeptides in the regulation of islet cell secretion is not clear. The islets can be easily identified with various histological stains, such as haematoxylin and eosin with which the cells react less intensely than do the surrounding endocrine tissues. The different cell types can be identified in various ways, including immuno-staining technique, *in situ* hybridization for their hormone products (using nucleotide probes comple-mentary to the target mRNA) and the electron-microscope appearance of their secretory granules. The β cells are located mainly in the core of the islets while α and δ cells are located at the periphery (Fig. 24.1.2).

The islet cells interact with each other through the direct contact and through their product (e.g. glucagon stimulates insulin secretion while somatostatin inhibits insulin and glucagon secretion). The blood supply within the islets is organized centrifugally so that the different cell types are supplied in sequence $\beta \rightarrow \alpha \rightarrow \delta$. Insulin also has an autocrine (self regulating) effect that alters the transcription of insulin and glucokinase genes in the cells (Fig. 24.1.3). Insulin, IGF-1 and IGF-2 play a definite role in the growth of β-cell in early postnatal period.

HORMONES OF PANCREAS

Insulin, glucagon, somatostatin, gastrin and polypeptide are the main pancreatic hormones. Pancreatic hormones other than insulin are described in Section 10.

Insulin

In 1869, a German medical student Paul Langerhans noted that pancreas contains two distinct groups of cells—the acinar cells and clusters of cells in islets or islands. In 1889, Oskar Minkowski and Joseph van Mering showed that dogs from whom pancreas had been removed exhibit a syndrome similar to diabetes mellitus in human beings.

In early 1900, Gurg Ludwig Zualzer, an internist in Berlin attempted to treat a dying diabetic patient with pancreatic extracts. The patient improved but later on when extract was exhausted he died. EL Scott, a student at the University of Chicago tried to isolate an active principle in 1911. Scott treated several diabetic dogs with encouraging results, his professor, however, considered the results inconclusive. Between 1916 and 1920, a Romanian physiologist, Nicolas Paolesco conducted a number of experiments where he found that pancreatic extract injection reduced urinary sugar and ketones in diabetics.

Unaware of the previous work, in 1921 Frederick Grant Banting, a young Canadian surgeon requested professor of physiology in Toranto, JJR Macleod to allow him to use his laboratory to search for antidiabetic principle of the pancreas. Together with Charles H Best a 4th year medical student, he was able to extract with ethanol and acid, pancreatic islets and use them as an effective agent to control blood sugar in diabetic dogs. The first patient to receive the active extract prepared by Banting and Best was Leonard Thompson aged 14 years. Banting, next year involved JB Collip, a brilliant chemist with expertise in extraction and purification of epine-phrine to help obtain active extracts. Collip purified the extract and made it suitable for human use. Ultimately within a year, many patients from various parts of North America were treated with insulin from porcine and bovine sources.

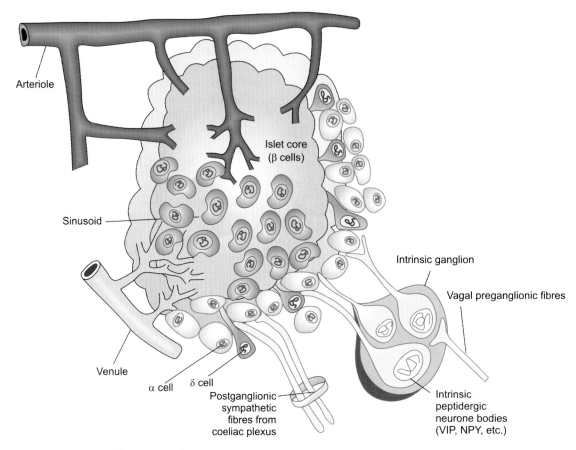

Fig. 24.1.2: Schematic representation of a pancreatic islet structure showing the anatomical location of β, α and δ cells

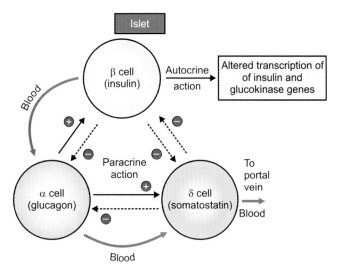

Fig. 24.1.3: Shows paracrine and autocrine action of secretory products of major islet cells (β, α and δ). Red lines indicate the direction of blood flow within the islets

Nobel prize in medicine/physics was awarded to Banting and Macleod in 1923. This resulted in uproar in the society which led to Banting sharing his prize with Best and Macleod with Collip.

Insulin is a small polypeptide with a molecular weight of about 6000 in the monomer form and is composed of two chains: A (glycyl) chain with 21 amino acids and B (phenylalanyl) chain with 30 amino acids held together by disulphide linkages. The structure of the molecule, as shown in Figure 24.1.4 was established in 1956 by Sanger and by 1964 its synthesis was achieved by Katsoyannis.

Insulin gene is located on chromosome 11 and contains three exons and two introns. The human, bovine and porcine insulin differ from one another (Fig. 24.1.5). Insulin from animal origin invariably results in production of antibodies in patients treated with these types of insulin. Human insulin also produces antibodies but to a lesser extent.

Commercially available human insulin is manufactured by different ways. The insulin obtained by each of these methods is identical to the human pancreatic insulin. The different procedures used are:

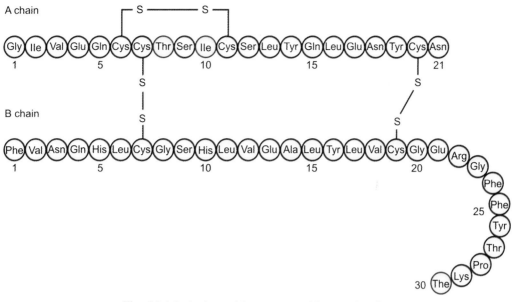

Fig. 24.1.4: Amino acid sequence of human insulin

	CHAIN A			CHAIN B
Position	8	9	10	30
Man	Thr	Ser	Ileu	Thr
Pig	Thr	Ser	Ileu	Ala
Beef	Ala	Ser	Val	Ala
Rabbit	Thr	Ser	Ileu	Ser

Fig. 24.1.5: The differences in human and animal insulin molecules

a. *Semisynthetic human insulin/human insulin emp (enzyme modified pork):* In this method, porcine insulin is converted to human insulin by enzymatically cleaving the beta-terminal amino acid, alanine and replacing it with threonine.

b. *Biosynthetic human insulin:* This is achieved by genetic engineering. Genetic engineering is a process by which genetic characteristic of a selected micro-organism are altered by inserting foreign DNA sequences (gene). Using this method, human insulin is produced in different ways. The two methods commonly used are:

    i. In one method, two sets of *E. coli* bacteria coded to produce either 'A' chain or 'B' chain are used. These chains are later extracted and chemically combined by inserting disulphide bridges.

    ii. In this method which has largely replaced other methods, human proinsulin or human miniproinsulin is produced by a genetically engineered *E. coli* or *Saccharomyces cervisae* (ordinary Baker's yeast). The proinsulin thus produced is then enzymatically cleaved and is purified to obtain human insulin.

Proinsulin

The preproinsulin (or insulin) gene is located on the short arm of chromosome 11. Transcription leads to production of preproinsulin which is a single chain 86 amino acids polypeptide and is converted to proinsulin in the endoplasmic reticulum of β cells by a protease enzyme. Proinsulin is structurally related to insulin like growth hormones I and II (IGFI and II). Proinsulin is packaged into vesicles and transported to the Golgi apparatus. It is a normal constituent of all insulin secreting cells. Human proinsulin is a single chain polypeptide with a molecular weight of about 9000 (Fig 24.1.6). Insulin, a two chain structure, is split-off by a trypsin-like enzyme from the single-chain proinsulin. This happens in the endoplasmic reticulum of β cells (Fig. 24.1.7). Since proinsulin contains the intact amino acid sequence of the insulin molecule, it cross reacts with antibodies of various species of insulin and may interfere with insulin RIA. Proinsulin exerts an insulin-like effect *in vitro* and *in vivo*. Its activity, however, is considerably less than that of insulin. The composition of the connecting peptide, which connects the N-terminal of the A chain to the C-terminal of the B chain varies greatly from species to species and may contain 30 to 40 amino acid residues. The terms connecting peptide and C-peptide are not synonymous. The C-peptide is proteolytically derived from the connecting peptide during the formation of insulin and has four basic residues less in its structure than the connecting peptide. Human C-peptide contains 31 amino acids and has a

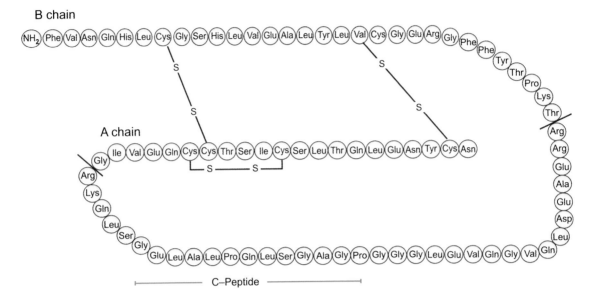

Fig. 24.1.6: The structure of human proinsulin

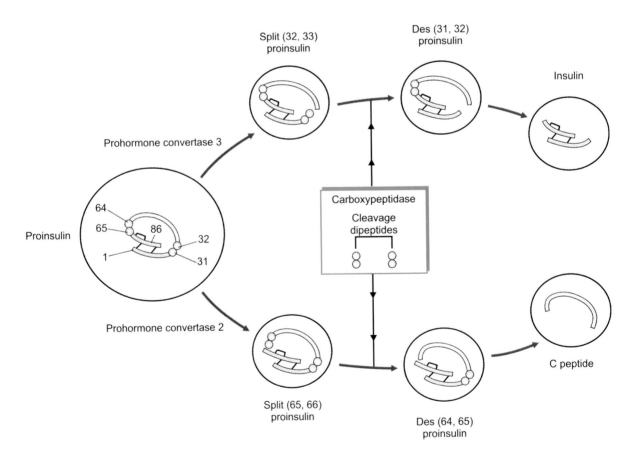

Fig. 24.1.7: Insulin biosynthesis from proinsulin. Proinsulin is cleaved on the C-terminal side of two dipeptides yielding the 'split' proinsulin products and ultimately insulin and C peptide

molecular weight of 3021. The C-peptide is biologically inactive.

The fasting concentration of proinsulin in normal subjects ranges from 0 to 0.4 ng/ml and represents 0 to 40% of the insulin concentration. The percentage of proinsulin in the pancreas is much less (1 to 2%). Plasma concentration of proinsulin, like that of insulin, rises after oral glucose or other (tolbutamide) stimulation. However, proinsulin and insulin ratio remains the same. Absolute increase in the plasma proinsulin level (>0.6 ng/ml) is seen only in islet cell tumours. Incretins (GLP-1 and GIP) stimulate proinsulin biosynthesis.

Secretion of Insulin

Normal insulin secretion is 30 to 50 units per day. Glucose is the key regulator of insulin secretion by the pancreatic beta cells. The amino acids, ketones, various nutrients, gastrointestinal peptides, and neurotransmitters also affect its secretion. Insulin release from the β cells in response to glucose is in a characteristic biphasic pattern—an acute first phase that lasts only a few minutes, followed by a more sustained second phase (Fig. 24.1.8) which lasts as long as the stimulus. Glucose level below 72 mg/dl (4 mmol/L) does not induce insulin release; half-maximum stimulation occurs at about 144 mg/dl (8 mmol/L).

Glucose must be metabolized within the β cells to stimulate insulin secretion. This is achieved through a series of regulatory steps that begin with its entry into the β cells (Fig. 24.1.9) via the GLUT-2 transporter and is then phosphorylated by the glucokinase which acts as a glucose sensor and matches insulin secretion to the prevailing glucose level. The activity of glucokinase is the rate-limiting step for glucose metabolism in the beta cell. Further metabolism of glucose-6-phosphate via

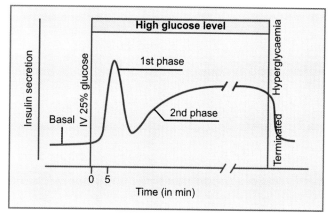

Fig. 24.1.8: The biphasic glucose-stimulated release of insulin from the beta cells of Langerhans

glycolysis and mitochondrial metabolism produces adenosine triphosphatase (ATP) which closes ATP-sensitive potassium (K_{ATP}) channels. This causes depolarization of the β cell plasma membrane, which leads to an influx of extracellular calcium through voltage-gated channels in the membrane. The increase in cytosolic calcium triggers insulin secretion. The newly secreted insulin is stored in the β cell granules. To facilitate insulin release, these granules migrate to the periphery of the cell, guided by a system of microtubules formed of polymerized tubulin and the sac in which they are enclosed fuses with the cell membranes. The granules are released by migration and granule extrusion, a process called 'emiocytosis.' The microfilaments of actin, interacting with myosin and other motor proteins such as kinesin, provide the motive force that propels granules along the tubules. This 'regulated pathway' with almost complete cleavage of proinsulin to insulin, normally carries about 95% of the β cell insulin production. In insulinoma and type 2 DM, an alternative 'constitutive'

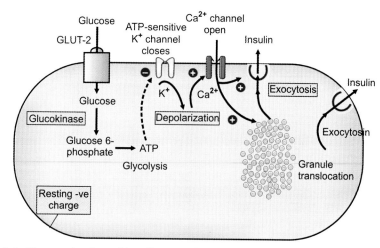

Fig. 24.1.9: The mechanism of insulin secretion from the β-cell as a response to glucose

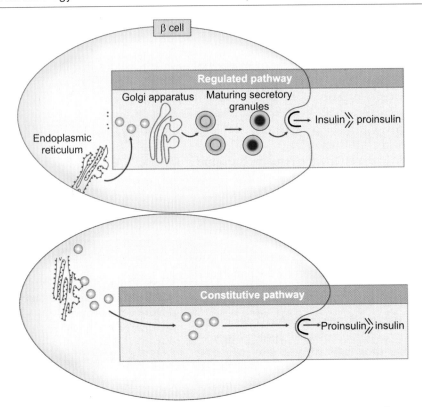

Fig. 24.1.10A: The regulated (normal) and constitutive (active in T2DM) pathways of insulin processing

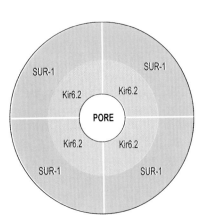

Fig. 24.1.10B: The structure of the K_{ATP} channel

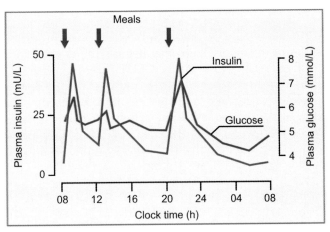

Fig. 24.1.10C: A 24-hour profile of plasma glucose and insulin concentrations in healthy (non-diabetic) individuals

pathway operates, in which larger amounts of un-processed proinsulin and intermediate insulin precursors (split proinsulin) are released directly from vesicles that originate from the endoplasmic reticulum (Fig. 24.1.10A).

The K_{ATP} channel is an octamer that consists of four K^+ channel subunits (called $K_{IR}6.2$) and four SUR-1 channels (Fig. 24.1.10B). The sulphonylureas (and miglinitide) stimulate insulin secretion by binding to SUR-1 component (sulphonylurea receptor) of the K_{ATP} channel and closing it.

Careful studies of insulin secretory profiles reveal pulsatile pattern of hormone release with small secretory bursts occurring about every 10 minutes superimposed upon greater amplitude oscillation of about 80 to 150 minutes. Meals and other major stimulants of insulin secretion induce large (4- to 5-fold) bursts of insulin secretion that usually last for 2 to 3 hours before returning to baseline (Fig. 24.1.10 C). Derangements in these normal secretory patterns are one of the earliest signs of beta cell dysfunction in diabetes mellitus.

Factors Stimulating Pancreatic Insulin Release (Fig. 24.1.11)

- *Hyperglycaemia:* Glucose stimulates the synthesis and release of insulin.
- *Amino acids:* Leucine, arginine, lysine and phenyl-alanine stimulate insulin release.
- *Glucagon:* It stimulates release of insulin by its direct action on the pancreas as well as by hyperglycaemia which results by glucagon.
- *Gut hormones (entero-humoral factors):* Secretin, pancre-ozymin and gastrin stimulate insulin secretion.
- *Neurogenic control of insulin release and neurotrans-mitters:* The pancreas is innervated by the sympathetic nervous system and by branches of the right vagus nerve. Insulin-induced hypoglycaemia results from right vagal stimulation. Insulin is also released under vagal stimulation during severe stress. Gastrin releasing polypeptide (GRP), VIP and pituitary adenylate cyclase activating polypeptides (PACAP) localized to parasympathetic nerve endings stimulate insulin secretion.

Factors Inhibiting Insulin Release

- Adrenaline inhibits insulin release through its alpha effects (In pancreatic islet cells alpha receptor mechanism predominates) and results in elevated blood glucose levels. Galanin and neuropeptide Y (NPY) localized to sympathetic nerve endings inhibit insulin secretion.
- Diazoxide (a benzothiadiazine compound) inhibits insulin release by reducing islet cell concentration of cyclic AMP and by promoting adrenaline release. The drug is, thus, diabetogenic. Other thiazide diuretics have a definite but milder diabetogenic action.

Actions of Insulin

Once insulin is secreted into the portal vein, 50% is removed and downgraded by the liver. Unextracted insulin enters into the systemic circulation and binds to its receptor at target sites. The insulin receptor is a cell-surface receptor, a glycoprotein that consists of two extra-cellular α subunits and two β subunits that span the cell membrane. The insulin receptor has tyrosine kinase enzyme activity which resides in the β subunit, (see Fig. 25.2.3). Insulin binding to the receptor stimulates intrinsic kinase activity, leading to receptor auto-phosphorylation and recruitment of intracellular signalling molecules such as insulin receptor substrates (IRS) 1 and 2. These and other adaptor proteins initiate a complex cascade of post-receptor phosphorylation and dephosphorylation reactions ultimately resulting in the widespread metabolic and mitogenic effects of insulin

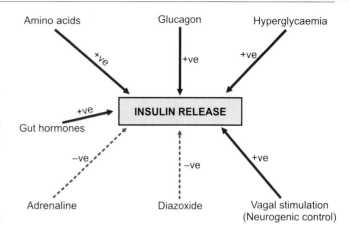

Fig. 24.1.11: Factors regulating insulin release

(Fig. 24.1.12) like translocation of glucose transporters (GLUT-4) to the cell surface (this event is crucial for glucose uptake, by the skeletal muscle), glycogen synthesis, protein synthesis, lipogenesis and regulation of various genes in insulin responsive cells. After binding of insulin to its receptor, the insulin-receptor complex is internalized by the surrounding membrane invaginating to form an 'endosome.' The protein 'clathrin' plays a key role in the endosome formation (Fig. 24.1.13). After internalization, the receptors are recycled to the cell surface, but insulin is degraded inside the cell by lysosomes. Elevated insulin levels (as seen in obesity and type 2 DM) lead to 'down-regulation' of the receptor, whereby internalization results in decreased number of receptors at the cell surface.

Glucose Transporters (GLUTS)

Glucose is carried across the cell membranes into the cells by a family of specialized transporter proteins called glucose transporters (GLUTS). The process is energy independent. The best characterized GLUTS are:
- GLUT-1. It is ubiquitously expressed and is probably responsible for basal non-insulin mediated glucose uptake.
- GLUT-2. It is present in the β cells and also in the liver, intestine and kidney. Together with gluco-kinase, it forms the β cells' glucose sensor and allows glucose to enter the β cell at a rate proportionate to the extracellular glucose level.
- GLUT-3. It is involved, along with GLUT-1, in non-insulin mediated glucose uptake in the brain.
- GLUT-4. It is responsible for insulin-stimulated glucose uptake in muscle and adipose tissue resulting in the classic hypoglycaemic action of insulin.
- GLUT-8. It is important in blastocyst development.
- GLUT-9 and GLUT 10. Their significance is not clear.

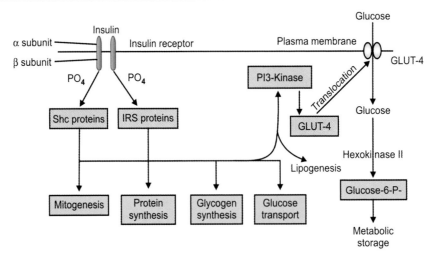

Fig. 24.1.12: Insulin signal transduction pathway

- Shc and IRS proteins are insulin receptor substrates proteins
- A number of docking proteins combine with these cellular proteins and initiate various metabolic effects of insulin
- Insulin increases glucose transport through PI 3-kinase which promotes the translocation of intracellular vesicles containing GLUT-4 glucose transporter to the plasma membrane

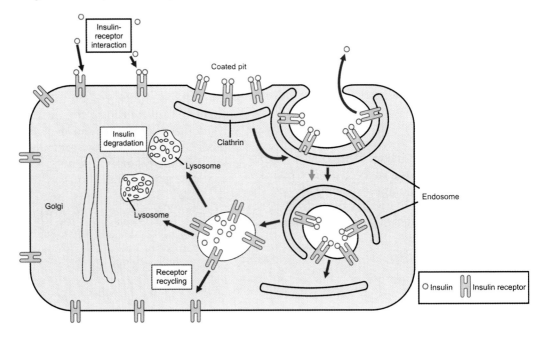

Fig. 24.1.13: Insulin receptor internalization

Most of the other GLUTS are present at the cell surface, but in the basal state GLUT-4 is sequestered within vesicles in the cytoplasm. Insulin causes the vesicles to be transported to the cell surface where they fuse with the membrane and the inserted GLUT-4 unit functions as a pore that allows glucose entry. The process is reversible. When insulin level falls, the plasma membrane GLUT-4 is removed by endocytosis and recycled back to vesicles for storage (Fig. 24.1.14).

Glucose homeostasis reflects a precise balance between hepatic glucose production and peripheral glucose uptake and utilization. Insulin is the most important regulator (see Fig. 24.1.11). Other contributory factors are neural inputs, metabolic signals and various hormones like glucagon, cortisol, growth hormone, thyroxine and adrenaline. Low insulin levels decrease glucose synthesis, reduce glucose uptake and promote mobilization of stored precursors.

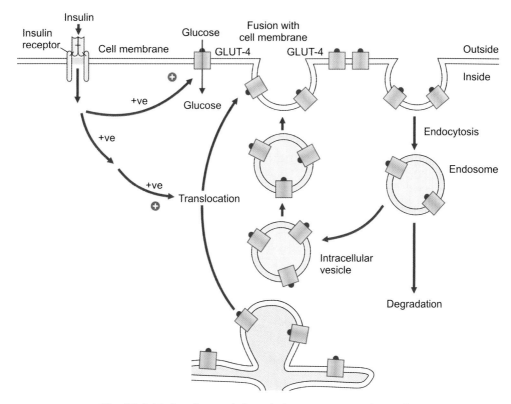

Fig. 24.1.14: Insulin regulation of glucose transport into cells

Unopposed glucagon stimulates glycogenolysis and gluconeogenesis by the liver and renal medulla. These processes are of great importance to ensure an adequate glucose supply for the brain. Glucose is carried both by plasma and RBCs.

Postprandial (PP) large glucose load elicits a rise in insulin and fall in glucagon leading to a reversal of these processes. The major portion of PP glucose is utilized by the skeletal muscle. Other tissues, most notably the brain, utilize glucose in an insulin-independent fashion. Besides brain, in liver, kidney, intestines and placenta the glucose uptake is insulin independent. In adipose tissue, skeletal and heart muscle, it is insulin dependent.

SUMMARY

Pancreas is an elongated flat racemose gland. It weighs about 80 G with approximately 1 G of the islet tissue. The beta islet cells secrete insulin. Insulin is a small polypeptide having 'A' chain with 21 amino acids and 'B' chain with 30 amino acids. Preproinsulin gene is located on the short arm of chromosome 11. Preproinsulin is a single chain 86 amino acids polypeptide. Human proinsulin is also a single chain polypeptide. The cleavage of proinsulin to insulin takes place in 'regulated

pathways' where the process is almost completed. In type 2 DM, an alternative 'constitutive pathway' operates where cleavage of proinsulin to insulin is not that effective and large quantity of proinsulin may be released.

Glucose is the key regulator of insulin secretion. It must be metabolized in the β cells to stimulate insulin secretion. This is achieved by a series of regulatory steps.

The role of Insulin receptor, glucose transporters (GLUTS) and various factors affecting insulin secretion and action is described in brief.

FURTHER READING

1. Ahuja MMS, Shah Pankaj. Seventy-five years of insulin user. National Medical Jr Ind 1997;10:1-2.
2. Banting FG, Best CH. Pancreatic extracts. J Lab Clin Med 1922;7: 464-72.
3. Mitrakov A, Kelley D, Veneman T, et al. Contribution of abnormal muscle and liver glucose metabolism to postprandial hyperglycaemia in NIDDM. Diabetes 1990;39:1381-90.
4. Reimann F, Gribble FM, Ashcroft FM. Differential response of K (ATP) channels containing SUR 2A or SUR B subunits to nucleotides and pinacidil. Mol Pharmacol 2000;58:1318-25.
5. William Gareth, Pickup C John. Normal physiology of insulin secretion and action. In Handbook of Diabetes. Oxford: Blackwell Publishing 2004;27-38.

24.2 Glucose Homeostasis

Y Sachdev

INTRODUCTION

Plasma glucose is the predominant metabolic fuel utilized by the central nervous system (CNS). Therefore, an adequate plasma glucose concentration is critical to sustain life. This is critical as central nervous system cannot:
- Synthesize glucose
- Store more than a few minutes' supply of glucose, and
- Concentrate glucose from the circulation.

Thus a brief period of hypoglycaemia can result in profound brain dysfunction while prolonged and severe hypoglycaemia causes brain death. The fasting plasma glucose concentration is usually maintained within a relatively narrow range of 60 to 126 mg/dl (3.5 to 7 mmol/L) (Fig. 24.2.1) despite wide variations in glucose influx and efflux such are seen after meals and during exercise. Sometimes, however fasting plasma glucose level may reach as low as 50 mg/dl (2.8 mmol/L). This narrow range is achieved by an extremely effective glucose regulatory (and counterregulatory) system. Insulin counterregulation is entrusted to several hormones and the entire hormonal system is considered to be the best in metabolism and one of the best known in human physiology.

SOURCES OF GLUCOSE

Glucose in the body comes from three sources:
- Intestinal absorption following digestion of dietary carbohydrates.
- Glycogenolysis—break down of glycogen (the poly-merized storage form of glucose), and
- Gluconeogenesis—the formation of glucose from lactate, pyruvate, amino acids especially alanine and to a lesser extent glycerol.

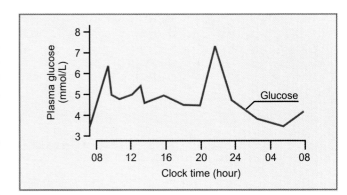

Fig. 24.2.1: Profile of plasma glucose values. Fasting glucose level is maintained in a narrow range of 3.5 to 7 mmol/L

Most tissues have the enzyme systems required to synthesize and hydrolyze glycogen (glycogen synthase and phosphorylase) but it is only liver and kidney which contain glucose-6-phosphatase, the enzyme necessary for the release of glucose into the circulation. These two organs (liver and kidney) also contain the enzymes necessary for gluconeogenesis (pyruvate carboxylase, phosphoenolpyruvate carboxykinase and fructose 1,6 bisphosphatase).

INTRACELLULAR GLUCOSE METABOLISM

The glucose transported into the cell may be dealt with as follows (Fig. 24.2.2):
- Stored as glycogen
- Undergo glycolysis to pyruvate (which can be reduced to lactate or transaminated to form alanine or converted to acetyl-CoA, which, in turn, can be oxidized to CO_2 and H_2O via the tricarboxylic acid cycle, converted to fatty acids (and stored as

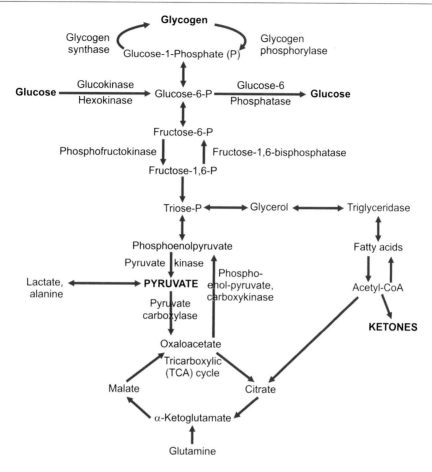

Fig. 24.2.2: Schematic representation of glucose metabolism

triglycerides or utilized for ketone body synthesis) or
• Released into the circulation.

ENDOGENOUS GLUCOSE PRODUCTION

The liver for all practical purposes is the sole source of endogenous glucose production. Renal gluconeogenesis and glucose release assume significance only during prolonged starvation. Under conditions of high glucose output, the energy needs of the liver are largely provided by the β-oxidation of fatty acids. The liver is also an organ of net glucose uptake where it can be stored as glycogen, undergo oxidation for energy and conversion to fat which can either remain in the liver or be transported to other tissues as very low density lipoproteins (VLDL).

Muscles can store and utilize glucose. The glucose utilization in the muscle is through glycolysis to pyruvate which is further reduced to lactate or transaminated to form alanine.

Adipose tissue can also utilize glucose for fatty acid synthesis or oxidation to glycerol-3-phosphate which can then esterify fatty acids (derived from circulating very low density lipoproteins) to form triglycerides (Fig. 24.2.3).

Recent observations have proved that adipose tissue is not simply an inert storage depot for lipids. The adipocyte secretes various bioactive proteins into the circulation. These proteins are collectively called 'adipocytokines' and include leptin, tumour necrosis factor α (TNF α), plasminogen-activator inhibitor type- 1 (PAI- 1), adipsin, resistin and adiponectin.

Adiponectin, the gene product of the adipose most abundant gene transcript 1 (apm 1), is an important member of the adipocytokine family. It is a collegen like protein that is exclusively synthesized in white adipose tissue and circulates at relatively high (μg/ml) concentrations in the serum.

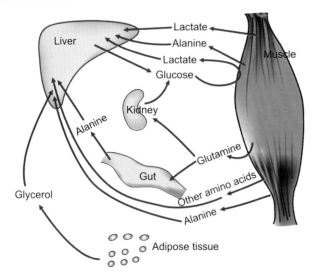

Fig. 24.2.3: The metabolism of substrates (lactate, glucogenic amino acids, glycerol) for gluconeogenesis

TABLE 24.2.1

Sites	Changes
A. Liver	↑ Glycogenolysis (initial)
	↑ Gluconeogenesis (later)
(Concomitantly)	↓ Utilization of glucose by tissues like brain.
B. Adipose tissue	↑ Lipolysis leading to
	↑ FFA, glycerol which results in ↑ Glucose
C. Muscle	↑ Proteolysis leading to
	↑ Alanine
	↑ Pyruvate
	↑ Lactate
D. Hormonal changes	↓ Insulin
	↑ Glucagon
	↑ Epinephrine
	↑ Cortisol
	↑ Growth hormone

Metabolic and hormonal changes to maintain glucose homeostasis during fasting

Adiponectin is a protein of 247 amino acids consisting of four domains (an amino-terminal signal sequence, a variable region, a collagenous domain and a carboxy-terminal globular domain).

Adiponectin plays an important role in glucose and lipid metabolism in insulin sensitive tissues. Its decreased level has been seen in obesity and insulin resistant states like type 2 DM. It is increased by administration of insulin sensitizers (like thiazoledinedione TZD). It appears to have antiatherogenic properties as well as anti-inflammatory properties including suppression of macrophage phagocytosis, TNF α secretion and blockage of monocyte adhesion to endothelial cells *in vitro*.

BLOOD GLUCOSE HOMEOSTASIS DURING POST-ABSORPTIVE OR FASTING PHASE

- In fasting state, 70% of glucose uptake is by insulin-independent tissues (mainly brain).
- In insulin-independent tissues, increased insulin level does not affect glucose metabolism but insulin lack may decrease the glucose utilization speed. Fat is preferred substrate of insulin dependent tissues in basal state. Over 50% of basal energy production relies on fat oxidation.

Immediately following a meal, the blood concentration of insulin and glucose are high and most body tissues utilize glucose energy as their body fuel. As the time passes after food ingestion, the fatty acids and ketone bodies metabolism overtakes that of glucose. This change to metabolism of lipid fuel is well advanced after an over night fast. However, even at this stage, certain tissues must have glucose available to them. These tissues include central and peripheral nervous system, red and white blood cells, fibroblasts, testes and renal medulla. Daily glucose requirement for these tissues is around 160 G (0.89 mol) for a 70 kg man. This glucose is provided by the liver and the kidneys, the only organs which have the enzyme glucose-6-phosphatase which allows glucose to be formed and released into the circulation. After an overnight fast, 75% of glucose released by the liver is derived from glycogenolysis and 25% from gluconeogenesis. As at this time liver contains only 70 to 80 G of glycogen, it gets exhausted over 24 hours. In man, liver glycogen is not reformed, therefore if fasting continues the process of gluconeogenesis becomes a prominent source of glucose production (Table 24.2.1).

With prolonged fasting, the obligatory glucose requirements decrease and after 6 weeks starvation, the daily glucose production comes down to mere 40 G (0.22 mol). This is supplied by gluconeogenesis. The decrease results partly from the adaptation of the brain to the metabolism of the ketone bodies so that in prolonged fasting 75% of its energy requirements are derived from this source. In addition, as circulating non-esterified fatty acids (NEFA) and ketone bodies concentration rises, muscle glucose utilization diminishes and glucose is further spared. During prolonged fasting the low circulating insulin concentration further decreases and becomes from low to very low. This level of insulin has no direct effect on glucose utilization at the periphery. Moreover, very low level of insulin results in increase in lipolysis and NEFA concentration. Both brain and muscle increase their ketone body metabolism and reduce glucose oxidation under these circumstances. Although during fasting and starvation time, gluconeogenesis increases, the quantity of glucose supplied by this process is always less (40 G/day at 6 weeks starvation) than glucose supplied from glycogenolysis in the over night-fasted state (160 G/day).

In diabetes where there is insulin deficiency or inefficiency, the liver functions as in a fasted state with a preferential activation of gluconeogenesis and glycogenolysis. The patients with poorly controlled T1DM exhibit a gross defect in suppression of hepatic glucose production following glucose ingestion, along with a failure to take up glucose and store as glycogen. In T2DM where insulin levels and action are partially retained, defects in suppression of hepatic glucose production and liver glycogen storage are also seen but to a lesser extent. Thus these defects (imbalance in hepatic glucose production and disposal) are two major contributory factors in development of hyperglycaemia and other disturbances in fuel homeostasis.

GLUCONEOGENESIS

Substrates for Gluconeogenesis

The principal gluconeogenic precursors are lactate (and pyruvate), the glucogenic amino acids and glycerol. After an overnight fast, lactate is more important substrate as it provides nearly half of the total substrate. Total lactate turnover is estimated at 140 G/day (1.6 mol/day) but more than half of this is derived from the glucose metabolism in extrahepatic tissues (the Cori cycle) and from the muscle glycogen.

Glycerol is released from the adipose tissue on hydrolysis of triglycerides. Further metabolism requires its phosphorylation in the liver under the influence of glycerol kinase. In an overnight fasted man, glycerol contributes less than 10% of glucose production by gluconeogenesis.

Amino acids are quantitatively the most important precursor for *de novo* glucose synthesis from gluconeogenesis. They contribute 6 to 12% of total glucose production after an overnight fast. Alanine and glutamine predominate and account for more than 50% of the amino acids released from the muscle into the circulation. Alanine serves primarily as a substrate for hepatic gluconeogenesis. Glutamine serves also as a

precursor for renal ammonia synthesis and as an energy source for the gut. After an overnight fast, most of the glutamine released by the muscle is taken up by the gastrointestinal tract. The gut readily converts glutamine to alanine which is released into portal circulation and taken up by the liver. Glutamine is also extracted by the kidney for ammonia production. As fasting continues for several days, the kidney becomes more important as a gluconeogenic organ and after several weeks, its contribution equals that of liver. The increased loss of ketone bodies in the urine in prolonged starvation is matched by an increase in ammonia excretion as the principal cation. Glutamine uptake by the kidney is increased, providing both the nitrogen for ammonia and glutamate for renal gluconeogenesis.

Alanine release by the muscle increases in the first few days of starvation, but as fasting continues, its release declines by more than 70%. In consequence, circulating alanine levels decrease and this may be a major factor limiting glucose production. In prolonged starvation, the production of glucose derived from glycerol increases to 20 to 80%. In contrast the relative importance of lactate as gluconeogenic substrate declines in prolonged starvation even though it still remains a significant substrate for glucose synthesis.

Regulation of Gluconeogenesis

The major factors which control gluconeogenesis are:
- Supply of substrate, and
- Hormonal regulatory status.

Gluconeogenesis in human liver increases as substrate supply rises. This assumes importance during starvation when gluconeogenesis uses increased amount of available glycerol. Concentration of other major gluconeogenic substrates, lactate and alanine falls with fasting. Despite this fall, gluconeogenesis from alanine and lactate increases making it clear that factors other than substrate supply are also very important. These factors are the hormones which regulate gluconeogenesis.

Hormonal Regulation of Gluconeogenesis

This is exercised by insulin, glucagon, cortisol, GH, catecholamines and sympathetic nervous system.

Insulin and Glucagon

These two hormones have opposing actions on gluconeogenesis exercised by:

- Substrate release from the peripheral tissues
- Substrate uptake by the liver
- Substrate utilization within the liver.

Substrate release from the peripheral tissues Insulin decreases release of amino acids from the muscle. It inhibits lipolysis resulting in diminished peripheral release of glycerol. The effect of insulin on lactate is complex and is determined by the ambient blood glucose concentration.

Glucagon, on the other hand, has no major effect on the release of substrates for gluconeogenesis. Alanine release, release of other amino acids and the release of lactate, stay unaffected by glucagon at physiological concentrations. However, in pharmacological doses, glucagon has lipolytic effect *in vitro* which is seen in man only when there is severe insulin deficiency, resulting in release of glycerol from adipose tissue triglycerides.

Substrate uptake by the liver Amino acids uptake by the liver is stimulated by both insulin and glucagon. Hepatic uptake of lactate, pyruvate and glycerol is not affected by hormones.

Substrate utilization within the liver Glucagon stimulates gluconeogenesis. It increases the activity of pyruvate carboxylase and decreases pyruvate kinase activity. It also increases fructose-1, 6-bisphosphatase and decreases 6-phosphofructokinase activities through decreased production of their intracellular regulator, fructose-1, 6-bisphosphate. The net result of these changes is stimulation of gluconeogenesis and inhibition of hepatic glycolysis.

Insulin inhibits glucagon-stimulated gluconeogenesis. It antagonizes the effects of glucagon on the activities of enzymes pyruvate kinase, fructose-1, 6-bisphosphatase and 6-phosphofructokinase. Insulin has no effect on gluconeogenesis in the absence of glucagon.

Role of Cortisol on Gluconeogenesis

Glucocorticoids increase gluconeogenic substrate delivery from peripheral tissues and they enhance glucose formation from these substrates in the liver. The release of glucogenic amino acids and lactate from the peripheral tissues is increased. The hepatic capacity for gluconeogenesis also rises. These changes occur due to induction of liver enzymes by glucocorticoids and begin in the first hour after glucocorticoid administration and extend to increasing number of enzymes over following days. The synthesis of phosphoenolpyruvate carboxykinase, fructose-1, 6-bisphosphatase and glucose-6-phosphatase increases. In addition, glucocorticoids have permissive effect on the actions of glucagon and catecholamines.

Role of Growth Hormone (GH)

GH has dual effect on blood glucose—an early insulin like action followed by a sustained diabetogenic effect. The insulin-like action of GH reflects both increased peripheral glucose utilization and decreased splanchnic glucose production. The diabetogenic effect of GH is the more important and persistent action.

Catecholamines and Sympathetic Nervous System

Both adrenaline and noradrenaline stimulate gluconeogenesis. Stimulation of both α and β adrenergic fibres causes an increase in gluconeogenesis. In addition catecholamines suppress insulin secretion and stimulate glucagon release. Human liver is rich in sympathetic nerve supply and hepatic sympathetic stimulation increases hepatic glucose output.

Figure 24.2.4 represents the main regulatory steps in gluconeogenesis.

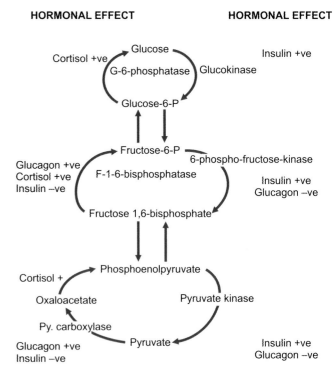

Fig. 24.2.4: Enzymatic and hormonal regulatory steps in gluconeogenesis

Regulation of Hepatic Glycogenolysis

The principal function of liver glycogen is to provide an immediate source of glucose for utilization by other tissues in short-term starvation, stress and exercise. Glycogen is broken down by phosphorylase which exists in highly active (α) and a less active (β) form while its synthesis is controlled by glycogen synthase (synthase D is active form and synthase 1 is inactive form). Protein kinase catalyses phosphorylation and activation of phosphorylase β and inactivation of glycogen synthase.

Glucose suppresses gluconeogenesis in the liver by inactivating phosphorylase α as well as by a separate mechanism which requires insulin.

Insulin and Glucagon

Glucagon causes a rapid increase in glycogenolysis through its action on cyclic AMP. Cyclic AMP increases the available phosphorylase α level. The glycogenolytic effect of glucagon in liver is inhibited by insulin.

Cortisol

Glucocorticoids stimulate hepatic glycogen synthesis *in vivo*. Glucocorticoids also have a permissive effect on glycogen degradation affected by glucagon and adrenaline.

Growth Hormone (GH)

Prolonged GH excess leads to inappropriately high rate of hepatic glucose production. This is affected through glycogen degradation as well as gluconeogenesis.

Catecholamines

The catecholamines have a gylcogenolytic effect mediated by α and β-adrenergic receptors.

Other Hormones

Vasopressin, oxytocin and angiotensin II have glycogenolysis effect. The exact importance of these hormones during starvation is uncertain.

POSTPRANDIAL BLOOD SUGAR HOMEOSTASIS

The principal carbohydrates ingested by man are:
- Sucrose which is hydrolysed to glucose and fructose in equimolar amounts,
- Lactose which yields glucose and galactose, and
- Starch which is broken in the gut to glucose.

Quantitatively glucose and fructose are the most important. Most of the ingested fructose is taken up by the liver and phosphorylated to fructose-1-phosphate which enters the glycolytic pathway. Besides conversion to glycogen, a large percentage of fructose load appears in the circulation as lactate. Dietary fructose therefore contributes little to the glucose rise seen after carbohydrate containing meals. Galactose is also metabolized almost exclusively by the liver and is converted to glycogen or glucose. As carbohydrate absorption is almost 100% and as most dietary glucose is absorbed as glucose, the nature provides an efficient mechanism for glucose disposal by the liver and peripheral tissues.

Liver and Glucose Disposal

When the portal venous glucose concentration is low, the liver releases glucose and when glucose concentration is high, there is net hepatic glucose uptake. This regulation of glucose release and uptake occurs independently of hormonal regulation though prior exposure to insulin is necessary for this hepatic glucose autoregulation.

Glucose uptake by the hepatocyte is so rapid that the intracellular glucose levels are very similar to extracellular concentrations. The phosphorylation of glucose to glucose-6-phosphate is a regulatory step in hepatic glucose uptake, and the quantity of glucokinase, the enzyme responsible, is increased by insulin. When glucose is abundant, hepatic glycogen synthesis is favoured and glycogenolysis is suppressed. Glucose itself also contributes to this control of glycogen metabolism. Glucose inhibits the activity of glycogen phosphorylase α and thereby reduces glycogenolysis. Moreover, as phosphorylase α inhibits glycogen synthase, glucose indirectly increases glycogen synthesis. Glucose also increases glycogen synthase phosphatase thereby increasing synthase activity.

In man after ingestion of say 100 G of oral glucose, nearly 8 to 10% of the glucose load is taken up by the liver in first pass and 90 to 92% reaches the peripheral circulation. The net uptake of the glucose by the liver after first and subsequent passes ranges from 20 to 60%. Insulin on its own has no direct action on hepatic glycogen synthesis. Glucagon inhibits glycogen formation. This action of glucagon is antagonized by insulin. After a carbohydrate rich meal, the rise in insulin secretion and fall in glycogen release favour glucagon formation.

Peripheral Tissue and Glucose Disposal

During starvation, the muscle glycogen stores are progressively depleted and are utilized for total oxidation or for glycogenolysis to lactate which then takes part in the Cori cycle. When an individual is refed, much of the glucose taken up by the peripheral tissues is utilized to replenish muscle glycogen. Glucose uptake directly by adipose tissue is only about 2% of the total body glucose disposal. Insulin is the main hormone responsible for peripheral glucose disposal. Circulating insulin levels increase after a substantial mixed meal or oral glucose load. The elevated insulin values stimulate membrane transport of glucose in muscle and adipose tissue. Insulin also stimulates glycogen synthesis by an increase in the activity of muscle glycogen synthase. It inhibits lipolysis

so that NEFA and ketone bodies concentrations fall. This indirectly stimulates the uptake of the glucose by the muscles through the glucose-fatty acid-ketone body cycle. The last mechanism appears to be the major step for stimulating glucose utilization in the periphery after small meals which result in a lesser increase in insulin secretion. Other hormones do not appear to play any significant role in a normal healthy man. In a stressed man, however, raised levels of circulating cortisol, adrenaline and GH may impair peripheral glucose utilization. Table 24.2.2 gives major effects of various hormones on glucose metabolism.

TABLE 24.2.2

| Hormone | Effect on blood glucose | Hepatic glucose output | | | | | Glucose uptake | | | | Other actions |
| | | Gluconeogenesis | | | Glycogenolysis | | Liver | | Muscle | | |
		Effect	Hepatic actions	Substrate supply	Effect	Hepatic actions	Effect	Hepatic actions	Effect	Actions	
Insulin	↓	↓	Inhibits glucagon effect (↑alanine uptake)	↓Amino acid release from muscles ↓glycerol release from adipose tissue	↓	Inhibits glucagon effects	↑	↑glucokinase permits autoregulation of glucose uptake	↑	↑membrane transport, ↑glycolysis, ↑glycogen synthase	↓Plasma NEFA and ketone bodies may increase muscle glucose
Glucagon	↑	↑	↑alanine uptake ↑pyruvate carboxylase ↓pyruvate kinase ↓6-phospho-fructokinase ↑fructose-1,6-bisphosphatase	Nil	↑	↑phosphorylase α synthase ↓synthase ↓glycogen synthase	Nil	–	Nil	–	–
Cortisol	↑	↑	↑PEP carboxy-kinase ↑fructose-1,6-bisphosphatase ↑glucose-6-phosphatase	↑amino acid and lactate release from muscle	↓	Secondary ↑glycogen synthase and ↓phosphorylase	?	–	↓	↓basal and insulin stimulated glucose uptake	Permissive and poten-tiating effects for glucagon and cate-cholamine
GH	↑ (↓)				?		?		↓ (↑)	↓ due to ↑plasma NEFA	
Catechola-mine	↑	↑	↑α and β media-ted fructose-1,6-bisphosphatase ↓6-phospho-fructokinase ↓pyruvate kinase ↓glucokinase ↑amino acid uptake	↑glycerol release from adipose tissue	↑	↑ α and β meliated phosphory-lase	?		↓	Adrenaline induced β-adrenergic mediated	↓insulin secretion ↑glucagon secretion

Hormonal influences on glucose metabolism

FATTY ACID AND KETONE BODY METABOLISM

The control of fatty acid mobilization from peripheral triacylglycerol stores is a major regulatory step in the control of ketogenesis. In normal man, fatty acid is released from adipose tissue at a rate of 6 μmol/kg/minute (600 mmol/24 hours for a 74 kg man). The fatty acid mobilization is modified by changes in:
• The rate of lipolysis
• Rate of esterification
• Both

Triacylglycerol is cleaved initially to diacylglycerol and then to monoacylglycerol and subsequently to glycerol. NEFA are released at every step. The rate-limiting enzyme in lipolysis is triacyl glycerol lipase. This enzyme is activated by phosphorylation by cyclic AMP-dependent protein kinase. Insulin is the major hormone which inhibits fatty acid mobilization in man. Insulin inhibits fatty acid mobilization both by an increase in esterification and a decrease in lipolysis. Insulin deficiency as seen in type 1 diabetes mellitus results in a brisk increase in fatty acid mobilization (Fig. 24.2.5). Sympathetic nervous activity and circulating catechola-

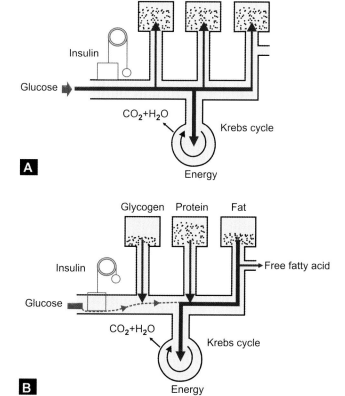

Figs 24.2.5A and B: (A) Normal glucose metabolism, (B) Glucose metabolism in absence of insulin. Insulin deficiency results in increased fatty acid mobilization

TABLE 24.2.3

Hormones	Effect on blood ketone bodies	Ketone body production	Ketone body utilization
Insulin	↓	↓	↓
Glucagon	↑ (Insulin deficiency)	↑	Nil
Cortisol	↑ (Insulin deficiency)	↑	Nil
Growth hormone	↑	↑	?
Catecholamines	↑	↑	?

Hormonal effects on ketone body metabolism

mines are the dominant factors which increase fatty acid release. The lipolytic effects of catecholamines are mediated through beta-adrenergic receptors. The dominant beta receptor in human adipose tissue is of the β_1 type. Alpha adrenergic stimulation in man is anti-lipolytic. Glucagon's lipolytic action becomes evident only in absolute insulin deficiency. GH causes an increase in lipolysis while glucocorticoids play a permissive effect for GH and catecholamines. Table 24.2.3 summarises the hormonal effects on ketone body metabolism.

Intrahepatic Control of Ketogenesis

The uptake of non-esterified fatty acid (NEFA) by the liver is concentration-dependent. Once in the hepatocyte, NEFA follows one of the two pathways:
• They may be esterified in the cell cytosol to triglyceride, or
• They may enter mitochondria for β-oxidation.

Inside the mitochondria, the acetyl CoA produced as a result of fatty acid oxidation, combines with oxaloacetate to form citrate in the tricarboxylic acid (TCA) cycle or alternatively acetyl CoA may be converted to the ketone bodies (see Fig. 24.2.2).

In the hepatocyte, NEFA are first converted to the fatty acyl CoA derivative. The transfer of fatty acyl CoA across the mitochondrial membrane is the major regulatory step for ketogenesis. The inner mitochondrial membrane is impermeable to long-chain fatty acyl CoA, which must be converted to fatty acyl carnitine by carnitine acyl transferase I (CATI). Fatty acyl carnitine crosses the membrane and fatty acyl CoA is reformed inside the mitochondria under the influence of carnitine acyl transferase II (CAT II).

Inside mitochondria, the ketone bodies are formed through the hydroxyl methyl glutaryl CoA (HMG-CoA) cycle.

Ketone Body Utilization

Ketone body utilization occurs in the mitochondria of extrahepatic tissues where they undergo oxidation. Utilization is concentration dependent and it inhibits uptake of glucose by the muscle and other tissues.

Effects of Hormones (Table 24.2.3)

Insulin inhibits the ketogenic effects of glucagon and diverts hepatic fatty acid metabolism away from ketogenesis and towards triglyceride synthesis. Insulin-deprived diabetic rapidly mobilizes fatty acid and develops ketosis. In established diabetic ketoacidosis, there is a major defect in ketone body utilization also. Glucagon stimulates ketogenesis and inhibits hepatic fatty acid synthesis. Glucocorticoids enhance hepatic triglyceride synthesis and VLDL secretion. GH, catecholamines, and thyroid hormone enhance ketogenesis while vasopressin inhibits it.

SUMMARY

Plasma glucose is normally maintained within a relatively narrow range by an extremely effective glucose regulatory mechanism. The regulatory control is exercised through various hormones and sympathetic nervous system. The main processes involved are glucose utilization for energy, its conversion to glycogen, gluconeogenesis and glycogenolysis. Closely connected with glucose metabolism is that of fatty acids and ketone bodies which are used for energy purposes during starvation period. This chapter deals with the role played by various hormones in glucohomeostasis.

FURTHER READING

1. Boden G, Chen X, Ruiz J, et al. Mechanisms of fatty acid induced inhibition of glucose uptake. J Clin Invest 1994;93:2438-46.
2. Ferrannini E, Barrett E J, Bevilac QVA S, et al. Effect of fatty acids on glucose production and utilization in man. J Clin Invest 1983; 72:1737-47.
3. Goldfine AB, Kohn RC. Adiponectin: linking the fat cell to insulin sensitivity. Lancet 2003;362:1431-2.
4. Maeda K, Okubo K, Shimomura I, Funahashi T, Matsuzawa YMatsubara K. cDNA cloning and expression of a novel adipose specific collagen-like factor, apMi (adipose most abundant gene transcript. Biochem Biophys Res Common 1996;221:280-9.
5. Steppan CM, Bailey ST, Bhat S, Brown EJ, Banarjee RR, Wright CM, et al. The hormone resistin links obesity in diabetes. Nature 2001; 409:307-12.
6. Valsamakis G, Chetty R, McTernan PG, Al-Daghri NM, Bamett AH, Kumar S. Fasting serum adiponectin concentration is reduced in Indo-Asian subjects and is related to HDL cholesterol. Diabetes Obes Metab 2003;5:131-5.

24.3 Hypoglycaemia

Y Sachdev

- Definition
- Symptoms
- Clinical Signs
- Aetiopathogenesis
  - Islet Cell Tumours, Islet Cell Hyperplasia, Reactive, Functional, Alcohol Induced and Leucine Sensitivity Hypoglycaemia, Hypoglycaemia due to Non-beta Cell Tumours, Autoimmune Hypoglycaemia, Pseudo-hypoglycaemia, Somogyi Effect
- Diagnosis
- Treatment
- Risk Factors and Prevention

- Hypoglycaemia in Children
  - Neonatal Hypoglycaemia
  - Neonates of Diabetic Mothers
  - Nesidioblastosis
  - Persistent Hyperinsulinaemic Hypoglycaemia of Infancy
  - Beckwith-Wiedemann Syndrome
  - Idiopathic Hypoglycaemia of Childhood
  - Ketotic Hypoglycaemia
  - Islet Cell Tumour
  - Prediabetics
  - Miscellaneous Causes
  - Summary

DEFINITION

The normal venous blood glucose value ranges between 50 to 90 mg/dl (2.8 to 5.0 mmol/L). The venous blood glucose value less than 40 mg/dl (2.2 mmol/L) is termed as hypoglycaemia. However, the hypoglycaemic symptoms and signs may occur at much higher level in a chronic hyperglycaemic patient if the fall in blood glucose occurs rapidly. On the other hand, a patient with recurrent episodes of hypoglycaemia as seen in a tight-control diabetes mellitus or if the low glucose level is sustained for sometime as seen in insulinoma may stay symptom-free even when the blood glucose level is much lower than 40 mg/dl.

SYMPTOMS

The symptoms can be divided into two groups:
- Due to adrenaline release (also called neurogenic or autonomic symptoms).

  These are early symptoms and are most frequently seen when there is rapid fall in blood glucose level. The main symptoms are palpitation, nervousness, anxiety, apprehension (all due to epinephrine release), tremors (due to norepinephrine release), sweating (cholinergic stimulation), hunger and paraesthesias. Headache is another common symptom and may be very severe.

  Sometimes the adrenaline response is sufficient to raise the blood sugar level and the next (neuro-glycopenic) group of symptoms may not appear at all. In other patients who have been having persistently low blood glucose levels (Type I DM patients, or spontaneous hypoglycaemic patient) the adrenergic symptoms may be very mild or even absent. These symptoms also disappear in a diabetic patient with autonomic neuropathy (Fig. 24.3.1).

- Neuroglycopenic symptoms due to glucose deprivation of CNS and its neurones. These symptoms may, in part, be related to an increase in brain cell

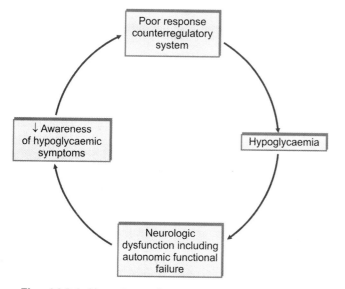

Fig. 24.3.1: Hypoglycaemia associated autonomic failure

osmolality caused by insulin itself. The main symptoms in this group are behaviour changes, confusion, fatigue, weakness, visual changes, seizures and even loss of consciousness and death when hypoglycaemia is prolonged and severe.

CLINICAL SIGNS

There is always some overlap between signs and symptoms due to adrenaline release and due to impaired nutrition of higher centres. The general clinical examination demonstrates pallor, profuse sweating, tachycardia and systolic hypertension.

The neuroglycopenic manifestations can be divided into two groups:

Psychiatric Signs

These include restlessness, mental instability, obstinacy, agitation, mental confusion, negativism, bizarre or psychiatric behaviour, incoherent speech, retrograde amnesia and delirium.

Neurological Signs

There may be diplopia, headache, aphasia or dysphagia. Circumoral paraesthesiae and numbness are common. Tremors and unsteady gait, convulsions and coma may also supervene if hypoglycaemia is prolonged. The other neurological signs are protean-hyperreflexia, transient hemiparesis, paraplegia, and monoplegia.

Extensor planter response, permanent neurological deficits and stertuous breathing may be seen in severe and prolonged hypoglycaemic patients some of whom may lapse into irreversible brain damage, coma and decerebrate state.

The clinical manifestations of hypoglycaemia are episodic and usually follow the same pattern in an individual patient though change in their character from time to time in the same individual has also been seen.

The effects of hypoglycaemia are more severe in elderly, atherosclerotic and alcoholics. Permanent myocardial damage may also occur especially in those with ischaemic heart disease as prolonged hypo-glycaemic episode leads to mobilization of glycogen from the cardiac muscle. Even after short duration hypo-glycaemia, focal neurological signs may persist for hours or even days. Recurrent episodes even when promptly treated can lead to mental and neurological deterioration with wide-spread degeneration and necrosis of cortical cells and reduction in their population.

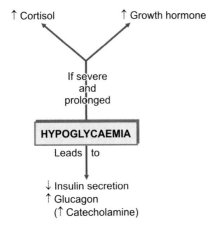

Fig. 24.3.2: Physiological response to hypoglycaemia

AETIOPATHOGENESIS

A normal healthy subject may fast for a period of 48 hours and then indulge in violent physical exertion without becoming hypoglycaemic. An obese subject on the other hand can fast for a considerable longer period without hypoglycaemia. In both instances, glycogenolysis and gluconeogenesis are sufficient to maintain the blood glucose level in the low normal range. Therefore the presence of hypoglycaemia indicates that the body is not able to initiate or sustain normal counterregulatory mechanism which normally happens on the fall of blood glucose level. In a healthy individual, physiological response to decrease in blood glucose level is fall in insulin secretion. If the decrease in blood glucose is substantial or sudden then besides proportionate fall in insulin secretion, glucose counterregulatory hormones system gets activated. In this system glucagon plays a dominant role while epinephrine assumes significance in its absence. Other hormones like growth hormone and cortisol get involved if hypoglycaemia is severe and prolonged (Fig. 24.3.2).

Causes

Main Causes

The main causes of hypoglycaemia are enumerated in Table 24.3.1. Some of these are described in brief. Some individuals may have more than one factor responsible for hypoglycaemia as is seen in cirrhotic patients with hepatocellular damage and alcohol consumption.

Factitious Hypoglycaemia

It is seen many a time in patients having insulin or oral hypoglycaemic agents. The hypoglycaemia due to exogenous insulin administration is diagnosed on a triad

TABLE 24.3.1

1. Iatrogenic
   Inappropriate insulin /oral hypoglycaemic drugs administration
2. Other drugs: Pentamidine, non-selective beta blocking agents, salicylates, clofibrate, azopropazone phenylbutazone group, isoniazid, pencillamine, quinine, chloromycetin, monoamine oxidase inhibitors, antihistamines, Amanita Palloides, ackee poisoning
3. Factitious
4. Spontaneous hypoglycaemia
   A. Fasting hypoglycaemia: due to
      a. Beta cell hyperplasia: benign or malignant neoplasms, islet cell microadenomatosis, nesidioblastosis, islet cell hyperplasia (infants of diabetic mothers), neonatal islet cell hyperfunction.
      b. Idiopathic hypoglycaemia of childhood.
      c. Leucine and fructose sensitivity.
      d. Galactosaemia.
      e. Extensive liver disease—hepatocellular, hepatoma, acute hepatic necrosis.
      f. Endocrine disease—hypopituitarism, Addison's disease, neuroblastomas.
      g. Glycogen storage disease.
      h. Nonpancreatic neoplasms—retroperitoneal sarcoma, rarely in bronchogenic and other carcinomas.
   B. Reactive hypoglycaemia due to
      a. Glucose:
         • Functional
         • Postgastrectomy and postgastroenterostomy
         • Potential diabetes
      b. Other substances:
         • Leucine, fructose, galactose sensitivity
         • Alcohol (it inhibits gluconeogenesis)
         • Tobacco
5. Due to excessive loss or utilization of glucose with relative failure of compensatory mechanism (very rare)
   • Prolonged starvation
   • Prolonged exercise
   • Pregnancy and lactation
   • Renal glucosuria

Main causes of hypoglycaemia

of low blood sugar, high IRI and low C-peptide value. Certain drugs like beta blockers, clofibrate, etc. potentiate the action of insulin and sulphonylureas and may cause hypoglycaemia by inhibiting the compensatory mechanism. Diabetics who have impaired renal or hepatic functions show markedly increased sensitivity to insulin and sulphonylureas and may go to prolonged, recurrent and sometimes fatal hypoglycaemia. When sulphonylureas are suspected to be responsible, a chemical test of the plasma to detect the drug may be required to confirm the diagnosis.

Islet Cell Tumours

These are the most important cause of spontaneous hypoglycaemia. As the clinical presentation is bizarre, the diagnosis may be delayed for years. A vast majority of patients present themselves initially to the neuro-physician or the psychiatrist. Therefore, this entity must be considered in differential diagnosis if a patient presents with protean symptomatology relating to psychiatric behaviour, intermittent neurological manifestations or focal neurological findings or episode of convulsive seizures. A detailed clinical history with relationship of symptoms with fasting/exercise must be sought and recorded. Usually in initial stages, hypo-glycaemic episodes/ symptoms are seen in the morning or after exertion and relieved by glucose. However, in certain patients hypoglycaemia may be reactive. Hunger and weight gain are two important features of islet cell tumours. This is particularly so in those patients whose symptoms disappear with ingestion of sugar/food.

The blood sugar fall in islet cell tumours is slow and not sudden, therefore sweating is usually less prominent in hypoglycaemic episodes. Family history of diabetes mellitus is present in about 20% patients and approxi-mately 10% of the islet cell tumours are malignant. Again in about 10% patients, the islet cell tumours are in a form of multiple, scattered microadenomas. Some of the islet cell tumours may also be associated with other endocrine gland adenomas or gut hormone secreting tumours.

Islet Cell Hyperplasia

It is commonly seen in the neonatal period in infants born of diabetic mothers and is discussed separately.

Reactive Hypoglycaemia

It is usually seen after partial gastrectomy and may occur several hours after a meal. An oral glucose tolerance test will show a typical 'lag curve'—with a high peak and a fall to hypoglycaemic level 2 to 4 hours after the test meal (75 G glucose).

Rapid gastric emptying in post-gastric surgery results in brisk glucose absorption, excessive insulin release and reactive hypoglycaemia.

In early stages of diabetes with partial decompensa-tion, there is initial β-cell inertia and insulin is not released till glucose level reaches 200 mg/dl or above. Thereafter the sudden release of insulin is liable to precipitate hypoglycaemia.

Nonspecific reactive hypoglycaemia may also be associated with anxiety.

Functional Hypoglycaemia

Patients with functional hypoglycaemia experience irregular and variable symptoms due to adrenaline release or acute neuroglycopenia. The symptoms typi-cally occur 2 to 4 hours after oral ingestion of carbo-hydrates. Such patients rarely become comatose. During 'attacks' there may be vague, nonspecific and often bizarre symptoms including hyperventilation. The patient is usually hypersensitive and emotionally labile. Some of the patients have a family history of diabetes and they themselves might be potential diabetics.

Alcohol-induced Hypoglycaemia

It is a genuine entity and follows ingestion of moderate or large amounts of alcohol. Children are particularly prone to it. The neuroglycopenic symptoms may occur shortly after the ingestion of alcohol and may be mild; while in others, especially who are undernourished, the symptoms may be delayed for hours and are profound leading to unconciousness and coma. In the latter group the diagnosis is liable to be missed and delayed. Hypothermia is a prominent feature especially in adults.

The condition appears to be due to direct slowing of Kreb's cycle, inhibition of gluconeogenesis as well as impairment of hypothalamic-pituitary axis by alcohol (as otherwise insulin secretion and peripheral glucose utilization are depressed during alcohol-induced hypoglycaemia). Response to intravenous glucose is prompt and impressive.

The diabetics who are on insulin or oral hypo-glycaemic agents (OHA) and consume a high alcohol intake are particularly at risk.

Alcohol induced hypoglycaemia is rare in well nourished individuals with abundant hepatic glycogen.

Leucine Sensitivity

Leucine stimulates insulin secretion and a large number of patients with islet cell adenomas are leucine sensitive. The leucine sensitivity does not exist as a specific sensitivity in adults. In susceptible children, leucine administration decreases blood glucose level in 20 to 30 minutes, raises insulin level and may cause hypogly-caemia and convulsions. It is a self-limiting sensitivity and disappears by 5 to 6 months age.

In our clinical practice more common causes of hypo-glycaemia are iatrogenic, drugs, reactive hypoglycaemia, ethanol intoxication, liver disease, islet cell tumours, large mesenchymal tumours, Addison's disease, sepsis, critical illness and inherited metabolic disorders. In liver disease, hypoglycaemia results when the glycogen stores are reduced and insulin destroying complex (insulinase) is deficient.

Hypoglycaemia due to Non-beta Cell Tumours

The most important non-beta cell tumours which cause hypoglycaemia are large retroperitoneal intraabdominal or intrathoracic tumours. The common epithelial tumours that cause hypoglycaemia are hepatoma, adrenocortical carcinoma and carcinoid tumours. More common carcinomas, lymphomas and haematological malignancies rarely cause hypoglycaemia. In vast majority of these patients IRI and C-peptide values are proportionately depressed with hypoglycaemia though a few cases have been reported with ectopic insulin production. Insulin-like growth factor I (IGF-I) is typically suppressed while IGF- II (especially big-IGF-II form) is increased and is responsible for hypoglycaemia. The diagnosis is usually clear on the basis of clinical examination, low insulin, proinsulin and C-peptide values while IGF-II and pro-IGF-II values are raised and IGF-II:IGF-I ratio is elevated.

Treatment of this type of hypoglycaemia is supportive and symptomatic with glucocorticoids or GH. The glucocorticoids (unlike GH) reduce IGF-II levels. Definitive treatment in the form of surgery, radio- or chemotherapy will depend upon the nature and extent of the tumour.

Autoimmune Hypoglycaemia

It is a rare condition. It may be associated with insulin antibodies or insulin receptors antibodies. The age of onset may be from a few days to an advanced age. Hypoglycaemia occurs at any time. Most of these patients have pre-existing insulin resistance and evidence of other autoimmune diseases before developing hypoglycaemia. Treatment with glucocorticoids and immunosuppressive therapy is helpful.

Autoimmune hypoglycaemia may also be associated with β-cell stimulating antibodies resulting in endogenous hyperinsulinaemia where insulin concentration may go beyond 6 µU/ml; C-peptide >0.6 ng/ml and glucose less than 45 mg/dl. Similar laboratory findings are also seen in insulinoma and sulphonylurea overdose.

Pseudo-hypoglycaemia

It is seen in certain leukaemias when the leucocyte counts are markedly elevated. It reflects utilization of glucose by leucocytes after the blood sample has been withdrawn. Artefactual hypoglycaemia may also be seen with improper sample collection or storage and errors in laboratory methodology.

Somogyi Effect

Insulin treated diabetic patients show a rapid swing to hyperglycaemia after episodes of hypoglycaemia. This rebound hyperglycaemia or Somogyi effect is considered to be caused by glucose counterregulatory hormones system.

DIAGNOSIS

It depends upon establishing that:
a. The hypoglycaemia, in fact, does exist in the given patient, and
b. Its real aetiological cause.

As the spontaneous hypoglycaemia is intermittent, one time blood glucose test may not be of much help unless it is done during an episode. Moreover, there are many disease entities which may mimic nonspecific hypoglycaemic symptoms, e.g. phaeochromocytoma, thyrotoxicosis, anxiety neurosis, vertebrobasilar ischaemia and cardiac dysarrhythmias. Therfore a detailed clinical examination is mandatory in all cases of spontaneous hypoglycaemia. A special attention should be directed towards liver and adrenocortical disorders, anterior pituitary problems, malignancies and metastatic deposits (Fig. 24.3.3).

Laboratory Investigations

The laboratory investigations which are helpful are:
- Blood glucose, insulin, C-peptide and proinsulin values (fasting, casual and during episodes).
- A 48 to 72 hours fast.
- A prolonged (4 hours) oral glucose tolerance test.
- Measurement of serum insulin-like growth factor (IGH-I, IGF-II) and binding protein1 (IGFBP-1).
- Imaging (X-ray, CT, MRI) of the brain and barium meal follow through studies to rule out pathological lesions responsible for hypoglycaemia.
- Other special investigations like tolbutamide, glucagon, leucine, fish insulin and ethanol or calcium gluconate infusion tests.

Blood Glucose and Insulin Estimation

If this test is done during 'an attack' then it will refute/confirm the existence of hypoglycaemia. If the insulin value (IRI) is inappropriately high (6 µU/ml or above) in association with low blood glucose value (less than 40 mg/dl) then the possibility of insulin-producing tumour is very strong. On the other hand if IRI values are at the lowest level of normal range or undetectable,

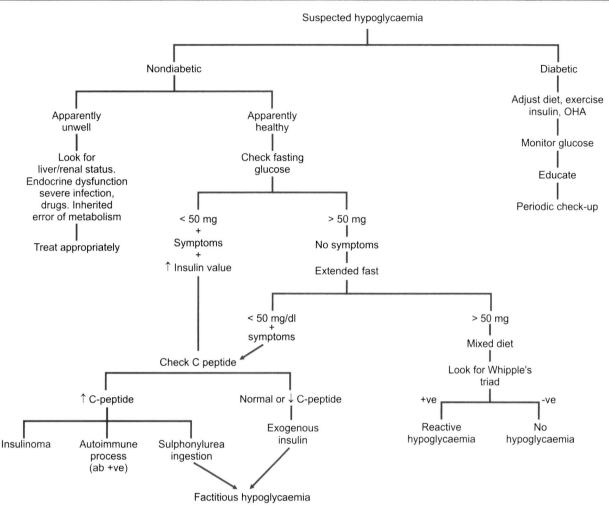

Fig. 24.3.3: Diagnostic approach in hypoglycaemia

insulinoma is more or less ruled out. In a large majority of patients with insulinoma, an overnight fast (10 to 12 hours) always reveals hypoglycaemia in one or more of the three consecutive blood glucose estimations. On the other hand, the fasting blood glucose level is invariably normal in patients with reactive hypoglycaemia. Thus this is another test which is extremely helpful.

48 to 72 Hours Fast

If a simple overnight fast does not confirm hypoglycaemia, then a 48 hours (sometimes extended to 72 hours) fast is the most useful diagnostic test. The test is conducted in a hospital under direct medical supervision. Only unsweetened oral liquids are permitted. Blood is tested for glucose and insulin every 8 hours and when symptoms of hypoglycaemia appear, the fast is terminated by giving glucose. Most patients with islet cell

tumours develop symptoms of neuroglycopenia well within 48 hours and the blood glucose level invariably falls to less than 30 mg/dl (1.7 mmol/L). Only rarely, one has to extend the fast beyond 48 hours. If even after 72 hours hypoglycaemia does not occur and neuroglycopenic symptoms do not appear and serum insulin value stays low or undetectable, it is almost certain that islet cell tumour does not exist.

Normal subjects and patients with reactive hypoglycaemia will stay normoglycaemic during 48 to 72 hours fast. The insulin/glucose ratio is always less than 0.04 in normal persons. In insulinomas it is greater than 0.04 and is often above 1.0.

It has been seen that all cases of insulinoma may not show elevated fasting insulin value. Therefore, if an inappropriate high insulin value (even though within normal limit) for the blood sugar level is observed, it favours the diagnosis of islet cell tumour. Such patients also demonstrate rapid spontaneous fluctuations in the serum insulin values. Therefore, multiple sampling is required.

The prolonged fast aims to demonstrate Whipple's classical triad, i.e. (a) symptoms are induced by fasting (b) symptoms are due to hypoglycaemia and (c) symptoms are reversed after glucose administration.

Glucose Tolerance Test (GTT)

A 4-hour extended GTT is very helpful in cases of reactive hypoglycaemia. The test, however, is not of much value in diagnosis of islet cell tumour.

C-Peptide Assay

Estimation of C-peptide concentration in serum reflects the secretion of proinsulin and hence of insulin. The endogenous secretion of insulin (and hence of C-peptide) is not diminished in insulinoma even when hypoglycaemia is produced by porcine or bovine insulin injection. This lack of suppressibility of C-peptide levels during insulin-induced hypoglycaemia is a better diagnostic finding than the absolute C-peptide value unless of course it is exceptionally high.

Plasma Proinsulin Levels

In a normal healthy individual plasma proinsulin represents 25% of the total immunoreactive insulin (IRI). Its hypoglycaemic effect is less than 10% of that of insulin. Proinsulin is secreted in excessive amount by insulinoma and undifferentiated islet cell tumours where it has very high proportion compared to insulin.

Measurement of Serum Insulin-like Growth Factor (IGF-I, IGF-II) and IGF Binding Protein1 (IGFBP-1)

The secretion of IGFBP-1 is acutely inhibited by insulin. Consequently IGFBP-1 is low in hyperinsulin-induced hypoglycaemia whereas in spontaneous, ketotonic or fasting hypoglycaemia where insulin level is low, IGFBP-1 levels are significantly high. Estimation of IGF-I and IGF-II is helpful in diagnosis of non-beta cell tumours.

Imaging of Chest, Pituitary Area and Abdomen

Imaging of chest, pituitary area and abdomen for bronchogenic carcinoma, pituitary and adrenal tumours are of diagnostic help if such problems are suspected. Contrast enhanced CT scan of the abdomen usually demonstrates the pancreatic tumours and metastases. Retroperitoneal tumours can also be seen by this technique.

Tolbutamide, Glucagon and Leucine Tests

These tests are no longer in use as very often false negative results are obtained. Other tests like infusion of ethanol or calcium gluconate again have limited utility though it is seen that they stimulate insulin release and produce hypoglycaemia in patients with insulinoma.

Therefore, the two tests which are reliable and are often used for diagnosis of insulinoma are:
a. Overnight fast.
b   Prolonged fast.

An extended (4-hour) oral glucose tolerance test is useful in diagnosis of reactive hypoglycaemia.

Localization of the Tumour

Once the possibility of insulinoma is established on clinical and laboratory evidence, it is imperative that an endeavour is made to localize the tumour preoperatively as surgeon may not be able to palpate small tumours (< 0.5 cm) on the table. Abdominal ultrasound, CT scan, selective abdominal angiography, MRI, hepatic venous sampling for insulin after intra-arterial injection of calcium, etc. are all useful methods to localize the tumour. Out of all these procedures, following are being preferred as they have higher positive percentage:

Ultrasound		
CT scan,	30 to 45 % positive	
MRI	(relatively less sensitive)	
Selective abdominal angiography (many false results)	60%	
Selective portal venous sampling (PVS) for insulin	80%	More
Intraoperative ultrasound	89%	sensitive
Endoscopic ultrasound	82%	methods
Hepatic venous sampling for insulin after calcium injection	94 %	

TREATMENT OF HYPOGLYCAEMIA

The definitive treatment will depend upon the underlying causative factor (see Fig. 24.3.3). The emergency treatment consists in making the patient normoglycaemic as promptly as possible. Intravenous glucose (10 to 25%) is infused rapidly after an initial bolus. If patient is conscious and able to swallow, then he is asked to swallow glucose, biscuits, sweets, etc. In severe cases intravenous hydrocortisone hemisuccinate and IM or subcutaneous glucagon (200 mg 4 to 6 hourly and 1 mg respectively) may be given to help raise the blood sugar (Table 24.3.2). In severe hypoglycaemia, glucagon (1 mg) may have to be given intravenously.

TABLE 24.3.2

Immediate	
Patient able to swallow and conscious	Oral glucose/sucrose (20 to 30 G)
Patient unable to swallow/unconscious	IV 25% 100 ml or 50% 50 ml ± IM/SC glucagon 1 mg (0.5 mg children)
Thereafter	Check plasma glucose after 15 to 20 minutes and maintain its level above 5 mmol/L (90 mg/dl)
On recovery	Search and delineate the cause, educate the patient to avoid recurrences
If recovery delayed	Set up 10% dextrose drip IV Hydrocortisone hemisuccinate 100 mg × 6 hourly When conscious, institute oral glucose, biscuits, etc.

Treatment of hypoglycaemia

In cases of repeated hypoglycaemia, octapeptide octreotide (long acting analogue of somatostatin) may be used 50 to 100 μg 8 hourly to reduce the insulin release from the pancreatic and extrapancreatic sources. Octreotide also inhibits growth hormone and various gut hormone secretions.

Diazoxide, a nondiuretic benzothiadiazine hypoglycaemic agent, is another drug that is useful in controlling the symptoms of hypoglycaemia. It inhibits pancreatic insulin secretion and facilitates hepatic gluconeogenesis. Its oral daily dose is 5 to 15 mg/kg body weight. It may be combined with a thiazide diuretic for greater effect. Diazoxide is liable to cause nausea, vomiting (especially, if the daily dose is over 200 mg), excessive hair growth, especially in females, and fluid retention with dependent oedema. Therefore, its use should be limited to those situations only where other measures fail. It has a proven utility in post-gastrectomy syndrome, islet cell carcinoma and idiopathic hypoglycaemia of infancy.

In case of reactive hypoglycaemia, precipitating factors like fructose, leucine, galactose should be avoided. Leucine rich diets like ragi, bajra, jawar, eggs, pork, milk and milk products should be omitted/given with caution. In some cases diazoxide therapy may have to be used. If hypoglycaemia is induced by carbohydrates then we recommend small frequent feeds which are rich in proteins and fats but low in carbohydrates. Administration of a α-glucosidase inhibitor, which delays carbohydrate digestion and subsequently its absorption from the intestines, has been used in treatment of reactive hypoglycaemia with beneficial effect in certain patients. Anticholinergic drugs like probanthine 15 mg × thrice daily may help in prolonging the gastric emptying time.

In patients where hypoglycaemia is a result of Addison's disease or hypopituitarism, therapeutic approach is well defined once a diagnosis is confirmed. When hypoglycaemia is due to inborn errors of metabolism in children, nonpancreatic neoplasm or advanced liver disease, curative management may not be possible. Symptomatic treatment is offered to alleviate patient's sufferings.

The treatment of insulinoma is surgical unless contraindicated due to other health problems. Once the diagnosis of insulinoma is confirmed, it is usual to initiate treatment with diazoxide or somatostatin analogue until the operation is carried out. The medical treatment helps make the patient normoglycaemic, minimize hypoglycaemic episodes, and fit to stand the surgical stress.

The insulinomas are almost always very small tumours and rarely exceed 3 cm diameter. Usually they measure only a few millimeter. More than 98% are in pancreas or are attached to it. They are usually solitary. Only less than ten per cent (10%) insulinoma are multiple and nearly 10% are malignant. Multiple insulinoma are indicative of MEN-I syndrome. Although pancreatic tail contains more beta cells than the head, the tumour occurs with equal frequency in all parts of the pancreas. They are usually well encapsulated, firmer than normal pancreas and highly vascular. The tumour may also be extrapancreatic in the duodenal wall, splenic hilum, in Meckel's diverticulum. Islet cell adenomatosis is uncommon and usually a part of MEN-I syndrome and requires resection of the pancreatic body and tail.

Sometimes with the very best efforts, tumour site is not localized. In such situations some surgeons close the abdomen, treat symptoms with pharmacotherapy and wait till the tumour becomes large while others remove both tail and the body of the pancreas providing relief in about 30% cases by this approach.

IV dextrose infusion is continued before and during operation to maintain blood glucose value 80 to 100 mg/dl (4.4 to 5.6 mmol/L). Serial blood sugar monitoring is mandatory and a sharp rise of blood glucose is observed usually within 20 to 30 minutes of removal of the tumour. Postoperatively insulin will be required to control hyperglycaemia.

If malignant islet cell tumour is found, radical surgery is ideal. This, however, is not always possible as by the time diagnosis is made, there are hepatic and distant metastases. In such cases chemotherapy is given. The current recommended choice is combination of streptozotocin and doxorubicin. Other combination is streptozotocin and 5-fluorouracil but the results with this combination are inferior to the recommended regimen. Streptozotocin causes nausea and vomiting in almost all patients, dose-related transient renal dysfunction including proteinuria, hepatic function abnormalities, leucopenia and thrombocytopenia. Chlorozotocin which is closely related to streptozotocin, gives similar results as streptozotocin when used singly or in combination and causes less nausea and vomiting. Single drug has limited effect hence it is better to use two drugs combination.

RISK FACTORS FOR HYPOGLYCAEMIA

Some of the common risk factors are:
- Relative or absolute insulin excess as seen by inappropriate and ill-timed exogenous insulin or oral hypoglycaemic agents administration.
- Exogenous glucose supply is reduced as during fasting, missed meals/snacks, overnight fast.
- Insulin-independent glucose utilization is increased, e.g. during exercise.
- Endogenous glucose production is reduced, e.g. after alcohol intake.
- Insulin clearance is reduced, e.g. in chronic renal failure.
- Miscellaneous causes like sepsis, unawareness of hypoglycaemia and absence of appropriate responses like early decrease in insulin level and elevation of glucagon.
- Defective glucose counter-regulation as seen in T1DM. Here as insulin deficiency progresses over first few months/years of the disease, circulating insulin levels are no longer tightly coordinated with glucose level, with the result insulin level does not decline as glucose level falls. Later on even glucagon response to hypoglycaemia is also lost and still later there is also decrease in epinephrine response as well.

PREVENTION OF HYPOGLYCAEMIA

- This involves adequate education of the patients and their relatives so that hypoglycaemia is avoided. The knowledge dissemination programme must cover topics like value of proper nutrition, importance of regular meals, graduated daily exercise, proper technique of injections, harmful effects of smoking, tobacco chewing, excessive use of alcohol and punctuality in medication.

- The patients and their relatives must also know about the prodromal and classical signs of hypoglycaemia and emergency steps to manage it till a medical attendant arrives on the scene.
- The treating physician must appreciate that a very tight glycaemic control is bound to have some episodes of hypoglycaemia. Therefore, he must avoid a very tight glycaemic control among type 1 DM children who have impaired glucose counter-regulatory system, elderly and mentally subnormal persons. In such cases mild to moderate hyper-glycaemic may have to be accepted as it outweighs the risk of having hypoglycaemia.
- Enforcement of rapid tightening of the glycaemic control increases the vulnerability of hypoglycaemia and probably worsening of the established micro-angiotherapy in initial stage. Therefore, such a schedule should be enforced gradually over a period of few weeks.
- Intensive insulin therapy again is not very desirable in very young children and in infants.
- If hypoglycaemia is associated with insulin antibodies, the use of human insulin should help reduce the number of episodes and their severity.
- In diabetic patients with autonomic neuropathy, the targets of glycaemic control may have to be modified in view of the possibility of their having unawareness about hypoglycaemia.

PAEDIATRIC HYPOGLYCAEMIA

The causes of hypoglycaemia and its manifestations in a child differ substantially from those seen in adults (Tables 24.3.3 and 24.3.4). Some of the more common conditions are described briefly.

Neonatal Hypoglycaemia

The foetus depends on the maternal blood sugar for continuous supply of glucose. After birth, the neonate relies on endogenous glucose production with only intermittent exogenous glucose delivery. Endogenous glucose production is achieved by gluconeogenesis for the first 4 to 6 hours after birth as mobilizable glycogen stores are limited. Therefore, normal glucose regulatory and counterregulatory hormone system, healthy liver (and kidney) status and availability of gluconeogenic precursors are essential to maintain normal blood sugar level in a newborn.

The umbilical cord blood glucose value ranges between 50 and 70 mg/dl. It is 10 to 15% higher if serum or plasma is used for estimation. The factors which

TABLE 24.3.3

Neonatal hypoglycaemia
- Prematurity
- Small for dates neonates
- Smaller of the twins
- Birth asphyxia
- Neonates born of toxaemic mother
- Neonates born of diabetic mother

Neonatal, infantile and childhood hypoglycaemia
- Hyperinsulinism, hypopituitarism, Addison's disease, gluconeogenesis and glycogenolysis defects, fatty acid oxidation defect and carnitine deficiency
- Ketotonic hypoglycaemia
- Poisoning—alcohol, salicylates, oral hypoglycaemic agents, propranolol, pentamidine, quinine, ackee fruit, vacor (rat poison), etc.
- Liver disorders: hepatitis, cirrhosis
- Amino acid disorders

    Maple syrup urine disease

    Tyrosinosis
- Systemic disorders, sepsis, heart failure, malabsorption, malnutrition, burns, diarrhoea, renal failure, shock, falciparum malaria
- Factitious

    Iatrogenic—excessive insulin therapy, less food intake, excessive exercise in a diabetic child

Common causes of hypoglycaemia in infants and children

TABLE 24.3.4

• Asymptomatic	• Tremors
• Poor feeding	• Irregular breathing
• Hypothermia	• Apnoea
• Hypotonia	• Cyanosis
• Tachycardia	• Sudden infant death
• Lethargy	• Convulsions
• Somnolence	• Coma

Clinical manifestations of neonatal hypoglycaemia

influence this value are the maternal blood glucose level, gestational age, duration of labour, nature of delivery (normal or complicated), weight and head circumference of the newborn. The rate of glucose utilization in infants is approximately 3 times higher than in adults (when expressed per unit of body weight) due to their large brain size relative to their body weight. The blood glucose value falls after birth and reaches its lowest level approximately 2 to 4 hours after delivery. This is a transient phenomenon and blood glucose values return to normal over the next 3 to 5 days. In some neonates, this fall in blood glucose may be excessive and prolonged

and hypoglycaemic symptoms may be observed during 2nd or 3rd day after the birth. The symptoms observed include poor feeding, hypothermia, hypotonia, lethargy or tremors (the jittery baby), attacks of apnoea and cyanosis followed by convulsions and coma in severe cases. Hypocalcaemia may also occur. The cause of this syndrome seen in infants of nondiabetic mothers is unknown. Probably it is nothing more than an exaggeration of the normal postpartum blood glucose decrease. Neonates with low birth weight, particularly small-for-dates and smaller of twins are at greater risk. Neonatal hypoglycaemia may be symptomatic or asymptomatic but it must be treated promptly and effectively initially with intravenous dextrose and later if necessary with hydrocortisone hemisuccinate.

The blood glucose value diagnostic of neonatal hypoglycaemia varies with new born's status at birth as under:
a. In full term infants, it is less than 40 mg/dl (2.2 mmol/L) while.
b. in low birth weight (less than 2500 G) it is less than 30 mg/dl (1.7 mmol/L).

However, out of concern for possible late neurological and psychological sequelae, any value less than 50 mg/dl in neonates 2 to 3 hours after birth, should be viewed with suspicion and treated.

Hypoglycaemia persisting beyond the neonatal period is usually due to hepatic or endocrine problems which need proper investigations and management to avoid possible residual mental subnormality.

Hypoglycaemia in Neonates Born to Diabetic Mothers

These newborns tend to be large and have a higher perinatal and neonatal mortality and morbidity. There is islet cells hyperplasia and hyperinsulinaemia (Fig. 24.3.4) which is due to maternal hyperglycaemia. It is seen the better the maternal diabetic control, the greater the potential for a normal infant.

Symptoms begin a little earlier than in normal neonatal hypoglycaemia and are usually seen within a few hours of the birth. Glucose is given during first 24 hours to treat the condition. After 24 hours, fructose is employed instead of glucose since fructose, unlike glucose, does not increase hyperinsulinaemia. Fructose is not employed during first 24 hours as during this period there is transient fructose intolerance which may further lower blood glucose level through unknown mechanisms. Breast-feeding is encouraged.

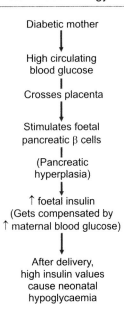

Fig. 24.3.4: Hypoglycaemia in a neonate born of diabetic mother

Hypoglycaemia in neonates of diabetic mothers rarely persists beyond a few days (3 to 4 days). Neonatal hypoglycaemia associated with islet cell hyperplasia is also a feature of erythroblastosis foetalis. This too is a transient condition.

Persistent Hyperinsulinaemic Hypoglycaemia of Infancy (PHHI)

It is caused by mutations in the potassium channel involved in insulin secretion by the β-cells. It is inherited in an autosomal recessive pattern. Hypoglycaemia is seen in immediate newborn period. The neonate is usually macrosomic and birth weight is excessive (over 4 kg). Usual drug therapy and infusion do not work adequately and pancreatectomy is strongly advised to avoid problems of persistent hypoglycaemia.

Beckwith-Wiedemann Syndrome

This syndrome manifests as persistent hyperinsulinaemic hypoglycaemia of infancy. It is characterized by duplicating/imprinting in chromosome at 11p15.1 (This is the region that encodes IGF-11 gene). The neonate is macrosomic at birth and suffers from moderate hypoglycaemia. There is no positive family history. Response to medical treatment is good. Spontaneous recovery is seen by 6 to 8 months. Some neonates may have other associated features like macroglossia, hemi-hypertrophy and omphalocoele.

Nesidioblastosis

Nesidioblasts are the cells that differentiate out of the duct epithelium to form islets. In nesidioblastosis, there is diffuse proliferation of the islet cells. All pancreatic endocrine cells (α, β, δ, PP) show proliferation on histological examination.

Nesidioblast is an unusual but important cause of neonatal hypoglycaemia. It is the commonest cause of postnatal hypoglycaemia in children under the age of one year. Symptoms appear in most cases before the age of 6 months and in many children start in the neonatal period often in the first few hours of life. The condition is liable to result in sudden infant death syndrome. Typical features include tachycardia, ataxia, somnolence, convulsions and coma. Symptoms are more prominent or appear before feeds/meals. The condition does not undergo spontaneous improvement though temporary remissions may occur.

Fasting hypoglycaemia with inappropriately high values of insulin (proinsulin and C-peptide) are confirmatory diagnostic findings. The condition produces recurrent and repeated hypoglycaemic attacks and needs frequent feeding; IV bolus (2 ml/kg) of 10% glucose followed by, glucose infusion of 5 to 8 mg/kg or even more of glucose/minute so as to achieve normal glucose levels. Central venous or umbilical venous catheter may be used to administer 15 to 20% glucose solution. IM or IV hydrocortisone 5 mg/kg/24 hrs or in 8 hourly doses or prednisolone 1 to 2 mg/kg/24 hr in 6 to 12 hourly dose may also be needed. Growth hormone 1 mg/24 hours may be added if hypoglycaemia persists inspite of IV dextrose. If above treatment is ineffective even after 3 to 5 days then diazoxide (10 to 25 mg/kg/24 hr), glucagon (1 mg IM) and octreotide therapy (10 to 25 mg/kg/24 hours) may be tried to control hypoglycaemia. These pharmacotherapeutic measures succeed in many cases especially of later onset. However, as the repeated episodes of hypoglycaemia are liable to result in brain damage, the treatment of choice is the surgical resection of the pancreas where partial or total pancreas is removed depending upon the severity of the symptoms.

Idiopathic Hypoglycaemia of Childhood

The condition is usually seen before the age of two years and almost always before five years. It may also be present at birth. The symptoms are usually mild and clinical signs are minimal or absent and there is tendency to spontaneous recovery. In some cases positive family history is forthcoming.

Ketotic Hypoglycaemia

This is the most common form of childhood hypoglycaemia. It is usually seen between 1 and 5 years and remits spontaneously by the age of 8 to 9 years. Hypoglycaemic episodes usually occur when food intake gets limited as during illness or when evening meal is missed and overnight fast gets prolonged.

At the time of hypoglycaemia, there is associated ketonuria, ketonaemia and low plasma insulin level. A susceptible child will develop this type of hypoglycaemia if child is fasted even for 12 to 18 hours whereas a normal child can stand a fast of this duration without any symptoms.

The aetiology of ketotic hypoglycaemia may be a defect in any of the complex steps involved in protein catabolism, oxidative deamination of amino acids, transamination, alanine synthesis or alanine efflux from muscles.

Children with ketotic hypoglycaemia have low plasma alanine values and an infusion of alanine (250 mg/kg) produces a rapid rise in plasma glucose value indicating the deficiency of this substrate as the cause of hypoglycaemia. IGFBP-1 concentration is significantly elevated.

As the condition usually remits on its own, the treatment consists in frequent feeding with high protein, high carbohydrate diet. During illness, child's urine must be tested for the presence of ketones as it becomes positive several hours before hypoglycaemia appears.

If ketonuria is present, high carbohydrate liquids should be given if tolerated. Otherwise, a short course of corticosteroids should be administered. If this does not help, child should be admitted to the hospital and IV glucose given.

Islet Cell Tumour

This is extremely rare in childhood. Convulsion and coma occur frequently in this condition. Fasting insulin values are high. Table 24.3.5 enumerates some of the laboratory criteria of hyperinsulinaemia due to any cause.

Prediabetes

Symptoms of hypoglycaemia are sometimes seen in children who are prone to develop diabetes in later life. Glycosuria and glucose intolerance develop after a variable (usually short) period of time. These children

TABLE 24.3.5

Plasma glucose	< 50 mg/dl
Hyperinsulinaemia	Plasma insulin >2 µU/ml
Hypofattyacidaemia	Plasma FFA <1.5 mmol/L
Hypoketonaemia	Plasma β-hydroxybutyrate < 2.0 mmol/L
Glucagon response (30 minutes after (1 mg/IV))	Inappropriate (Rise in glucose less than 40 mg/dl)

Some of the laboratory criteria in hyperinsulinaemia

have a very strong family history of diabetes and hypoglycaemic symptoms usually appear after a carbohydrate meal. The symptoms are usually mild though seizures and unconsciousness have also been seen in this, rather, uncommon condition

Miscellaneous Causes

Hypoglycaemia in childhood is also seen in some types of glycogen storage disease where hepatic glycogen cannot be converted to glucose, e.g. galactosaemia, hereditary fructose intolerance. familial fructose and galactose intolerance (Dormandy's syndrome).

SUMMARY

Hypoglycaemia is a very common emergency for a diabetologist as well as a neonatologist. The clinical manifestation of hypoglycaemia are palpitations, nervousness, anxiety, heavy head, hunger and sweating. If it remains unaltered, convulsive seizures and coma may also develop.

The more common causes of hypoglycaemia in our clinical practice are the inappropriate dose of insulin/OHA, missed meals, alcohol abuse, liver disease, reactive hypoglycaemia, islet cell tumours and adrenal disease. In neonates the common causes are prematurity, small for dates neonates, neonates born to a diabetic mother and birth asphyxia; while in childhood, idiopathic hypoglcaemia of childhood and ketotic hypoglycaemia are the most common forms of childhood hypoglycaemia.

The chapter discusses in details the, clinical presentation, risk factors, preventive measures, investigations and management of various diseases which may lead to this common endocrine emergency. It stresses the role of intravenous dextrose, glucagon, glucocorticoids, growth hormone, octreotide, diazoxide and surgery (in pancreatic and non-pancreatic tumours) to control repeated episodes of hypoglycaemia.

FURTHER READING

1. Banarer S, Mc Greger VP, Cryer PE. Intra islet hyperinsulinaemia prevents the glucagons response to hypoglycaemia despite an intact autonomic response. Diabetes 2002;15:958-65.
2. Cornblath M, Hawdon JM, William AF, et al. Controversies regarding definition of neonatal hypoglycaemia: suggested operational thresholds. Paediatrics 2000;105:1141-5.
3. Crayer PE. Hypoglycaemia: Pathophysiology diagnosis and treatment. New York. Oxford University Press 1997.
4. Crayer PE. Hypoglycaemia. The limiting factor in the glycaemic management of the type I and type II diabetes. Diabetologia 2002; 45:937-46.
5. Kane C, Lindleyk J, Johnson PRV, et al. Therapy for persistent hyperinsulinaemic hypoglycaemia of infancy. J Clin Invest 1997;100:188-93.
6. Meissner T, Otonkoski T, Feneberg R, et al. Exercise induced hypoglycaemic hyperinsulinism. Arch Dis Child 2001;84:254-7.
7. Sperling MA, Menon RK. Hperinsulinaemic hypoglycaemia in infancy. Endocrinol Metab Clin North Am 1999;28:695-708.

SECTION

25

DIABETES MELLITUS AND INSULIN RESISTANCE

25.1 Epidemiology and Aetiopathogenesis

Y Sachdev

DEFINITION

Diabetes mellitus (DM) is a complex metabolic syndrome with an absolute or relative deficiency or inefficiency of insulin. The absolute or relative lack of insulin results in disturbed intermediary metabolism manifesting as:
- Chronic sustained hyperglycaemia
- Glycosuria, ketonaemia, ketonuria
- Dyslipidaemia, and
- Progressive tissue damage with microvascular and macrovascular complications.

DM affects all body systems though the main brunt is borne by the eyes, kidneys, skin and nerves.

EPIDEMIOLOGY

With the ever increasing incidence of DM, it has become one of the major global and national health problems. In 1970-1972, in an urban and semiurban community survey in Maharashtra, we found its prevalence as 1.4%. Nearly similar (1.2%) prevalence was quoted by Tripathy et al from Orissa while Indian Council of Medical Research (ICMR) reported it as 2.3%. In 1984-85, in another community survey in Uttar Pradesh (UP) the author reported its prevalence as 4.8% while in 1998-99, in Delhi and surrounding areas, he observed it to be 8.2%. Presently, its prevalence has been reported as 13 to 15% in urban areas by various Indian workers. Possibly the prevalence is higher than quoted as in this huge Indian subcontinent with less than ideal health care system, there are many individuals who stay undiagnosed for a long time. Some workers believe that nearly equal number of undiagnosed diabetics are present in India; while others have reported nearly 12% yearly increase

in diagnosed diabetics in our country. Factors responsible for this ever-increasing prevalence are better diagnostic criteria, improved laboratory facilities, urbanization, erratic eating habits, inactivity, central obesity and diminished physical exercise. The World Health Organisation (WHO) estimates that by 2025 World wide there will be 300 million diabetics (5.4%). India, by then, will be a home to more than 57 million diabetics. This will be the largest number compared to other countries world over. Presently the diabetic population in India is estimated to be approximately 32 millions. Thus the increase will be much more compared to other countries. Genetic predisposition, inherent ethnicity, consanguinity in marriages, increased waist to hip ratio, overweight/ obesity, malnutrition and increased body mass index (BMI), insulin resistance, malnutrition, low birth weight and migration to urban slums from rural areas are blamed for this difference. Type 2 DM is the commonest type of DM and accounts for almost 90% of diabetics (Figs 25.1.1A to C).

Type 1 DM (T1DM)

The exact incidence of T1DM in India is not known. According to available data, it is nearly 5% of the diabetic population and is less than that seen in the Western countries. T1DM is seen in younger age group, usually makes a sudden appearance with classical symptoms of polyuria, polydipsia, polyphagia and unusual loss of body weight. The individual is usually thin and lean. Its incidence is at its peak around puberty when the body is facing hormonal stress. Finland reports an annual incidence of 45 to 49 cases per 100,000 children while the

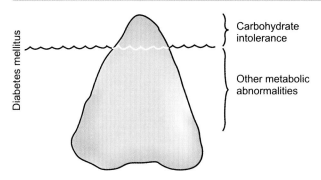

Fig. 25.1.1A: Hyperglycaemia is one of the metabolic abnormalities seen in diabetes mellitus syndrome and can be compared to the tip of the iceberg as many more metabolic abnormalities are present in this syndrome

oriental population like China, Ukraine, Venezuala has its incidence as low as 0.1 to 1 per 1000,000 children population. Marked variations in the incidence are seen not only between populations but also within populations. Winter and cold autumn months record higher incidence in some communities and is thought to reflect exposure to viruses. All these differences go to prove that environmental and ethnic factors are as important (if not more) as genetic factors in triggering T1DM. Interestingly, people who migrate from an area of low incidence of T1DM to an area of high risk seem to adopt the same level of risk as the population to which they have moved.

Type 2 DM (T2DM)

Type 2 DM is showing a progressive increase world over (Table 25.1.1, Fig. 25.1.2). In India, the increase is more obvious especially in urban areas. A similar increase,

TABLE 25.1.1

	No. in million	
Countries	Year 1995	Year 2025
India	19.4	57.2
Brazil	4.9	11.6
China	16.0	37.6
Indonesia	4.5	12.4
Japan	6.3	8.5
Mexico	3.8	11.7
Pakistan	4.3	14.5
Russian Federation	8.9	12.9
USA	13.9	21.9

Approximate and projected diabetic population in some of the countries

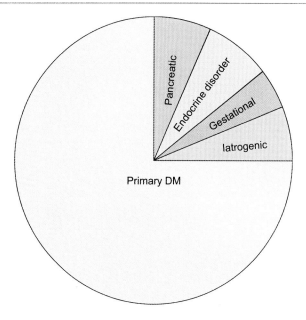

Fig. 25.1.1B: Diabetes mellitus and its subtypes

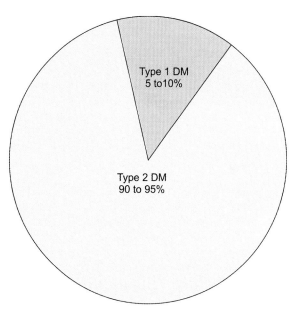

Fig. 25.1.1C: Shows relative percentages of T1DM and T2DM in India

though less marked, is noted in rural areas also. Compared to European and American population, Indians develop T2DM approximately 10 years early in their life. With this early onset, the risk of developing long-term diabetic complications increases. In order to guard against these complications, it is obligatory to conduct holistic and thorough clinical evaluation to ensure early detection of complications if any, and to provide specific management and a tight glycaemic control. These endeavours are

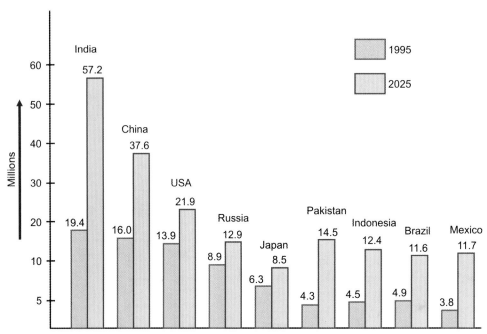

Fig. 25.1.2: Approximate and projected diabetic population in some of the countries
(World Diabetic Population: year 1995—135 million; year 2025—300 million)

greatly helped by educating the community and increasing their awareness for self care and self monitoring of the blood glucose. Our clinical data show that among T2DM patients, hypertension is present in approximately 40%, retinopathy 25%, coronary artery disease (CAD) 15%, autonomic neuropathy 33%, peripheral neuropathy 30% and nephropathy (all grades) in nearly 10%. It is also seen that well informed knowledgeable patient lives longer than ill-informed ignorant individual who dies and suffers much more.

The importance of tight glycaemic control to avoid diabetic complications was well recognized by senior diabetologists and was always stressed in 1960s. Unfortunately, over period of years, this fact was lost sight of somewhere midway. Its significance was once again brought home by various well conducted experimental and epidemiological studies and was highlighted by some of the recent mega trials like Diabetes Control and Complications Treatment (DCCT), Kumomoto and UK prospective diabetes Study (UKPDS). DCCT study covered over 1400 T1DM North Americans over a period of 12 years while UKPDS spent over 20 years and covered 5000 T2DM.

HISTORICAL ASPECTS

Egyptian literature, Ebers papyrus (15th century BC) contains the earliest reference to clinical polyuric states resembling diabetes mellitus. The Sanskrit literature of

Charaka and Sushruta era (400 BC) have vivid description of diabetes mellitus. These two great sages recognized the differences between the two main types of the diabetes syndrome: One associated with emaciation, dehydration, polyuria and lassitude; the other associated with stout built, obesity and sleeplessness. Aretaeus of Coppadocia (2nd century AD) was the first to use the word 'Diabetes'. It comes from the Greek, meaning siphon. He gave a detailed clinical description noting increased urine flow, thirst and weight loss. He described diabetes as a dreadful affliction being a melting down of the flesh and limbs into urine.

It was in 19th century (1869) when the German scientist Paul Langerhans recognized and isolated pancreatic islets that the role of pancreas in DM was appreciated. Thereafter in 20th century rapid strides were made towards the understanding of aetiopathogenesis, clinical expression and variations in presentation along with therapeutic management. Later, the molecular and genetic advances led to the discovery of insulin and glucagon molecule, insulin receptors and cloning of insulin gene. Table 25.1.2 gives some of the important historic milestones of diabetes mellitus.

CLASSIFICATION OF DIABETES MELLITUS

Diabetes Mellitus is a heterogeneous metabolic syndrome with wide variations in its presentation, clinical course and complications. Different classifications have been

TABLE 25.1.2

Authors/literatures	Years	Observations
Ebers Papyrus (Egypt)	1500 BC	Clinical polyuric states
Charaka and Sushruta (India)	400 BC	Main types of DM
Aretaeus (Greek)	2nd century AD	Name 'Diabetes' used for the first time
John Rollo	18th century	First to apply the adjective mellitus to the disease (Greek and Latin for honey)
Paul Langerhans (Germany)	1869	Isolation of pancreatic islets
Claude Bernard (French)	1870	Glucose stored in the body as glycogen
Oskar Minowaski and Josef von Mering (Germany)	1889	Pancreatectomy in dog results in DM
George Zuelzer (Germany), Nicolas Paulesco (Romania), Ernest Scott and Israel Kleiner (USA)	19th century AD	Impure hypoglycaemic extracts from pancreas
Jean de Meyer (Belgium)	1909	Glucose lowering agent named insulin
Banting, Best, Collip, Macleod (Canada)	1921	Insulin isolation and its clinical trials
JR Murlin (America)	1923	Glucagon discovered
Frederick Sanger (England)	1955	Sequencing of insulin
Dorothy Hodgkin (England)	1969	Three-dimensional structure of insulin by X-ray crystallography
Roth et al	1971	Insulin receptor discovery
Ulrich et al	1977	Insulin gene cloned

Some of the historical milestones in the story of diabetes mellitus

offered from time to time. In early 19th century, its two main types were called:
- Diabetes maigre, and
- Diabetes gras

In early 20th century these two types were named:
- Juvenile onset, and
- Maturity onset diabetes mellitus.

In later years these two types came to be known as insulin dependent and non-insulin dependent diabetes mellitus (IDDM and NIDDM). Presently the nomenclature has further changed and we call them type 1 and type 2 diabetes mellitus (T1DM, T2DM).

T1DM is not a single entity. It is a heterogeneous group of disorders with distinct genetic patterns and other aetiological and pathophysiological mechanisms that leads to impairment of glucose tolerance. Table 25.1.3 gives the present day classification. This classification is based on the pathogenesis responsible for hyperglycaemia unlike earlier classifications which were based on the age of the individual or the treatment given.

TABLE 25.1.3

Type 1 Diabetes
(β cell destruction often leading to absolute insulin deficiency)
- Immune-mediated   (1A DM)
- Idiopathic   (1B DM)

Type 2 Diabetes
- Insulin resistance + relative insulin deficiency
- Insulin secretory defect + insulin resistance

Other specific types of diabetes
(A) Genetic defects of β cell function characterized by mutations in:
  - Hepatocyte nuclear transcription factor (HNF) 4α (MODY 1)
  - Glucokinase (MODY 2)
  - HNF-1α (MODY 3)
  - Insulin promoter factor (IPF) (MODY 4)
  - HNF-1β (MODY 5)
  - Neurod-1 (MODY 6)
  - Mitochondria DNA
  - Proinsulin or insulin conversion
(B) Genetic defects in insulin action:
  - Type A insulin resistance
  - Leprechaunism
  - Rabson-Mendenhall syndrome
  - Lipoatrophic diabetes
(C) Disease of exocrine pancreas:
  - Pancreatitis, pancreatectomy, neoplasia, cystic fibrosis
  - Haemochromatosis, fibrocalculous pancreatopathy
(D) Endocrine disorders: Acromegaly, Cushing's syndrome, glucagonoma, phaeochromocytoma, hyperthyroidism, somatostatinoma.
(E) Drug induced: Vacor, pentamidine, nicotinic acid, glucocorticoids, thyroid hormone, diazoxide, β adrenergic agonists, thiazides, phenytoin, β-interferon, protease inhibitors, clozapine, β-blockers.
(F) Infections: Congenital rubella, cytomegalovirus, coxsackie.
(G) Uncommon forms of immune-mediated diabetes. Stiff-Man syndrome, anti-insulin receptor antibodies
(H) Other genetic syndromes sometimes associated with diabetes:
  - Down's, Klinefelter's, Turner's, Wolfman's syndrome, Frederich's ataxia, Huntington's chorea, Laurence-Moon–Biedl syndrome, Prader–Willi syndrome, porphyria, myotonic dystrophy

Gestational diabetes mellitus

Aetiological classification of diabetes mellitus

With the advancement of our knowledge regarding its aetiopathogenesis, type 1DM is further subdivided into type 1A and type 1B.

Secondary Diabetes Mellitus

When hyperglycaemia is the result of known endocrinopathies or a part of a genetic syndrome or disease of exocrine pancreas, it is called secondary diabetes mellitus.

Whatever the underlying aetiopathogenesis, the resultant consequence is the inadequacy or inefficiency of insulin leading to counter-regulatory hormones (glucagon, cortisol, GH, catecholamines) taking an upper hand and aggravating the metabolic scenario created by the insulin deficiency (Fig. 25.1.3).

AETIOPATHOGENESIS

Type 1A DM

Type 1A DM or immune mediated type 1 DM is the most common form of T1DM (over 90%). It is a result of cellular mediated autoimmune destructive process which ultimately destroys the beta cells and leads to insulin deficiency most of the time. The markers of immune destruction of the beta cells like islet cell antibodies (ICAs), autoantibodies to insulin (IAA), autoantibodies to glutamic acid decarboxylase (GAD) 65 and antibodies to tyrosine phosphates, 1A-2 and 1A-2B are present much before the disease manifests clinically and can be demonstrated. As is typical with all autoimmune disorders, this type of DM has strong histocompatibility complex (HLA) association. The rate of beta cell destruction is quite variable. It is rapid in infants and children while it is slow in adults. It is probable that environmental factors trigger the onset in individuals with inherited predisposition (Fig. 25.1.4).

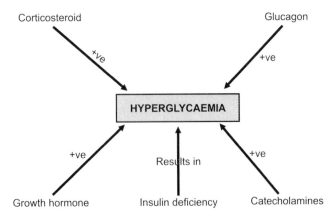

Fig. 25.1.3: Insulin deficiency and role of counterregulatory hormones in hyperglycaemia

Type 1B DM

It is also characterized by insulin deficiency but the immunological markers indicative of autoimmune destruction of beta cells are absent. The exact mechanism responsible for beta cell destruction in this type is unknown. Hence, this is also called Idiopathic T1DM. Relatively few patients belong to this category and are mostly of African or Asian origin. Individuals with this type of DM exhibit varying degrees of insulin deficiency and are not HLA associated. This form of diabetes is strongly inherited.

Both type 1A and 1B are prone to ketosis and need insulin for survival. Although T1DM most commonly develops before 30 years, an autoimmune beta destruction can develop at any age and we do see some cases of T1DM after 30 years (5 to 10%). Similarly T2DM has been seen in some obese children.

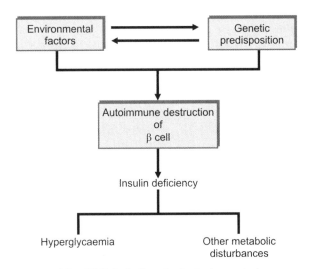

Fig. 25.1.4: Aetiopathological events in immune-mediated T1DM

Development of Florid Type 1 Diabetes Mellitus (Fig. 25.1.5)

There appear to be several stages in the development of florid type 1DM (Fig. 25.1.6)
- Genetic susceptibility.
- Induction and advent of autoimmunity.
- Decline in beta cell mass and function.
- Development of florid diabetes, and
- Complete loss of insulin secretion.

The duration of these stages is variable in affected individuals.

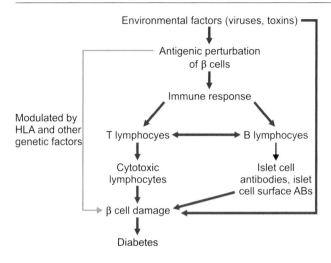

Fig. 25.1.5: Possible pathogenesis of insulin dependent DM (T1DM)

Genetic Susceptibility

The genetic background of type 1 DM is highly complex and the syndrome is best described as of multigenic origin. Familial occurrence is also variable (10 to 15%) and most cases are of sporadic nature. Paternal inheritance is about 5 times that of maternal inheritance. If both parents have type 1 DM, then 6 to 8% of their offsprings appear to be vulnerable. In monozygotic twins, concordance rate ranges from 30 to 50%, while in fraternal twins, the incidence is same (about 7%) as among other siblings.

Genes for type 1 DM provide susceptibility as well as protection. The most important genes are located within the major histocompatibility complex (MHC) HLA class 11 region on the chromosome 6 p21; (formerly termed 1DDM 1 locus) and account for about 60% genetic susceptibility for the disease. The risk for the disease is associated with HLA-DR3, HLA-DR4, DQ α-chains and DQβ-chains.

Inheritance of HLA-DR3 or DR4 antigens appears to confer a 2- to 3-fold increased risk for the development of type 1 DM. When both DR3 and DR4 are inherited, the relative risk for the development of diabetes is 7 to 10 times. The homozygous absence of aspartic acid at position 57 of the HLA DQβ-chain confers an approximately 100-fold relative risk for the development of type 1 diabetes. The heterozygous absence of aspartic acid at position 57 is only marginally more susceptible than individuals who have aspartic acid at both DQβ-chains. Thus the presence of aspartic acid at one or both alleles of DQβ-chain protects against the development of autoimmune diabetes. The incidence of type 1 diabetes in any given population appears to be proportional to the gene frequency of the non-ASP (aspartic acid) alleles in that population.

Besides this, arginine at position 52 of DQβ-chain confers marked susceptibility to type 1 DM. The 52 and 57 positions of DQB appear to be critical locations of the HLA molecules that permit or prevent antigen presentation to T-cell receptors and activate the autoimmune cascade.

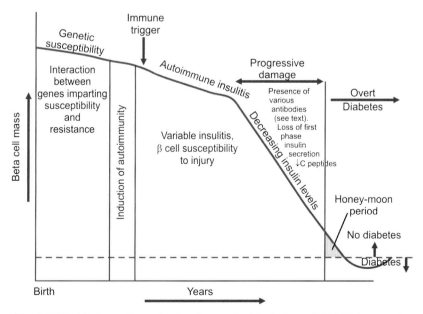

Fig. 25.1.6: Various stages in development of florid type 1 DM (A temporal model)

The MHC haplotypes which provide protection are:
HLA-DRβ 1.0403,
HLA- DQβ 1.0602,
HLA-DQA 1.0102,

whereas susceptibility is provided by the presence of
HLA-DRβ 1.0301,
HLA-DRβ 1.0401,
HLA-DQβ 1.0302,
HLA-DQA 1.0301.

Interestingly, in spite of prevalence being 15 to 20 times higher than in general population, only 10% of subjects with DR3/DR4 HLA are vulnerable. This confirms that other genetic and environmental factors are also involved. There appear to be some 17 non-HLA genes which contribute towards the development of type 1 DM. Among them, IDDM 12 corresponds to the insulin gene locus on chromosome 11. It has a smaller role than IDDM 1; acts independently and appears to be an associate in type IB diabetes. Somatic mutations involving genes for T cell receptors often create variance in the genetic fabric of monozygotic twins. Two candidate genes that are associated with susceptibility to T1DM have been identified-one is a variable number of tandem repeats (VNTR) upstream of insulin; the other is a splice variant of CTLA-4, a regulator of T-cell function.

Induction of Autoimmunity

Injury to β cells by several agents like viruses, biological/chemical toxins, food contaminants, nitroso compounds such as vacor may lead to release of auto-antigenic components on the surface of the cells. Surprisingly, other cells—α, δ or PP cells though functionally and embryologically similar to beta cells, are spared from the autoimmune process. Inter reactions among the genetic promoters may also serve as a trigger to induce autoimmune reactions. Among viruses, those of rubella, mumps, coxsackie B, cytomegaloviruses, reo and herpes viruses have been implicated. Most significant of all these appears to be congenital rubella infection. Viruses may target the β cells and destroy them directly through a cytolytic effect, or by triggering an autoimmune attack against β cell. Autoimmune mechanism may include 'molecular mimicry', i.e. immune responses against a viral antigen that cross-react with a β cell antigen. Recently a viral protein homologous to KD 52 antigen in β cell has been identified. Moreover in about 75% of T1DM cases, anti-insulin antibodies cross-react with the retroviral p23 antigen.

Alternately, viral damage may release sequestered islet antigens and thus restimulate resting autoreactive T cells,

previously sensitized against β cell antigens ('bystander activation'). Persistent viral infection may also stimulate interferon-α synthesis and hyper-expression of HLA class 1 antigens and secretion of chemokines that recreate activated macrophages and cytotoxic T cells (Fig. 25.1.7). Some percentage (15 to 20%) of type 1 DM develop both islet cell and thyroid antibodies over a period of time.

The incidence of type 1 DM is increasing in many countries. It is particularly notable under the age of 5 years. This rise in frequency is considered a pointer towards changing environmental factors that operate, these days, in early life rather than any influence by the genetic pattern.

Advent of Autoimmunity

The injured β cells initiate the process of autoimmunity by shedding the antigen which induces β lymphocytes to multiple and process the autoantibodies corresponding to the β cell-derived antigens. These antibodies are released to the circulation and, under appropriate conditions, may react with antigens present in the β cells.

However, it is to be appreciated, that cell-mediated autoimmune reaction is the predominant pathological process. Mononuclear cell infiltration of the islets is the major feature of insulitis where activated CD8+ T cells constitute the majority of the cell population.

Following abnormalities are recognized in both humoral and cellular arms of the immune system:
- Islet cell autoantibodies.
- Activated lymphocytes in the islets and systemic circulation.
- T lymphocytes that proliferate when stimulated with islet proteins, and
- Release of cytokines within the insulitis.

B cells are particularly susceptible to the toxic effects of some cytokines (tumour necrosis factor α, interferon γ and interleukin 1).

Most useful markers of type 1 DM are islet cell antibodies (ICA), insulin antibodies (IAA), glutamic acid decarboxylase (GAD) 65, and autoantibodies to 1A-2 (protein tyrosine phosphatase), its fractions 1CA512 and 1A2b (phogrin, insulin granule protein). If the presence of these antibodies is considered individually, then the predictive value is quite low-less than 10%. Their significance is enhanced only if 2 or more of them are present. In the absence of protective HLA DQB1.0602 gene, nearly 70% individuals develop type 1 DM over a period of 6 years. The presence of GAD65ab is particularly useful in recognizing type 1 DM when it is detected in adults with apparent type 2 DM, some call such adults as type

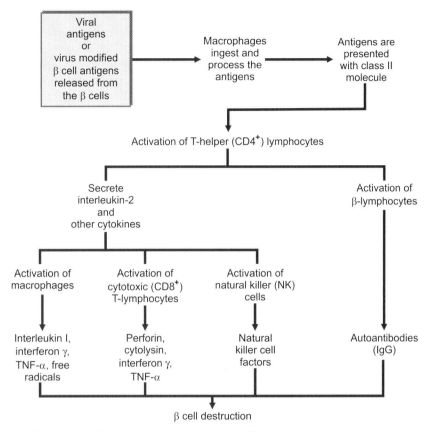

Fig. 25.1.7: Probable course of events in β-cell destruction by viruses

1.5 DM or latent autoimmune disease in adults (LADA). Islet cell antibodies (ICAs) are a composite of several different antibodies such as GAD, insulin, 1A-2/CA512, and an islet ganglioside and serve as a marker of the autoimmune process of type 1 DM. ICAs are present in over 75% of new onset type 1 DM. Therefore their presence should help in the diagnosis. However, they are also present in a few cases of newly diagnosed type 2 DM and occasionally (5%) in individuals with gestational DM (GDM). As such presently, ICAs are used only in research studies and not in clinical practice. Patients with islet cell antibodies (ICAs) are more prone to develop isolated autoimmune endocrine disorders, coeliac disease, vitiligo and pernicious anaemia.

Type 1 DM may also be a component of autoimmune polyendocrine syndrome (APS) 11.

Decline/Destruction of β Cell Mass and Function

The development of type 1 DM is stochastic and is programmed by multiple variables. Putative environmental triggers include viruses, early exposure to bovine milk protein and nitroso urea compounds. Surveys have shown association between consumption of bovine milk protein and a low prevalence of breast-feeding with type 1 diabetes. It has been suggested that antibodies against bovine albumin may cross-react with an islet antigen (ICA 69). The studies are inconclusive and the suggestion remains controversial. A single factor like genetic susceptibility or even appearance of autoantibodies is not enough to ensure progressive β cell destruction. Cytotoxic T cells are considered to be the major factor in the destruction of β cells. Killer and natural killer lymphocytes also contribute to this process. Humoral factors like nitric oxide (NO) and oxygen free radicals (O_2) have also been implicated in the process of β cell destruction.

Another model of β-cell destruction is by the process of 'apoptosis' or 'programmed cell death.' This is affected by the activation of cellular caspase enzymes triggered by:
• Intersection of cell surface Fas (the death-signalling molecule) with its ligand FasL on the surface of the infiltrating cells
• Macrophage-derived nitric oxide (NO)
• Toxic free radicals,
• Disruption of the cell membrane by cytotoxic T cells (T-cell cytokines, (interleukin 1, interferon γ, the tumour necrosis factor α), perforin and granzyme β produced by these cells).

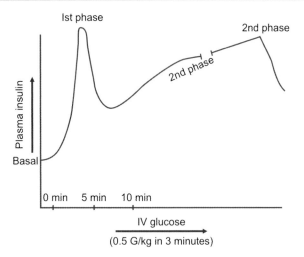

Fig. 25.1.8: Biphasic normal insulin response to IV glucose

Clinically, the effect of β cell damage is seen initially as decrease in the first phase of insulin response (FPIR) to IV glucose (Fig. 25.1.8). Later on, one finds reduction in fasting and PP insulin, and C-peptide values. The plasma glucose values remain within normal range initially, though later on glucose intolerance and ultimately persistent hyperglycaemia prevail. Frank and florid diabetes appears when over 80% of β cells have been destroyed.

Type 2 Diabetes Mellitus (Fig. 25.1.9)

Till 1979 it was called maturity onset diabetes mellitus, thereafter the name 'non-insulin diabetes mellitus (NIDDM)' was given to it. Presently, it is known as type 2 diabetes mellitus (T2DM). It constitutes nearly 85 to 95% of all patients with diabetes mellitus. Various risk factors associated with the disease are increasing age, obesity, reduced physical activity, positive family history, previous history of gestational diabetes and racial factor. The disease has a slow and insidious onset with a prolonged (years) subclinical course. India has the highest number of diabetic population and Indian migrants in various parts of the world have a higher frequency of diabetes than the indigenous population. It is more common in urban than in rural areas. Social deprivation, poverty in city slums, and diabetogenic lifestyle appear to be responsible. The peak age of T2DM in India is 10 to 15 years earlier than western countries and presently one does come across this disease even in obese children and adolescents with a positive family history. Its pathogenesis is varied and complex. Two factors, however work in tandem in the evolution of this syndrome. Insulin resistance and decline in insulin secretion; both these factors, are central to the development of T2DM. At the time of diagnosis, β-cell function is usually already reduced by over 50 per cent. Most studies support the view that insulin resistance precedes the insulin secretory defect. Thus, there are many families where insulin resistance is seen without abnormal insulin secretion which develops in later stages. Both insulin resistance and abnormal insulin secretion appear to be modulated by heredity and environmental factors.

Genes and Type 2 Diabetes Mellitus

Type 2 DM is not associated with genes in the HLA region. It is probably associated with different combinations of possible gene defects. Candidate genes tested and identified as having association are insulin promoter, Transcription factors (e.g. hepatic nuclear factor 4 α), Peroxisome proliferation activated receptor-γ (PPAR-γ) and insulin receptor substrata-1 (IRS-1).

No genes have been identified, till date, that have a moderate or major effect on the disease.

Influence of Intrauterine and Neonatal Nutrition on Type 2 Diabetes Mellitus

Since early 1900s it has been observed that low birth weight children have the highest frequency of diabetes and IGT in adult life. It has been proposed, that foetal and early childhood malnutrition programmes the child's metabolism by impairing β-cell development and inducing insulin resistance. If nutrition is abundant in adult life leading to obesity, then IGT and diabetes result. This is called the 'thrifty phenotype' hypothesis (Fig. 25.1.10). Studies have shown that low birth weight is also associated with other features of metabolic syndrome.

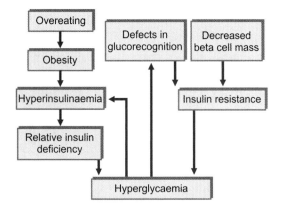

Fig. 25.1.9: Possible pathogenesis of T2DM

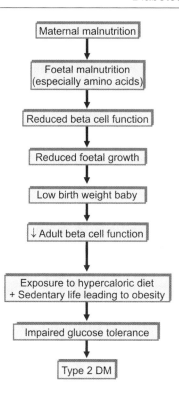

Fig. 25.1.10: The 'thrifty phenotype' hypothesis

Insulin Secretion in Type 2 Diabetes Mellitus

Insulin secretory function in type 2 DM shows a wide heterogeneity and is reflected in varying insulin levels in different patients. The insulin values are usually high in obese prospective diabetes patients especially when they demonstrate an impaired glucose tolerance (IGT), whereas those values may be low in non-obese IGT diabetics. Beta cell function is measured by the homeostasis model assessment (HOMA) which is calculated from the fasting blood glucose and insulin values.

Approximately 20 to 80% (mean 50%) of insulin released by the β cells are extracted by the liver from portal blood. This does not happen to C-peptide fraction of proinsulin. Half-life of insulin in the peripheral blood is very short (20 minutes). C-peptide, on the other hand, has a much longer half-life. The ideal way to assess the insulin secretion is by analysis of the portal blood: but this is a very difficult proposition in clinical practice.

Populations like Pima Indians, Mexican Americans and Pacific islanders demonstrate hypersecretory state of β cells with elevated values of plasma insulin at fasting and 2 hours after the glucose load at prediabetic IGT and close to onset of type 2 diabetes. In type 2 DM there is reduction or loss of first phase of insulin secretion and

prolongation of the second phase. Plasma insulin and C-peptide values are low in the initial 20 to 30 minutes of the test meal but are higher at 2nd or 3rd hour after the meal. Secondly, the pulsatile characteristics of insulin secretion is lost quite early in T2DM. This fact is seen even at IGT stage of T2DM. Leaner type 2 diabetics have lower insulin value than the obese patients. Lean diabetics have normal fasting insulin values but postprandial insulin values are relatively always low. In obese patients, the insulin resistance demonstrates best relationship with the visceral fat which liberates large amounts of non-esterfied fatty acids (NEFAs), increasing gluconeogenesis in the liver and impaired glucose uptake and utilization in the muscle.

Factors responsible for impaired β cell function are both genetic and environmental (Fig. 25.1.11). So far monogenic mutations leading to defects in insulin secretion have been seen in five sub-types of maturity onset type of diabetes in the young (MODY) and two clusters with mitochondrial DNA mutations. Specifications of genetic loci in the rest is continuing and surely our knowledge will progressively increase in this respect.

Association of foetal undernutrition (low birth weight) and development of type 2 DM in adult life is attributed to raised insulin resistance rather than impaired β cell function. Unequivocal β cell dysfunction, however, is clearly documented in marasmus, kwashiorkor and malnutrition-modulated diabetes mellitus (MMDM).

Glucotoxicity (sustained hyperglycaemia) and lipotoxicity [elevated levels of free fatty acids (FFA)] are the two main factors responsible for inducing acquired defect in β cell function and its progression towards frank

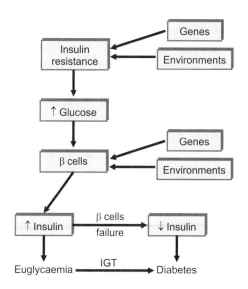

Fig. 25.1.11: Genetic and environmental factors in pathogenesis of type 2 diabetes mellitus

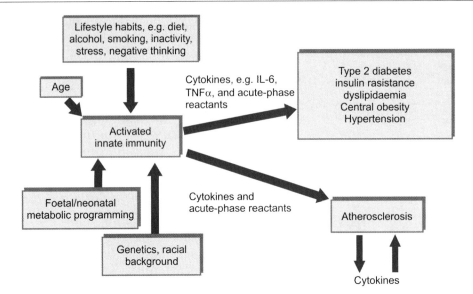

Fig. 25.1.12: Various factors which result in insulin resistance, T2DM and other components of insulin resistance or metabolic syndrome

diabetes mellitus. In the uncontrolled diabetes, β cell response to glucose is grossly impaired—this impairment is much more severe as compared to other secretagogues such as arginine or glucagon. Chronically raised FFA block glucose utilization by the muscle. FFA also increase gluconeogenesis in the liver.

Randle and associates (1963) were the first to highlight the interrelationship between free fatty acids (FFA) and glucose. The adverse metabolic effects of glucose and FFA are together known as glucolipotoxicity.

The main histological abnormality in the islets of type 2 DM is the presence of amyloid, insoluble fibrils that lie outside the cells and derive from islet amyloid polypeptide (IAPP, also known as amylin). IAPP is co-secreted with insulin in a molar ratio of 1:10 to 90. Its presence impairs insulin secretion and it is considered toxic to the β-cells. Even then it does not appear to play a big role in pathogenesis of type 2 DM and its deposits are found in 20% of elderly subjects having normal glucose tolerance.

In most of the type 2 DM, the β-cell mass is reduced by only 20 to 40% while their functional capacity (insulin secretion) may be reduced up to 50% or even more. This is thought to be due to glucolipotoxicity and offset of IAPP oversecretion.

5 to 10% of type 2 DM are due to autoimmune process. Such patients are usually thin and are positive for GAD antibodies. They require insulin within 3 to 10 years of follow up and slowly progress towards type 1 DM. This variant is sometimes called 'latent autoimmune disease of adults (LADA)' or 'slowly progressive type 1 DM' or even 'type 1.5 DM.'

Markers of Type 2 Diabetes Mellitus

Raised levels of C-reactive protein (CRP), and sialic acid (which are part of acute-phase response to innate immune syndrome), and 1L-6 in non-diabetic subjects predict the later development of T2DM. On the basis of this, it has been hypothesized that activated innate immunity or chronic low grade inflammation may play a role in the pathogenesis of T2DM. The innate or natural immune system is the body's rapid first-line defence against environmental threats like infections, physical or chemical injury, etc. It goes to the credit of Schmidt and associates who demonstrated a number of inflammatory markers (↑TLC, low serum albumin, α1-acid glycoprotein, fibrinogen, sialic acid and CRP) that predicted development of T2DM in a middle-aged population. Since then there has been explosion of interest in the belief that chronic low grade inflammation and activation of innate immune system are closely involved in the pathogenesis of T2DM. Figure 25.1.12 summarises several factors concerned with the pathogenesis of T2DM.

SUMMARY

There is a progressive and persistence increase in the prevalence and incidence of the diabetes mellitus. 13 to 15% of Indian population is estimated to be diabetic and it seems to register a 12% yearly increase. T1DM forms nearly 5% of total Indian diabetic population whereas

T2M is between 90 and 95%. An interplay between genetic (especially T1 DM) and environmental factors results in β cell damage leading to this syndrome.

Autoimmune dysfunction usually triggered by viral infection plays a highly significant role in T1DM. In T2DM, monogenic defects and environmental factors like obesity, overeating, inactivity, abdominal fat, foetal under-nourishment and urbanization are responsible for the problem. In nearly 5 to 10% T2DM, autoimmunity plays a major role. Such patients are positive for GAD antibodies.

Hyperglycaemia may also be the result of other endocrine or exocrine organs when it is called 'Secondary Diabetes.' Persistent hyperglycaemia and resultant hyperlipidaemia (glucolipotoxicity) further damage the beta cells thus aggravating the problem.

FURTHER READING

1. Ahuja MMS. Epidemiological status in diabetes mellitus in India. In Ahuja MMS (Ed): Epidemiology of Diabetes Mellitus in Developing Countries, New Delhi: Interprint, 1979.
2. American Diabetic Association. Clinical practice recommendations 2002. Diabetes Care 2004;27:51.
3. Duncan BB, Schmidt MI, et al. Factor VIII and other homeostasis variables are related to incident diabetes in adults. The atherosclerosis risk in communities (ARIC) study. Diabetes Care 1999; 20: 767-72.
4. Expert Committee on the diagnosis and classification of diabetes mellitus. American Diabetes Association. Diabetes Care 2002;25 (suppl 1): S5-S20.
5. Prospective Diabetes Study Group. Intensive blood glucose control with sulphonylureas or insulin compared with conventional treatment and risk of complications in patients with Type 2 diabetes (UKPDS). Lancet 1998;352:854-65.
6. Ramachandran A, Snehalatha C, et al. Impact of urbanization on the lifestyle and on the prevalence of diabetes in native Asian Indian population. Diab Res Clin Prac 1999;44:207-13.
7. Ramachandran A, Snehalatha C, Latha E, et al. Rising prevalence of NIDDM in an urban population in India. Diabetology 1997; 40:232-7.
8. Schmidt MI, Duncan BB, Sharrett AR, et al. Markers of inflammation and prediction of diabetes mellitus in adults (Atherosclerosis risk in communities study): a cohort study. Lancet 1999;353:1649-52.
9. The effect of intensive treatment of diabetes on the development and progression of long term complications in insulin dependent diabetes mellitus. The Diabetic Control and Complications Trial research Group. NEJM 1993;329:977-86.
10. The Writing Team for the diabetes control and complications trial/epidemiology of the diabetes, interventions and complications research group—Effects of intensive therapy on the microvascular complications of type 1 diabetes mellitus. JAMA. 2002;287:2563.
11. Zimmet PZ. Challenge in diabetes epidemiology. From West to the Rest. Diabetes Care 1992;15:132-52.
12. Zimmet P, Alberti KGi, Shaw J. Global and societal implications of the diabetic epidemic. Nature 2001;414:782-7.

25.2 Insulin Resistance

Y Sachdev

- Definition
- Measurement of Insulin Resistance
  - Clinical
  - Biochemical
  - Euglycaemic Hyperinsulinaemic Clamp Studies
  - Minimal and HOMA Models and Other Methods
- Sites of Insulin Resistance
  - Muscles
- Adipose Tissue
- Liver
- Cellular Mechanism of Insulin Resistance
- Insulin Resistance Syndrome
  - Clinical Associations
  - Aggravating Factors
  - Biochemical Associations
  - Management

DEFINITION

Insulin resistance (IR) implies there is target level resistance to the physiological actions of insulin. This resistance is seen at peripheral tissues especially muscle, adipose tissue and liver. The end results of IR are:
- Decreased peripheral uptake of glucose.
- Inadequate suppression of hepatic glucose production, and
- Increased lipolysis.

MEASUREMENT OF IR

Clinically, the IR is apparent when an appropriate dose of insulin fails to lower plasma glucose to the same extent as seen in controls. Biochemically, the presence of relatively higher fasting and post-secretagogue insulin values are indicative of IR. The impairment of insulin action can be measured by euglycaemic hyperinsulinaemic clamp studies as well as the minimal and homeostasis model assessment (HOMA) methods. In euglycaemic hyper-insulinaemic clamp, a fixed amount of insulin is infused intravenously and a titrated infusion of intravenous glucose is administrated to maintain normoglycaemia. A low rate of exogenous glucose infusion indicates insulin resistance. Glucose disposal in clamp studies typically measures up to 7 mg/kg/min in controls while in overweight T2 DM it is observed to be much lower, (around 2.5 mg/kg/min.). Table 25.2.1 enumerates other tests for measuring IR. The author recommends 2 (a) and 3 as simple, easy and reliable tests for use in clinical practice and are described in the appendix at the end of this subsection.

SITES OF INSULIN RESISTANCE

Muscles

The skeletal muscles (like adipose tissue) require insulin for optimal glucose uptake and utilization. In T2DM, available insulin fails to recruit more GLUT-4 for facilitated glucose transportation across the cell membrane (Fig. 25.2.1). Therefore, the entry of glucose into the myocytes is only through mass action. This results in reduction in glucose uptake from the standard 60 G to 44 G in 3 to 5 hours after a stipulated glucose load. The insulin mediated glucose utilization by the muscles is also impaired in T2DM. Both these factors combined together contribute to the elevated postprandial blood glucose levels seen so frequently in early stages of T2DM.

Adipose Tissue

The resistance of adipocytes to insulin action leads to increased lipolysis resulting in elevated FFAs in

TABLE 25.2.1

1. *Dynamic tests*		
	a. Hyperinsulinaemic euglycaemic clamp technique	a. 'Gold standard' test
	b. Insulin tolerance test	b. 15 minutes test 0.05 U/kg IV infusion Satisfactory results
	c. Insulin sensitivity test	c. 3 hours test Fixed rate of insulin infusion + Defined glucose load + Somatostatin Correlates with (a)
	d. Low dose insulin and glucose insulin test	d. Simple alternative to (a) Useful for community survey
2. *Minimal models*		
	a. Frequently sampled IV glucose tolerance test	Glucose bolus 0.3 G/kg IV over 1 minute ± tolbutamine Reliable test
	b. Continuous infusion of glucose with model assessment	Not very reliable
3. *Oral glucose tolerance test*		Several investigators use different indices; Easy and useful.
4. *Mathematical calculations (Homeostatic models)*		
	a. Fasting insulin level	Not very reliable
	b. Glucose/insulin ratio	Efficacy disputed
	c. Homeostatic model assessment (HOMA)	
	d. Quantitative insulin sensitivity check index (QUICKI)	Useful for large population studies

Techniques used for measurement of insulin resistant

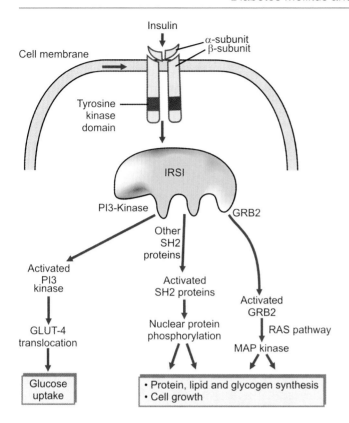

Fig. 25.2.1: Shows various steps through which insulin exerts its biochemical effects

Insulin resistance could be the result of defect in insulin receptor, IRSI; decline in release of tyrosine kinase; lowering of PI 3-K; defect in GLUTS molecule, and other factors (see text)

circulation and tissues. Leptin is a protein secreted by adipose tissue. In rodents it inhibits neuropeptide neurones, (they stimulate feeding) to the hypothalamus. Its defects give rise to over feeding and obesity in rodents. The role of leptin in human T2DM is unclear.

Adipose tissue also secretes the cytokine TNFα, which may cause insulin resistance by inhibiting tyrosine kinase activity of the insulin receptor and decreasing the expression of glucose transporter (GLUT-4). IL-6 secreted by adipose tissue and other cells also induces insulin resistance. The protein adiponectin is secreted by fat cells and ameliorates insulin resistance probably by increasing fat oxidation. Its level is low in obesity. The role of the protein resistin which is also secreted by adipocytes and implicated in IR is not very clear as yet. Moreover, in obesity there is often an increased sympathetic over activity which leads to increased lipolysis, reduced muscle blood flow and thus decreased glucose delivery (Fig. 25.2.2). Recently it has been observed that foetal and postnatal overnutrition in the first 5 to 10 years which leads to obesity results in IR and metabolic syndrome in later life.

Liver

Both glycogenolysis and gluconeogenesis are under the influence of insulin. In patients with IR, there is impaired restraining effect of insulin on gluconeogenesis and hepatic glucose production (HGP). In T2DM, the requirement of insulin for the control of HGP is nearly double the amount required in normal subjects. Moreover, loss of first phase of insulin secretion seen even at the

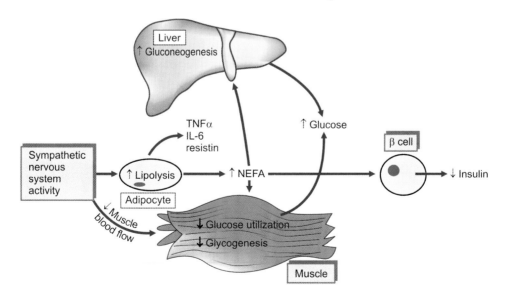

Fig. 25.2.2: Mechanism of insulin resistance in T2DM

TNFα, IL-6 and adiponectin all increase insulin resistance. Tyrosine kinase activity and GLUT-4 expression are inhibited

TABLE 25.2.2

Prereceptor sites	Receptor sites	Postreceptor sites
• Abnormal insulin	• Reduction in the number of receptors	• Defect in internalization
		• Defect in recycling of receptor
• Insulin antibodies	• Reduction in affinity of receptors	• Decline in release of tyrosine kinase
		• Lowing of post-binding signal transducer, PI 3-K
	• Mutation in receptor gene at chromosome 19	• Defect in phosphorylation of glucose and glycogen synthesis
		• Defect in GLUT-4 molecule

Cellular mechanism of insulin resistance

stage of IGT also contributes to the failure of prompt post-load suppression of gluconeogenesis. The end result is elevated post-absorptive (fasting) and postprandial (PP) blood sugar values.

CELLULAR MECHANISM OF INSULIN RESISTANCE (TABLE 25.2.2)

Impairment of insulin action can occur at:
a. Pre-receptor site due to: abnormal insulin or insulin antibodies, or
b. At the receptor site (Fig. 25.2.3) where it could be due to:
   - Reduction in the number of receptors
   - Reduction in affinity of receptors
   - Mutation in receptor gene at chromosome 19 or
c. As a postreceptor event where it could be due to:
   - Defect in internalization
   - Defect in recycling of receptor
   - Decline in release of tyrosine kinase
   - Lowering of post-binding signal transducer PI 3-K
   - Defect in phosphorylation of glucose and glycogen synthesis or
   - Defect in glucose transporter (GLUT-4) molecule.

INSULIN RESISTANCE SYNDROME

The concept of insulin resistance syndrome (IR) was published as early as 1936 in the 'Lancet' by Himsworth wherein he divided diabetes mellitus into insulin sensitive and insulin insensitive types. Later in 1985, Modan described the deleterious effects of IR. However, it goes to the credit of Reaven who in 1988 during 'Banting' oration correlated IR, glucose intolerance, hyperinsulinaemia, hypertension, elevated triglyceride, VLDL and low HDL cholesterol and termed it as syndrome X. Reaven's description pertained to lean diabetics, though later on, it was appreciated that IR is much more common in obese diabetics. Syndrome X is present in both lean and obese diabetics though it is more common in the latter group. IR is also seen in obese individuals without diabetes mellitus. These individuals demonstrate high insulin levels to

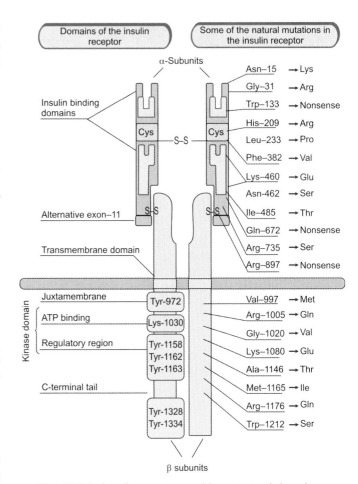

Fig. 25.2.3: Insulin receptor and its structural domains
Mutations in the receptor interfere with insulin actions as well as cause insulin resistance

maintain euglycaemic status. The syndrome X is also known as Reaven's syndrome, metabolic syndrome, deadly quartet, CHOAS, New World syndrome and civilization syndrome. The lipid abnormality of low HDL and high triglyceride is characteristic of type 2 DM (and not type 1 DM) and is known as 'diabetic dyslipidaemia'.

Presently, it is recognized that android type of truncal adiposity (abdominal fat), tendency to atherosclerotic disorders especially coronary heart disease (CAD), elevated apolipoproteins B, excess of small dense LDL cholesterol, microalbuminuria, raised plasminogen activator inhibitor-1 (PA1-1), nonalcoholic steatohepatitis (NASH) and polycystic ovarian syndrome are some of the other features and associations of this syndrome. Classically, the syndrome represents a complex inter-relationship of metabolic abnormalities, namely hyper-insulinaemia, hypertension, dyslipidaemia, central obesity and glucose intolerance. The combination of these meta-bolic abnormalities is associated with an increased risk of CAD in T2DM (Fig. 25.2.4).

Aggravating Factors of IR

Insulin resistance is aggravated by:
- Diets, which are rich in saturated fats, or have highly disproportionate omega 6 polyunsaturated acid relative to omega 3, promote insulin resistance
- Vitamin C and E deficiency and oxidant strain also increase IR
- Reduced physical activity with low maximum aerobic power
- Ageing has a relatively minor role
- Excessive and habitual tobacco smoking
- Atmospheric pollution
- Android type of central obesity. Large adipocytes in the truncal subcutaneous tissue secrete excess of TNF-α, IL-6, and leptin.

Biochemical Changes Associated with IR

- Hyperinsulinaemia
- Elevated TNF alpha

- Reduced adiponectin
- Elevated NEFA, triglycerides
- Reduced HDL-cholesterol, and
- Normal or slightly elevated LDL-cholesterol.

Associations of Insulin Resistance (Table 25.2.3)

Hypertension and IR

Nearly 50% of hypertensives have IR and raised insulin values. IR and elevated insulin values have been documented even in lean hypertensives who are not diabetic. This association could be explained:
a. As outlined in the Figure 25.2.4.
b. Hyperinsulinaemia may also produce hypertension by causing cell membrane defect and modifying the ion transportation across the cell membrane and resulting in increase in cytosolic calcium.
c. Hyperinsulinaemia also augments the pressor and aldosterone response to angiotensin II (Fig. 25.2.5).

Hyperinsulinaemia and Dyslipidaemia

a. It is obvious that due to insulin resistance at the adipose tissue level, there is impairment of normal suppression of FFA release from the adipose tissue in the post-prandial period. Increased quantity of FFA is thus released from the abdominal adipose tissue and delivered to the liver by the portal circulation. This results in increased triglyceride synthesis and production of VLDL cholesterol.
b. Hyperinsulinaemia also down-regulates the activity of lipoprotein lipase—an enzyme which is important in VLDL cholesterol metabolism. There is also increased oxidation of LDL cholesterol.

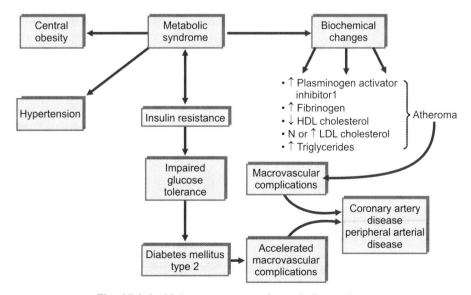

Fig. 25.2.4: Main components of metabolic syndrome

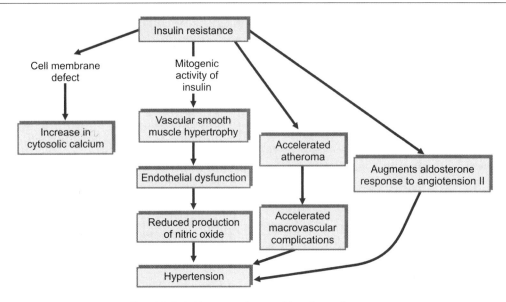

Fig. 25.2.5: Hypertension and insulin resistance

TABLE 25.2.3

1. *Hypertension*
   • 50 % of hypertension have IR and↑ insulin values
   • IR is present in hypertensives even when they are not diabetic
2. *Dyslipidaemia*
   • ↑ FFA release from the adipose tissue
   • ↑ Triglycerides synthesis
   • ↑ VLDL cholesterol production
   • ↓ HDL cholesterol
   • ↑Insulin down regulates the activity of lipoprotein lipase
   • ↑ TNFα
3. *Polycystic ovary syndrome*
   • Polycystic ovaries
   • Irregular menses
   • Chronic anovulation
   • Obesity
   • Hperandrogenism
   • Hyperprolactinaemia (30%)
4. *Coronary artery disease*
   Hyperinsulinaemia promotes
   • Smooth muscle proliferation
   • Growth factors
   • Connective tissue production
   • LDL receptor activity
   • Cholesterol synthesis
5. *Other associations*
   • Elevated PAI-1, elevated fibrinogen, VWF, factor X
   • Reduced nitric oxide (NO)
   • Reduced adiponectin
   • Acanthosis nigricans
   • Non-alcoholic steatohepatitis (NASH)
   • Various syndromes (see next subsection)

Common associations of IR

c. All these changes result in increased atherogenicity, endothelial dysfunction and exaggerated smooth muscle growth.

Polycystic Ovary Syndrome and IR

The association of IRS with polycystic ovarian syndrome (PCOS) affects 5 to 10% of premenopausal women and is characterized by:
• Polycystic ovaries
• Irregular periods
• Chronic anovulation
• Hyperandrogenism
• Prolactinaemia (30%).

Most of these women are obese and the obesity is mostly central. The degree of IR is similar as seen in type 2 DM. Interestingly, ovulation may be induced by decreasing the IR.

Insulin Resistance and Coronary Artery Disease

Hyperinsulinaemia has deleterious effect on arterial wall. It promotes:
• Proliferation of smooth muscle cells
• Stimulation of growth factors
• Connective tissue production
• Enhancement of LDL receptor activity
• Cholesterol synthesis.

All these factors promote increased formation and decreased regression of lipid plaques. Hyperinsulinism is supported in all its above mentioned actions by insulin-like molecules, namely proinsulin and 32-33 split proinsulin.

Other Associations

a. IR results in elevated plasminogen activor inhibitor 1, elevated fibrinogen, elevated von-Willibrand factor (VWF), and factor X resulting in alteration of normal fibrinolysis whereas endothelial dysfunction results in reduced nitric oxide secretion.
b. Insulin resistance and acanthosis nigricams (AN): AN is regarded as a clinical marker of IR. It presents as velvety, mossy, verrucous hyperpigmented skin lesions over the nape of the neck, axillae and beneath the breast
c. IR may also be a component of various genetic syndrome described in the next subsection.

Management of Insulin Resistance Syndrome

Most effective way to reduce IR is by weight loss and exercise. A lifestyle where there is increased physical activity, less of sedentary life and more of daily graduated exercise is seen to enhance insulin sensitivity.

There is close association of obesity with insulin resistance which has been recognized in all ethnic groups across full range of body weights, all ages and both sexes. Therefore, reduction of body weight by diet control and exercise improves insulin sensitivity. This effect is seen even when weight is reduced 5 to 10% only. Exercise and muscle contractions increase glucose transport by the translocation of intracellular GLUT-4 glucose transporter to the cell surface.

Elevated FFAs and triglycerides aggravate insulin resistance. A diet with restricted fat intake, is therefore, useful in management of IRS. Similarly accumulation of free radicals, glucotoxicity are harmful and increase IR. A diet rich in fresh fruits, vegetable, vitamin C, vitamin A with restricted fats should be encouraged. Some researchers have advocated a Mediterranean-type MUFA diet, (38% calories from fats: 10% saturated fat, 22% MUFA, 6% PUFA) to improve endothelial function. Drugs like metformin, pioglitazone also reduce insulin resistance. Thiazolidinediones (TZDs) directly inhibit aromatase activity in human ovarian granulosa cells. Their mode of action has been detailed in a separate chapter.

SUMMARY

Insulin resistance is a condition where target tissues response to insulin is reduced leading to various metabolic abnormalities. These metabolic anomalies have been grouped under the heading 'Insulin Resistance Syndrome (IRS)'. IRS has been discussed with its pathogenesis, clinical relevance and management.

APPENDIX

MEASUREMENT OF INSULIN RESISTANCE

Hyperinsulinaemic Euglycaemic Clamp Technique

Basal insulin and glucose levels are measured followed by a priming dose of insulin to increase the plasma insulin concentration to a supraphysiological level. The glucose levels are then maintained at basal levels by infusing glucose at varying rates while the insulin infusion is maintained at a predetermined rate. The plasma glucose and insulin levels are measured at fixed intervals (depending on the protocol) by drawing blood via an indwelling cannula. The glucose infusion rate is altered till a steady state is reached where the coefficient of variation is less than 5%. The amounts of glucose infused (μmol/kg/min) once the steady state is reached indicate the whole body glucose disposal (M value). The insulin sensitivity index (SI_{clamp}) is calculated by dividing the M value by the mean steady state insulin concentration (M/I). More the amount of glucose infused, more insulin sensitive is the individual. Conversely, less the amount of glucose infused, the more insulin resistant is the individual.

The advantages of the technique are that the confounding factors such as hypoglycaemic counter-regulation and endogenous insulin secretion are eliminated. Moreover, supraphysiological levels of insulin suppress hepatic glucose production (HGP).

However, the clamp technique also has its limitations. Firstly, it is extremely labour intensive and expensive hence it is clearly unsuitable for large epidemiological studies. Moreover, it does not represent physiological conditions. The multiple sampling (usually every 5 to 10 minutes depending on the protocol) and large amounts of blood drawn makes it unsuitable for clinical practice. It therefore remains a research tool.

Frequently Sampled Intravenous Glucose Tolerance Test (FS_{IVGTT})

Here, an intravenous injection of glucose bolus (0.3 g/kg) is infused over a minute to stimulate insulin secretion. Frequent samples (25 to 30 samples) are collected over the next 3 hours for the measurement of plasma glucose and insulin concentration. The insulin and glucose dynamics are then modelled using a computer programme, which provides an estimate of insulin sensitivity (SI_{IVGTT}). Secretogogues like tolbutamide are administered along with glucose in some cases. This method also correlates well with the euglycaemic clamp technique.

Indices from Oral Glucose Tolerance Test (OGTT)

Most commonly used test to confirm glucose intolerance, the GTT is also used to assess insulin sensitivity and secretion. In the standard OGTT, 75 gm glucose is given orally after 10-hour fast. Blood samples are collected at 30 minutes intervals after the glucose load for a period of 2 hours to determine plasma glucose and insulin levels. A number of modifications have been made in the OGTT procedure to measure insulin sensitivity more effectively. Certain investigators prefer an extended OGTT where samples are taken more frequently for 4 hours. As no intravenous access is required, OGTT remains the most popular technique. The various measures used to estimate insulin sensitivity based OGTT include insulin area under the curve ($AUC_{insulin}$), $AUC_{glucose}/AUC_{insulin}$ ratio and various indices proposed by different investigations depending on the sampling times.

FURTHER READING

1. Barker DJ, Osmond C, Golding J, et al. Growth in utero, blood pressure in childhood and adult life and mortality from cardiovascular disease. BMJ 1989;298:564-7.
2. Bhargava SK, Sachdeo HS, Fall CH, et al. Relation of serial changes in childhood body mass index to impaired glucose tolerance in young adulthood. N Engl J Med 2004;350(9):865-75.
3. Gerich JE. Contributions of insulin-resistance and insulin secretory defects to the pathogenesis of type 2 diabetes mellitus. Mayo Clin Proc 2003;8(4):447-56.
4. Himsworth H. Diabetes Mellitus: its differentiation into insulin sensitive and insulin insensitive types. Lancet 1936;1:127-30.
5. Martin BC, Warram JH, Krolewski AS, et al. Role of glucose and insulin in development of type 2 diabetes mellitus: results of a 25-year follow-up study. Lancet 1992;340:925-9.
6. Perez-Jimenez F, Castro P, Lopez-Meranda J, et al. Circulating levels of endothelial functions are modulated by dietary monounsaturated fat. Atherosclerosis 1999;145(2):351-8.
7. Reaven GM, Banting lecture 1988: role of insulin resistance in human disease. Diabetes 1988;37:1595-607.
8. Sandeep Sreedharan, Viswanathan Mohan. Assessing insulin resistance: an overview. Ind J Endocr Metab 2004;VI:24-31.
9. Yajnik CS, Lubree HG, Rege SS, et al. Adiposity and hyperinsulinaemia in Indians are present at birth. J Clin Endocrinol Metab 2002;87(12):5575-80.

25.3 Clinical Presentation

Y Sachdev

- Type 1 DM (T1DM)
- Type 2 DM (T2DM), Lean or Low Body Weight T2DM
- Other Types of Diabetes Mellitus
  - Malnutrition-modulated Diabetes Mellitus (MMDM)
    - Protein Deficient Diabetes Mellitus (PDDM)
    - Fibrocalculous Pancreatic Diabetes Mellitus (FCPDM)
  - Genetically Defined Monogenic Forms of Diabetes Mellitus
- Maturity Onset Diabetes of Young (MODY)
  - MODY 1,2,3,4,5,6
- Mitochondrial DNA (mt DNA) Defects
- Insulinopathies or Proinsulin/Insulin Conversion Defects
- Genetic Defects in Insulin Action
- Pancreatic Diabetes
- Endocrine Diabetes
- Gestational Diabetes

INTRODUCTION

Clinical presentation of diabetes varies with the type of diabetes and the age of the person. The lifestyle, knowledge and awareness of the patient and the family background play a big role in the clinical presentation and an early

diagnosis. The vague symptoms of general weakness, evening fatigue, headache, change in frequency of urine, increased desire for water, etc. are important pointers to a person who knows about diabetes or has the family history, otherwise these pointers are easily overlooked and diagnosis is delayed. The classical presenting features of polyuria, polyphagia and polydipsia are seen only in type 1 patients and that too not in all of them. Sir William Osler once said, 'If one has a chronic but a manageable disorder, one is most likely to lead a more hygienic and a more thoughtful existence and thus live longer than the apparently more healthy individuals'.

TYPE 1 DIABETES MELLITUS

In this type, the diagnosis is usually straight forward as onset is acute. In small children, the mother may bring the child for persistent bedwetting or enuresis. The diagnosis is obvious if this appears in a child who has already achieved toilet control. In such cases, a single blood sugar test is enough to confirm the diagnosis. In other patients the chief complaints may be osmotic symptoms like polyuria, polydipsia, polyphagia, blurred vision, constant headache, irritability, easy fatigability, muscle weakness and significant loss of body weight inspite of adequate food intake. Abdominal pain, persistent vomiting, dehydration, excessive weakness and prostration, are sinister signs and are indicative of very high degree of hyperglycaemia and ketosis. Such patients are liable to go into deep drowsiness and coma unless treated urgently. In many such patients clinical evidence of skin, chest and urinary tract infection may also be present.

T1DM patients are usually below 20 years, have low BMI and poor muscle mass. There is usually no family history. Some of them, however, may give history of other autoimmune disorders like Graves' disease, thyroiditis, Addison's disease, vitiligo and pernicious anaemia in first degree relatives and are prone to develop these problems themselves.

TYPE 2 DIABETES MELLITUS (T2DM)

This type of diabetes often stays unrecognized for many years as the hyperglycaemia develops gradually and there are no recognisable symptoms in early stages of the disease. The classical symptoms of T1DM are usually absent. Most of the time, the first time diagnosis is made only on a routine health check in an asymptomatic healthy man.

T2DM patients have insulin resistance and usually only relative (not absolute) insulin deficiency. Majority of T2DM are overweight and obese. Those who are overweight do have increased percentage of body fat. T2DM in not ketosis prone and they do not need insulin for survival. Spontaneous ketoacidosis is never seen in T2DM patients. Usually infections, severe mental stress, excessive carbohydrate intake, missing of medication,

myocardial infarction and stroke are responsible for ketoacidosis whenever it occurs. Many a time, the disease is suspected when an injury/wound takes a long time to heal or when there are frequent and repeated infections like boils, carbuncles, respiratory or urinary tract infections. Genital infections like balanitis, vulvovaginitis, premature cataract, and periarthritis of the big joints, especially shoulder joints demand blood sugar (F and PP) test to rule out T2DM. In some patients with insulin secretion dysfunction, there may be hypoglycaemic episodes 2 to 3 hours after meals which recover on their own.

Classically, T2DM is seen in patients above 30 years. Compared to Western countries, it occurs approximately 10 to 15 years earlier in Indian population. Probably genetic make-up has something to do with it. Some patients may even be below 20 years when they are detected to have T2DM.

Obesity is present only in about 50% (compared to Western population where it is about 80%) of our patients, the others are of normal weight or even underweight (10 to 25%).

Sometimes the patient may report with cardiac, ophthalmic, neurological, renal or skin manifestations where they are diagnosed for the first time. A few female patients may be picked up from the gynaecological OPD where they report with complaints of disordered uterine bleeding, amenorrhoea, or sexual problems. Table 25.3.1 gives a comparative statement of some of the clinical characteristics of these two main types of diabetes mellitus.

Lean or Low Body Weight Type 2 Diabetes Mellitus

Besides the above main types, there is another special type of diabetes mellitus—the lean type 2 DM which we see (10 to 25%) in our clinical practice. This is not associated with malnutrition or pancreatic fibrosis.

There is a significant prevalence of family history and majority of the patients come from middle socioeconomic class. There is substantial beta cell reserve and most patients respond satisfactorily to OHAs. Ketosis is usually absent inspite of high blood glucose values. Infections and peripheral neuropathy are the usual presenting features. Lipid disorders are less frequent and so are the macrovascular complications of T2DM.

OTHER TYPES OF DIABETES MELLITUS

Malnutrition-modulated Diabetes Mellitus (MMDM)

Malnutrition-modulated diabetes mellitus (MMDM) is seen only in poor and developing countries of tropics and

TABLE 25.3.1

Clinical signs	Type 1 DM	Type 2 DM
Age of onset	5 to 30 years	Over 30 years
Male: female ratio	1:1	M>F (c̄ f Western countries where F>M)
Prevalence	1 to 5 %	90-95% of all diabetes Urban > rural Low in tribals
Genetics	Heredity + HLA association	Heredity—strongly positive No HLA association
Body build	Normal	Often overweight and obese. Common in lean and thin Indians also
Mode of onset	Rapid	Slow and insidious
Severity	Severe	Usually mild
Ketosis	Prone	Not prone
Islet cell antibodies	Positive within 6 to 12 months	Absent
Insulin lack	Absolute	Relative
Insulin resistance	Rare	Very common and usual. More so in obese.
Insulin requirements	Always	May be required (<25%)
Insulin sensitivity	Sensitive	Less sensitive
Oral hypo-glycaemic agents	No response	Response is usually positive
Complications	• Nephropathy, coronary artery disease, ketoacidosis, hypoglycaemia • Very common (>90%)	Infections, coronary artery disease, nephropathy, neuropathy, stroke, peripheral arterial disease, gangrene Common and slow developing

Characteristics of type 1 and type 2 diabetes mellitus

subtropics. MMDM (Table 25.3.2) is further subdivided into:
a. Protein-deficient diabetes mellitus (PDDM), and
b. Fibrocalculous pancreatic diabetes (FCPD).

Protein-deficient Diabetes Mellitus (PDDM)

Protein-deficient diabetes mellitus (PDDM) is seen in children and young adults (10 to 30 years). The characteristic features are extreme thin body built (BMI <18.5 kg/M^2), severe hyperglycaemia not responding to

oral drugs and requiring high dose of insulin (over 2 units/kg body weight) but they are ketosis-resistant. Socioeconomic background of these patients is poor and there are clinical stigma of protein deficiency malnutrition from the early infancy. The nutritional supply *in utero* is also inadequate. Early life poor nutrition results in insulinopenia and concomitant insulin resistance leading to impaired glucose tolerance and frank diabetes mellitus ultimately.

Fibrocalculous Pancreatic Diabetes (FCPD)

Fibrocalculous pancreatic diabetes (FCPD) is mostly prevalent among adolescent and young adults. It has, however, been seen in some senior citizens as well as in very young children. The pancreatic size may be near normal or it may be totally shrunken to a fraction of its normal size. Its consistency is variable—firm at some places and cystic elsewhere. Pancreatic parenchyma shows varying degree of fibrosis with calculi of variable number and sizes. These calculi are present within irregularly dilated ducts leading to stasis of thick, mucinous, viscid and gritty acinar secretions in the ducts. At some places ductal saccules with large stones may be seen while other ductules and tributaries may have denuded epithelium. Inflammatory cells are also seen at different stages, Interacinar spaces are wide. Islets of Langerhans' are reduced in number.

The acinar, periacinar, interacinar and periductal fibrosis compromise the blood supply to the islets resulting in their functional loss and reduced insulin value. These patients may have additional complaints of steatorrhoea, frequent attacks of vague abnormal pain since childhood, diarrhoea and abnormal exocrine pancreatic function. These are also ketosis resistant. FCPD is secondary to chronic nonalcoholic calcific pancreatitis. Till date, the largest number have been reported from the southern Indian state of Kerala.

Genetic Defects of B-Cell Function Characterized by Mutations

Genetically Defined Monogenic Forms of Diabetes Mellitus

Maturity onset diabetes of young (MODY) comprises a phenotypically and genetically heterogeneous subtype of DM. Commonly it is due to mutations in the transcription factors or the glucokinase enzyme. Onset of this rare type of diabetes mellitus typically occurs between the ages of 10 and 25 years. Six variants of MODY have been recognized so far (Table 25.3.3). All are transmitted as

TABLE 25.3.2

Clinical parameters	Protein deficient diabetes mellitus (PDDM)	Score	Fibrocalculous pancreatic diabetes (FCPD)	Score
Age of onset	Children and young adults (10-30 years)	1	Adolescents and young adults (13 to 30 years)	1
MF ratio	More in male		More in male	
Prevalence	40 to 50% of young onset diabetes in tropical developing countries		More in Casava eating tropical countries	1
BMI	<19	2	<19	1
Genetics	? Non-contributory		? Non-contributory	
Body build	Poor and emaciated		Variable. May be thin and emaciated	
Childhood stigmata of malnutrition	Rural background stigmata +	12	H/O or stigmata of PEM	1
Mode of onset	Gradual and progressive	1	Slow with abdominal problems especially colics	1
			Absent H/o pancreatitis (Alcohol)	2
Hyperglycaemia >200 mg/dl	+	1	+	1
Ketosis proneness	Not prone even on withdrawal of insulin therapy	3	Not prone	1
Islet cell Antibodies	Absent		Absent	
Insulin lack	Usually moderate		Usually moderate	
Insulin resistance	Moderate to high		Moderate	
Insulin requirements	High (2 U/kg/day)	2	Moderate	
Calculi or pancreatic disease on U/S	Absent	2	Pancreatic stones present	4
			Ductal dialation and pancreatic fibrosis	2
Oral hyperglycaemic agents	No response		Usually no response	
Cause of death	Delayed and poor treatment, infections		Delayed and poor treatment	

(Suggestive score 10-11)
Clinical parameters of malnutrition-modulated diabetes mellitus (MMDM)

TABLE 25.3.3

Transcription factors	Extrapancreatic clinical features
HNF 1 α (MODY 3)	• Low renal threshold (Glycosuria)· • Sensitivity to insulin • Raised HDL
HNF 4 α (MODY 1)	• Low fasting triglycerides • Reduced apolipoproteins (apo A II, apo C III)
HNF 1 β (MODY 5)	• Renal cysts • Renal histology-Glomerulocystic kidney disease, renal dysplasia, oligomeganephronia • Renal impairment • Uterine and genital abnormalities • Hyperuricaemia • Short stature
IPF-1 (MODY 4)	• Pancreatic agenesis with homozygotic mutations
Neurod 1 (MODY 6)	?
Glucokinase gene (MODY 2)	?

Extrapancreatic features in MODY

autosomal dominant disorders. There is β-cell dysfunction but unlike T2DM, obesity and/or insulin resistance are rare. Table 25.3.4 gives the diagnostic criteria which help decide if diabetes patient has MODY.

MODY 2 which is the most common variant is caused by mutations in the glucokinase gene located on the short arm of chromosome 7. Over 100 different glucokinase mutations have been described. Physiologically glucokinase catalyzes the formation of glucose-6-phosphate from glucose, a reaction that is important for glucose sensing by the beta cells and for glucose utilization by the liver. In MODY 2, as a result of glucokinase mutations, higher glucose levels are required to elicit insulin secretory responses. This leads to elevation of the set-point for insulin secretion. Clinically, it presents as a mild stable fasting hyperglycaemia which occurs from birth. Postprandial hyperglycaemia is usually not there. It is treated with diet restriction. Complications are rare as the hyperglycaemia is mild.

TABLE 25.3.4

- Diagnosis of diabetes before 25 years in at least one or ideally two family members
- Absence of insulin requirement for at least 5 years of the diagnosis

  Or

- Significant C-peptide levels in a patient on insulin treatment
- Autosomal dominant inheritance in vertical transmission of diabetes through at least two generations. Ideally, it is three generations with a similar phenotype in first or second cousins.
- These patients are rarely obese.
- Insulin values are inappropriately low for the hyperglycaemia present meaning thereby that there is β cell dysfunction but no insulin resistance.

Diagnostic criteria for maturity onset diabetes of the young (MODY)

MODY 1, MODY 3 and MODY 5 are caused by mutations in the hepatocytes nuclear transcription factors, HNF-4α (located in the long arm of chromosome 20), HNF-1α (located on the long arm of chromosome 12) and HNF-1β respectively. The mechanism by which these mutations lead to DM is not known exactly. It is believed that these mutations affect the development of the islets or transcription of genes that are concerned with insulin secretion. MODY 3 (HNF 1α defect) is the most common type caused by transcription factors mutations. Subjects develop diabetes at 10 to 30 years of age. There is marked postprandial hyperglycaemia. It responds to oral hypoglycaemic sulphonylureas and insulin. Biguanides have a little effect.

MODY 4 is a rare variant caused by mutations in the insulin promoter factor (IPF-1). This is a transcription factor that regulates both pancreatic development and insulin gene transcription. Homozygous inactivating mutations lead to pancreatic agenesis while heterozygous mutations result in early onset of DM. The patients with maturity onset diabetes of the young (MODY) usually have a very strong family history running into three generations. Extrapancreatic clinical features (see Table 25.3.3) help in differential diagnosis of MODY.

Mitochondrial DNA Defect

Mutations in mitochondrial DNA (mt DNA) are associated with diabetes or IGT and are a cause of several syndromes. These mutations are inherited maternally and lead to impaired oxidative phosphorylation and β-cell dysfunction. The main clinical features of these syndromes include neurological abnormalities.

a. A point mutation in mt DNA encodes the transfer RNA for the amino acid leucine, leads to maternally transmitted diabetes with sensorineural deafness, and/or MELAS syndrome (myopathy, encephalopathy, lactic acidosis and stroke-like episodes).

b. Wolfram's syndrome or DIDMOAD (diabetes insipidus, diabetes mellitus, optic atrophy and deafness) results from both mt DNA mutations and a nuclear gene defect on chromosome 4. Diabetes mellitus usually appears first in childhood or early adult life and the other features develop later over several years in variable sequence.

Insulinopathies or Proinsulin/Insulin Conversion Defects

Insulinopathies are rare mutations in the human preproinsulin gene that leads to either incompletely cleaved proinsulin with 'C-peptide' still attached or a mutant insulin with diminished bioactivity. Since the individuals are heterozygous, both normal and abnormal insulin are present in the circulation.

Patients with insulinopathies have hyperproinsulinaemia, varying degrees of glucose intolerance (normal or frank diabetes) with a normal response to exogenous insulin. Glucose tolerance of affected subjects deteriorates with age due to superimposition of environmental and other genetic factors.

Genetic Defects in Insulin Action

There are several genetic and acquired syndromes of severe insulin resistance. Patients often present with marked postprandial hyperglycaemia but normal fasting blood glucose concentration. Clinical features often seen in these conditions are acanthosis nigricans and hyperandrogenism. Both of these are probably a result of action of compensatory hyperinsulinaemia on tissues and organs. Acanthosis nigricans comprises areas of hyperpigmented velvety skin, usually in flexures of the axillae, back of the neck and groin. Hyperandrogenism is common in postpubertal girls with these syndromes and is manifested as amenorrhoea or oligomenorrhoea, hirsutism, acne and polycystic ovaries. Examples of these rare genetic syndrome are as follows:

Type A Insulin Resistance

Type A insulin resistance almost always affects adolescent females. In nearly 25% of these patients there is mutation of the tyrosine kinase domain of the β subunit of the insulin receptor.

Leprechaunism (Donohue's Syndrome)

It is a rare congenital condition in which there is severe intrauterine and postnatal growth retardation. Patients have dysmorphic facies, acanthosis nigricans, little subcutaneous fat and severe insulin resistance. Mutations affect both alleles of the insulin receptor's 'α' subunit which results in complete loss of receptor function. Death usually occurs in childhood.

Robson-Mendenhall Syndrome

This syndrome is associated with 'α' subunit insulin-receptor mutations. It is associated with only partial loss of receptor and frank diabetes mellitus.

Lipoatrophic Diabetes

A number of congenital and acquired lipodystrophies are linked with severe insulin resistance. Berardinelli-Seip congenital lipodystrophy (BSCL) is an autosomal recessive inherited condition where there is generalized absence of metabolically active subcutaneous and visceral fat, hepatomegaly and acromegalic features, hypoglycaemia and elevated triglyceride. Due to lack of fat there is leptin deficiency, resulting in voracious appetite. The lipotrophy is apparent despite voracious appetite and adequate nutrition.

Type B Insulin Resistance

It is an acquired condition caused by immunoglobulin G (IgG) autoantibodies to the insulin receptor. It is seen mostly in females. As antibodies can be stimulatory or inhibitory there may be fluctuating hyper-and hypoglycaemia. Other immune disorders like arthritis, nephritis, vitiligo, alopecia areata, and systemic lupus erythematosus may also be seen.

Pancreatic Diabetes

Several pancreatic disorders result in glucose intolerance and diabetes mellitus. They account for only 1% or less of the total number of diabetes in India.

Acute Pancreatitis

Acute pancreatitis usually results in transient hyperglycaemia though permanent diabetes may be seen in 15% of patients. Elevated blood glucose levels may be accompanied by raised amylase and lipase values. Pancreas may show oedema and swelling on MRI/CAT scan.

Chronic Pancreatitis

Chronic pancreatitis leads to impaired glucose (IGT) or diabetes in 40 to 50% cases. Intraductal protein plugs, calcite stones, cysts and fibrosis may be detected on imaging (Fibrocalculous pancreatic diabetes). Sometimes very large pancreatic stones and steatorrhoea may be present.

Haemochromatosis

Genetic or primary haemochromatosis is an autosomal recessive inborn error of metabolism. It is usually caused by a mutation in the haemochromatosis gene, HFE, on chromosome 6. The HFE proteins expressed on duodenal enterocytes modulates iron uptake. Haemochromatosis is associated with increased iron absorption and tissue deposition of iron, notably in the liver, islets of pancreas, skin and pituitary gonadotrophs. The classical triad is hepatic cirrhosis, glucose intolerance and hyperpigmentation. Twenty-five per cent of these patients require insulin for proper control. Serum iron and ferritin levels are raised. It is also known as Bronzed diabetes.

Secondary Haemochromatosis

Secondary haemochromatosis may occur in patients who require frequent blood transfusions, e.g. in β-thalassaemia.

Pancreatic Carcinoma

It may be associated with T2DM and accounts for unexplained weight loss inspite of proper blood sugar control. Diabetes usually improves when the tumour is removed.

Endocrine Disorders Associated with Diabetes Mellitus

Several endocrine conditions are associated with diabetes mellitus. These are:

Cushing's Syndrome

It is due to excess of glucocorticoids due to any cause. Glucocorticoids cause insulin resistance which stimulates hepatic gluconeogenesis, adipose tissue lipolysis and non-esterified fatty acids release and inhibits peripheral glucose uptake. Most patients (75 to 80%) will have some degree of glucose intolerance but insulin requiring diabetes is seen only in 10 to 20% cases.

Acromegaly

Here excess of GH causes glucose intolerance by inducing insulin resistance due to decrease in receptor affinity and a postreceptor defect. Glucose intolerance of varying severity is seen in nearly 30% of acromegalic patients.

Glucose tolerance becomes normal once GH level is reduced.

Phaeochromocytoma

Nearly 75% of these patients have IGT or type 2 like diabetes. It is due to anti-insulin actions of catecholamines, namely inhibiting insulin secretion, stimulating glucagon secretion, liver and muscle glycogenolysis, and adipose tissue lipolysis. Elevated catecholamines also cause postreceptor resistance to insulin stimulated glucose uptake.

Glucagonomas

These are rare tumours of islet α cells. These tumours grow slowly but are usually malignant. They are common in postmenopausal women. The most striking clinical features are weight loss and a characteristic rash termed 'neurolytic migratory erythema'. The rash is commonly seen in groin, perineum and buttocks. There is also a tendency to thrombosis (pulmonary embolism is a common cause of death) and neuropsychiatric disturbances. Diabetes is due to gluconeogenesis and glycogenolysis induced by raised glucagon values. It is usually mild to moderate.

Other Endocrine Causes

Glucose intolerance is also seen in thyroid disorders, hyperaldosteronism, Verner-Morrison syndrome and carcinoid syndrome.

Gestational Diabetes Mellitus

Gestational diabetes mellitus (GDM) is defined as diabetes or abnormal GTT occurring for the first time during pregnancy. It excludes patients with pre-existing diabetes and those who had GDM in earlier pregnancies. Seshiah and associates have indicated GDM prevalence as 16.6% in our country. Table 25.3.5 enumerates some of the main risk factors for developing GDM.

Carbohydrate Metabolism in Pregnancy

A pregnant female needs increased calories and nutrients to meet the requirement of pregnancy. An increment of approximately 280 to 300 calories per day over and above the basic requirements is considered sufficient to meet the extrademand of the foetus.

During the initial few weeks of pregnancy, there is an increased secretion of both oestrogen and progesterone. This results in β-cell hyperplasia and enhanced insulin secretion. The maternal blood sugar values (both F and PP) fall by about 10 to 15%. In our laboratories, plasma glucose values during the first trimester have been observed as fasting 70.2 ± 9.8 and PP 110.3 ± 18.7 mg/dl.

TABLE 25.3.5

Obesity and over-weight
Previous history of diabetes with oral contraception/pregnancy
Previous history of heavy babies, unexplained stillbirth, low birth weight, neonatal death during previous pregnancies.
Glycosuria on two or more occasions during the current pregnancy
High risk ethnic group

Risk factors for gestational diabetes mellitus

During the latter half of pregnancy, maternal carbohydrate metabolism is stressed by the ever increasing levels of hCG and various other hormones secreted by the placenta.

Inspite of all these developments, the maternal blood glucose level is maintained within a narrow normal range throughout pregnancy. This is achieved by the already discussed hormonal adjustments. Abnormalities of glucose tolerance develop when there is reduced insulin secretion or there is increased insulin resistance (Insulin resistance is known to be present in pregnancy).

Diagnostic Criteria for GDM

There are known differences in diagnostic criteria of GDM in various countries. The guidelines issued by WHO and American Diabetic Association (ADA) are also at variance. WHO regards both IGT and diabetes occurring in pregnancy (GIGT, GDM) as one entity and advocates intervention. WHO recommends 75 G oral glucose tolerance test as the gold standard for confirming the diagnosis. The WHO recommended diagnostic criteria are F PG>126 mg/dl; 2 HPPG >140 mg/dl (same criteria as applied outside pregnancy). The ADA, on the other hand, recommends 100 G oral glucose tolerance test extended to 3 hours. The ADA diagnostic criteria are:

Fasting	95 mg/dl (<5.3 mmol/L)
One hour	180 mg/dl (10 mmol/L)
Two hours	155 mg/dl (8.6 mmol/L)
Three hours	140 mg/dl (7.8 mmol/L).

The diagnosis is confirmed if any two of the four plasma glucose values are equal or above the mentioned figures. ADA further recommends that all pregnant women between 24th and 28th weeks pregnancy should be subjected to a 'screening test' where 50 G of glucose is given without any regard to the time of the day or the last meal. Venous blood is tested for glucose after one hour. If the value is 140 mg/dl or above, it indicates GDM and a confirmatory 100 G glucose GTT for 3 hours may be carried out. The extended GTT is better conducted after 3 days of preparation with 300 G carbohydrates per day.

Screening of GDM (with 50 G glucose) may not be necessary if the pregnant female is young (less than 25 years), has normal body weight, normal blood pressure, with no family history of diabetes and does not belong to high risk ethnic community (Indians are high risk ethnic group).

Table 25.3.6 gives White's classification of diabetes in pregnancy.

Diagnostic Criteria at Our Clinic

On the very first visit of a pregnant female we conduct a thorough clinical examination to determine maternal and foetal health status. If the visit is with a prior appointment, she is instructed to report on an empty stomach. Her blood for biochemistry (LFT, lipids, BUN, creatinine, sugar), and urine (morning sample) are taken and she is given 75 G glucose. Two hour PP plasma glucose is again checked. If 2 H value is 140 mg/dl or above, GDM is confirmed. If it is less than 140 mg/dl but equal to or above 120 mg/dl, we level it as IGT.

In case the first visit is not planned, then casual plasma glucose in estimated. If it is above 140 mg/dl, diagnosis of GDM is confirmed.

In our clinic we take both IGT and DM (GIGT, GDM) as one entity and advise the patient appropriately to ensure normal maternal and foetal health, normal foetal development, normal pregnancy and delivery.

We advise GTT be carried out three times in the whole period of pregnancy so as not to miss GDM:

First	On very first visit (usually first trimester)
Second	24 to 28 weeks
Third	32 to 34 weeks

Management of GDM

Strict diet and glycaemic control are essential part of treatment. 30 to 35 calories per kilogram of present body weight is recommended with 50 to 55% carbohydrate, 20 to 25% protein and rest in the form of fat. The total calorie intake is split into 5 to 6 portions to reduce the load on β cells. GDM (like T2DM) patients are deficient in the first phase of insulin secretion. The deficiency is compensated when the quantum of food challenge at any one time is reduced.

Indian women gain 8 to 12 kg body weight by term and their weekly weight gain is about 200 to 300 G. The prescribed diet, therefore, must ensure proper growth and development of the foetus and placenta to avoid small for dates or heavy neonates.

Medication: It is necessary if diet control fails to achieve euglycaemic status. Human insulin (actrapid/premix) or

TABLE 25.3.6

Diabetes classes	Descriptions
A	Euglycaemia maintained by diet alone, diabetes may be of any duration and onset may have occurred at any age
B	Onset 20 yr/> and duration <10 yr
C	Onset 10 to 19 years and duration 10 to 19 yr
D	Onset < 10 yr and duration >10 yr (background retinopathy or hypertension)
F	Nephropathy with proteinuria > 500 mg/day
R	Proliferative retinopathy or vitreous haemorrhage
RF	Criteria for classes R and F coexist
H	Arteriosclerotic heart disease clinically evident
T	Prior to renal transplantation

White's classification of diabetes in pregnancy

its analogues are the ideal way to control hyperglycaemia in pregnancy. In clinical practice, however, we have seen that many diabetic women are on oral hypoglycaemic drug therapy when they miss their menstrual period and realize they are pregnant. In rural India and even in semi urban towns it may take anything from 8 to 12 weeks before pregnancy is confirmed. In such cases the female continues taking OHAs. We have not come across, in such cases any foetal or placental anomaly that could be attributed directly to consumption of OHAs. This aspect, however, needs looking into more closely and seriously to decide whether these drugs are safe and have any role during pregnancy. As for now, we advise immediate stopping of oral hypoglycaemic drugs and institution of insulin therapy for glycaemic control in GDM.

We aim to keep FPG around 85 mg/dl; 1 hour PP below 140 mg/dl and 2 hour PP less than 120 mg/dl. Such a tight control may require multiple insulin injection (Table 25.3.7). During labour blood glucose level should be kept below 100 mg/dl (80 to 100 mg/dl). Hypoglycaemic episode are an expected event with a tight glycaemic control. To guard against these episode, frequent diet intake as written above is very helpful and effective. In a few pregnant women with previously diabetes mellitus where we have used insulin pump therapy, we found better glycaemic control and higher level of patients satisfaction.

Physical exertion: Normal activity consistent with the stage of pregnancy plus graduated daily exercise like walking is advised. This helps glycaemic control.

Maternal parameters: Regular body weight and blood pressure charting, maternal Hb, HbA1C, biochemistry and

TABLE 25.3.7

S. No.	Insulin type	Before					
		Break fast	Midday snacks	Lunch	Evening tea	Dinner	Bed-time
1.	Plain insulin (short acting)	Short	—	Short	—	Short	—
2.	Plain insulin short	Short	Short	Short	Short	Short	—
3.	Mixed insulin (short + intermediate)	Mixed	—	—	—	Mixed	—
4.	Short acting + mixed insulin	Mixed	—	Short	—	Mixed	—
5.	Short + Long or (intermediate)	Short	—	Short	—	Short	Long or intermediate
6.	Short + Mixed	Shorrt	—	Short	—	Mixed	—
7.	Continuous insulin infusion pump						

Various insulin combinations to control hyperglycaemia in pregnancy

plasma glucose (self monitoring), periodic ophthalmic, cardiac and renal status assessment.

Foetal parameters: Foetal growth and development by clinical examination and ultrasonography. Detection of congenital anomalies, amniocentesis for karyotype, chromosomal abnormalities, alpha-foeto-proteins and hCG.

Determination of KAP of patient and her family: Education of the patient and her close family members regarding basic facts of GDM, role played by diet and activity in controlling hyperglycaemia, timely administration of medication, self monitoring of blood glucose, care of the newborn and regular visits to one's doctor for complete assessment are some of the important points on which detailed interactive discussion and knowledge dissemination sessions must be organized. The frequency of self monitoring of blood glucose (SMBG) will depend upon the degree of glycaemic control, number of daily insulin injection and hypoglycaemic events.

Ideal management approach: Management is best done by a team comprising a diabetologist, obstetrician, neonatologist, lady health visitor and educator, and a specialist neonatology nurse who has sufficient knowledge and experience of newborns of diabetic mothers. Some women become too apprehensive to interact with so many individuals. In such cases obstetrician may be asked to look after and seek advice when and if necessary.

Hazards of poor maternal glycaemic control: These are:
- Poor or excessive weight gain by the mother
- Abnormal foetal growth and development resulting in small for dates or heavy neonates
- Increased perinatal mortality/morbidity
- Increased number of abortions/miscarriages
- Increased placental and foetal anomalies
- Respiratory distress syndrome of the newborn.

Follow-up evaluation: GDM women must have an OGTT (75 G glucose) 6 to 8 weeks after delivery to define their glycaemic status (normal, impaired fasting glucose (IFG), impaired glucose tolerance (IGT), diabetes mellitus (DM). The newborn must be followed in the well baby centre of the neonatology paediatric department.

SUMMARY

Achieving and monitoring euglycaemia throughout pregnancy reduces the risk of adverse outcome for both the mother and the offspring. Combination of diet, exercise, intensive insulin therapy and multiple self monitored blood glucose determinations are extremely helpful approach. There are a number of oral agents available for treatment of diabetes mellitus, their safety in pregnancy is not fully tested and are not advised to be used.

FURTHER READING

1. American Diabetes Association: Clinical practice guidelines, gestational diabetes mellitus. Diabetes Care 2003;26(suppl):S 103-5.
2. Banerjee S, Ghosh US, Banerjee D. Effect of tight glycaemic control on foetal complications in diabetic pregnancies. JAPI 2004; 52:109-13.
3. Gabbe SG, Holing E, Temple P, Brown ZA. Benefits, risks, costs and patient satisfaction associated with insulin pump therapy for the pregnancy complicated by type 1 diabetes mellitus. Am Jr Obstetrics and Gynecology 2000;182(6):1283-91.
4. Kajos SI, Buchanan TA. Current concepts: gestational diabetes mellitus. New England Journal of Medicine 1999;341(23):1749-50.
5. Samanta A, Burden MI, Burden AC, Jones GR. Glucose intolerance during pregnancy in Asian women. Diabetes Research Clin Pract 1989;7:127-35.
6. Seshiah V, Balaji V, Madhuri S Dalaji. Sanjievi CB, Green A. Gestational diabetes mellitus in India. JAPI 2004;52:707-11.
7. Veciana M, Major CA, Morgan MA, Asrat T, Toohey JS, Lien JM, et al. Postprandial versus preprandial blood glucose, monitoring in women with gestational diabetes mellitus, requiring insulin therapy. New England Journal of Medicine 1995;333(19):1237-41.
8. White P. Pregnancy and diabetes. Medical aspects. Med Clin North Am 1965;49:1015-24.

SECTION

26

DIAGNOSIS AND MANAGEMENT OF DIABETES MELLITUS

26.1 Diagnosis of Diabetes Mellitus

Y Sachdev

- Diagnostic Criteria
  - Fasting and Casual (Random) Blood Glucose
  - Oral Glucose Tolerance Test (OGTT)
- Clinical Assessment
- Laboratory Investigations

- Haemogram, Glycosylated Hb
- Biochemistry, Imaging
- Ewing's Tests
- Insulin and Other Antibodies
- Other Endocrine Tests
- Cardiac Assessment Tests

DIAGNOSTIC CRITERIA

The diagnostic criteria for diabetes mellitus proposed by the World Health Organization (WHO) in 1979 were used till 1997. Thereafter, these criteria were changed by the American Diabetic Association (ADA) and were ratified by the WHO in 1999. The new diagnostic criteria are based on the epidemiological data of natural history of glucose intolerance particularly relationship of blood glucose concentrations with diabetes-specific micro-vascular complications. These criteria are summarized in Figure 26.1.1.

If a patient is symptomatic, the diagnosis is obvious and a single test is usually confirmatory. This is particularly applicable to T1DM where a vast majority of patients present with classical symptoms (Fig. 26.1.2) and in T2DM who report with chronic diabetic compli-

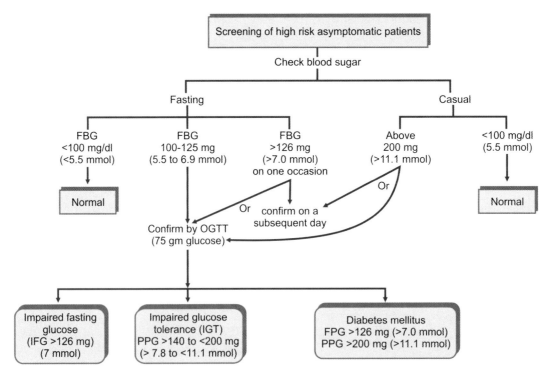

Fig. 26.1.1: American Diabetic Association, WHO and
Indian College of Physicians screening criteria of high-risk asymptomatic patients

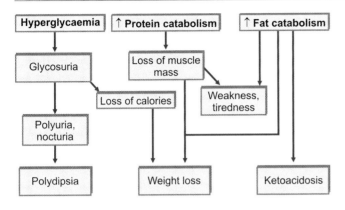

Fig. 26.1.2: Classical symptoms of T1DM

cations like retinopathy, nephropathy, neuropathy, frequent recurrent infections, etc. OGTT is not required if in a **symptomatic** patient blood glucose values are as shown in Table 26.1.1.

TABLE 26.1.1

	Whole blood		Plasma	
	Venous	*Capillary*	*Venous*	*Capillary*
Fasting	Over 110	Over 110	Over 126	Over 126
Casual	Over 180	Over 200	Over 200	Over 220

Fasting and casual blood glucose concentration (mg/dl) in diabetes mellitus

If only casual blood is tested and is abnormal/borderline, it is advisable to confirm it by testing fasting blood sugar as well.

In an asymptomatic patient, if fasting plasma glucose value is 126 mg/dl or above on more than one occasion, the diagnosis is confirmed. In other asymptomatic patients, who come for diabetes mellitus screening test and whose plasma fasting blood glucose level is below 126 mg/dl and between 90 and 125 mg/dl, OGTT must be done to reach a definite diagnosis.

It is to be remembered that
- Fasting is defined as no caloric intake for a minimum period of 10 hours
- Casual (or random as was called earlier) is defined as any time of 24 hours without any regard to the last meal. However, for correct appreciation of blood sugar, it is better if one knows the timing of the last meal
- Plasma glucose is 10 to 15 per cent higher than the whole blood glucose. Arterial glucose level is higher than capillary glucose which is higher than venous glucose level. The difference is variable and depends upon the circulatory region and on its rate of glucose utilization

- In fasting state, venous and capillary glucose is same but it differs in the postprandial state
- Enzymatic methods such as glucose oxidase, glucose dehydrogenase or hexokinase method are preferred to nonenzymatic methods for glucose estimation.

Oral Glucose Tolerance Test (OGTT)

As per WHO specifications, it is to be conducted as under:

The test must be done after at least 3 days (better 5 days) of unrestricted dietary intake containing over 300 gm carbohydrate daily and normal physical activity.

- The test must be preceded by an overnight fast of 10 to 16 hours during which only plain drinking water is permitted
- The test should be done in the morning in the resting patient
- Smoking is prohibited on the morning of the test as well as during the test
- After collecting the blood and urine samples for glucose levels, 75 gm of glucose (or 1.75 gm/kg in children if body weight is over 18 kg) dissolved in 250 ml of water is given to the individual who drinks it over about 5 minutes.
- Time is recorded when the drink is started/finished.

After the glucose load, four more samples of blood and urine should be collected every 30 minutes for two hours (Fig. 26.1.3). ADA and WHO, however, advocate only two samples to be collected, as their criteria stress only on fasting and 2 hours post-glucose load values for the diagnosis. The test is interpreted as shown in Table 26.1.2 and Figure 26.1.4. The author feels that if these criteria are applied in our Indian population, we are liable to miss many of the diabetics as the normal

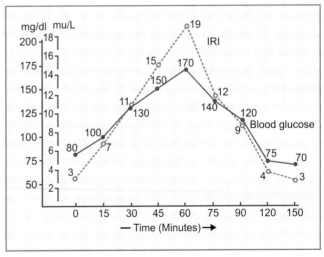

Fig. 26.1.3: Blood glucose and IRI values during OGTT in a normal healthy male of 25 years

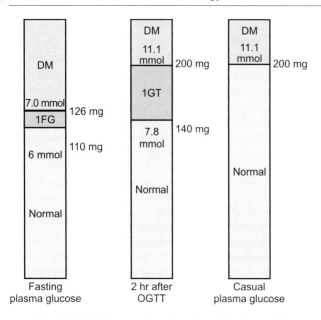

Fig. 26.1.4: Diagnostic values for diabetes mellitus

difference between our fasting and postprandial plasma glucose values is around 30 to 35 mg/dl (and not 80 to 90 mg/dl). Therefore, it might be better for us to remember this while interpreting the OGTT results. In our centre we regard following plasma glucose (venous) values as diabetic.

F	½ hr	1 hr	1½ hr	2 hr
> 100	>180	>200	>200	>140 mg/dl

Similarly, in Indian community, where most (82%) of our young adults between 18 and 25 years have fasting plasma glucose values between 60 and 85 mg/dl, it is better to be suspicious if the fasting glucose values (done twice after a gap of 2 to 3 days in between) are persistently above 95 mg/dl. In our experience, we find some of these individuals (18 to 19%) turn out to be impaired glucose tolerance or frank diabetes mellitus. Similarly, we find that adult values do not always apply to many of the elderlies above the age of 60 years. In such circumstances, availability of a nomogram depicting critical 2-hour PP blood glucose values in the different ages in the community is very helpful. We recommend all individuals whose values are above 90 percentile of the nomogram should be kept under observation and evaluated periodically. One such nomogram is given in Figure 26.1.5.

A reconstituted International Expert Committee (2003) reviewed the diabetes diagnostic criteria and suggested following alterations to be made in these criteria:

TABLE 26.1.2

Oral glucose tolerance test (OGTT)	Glucose value (mg/dl)		
	Whole blood		Plasma
	Venous	Capillary	Venous
Normal			
Fasting	<100	<100	<110
2 hr postprandial (PP)	<120	<140	<140
Diabetes mellitus			
F	>110	>110	>126
PP	>180	>200	>200
Impaired glucose tolerance			
(IGT)			
F	<110	<110	<126
PP	120-180	140-200	140-200
Impaired fasting glucose (IFG)			
F	101-110	101-110	111-125
PP	<120	<140	<140

ADA and WHO diagnostic values oral glucose tolerance test

Impaired fasting plasma glucose (IFG) should be > 100 mg/dl (100 to 125 mg/dl) and not 110 mg/dl (110 to 125 mg/dl) (Table 26.1.3).

The impaired glucose tolerance (IGT) and impaired fasting glycaemia (IFG) group of individuals are important, since they have higher risk of becoming frank diabetics and are prone to develop macrovascular complications.

TABLE 26.1.3

Clinical category	Fasting plasma glucose	2-hour post glucose
Normal	<100 mg/dl (<5.6 mmol/L)	<140 mg/dl (< 7.8 mmol/L)
IFG	100-125 mg/dl (5.6-6.9 mmol/L)	—
IGT	—	140-199 mg/dl (7.8 to 11.0 mmol/L)
Diabetes	>126 mg/dl (>7.0 mmol/L)	>200 mg/dl (>11.1 mmol/L)

Revised criteria (Expert Committee on the Diagnosis and Classification of Diabetes, 2003)

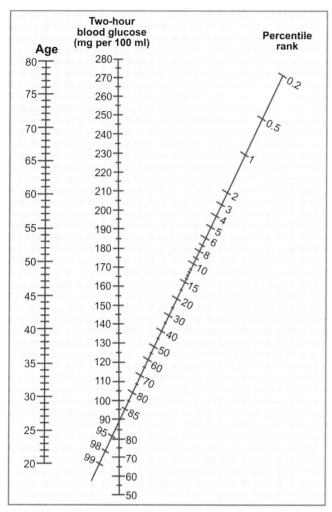

Fig. 26.1.5: A nomogram with two hours crtitical postprandial plasma glucose values (*Courtesy:* Andres R, Mayo Clinic Proc 1967;42:674)

CLINICAL ASSESSMENT FOR DIABETES MELLITUS

A thorough clinical assessment embraces a detailed record of:

1. *Personal history:* It covers age, sex, occupation, physical activity, exercise, diet intake, alcohol consumption, smoking, tobacco chewing, medication if any and symptoms (with duration) of diabetes mellitus. Enquiry should be made about unusual weight loss, generalized debility, muscle weakness and muscle mass wastage, periarthritis, delayed healing of injuries and wounds, visual problems, balanitis, vulvovaginitis and repeated recurrent infections especially UTI, skin and chest infection.

2. *Previous history:* It should include history of ketosis, hyperosmolar coma, hypoglycaemia, pancreatitis, cardiac problems and cerebrovascular complications.
3. *Family history:* It includes health and glycaemic status of all first degree relatives.
4. *Occupation:* It covers details of the job done by the individual. Cultural, psychosocial, educational, economic and activity status and exercise details must be noted down to get an impression about energy expenditure.
5. *Gestational history:* It includes details about pregnancies, toxaemias, stillbirths, premature deliveries, low and heavy birth weight babies, hydramnios and other complications of pregnancy.
6. *Treatment details:* These include previous and present treatment details and the documented effects on the symptomatology and disease process.
7. *Clinical examination:* It should include anthropometric measurements (body weight, height, waist-hip ratio, skin-fold thickness, BMI). A detailed general physical examination includes skin changes, hair texture, hair loss, prominent veins, callus formation, cracks, ulcers, fissure and foot deformity. Presence or otherwise of acanthosis deserves recording as it is an indicator of insulin resistance. Bilateral parotid enlargement, brown spots on the shins also are markers of diabetes.

Examination of peripheral pulsations (dorsalis pedis, posterior tibial, popliteal) heart rate, brachial-BP both supine and standing (after 1 minute) and ankle blood pressure recording with calculation of ankle-brachial index if needed, tendon reflexes, superficial and deep sensations, vibration sensation and sense of position, muscle mass and muscle power are other important clinical findings that require to be recorded.

Eye examination including eye movements, pupillary reflexes, corneal sensations, ulceration, lenticular opacities and retina/fundus examination must have a mention. Besides these, cranial nerves and special sensations like hearing, taste, etc. must be examined. One should also carry out detailed evaluation of autonomic neuropathy and look for evidence of other autoimmune disorders like thyroid dysfunction, vitiligo, Addison's disease, pernicious anaemia, etc. Details about sexual functions also have to be inquired. Bruit over carotid, aorta, iliac and femoral arteries and complete cardiac assessment should also be included.

As a matter of fact it is better to have a printed format for all these symptoms/signs so as not to miss any findings.

INVESTIGATIONS

Investigations include various laboratory, radiological and biochemical parameters which get affected by persistent hyperglycaemia. These are:

- *Haemogram* including ESR and peripheral blood smear examination
- *Glycosylated Hb:* It provides a retrospective index of glycaemic control over the preceding 8 to 12 weeks. It is a crucial investigation and should be performed 3 monthly. The test is affected by hyperlipidaemia, urea, aspirin, penicillin, anaemia, haemoglobinopathy and environmental temperature.
- *Fructosamine test:* Fructosamine estimation provides a retrospective index of glycaemic control over the preceding 4 weeks. It is most valuable if a rapid change in blood glucose results are expected as following a change in treatment strategy or if monitoring at short intervals (as in pregnancy) is required. It is a sensitive test requiring strict calibration. Its assay is affected by triglyceride, uric acid, bilirubin, heparin, EDTA and ascorbic acid.
  - Normal value is 1.7 to 2.8 mmol/L
  - Diabetic value is 2.6 to 5.0 mmol/L
- Fasting plasma glucose
- Liver function tests
- Lipid profile (complete)
- BUN, creatinine, uric acid
- Urine RE (morning sample) and ketonuria, if blood sugar value is over 250 mg/dl
- 24 hr urine for microalbuminuria
- X-ray chest PA view to rule out infection
- Sputum for AFB
- ECG, echocardiography
- Doppler studies for arterial pulsation in feet in selected cases
- Cardiac stress test
- Ultrasonography for pancreatic and KUB status
- Ewing's tests
- C-peptide stimulation tests
- Islet cell and other antibodies
- Various endocrine hormone estimation, wherever needed.

SUMMARY

The diagnostic criteria of diabetes mellitus as proposed ADA, WHO and later by the International Expert Group on diabetes are mentioned in this chapter along with the guidelines of Indian College of Physicians. The author has mentioned blood glucose values being followed at his diabetic centre and has recommended the importance of nomogram of the community, listing F and critical 2 hr postglucose values. He suggests keeping those above 90 centile under periodic observation. He stresses that in Indian youth (especially rural and semiurban) the mean blood glucose values are much lower than those seen in American and European populations and postprandial values are usually only 30 to 35 mg/dl higher than the fasting values.

FURTHER READING

1. The Decode Study Group on behalf of the European Diabetes Epidemiology Study Group. Will new diagnostic criteria for diabetes mellitus change phenotype of patients with diabetes? Reanalysis of European epidemiological data. BMJ 1998;317: 371-5.
2. The Expert Committee on the diagnosis and classification of diabetes mellitus. Report of the Expert Committee on the diagnosis and classification of diabetes mellitus. Diabetes Care 1997;20:1183-97.
3. World Health Organization: Definition, diagnosis and classification of diabetes mellitus and its complication: Report of WHO Consultation Part 1: Diagnosis and Classification of Diabetes Mellitus. Geneva, WHO 1999.
4. The Decode Study Group on behalf of the European Diabetes Epidemiology Group. Is the current definition for diabetes relevant to mortality risk from all causes and cardiovascular and nonvascular diseases. Diabetes Care 2003;26:688-96.
5. The Decode Study group, European Diabetes Epidemiology Group: Diabetes Epidemiology. Collaborative Analysis of Diagnostic Criteria in Europe. Glucose tolerance and mortality. Comaparison of WHO and American. Diabetes Association Diagnostic Criteria. Lancet 1999;354:617-21.
6. The Expert Committee on the Diagnosis and Classification of Diabetes Mellitus. Report of the Expert Committee on the Diagnosis and Classification of Diabetes Mellitus. Diabetes Care 2003;26(supp 1):3160-7.

26.2 Management of Diabetes Mellitus

Y Sachdev

- Holistic Approach
- Quantum of the Problem
- Strategy of Management
- Screening of High Risk Population
- Lifestyle Changes
- Patients' Education
- Nutrition and Diet

- Artificial Sweeteners
- Exercise
- Oral Hypoglycaemic Drugs
- Antiobesity Drugs (in Type 2 DM)
- Herbal Medicines and Dietary Supplements
- Management of Hypertension in T2DM

HOLISTIC APPROACH

The management of diabetes mellitus is not just control of blood sugar level. It is much more than that and comprises the management of several metabolic parameters including dyslipidaemia, maintenance of normotension, euglycaemic status with particular reference to postprandial blood sugar, avoidance of acute complications and prevention, control and regression of chronic complications.

To achieve this, a tight control of blood glucose is essential and a good doctor-patient professional understanding is necessary to fight it better. An earnest endeavour is required to bring the blood glucose to near normal values and maintain it there. This is achieved by diet control, physical exercise, other nonpharmacological measures like weight reduction, relaxation exercises, yoga, meditation, positive thinking and healthy lifestyle. It is possible to achieve glycaemic and other objectives of good diabetic control (Table 26.2.1) by these means in some (25 to 30%) diabetics particularly those who are obese while in others (45 to 50%) oral medication and/or insulin (20 to 30%) has to be added to attain the objective. Patient's education and family support are two highly significant factors that help reach the goal.

QUANTUM OF THE PROBLEM

Type 2 DM is becoming a progressively increasing menace. Its annual growth is estimated to be around 12 to 14 per cent. The increase is primarily due to ageing of the population, sedentary lifestyle and ever-increasing body weight and obesity. It is also getting aggravated by the high and middle class urban society's latest fad of consuming more and more simple sugars and high caloric-density food items.

TABLE 26.2.1

1. Patient's education and awareness about the disease process, proper diet intake, regular graduated exercise and healthy living style.
2. Maintenance of body weight. Aim is to keep body weight between 85 and 90% of ideal weight.
3. Achievement of euglycaemic status with normal fasting, pre-meal and postprandial blood sugar values.
4. Achievement of normal lipid profile.
5. Achievement of symptom-free active healthy life.
6. Maintenance of normal blood pressure.
7. Prevention of acute metabolic complications.
8. Avoidance/regression of chronic complications.
9. Establishment of medicosocial worker's activities regarding self monitoring, self care, etc.
10. Normalization of biochemistry especially blood glucose values as:
    - F <100 mg/dl; premeal < 130 mg/dl (preferably < 120 mg/dl)
    - Postmeal <160 mg/dl (preferable 140 mg/dl)
    - Glycoscylated Hb < 6.5%
    - Total cholesterol <180 mg
    - LDL < 100 mg; HDL > 40 mg; triglyceride <120 mg
    - BUN, creatinine, normal and urinary proteins <30 mg/24 hr

Objectives of good diabetic control

As the diabetes-related morbidity, mortality and associated expenses are indeed staggering, the management strategy recommended is as under.

STRATEGY OF MANAGEMENT

a. The best way to control the ever-increasing prevalence of type 2 DM and its complications is to ensure its:

i. Prevention (by education, knowledge dissemination and healthy lifestyle changes), and

ii. Early detection by screening the asymptomatic individuals belonging to high risk groups (Table 26.2.2).

TABLE 26.2.2

- History of DM in first degree relatives
- Overweight (BMI>25 kg/m^2)
- Habitual laziness and no exercise habits
- High risk ethnic background (like Asians including Indians)
- Previously diagnosed IFG/IGT
- High blood pressure (>140/90)
- Dyslipidaemia especially elevated triglycerides
- History of gestational diabetes/heavy babies/stillbirths/ prematurity
- Low birth weight children
- Artificial milk fed children
- Polycystic ovarian syndrome

High risk group for diabetes mellitus

b. The screening of other than high risk population is debatable as it involves heavy health care expenses which many developing countries can ill afford. All the same we do believe and recommend that all individuals above 40 years should undergo a screening test which, if normal, could be repeated every year.

c. A single fasting blood sugar estimation appears to be the most cost-effective screening test. If this is 95 mg/dl or above, on two occasions in Indian community, we recommend an oral glucose tolerance test (OGTT) and its interpretation by Indian standards.

d. If a nomogram of the community is available, fasting and PP blood sugar values (after 75 G glucose load) should suffice for screening purposes. Those above 90th centile are to be kept under observation and test to be repeated every 6 to 12 months.

e. Please ensure before an individual is labelled as diabetic that one of the three diagnostic criteria (namely fasting, casual and PP glucose values) is met on at least two separate occasions.

LIFESTYLE INTERVENTIONS

Lifestyle is a pattern of living which has four main components: physical, psychological, social and spiritual. These four components together make an individual a unique, unified biological entity—an absolutely individualized person who is different from others. Environments, nutrition, climate, social interaction, education, job requirements and economic status greatly influence our lifestyle. The ever-increasing industrialization and socioeconomic advancement have immensely affected our lifestyle making us lazy, sedentary, obese, materialistic and consumer of unhealthy high caloric fried fast food. This has resulted in phenomenal increase in 'lifestyle diseases' like obesity, diabetes mellitus, hypertension, coronary artery disease, peptic ulcers, non-specific colitis, endogenous depression, etc.

Lifestyle modification are, therefore, being advocated to affect a long-term positive influence on the ever-increasing prevalence of these diseases. As far as diabetes mellitus is concerned, lifestyle interventions include recommendations about patients' daily rituals, physical activity, graduated exercise, diet intake, alcohol and tobacco consumption, smoking, body weight control and recognition of risk factors.

Self control of anxiety, negative thinking, body and mental tensions by relaxations, meditation and yoga exercises make an important component of lifestyle interventions.

It has been documented that a lifestyle intervention, where sedentary life pattern is changed to an active routine, reducing overweight and lipid abnormality and patient adopts a healthy outlook, onset of diabetes is delayed and progression of IGT to frank diabetes markedly slowed down.

In view of linkage of artificial milk feeding and development of DM in later life, breast-feeding must be encouraged for all infants. This advice is based on the premise that there is 'molecular mimicry' between milk protein and β cell antigen.

PATIENT'S EDUCATION

Diabetes being a life long disease, it is essential that patient is aware and adheres to day-to-day treatment and adopts it as a routine. It is very difficult, if not impossible, for the health care provider to supervise the patient from close vicinity and render the guidance on daily basis. Therefore, it is imperative that the patient should be educated about his/her diet, exercise, self care, recognition of alarm signals, home management of minor crisis and seek medical advice at an early opportunity. It has been seen that 'foolish' diabetics die first. As such we recommend that diabetic self management education should include (Table 26.2.3):

- Basic pathophysiology of diabetic process
- Role of nutrition and diet management
- Distribution of dietary intake over 24 hours, importance of daily graduated exercise

TABLE 26.2.3

- Basic defect in human system resulting in diabetes mellitus
- Role of nutrition and diet in diabetes management
- Type of diet to be taken
- Dietary items to be avoided/deleted
- Distribution of dietary intake over 24 hours
- Importance of daily graduated exercise
- Ideal exercise to meet individual needs
- Timing of medication and its relation with food intake
- Self-monitoring of urine and blood glucose. The availability of reflectance meters (glucometers) has made it extremely easy
- Type of insulin (if being given), sites and correct technique of injections
- Recognition of acute complications
- Importance of regular medical consultation and clinic visits

Salient points of self management education to diabetic patients

- Ideal exercise to meet individual needs
- Timings of medication
- Self monitoring of urine and blood
- Minor adjustments of diet/medication/exercise as per self monitored blood result
- Sites and technique of injecting oneself
- Recognition of acute complications like hypoglycaemia, ketoacidosis, etc.
- Importance of periodic reviews by a doctor.

It is better if a small booklet containing essential information is given to the patient along with a note book to enter his/her complaints/observations/self monitoring results and other relevant information for perusal by the doctor and other health care personnel.

NUTRITION AND DIETARY INTAKE

WHO recommendations (1990) on diet in diabetes are:

Carbohydrates	50 to 60 per cent
Fats	30 per cent
Proteins	12 to 20 per cent of total energy requirements.

The American Diabetes Association (ADA) 1988 dietary recommendations are:

Proteins	0.8 gm/kg
Carbohydrates	55 to 60 per cent (with minimum 130 gm/day) and
Fats	20 to 30 per cent

The author believes that a comprehensive individualized plan for nutrition and diet intake is essential. The plan should be finalized after considering patient's home circumstances, preferences, cultural background, activity, body weight, blood pressure, blood glucose levels, haemoglobin and glycosylated Hb. Detailed discussion with the patient and close relatives staying with him/her will help understand patient's preferences and weaknesses. It is always better to involve a skilled dietician who has good understanding of human nutrition and diabetes.

If dietician is not available, a diabetologist can develop the dietary advice by asking the patient as to what all he/she eats and drinks throughout 24 hours. If this information noted correctly by the patient/close relative over a period of 2 to 3 days is made available to the diabetologist, it is highly useful. It is better if information is cross checked with the house keeper. True details of dietary intake give sufficient information to the doctor to calculate daily caloric intake. With this information and body weight and biochemistry picture available, the doctor can easily work out a healthy nutrition plan. The plan should be simple and easy to understand.

Plato has once said that 'elaborate food produces disease, simplicity in physical education produces health of the body'. Basic principle of giving 20 calories or less/kg/day in overweight and 35 to 40 calories per kg/day to underweight diabetics considering their active/sedentary lifestyle should not be lost sight of. In children up to 1 year, daily calorie requirements are 1000 calories and thereafter up to 12 years add 100 (for girls) and 120 (for boys) calories per year.

As a general rule, in a diabetic patient, considering his lifestyle and body weight we advise 1400 to 2000 caloric diet which is constituted by the following:

• Protein	10 to 15 % of total calories
• Fat	15 to 30% of total calories
• Saturated fatty acid	6 to 7% of total calories
• Polyunsaturated fatty acid	6 to 7% of total calories
• Monounsaturated fatty acid	6 to 7% of total calories
• Linoleic acid (LA/n6)	3 to 7% of total calories
• α-linolenic acid (αLNA/n3)	0.5 to <1% of total calories
• LA : αLNA ratio	5 to 7 : 1% of total calories
• Carbohydrate (Complex carbohydrates preferred)	60 to 65% of total calories
• Dietary fibre	40 gm/day

The above mentioned recommendations are based on the knowledge that besides n3 fatty acid, alpha linolenic acid, eicosapantanoic acid (EPA), and docosahexanoic acid (DHA) are also required for normal insulin action.

The 24 hours dietary intake is split into 6 to 7 portions as under:

Diatery intakes	Calories	
Morning tea at 0600 hr	70	
Morning breakfast at 0900 hr	360	500
Midday snacks	70	
Lunch	450	
Evening tea	50	500
Evening supper/dinner	400	
Night cap	50	450

The obese and overweight must be encouraged to reduce weight. An energy deficit of 500 calories/day will help most of the patients reduce approximately 1 kg in two weeks time.

Carbohydrate

Carbohydrates are that component of the diet which have the greatest influence on blood glucose level. These should be derived from whole grains, fruits, vegetables and low fat milk. It is the total quantity of carbohydrate and not that much the type and source which is important for the glycaemic effect of carbohydrate. The dose of medication especially short acting insulin must be adjusted according to the quantity of carbohydrate taken in a meal. It is important that daily intake especially of carbohydrate is consistently similar otherwise glycaemic control will not be ideal.

The preferred use of low glycaemic index (GI) foods (Table 26.2.4) will definitely reduce PP blood glucose values, though their long-term benefits are doubtful. One must use the principle of GI carefully as ice-cream has a very low glycaemic index but it is not a healthy food if taken in an unrestricted amount and is not recommended for diabetes. The glycaemic index is a measure of the change in blood glucose value following ingestion of carbohydrate-containing foods. GI is a ranking of carbohydrate exchanges according to their effect on postprandial glycaemia. Carbohydrates which produce gradual and smaller blood glucose peaks are preferred in diabetic diets.

Sucrose and sucrose-containing diets do not increase glycaemia to a greater extent than isocaloric amount of starch; even then their intake must be in the context of a healthy diet and should not be over 5 per cent of total carbohydrate intake.

We prefer to advise no free sugar though fruits are allowed. We, at our diabetic centre, do not recommend low carbohydrate diet as carbohydrates are affordable and are rich source of energy, water soluble vitamins and fibre.

Protein

0.8 to 0.9 gm/kg of protein intake should suffice for a normal weight diabetic. Intake requires to be increased in pregnancy, lactation and growing children. In such situations it could be as much as 1.2 to 1.5 gm/kg body weight. Pulses, lentils, cottage cheese, curd, soya, fish, chicken and egg white are important source of protein. Out of animal sources we advise to take fish and chicken. Beef, mutton, ham, bacon and organ meat should be avoided.

In case there is evidence of renal involvement, the protein intake should be curtailed to 0.8 gm/kg/day (30 to 50 gm per day) depending upon BUN and creatinine values. In protein-deficiency-mediated diabetes, protein intake should be generous and be related to plasma protein and serum albumin values.

Fats

15 to 30 per cent of total calories should come from fat intake. Thus in a 1800 calorie diabetic diet, 360 to 450 calorie should be from the fats (40 to 50 gm). While calculating fats, invisible fats in the diet should also be considered. It is a good policy to equally distribute the fat intake between saturated (6 to 7%), polyunsaturated (6 to 7%) and monounsaturated (6 to 7%) with omega 6 and omega 3 ratio between 5:1 to 7:1. The daily dietary cholesterol intake should be less than 300 mg.

Olive oil, canola, peanut or soya and mustard oil are the ones which should be preferred. No single oil is an ideal source of all the three types of fat, therefore a combination of at least two oils may be recommended.

Fibre

Dietary fibres are helpful in controlling sudden elevation in blood glucose levels. They also reduce VLDL and LDL cholesterol. An intake of 40 gm/day of natural sources fibre is ideal. Indian foods are rich in dietary fibres and we rarely require addition of fibre supplementation. The foods especially rich in dietary fibres are fresh green leafy vegetables, fruits, whole pulses, whole green cereals, salads, etc.

The dietary fibre derived from legumes and pulses is viscous and more effective than non-viscous fibre derived from wheat and rice. Guar gum (a product from cluster beans) is highly viscous and effective in reducing blood sugar to a much greater extent than other fibres.

TABLE 26.2.4

Low GI foods	GI (<40)	Moderate GI foods	GI (<70)	High GI foods	GI (>70)
				Bread white	70-79
				Bread brown	70-79
				Polished rice	70-79
—		—		Unpolished rice	60-67
				Wheat floor	70-79
				Millet	70-79
—		—		Upma	70-79
				Cornflakes	80-90
				Noodles	70-79
—		—		Paratha	70-79
Pulses/Dals/Legumes					
Bengal gram dal (Chana dal)	30-39	Green gram dal (Mung)	40-49		
Rajmah	20-29	Black gram dal (Urad)	40-49	Potato	80-90
Soya bean	10-19	Baked beals	40-49		
Lentil (Masur)	20-29	Sprouted green gram	60-69		
Vegetables					
Brinjal, tomato	10-19	Beet	60-69		
Green vegetables	10-19	Yam	50-59		
Fruits					
Apple	30-39	Orange	40-49		
		Banana	60-69		
		Orange juice	40-49		
Milk products					
Milk	30-39				
Curd	30-39				
Ice cream	30-39				
Miscellaneous					
Ground nut	10-19	Arrow root biscuits	50-59	Idli	70-79
		Potato chips	50-59	Honey	80-90
		Pongal	50-59	Chocolate bar	70-79
		Pesarattu	60-69	Colas	70-79
				Fructose	20
				Glucose	100
				Maltose beer	100
				Sucrose	59

Glycaemic index (GI) of common Indian foods

TABLE 26.2.5

- Drink plain water/sugar free liquids whenever thirsty
- Eat meals at regular time. Avoid fried and sugary food
- Eat plenty of vegetables, whole fresh fruits and sprouts. Avoid root vegetables, mangoes, banana, custard apple, dates, if your glyecaemic control is inadequate
- Consume high fibre and low glycaemic index foods. Include whole grains, legumes, brown rice in your main meals
- Avoid or limit intake of white bread, polished rice, mashed potatoes and other high glycaemic index food items
- Avoid or limit consumption of animal products with high content of cholesterol and saturated fat-red sausage, bacon, salami, pork, meat, egg yellow, organ meat (liver, kidney, brain) and high fat dairy products
- Eat lean meat, fish, poultry (without skin) and low fat dairy products
- For snacks, use nuts, salads, fruits. Avoid biscuits, cakes, confectionary which are rich in saturated and trans-fats and salt.
- Use refined vegetable oils for cooking and baking (Mustard, olive, corn oils)
- Better grill or stir fry than deep fry
- Use nonstick pans
- Limit cooking medium to 20 to 30 gm a day
- Use liberal amount of kitchen paper to absorb surface fat
- Roast in foil rather than in fat
- Take alcohol only if glycaemic control is satisfactory
- Limit alcohol to 1 to 1.5 units per day only
- Do not overeat
- Split 24-hour intake into 5 to 7 small frequent portions
- Keep a close watch on your body weight and biochemical parameters

General recommendation for diabetic patient diet

Fruits

Fresh fruits especially citrus, apples, papaya, guavas, 300 to 400 gm daily should form daily fixture of food intake. Table 26.2.5 enumerates general dietary recommendations for a diabetic patient.

Condiments and Spices

Condiments and spices are used as per taste. They are also a source for antioxidants, trace elements and omega 3 fatty acids. Green chillies are rich in vitamin C; black pepper reduces cholesterol while cumin seeds are rich in calcium and iron.

Sodium Chloride

Sodium chloride 6 gm/day is enough. It may have to be reduced to 4 gm or even less in presence of hypertension, renal failure and cardiac problems.

Tobacco

Tobacco consumption should be stopped completely as it enhances CAD risk in inhalers. Nicotine increases adrenaline level, heart rate and blood pressure. It reduces O_2 carrying capacity of blood and increases platelets density and size.

Alcohol

Alcohol in small quantities (1 to 1½ units/day) is protective for CAD as it increases HDL cholesterol, decreases coagulation factors and enhances insulin sensitivity. Excessive use, however, is harmful as it provides easily available calories without any nutritional value.

The snacks accompanying the drinks should be roasted food items rather than fried and greasy preparations. Alcohol and some of the hypoglycaemic agents (like chlorpropamide) produce flushing and palpitations and must be avoided.

Alcohol is liable to potentiate the hypoglycaemic effect of insulin/OHAs and should not be consumed by those who are liable to have hypoglycaemic episodes, have neuropathy, high triglycerides, hypertension, obesity, pancreatic/hepatic dysfunction and are pregnant.

Table 26.2.6 gives the caloric values of some of the common alcoholic drinks. Wines are considered better than spirits.

Special Indian Food Items

Sprouted lentils, beans, gram are rich in fibre and vitamin C and E. Bitters like juice of bitter gourd, neem leaves, fenugreek seeds, etc. are astringents and interfere with food absorption. Use of such items may reduce blood sugar by 10 to 15 per cent.

Tables 26.2.7 and 26.2.8 give the composition of some of the common Indian foods and cooking oils.

TABLE 26.2.6

Alcoholic beverages	Quantity (ml)	Calories
Beer	250	122
Brandy/rum	30	98
Whisky	30	91
Gin	30	85
Vodka	30	85
Champagne and bubbling wines		
Dry	135	105
Sweat	135	160
Other wines		
Red	100	82
White	100	75

Calorie values of alcoholic beverages

TABLE 26.2.7

Food items	Qty (gm)	Calorie	Protein (gm)	Fats (gm)				CHO
				Total	Saturated	Mono-unsaturated	Poly-unsaturated	
Milk								
3.3%	1 cup (244 gm)	150	8	8	5.1	2.1	0.2	11
1.0%	1 cup (244 gm)	100	8	3	1.6	0.7	0.1	12
Yogurt								
Low fat	227 gm	145	12	4	2.3	0.8	0.1	16
High fat	(8 ounces)	140	12	7	4.8	1.7	0.1	11
Butter milk	1 cup (245 gm)	100	8	2	1.3	0.5	Trace	12
1 egg								
whole	50 gm	80	6	6	4.8	1.7	0.1	11
white	33 gm	15	3	Trace	0	0	0	Trace
5TbSF butter	14 gm	100	Trace	12	7.2	2.9	0.3	Trace
1 TbSF Margarine	14 gm	100	Trace	12	2.1	5.3	3.1	Trace
Bread slice white	25 gm	70	2	1	0.2	0.3	0.3	13
Whole wheat flour	1 cup (100 gm)	400	16	2	0.4	0.2	1.0	85
Walnuts	1 cup (125 gm)	785	26	74	6.3	13.3	45.7	19
Cashew nuts Roasted	1 cup (140 gm)	785	24	64	12.9	36.8	10.2	41
Coconut-grated	1 cup (80 gm)	275	3	28	24.8	1.6	0.5	8
Dal cooked	1 cup (200 gm)	210	16	Trace	—	—	—	
Peanuts	1 cup (144 gm)	840	37	72	13.7	33.0	20.7	27
Honey	1 TbSF (21 gm)	65	Trace	0	0	0	0	17
1 Potato large	135 gm	105	3	—	—	—	—	23
Potato finger Chips (1 cup)	10-12 gm	12	0.1	<0.8	0.2	0.14	0.4	1.0
Papaya (1 cup)	140 gm	65	10	0	0.1	0	0	17
Peaches (1 peach)	87 gm	35	1.0	0	0	0	0	10
Peers (1 peer)	166 gm	100	1.0	0	0	0	0	25
Oranges (1 orange)	131	60	1.0	0	0	0	0	
Plaintains (1 cup)	179	220	2.0	0	0	0	0	57
Water melon (1 piece)	482	155	3	2	0.3	0.6	0.5	35
Rice (white, cooked 1 cup)	205	225	4	0	0	0	0	50
Jam and preserves (1 TbSF)	20	55	0	0	0	0	0	14
Raisins (1 cup)	145	435	5	1	0.2	0.4	0.4	115
Sugar (white granulated 1 cup)	200	770	0	0	0	0	0	199
Sugar (powedered sifted 1 cup)	100	385	0	0	0	0	0	100

Calories and composition of common Indian foods

TABLE 26.2.8

Oil/fat (100 gm)	Saturated fatty acid	Unsaturated fatty acid	
		Mono	Poly
Corn oil	12.7	24.6	57.4
Soya oil	15.0	22.8	50.8
Ground nut oil	17.4	45.6	31.0
Cotton seed oil	26.0	18.1	50.3
Til oil	13.0	49.3	37.7
Mustard oil	6.5	55.5	33.3
Coconut oil	86.3	5.6	1.8
Vanaspati	25.3	72.8	1.9
Ghee	64.2	33.2	Nil
Margarine (hard)	88.14	10.5	1.29
Palm oil	53.0	37.9	9.0
Butter	51.4	20.7	2.14
Margarine (soft)	15.0	37.85	22.14

Per cent composition of common cooking oils used in Indian households

Very Low Calories Diet or Microdiets

Very low calories diet or microdiets (with < 500 calories and < 300 calories respectively) are never recommended at our centre as we find they do not work ultimately.

Artificial Sweeteners

Glucose and sucrose are the common sweeteners that we use routinely. Their use adds to calories as well as rapid increase in blood sugar levels. Fructose which is present in honey and fruits may induce hyper-triglyceridaemia while sorbitol may cause sorbitol diarrhoea. Both contribute 4 calories per gram. Artificial sweeteners like saccharine, aspartame, acesulfame potassium and sucralose are non-nutritive and are acceptable. Their use makes it difficult if you want to re-educate your taste. Their use should be limited to maximum of 3 tablets/day. This should be stopped during pregnancy and lactation. Popular brands of aspartame (Sugar free, Aspa sweet, Equal) are easily available across the counter.

Commercial Enteral Nutrition Formulations

Most of these formulations (glucerna, etc.) have a high fat content (50%) out of which 10 per cent are saturated, 33 per cent are monounsaturated and 7 per cent are unsaturated fatty acids, 35 per cent carbohydrates and 15 per cent proteins. This composition is based on the observation of some research workers (Garg A et al; Bradley JE and associates) that partial replacement of dietary carbohydrate by monounsaturated fatty acids improves glycaemic control and triglycerides levels without increasing LDL cholesterol.

EXERCISE

Physical activity and graduated daily exercise are important factors in the management of diabetes mellitus. Physical activity is defined as body movements produced by the contraction of skeletal muscles, while exercise is a subset of physical activity which is planned, structured and performed by repetitive body movements. Exercise increases insulin sensitivity, helps lower sugar and body weight by burning energy, reduces tension and blood pressure, protects cardiovascular system and creates a sense of well-being and positive thinking. It also improves lipid profile, increases collaterals, improves cardiac dynamics, normalizes fuel-oxygen ratio and reduces calcium ion loss.

Exercise must be done on a relatively empty stomach and it must be graduated to be effective. It must be done every day more or less at the same time. Aerobic (isotonic) exercises like brisk walk, swim, cycle, badminton, basket ball are more effective than isometric exercises like weight lifting, sustained grip, etc. Aerobic exercise involves rhythmic, repeated, and continuous movements of the same group of large muscle. It is extremely useful when performed at sufficient intensity and frequency in a graduated manner.

It is imperative to render individualized advice regarding exercise. The factors to be considered are glycaemic status, body weight, daily routine and diet intake. A person who is not used to any exercise must have his cardiovascular check before indulging in any physical exertion. Initially 20 minutes daily walk which, after 5 to 7 days, is increased to 30 minutes and then to 40 and 60 minutes is sufficient. Thereafter the person picks up the speed so as to cover 3.5 to 4 km in 60 minutes.

In type 1 DM it is always better to reach glycaemic control before embarking on any exercise. If the glycaemic control is extremely satisfactory and exercise is expected to be strenuous, it is better to have a small pre-exercise carbohydrate snack. In such cases, a pre-exercise blood sugar test may be useful. Strenuous exercise, Valsalva manoeuvre and weight lifting are bad for those with proliferative retinopathy. Exercise may be discarded when metabolic control is poor and unsatisfactory.

A suggested exercise schedule recommended in our centre is given in Table 26.2.9. A few illustrations showing stretching and strengthening exercises for elderly diabetics are given in Figure 26.2.1 to 26.2.3.

TABLE 26.2.9

- Recommend exercise after determining cardiac status of your patients
- Recommend a individualized tailor-made exercise schedule for your patients
- Recommend a graduated daily exercise schedule which must be done at least 5 days a week
- Exercise must have a warming up and cooling down period of 5 to 7 minutes each
- Exercise must be aerobic type and initially must begin from 20 minutes daily
- It should be increased gradually to 60 minutes daily within 30 to 35 days
- Exercise must be done on an empty stomach or 3 to 4 hours after last meal
- For young patients and children, running, jogging, games, dancing, cycling may be recommended while for older diabetics, brisk walk golf or swimming are ideal
- Exercise recommend must be after due consideration to heart status, BP reading and blood glucose values (before and after exercise)
- Drugs taken by the patient and their effect on exercise must be known to the doctor and patient
- If necessary, pre-exercise snack (75 to 100 calories) may be prescribed for the patient
- Those with gross retinopathy, IHD, nephropathy, peripheral vascular disease, peripheral neuropathy and autonomic neuropathy should avoid strenuous exercise
- Exercise must be enjoyable
- Exercise must be at a convenient place and with convenient attire
- If blood pressure or blood sugar is high it must be controlled before exercise is recommended
- Proper record of blood pressure, blood glucose, HR, etc. before and after exercise, must be kept in elderly patients and those with compromised heart status

Recommended exercise schedule for diabetic patients

Besides graduated physical exercises, we also recommend yoga and relaxation exercises where a diabetic tries to relax his mind and body muscles. Yoga and relaxation (Tables 26.2.10 and 26.2.11) exercises also reduce mental stress, blood pressure, dyslipidaemia and insulin resistance.

TABLE 26.2.10

A. **Essentials**
- Select a quiet, comfortable place for meditation
- Select one good thought for meditation
- Close your eyes and breath normally in a rhythmic manner without any break or breath stopping
- Continue rhythmic breathing for about 2 to 3 minutes
- Try to concentrate your mind on one thought. If stray thoughts, bother you, try to remove them away from your mind and bring back the selected thought. This is a difficult task and will take a few days. Continue the process for about 10 to 15 minutes
- At the end of 15 minutes, again start rhythmic breathing lasting for another 2 to 3 minutes
- Thereafter open your eyes and leave the seat
- Meditation must be done effectively every day for a minimum period of 6 months before one can appreciate any change in oneself

B. **Benefits**
- Better awareness of surroundings
- More calmness of mind, and inner peace
- Less mental tension
- A better feeling of well-being and fellow-feeling
- Pain threshold, stress resistance are raised
- Helps in positive thinking
- Brings down BP, blood sugar, lipids and insulin resistance

Essentials and benefits of meditation

TABLE 26.2.11

- Identify stress and what situations cause it
- Know your personality, heart status and blood pressure
- Choose your response to stress purposely to avoid its bad effects
- Avoid getting worked-up
- Avoid getting overtired
- Ensure you do not have hypoglycaemia
- Ensure quality sleep
- Know your capabilities and limits
- Learn to say 'No' to extra-responsibilities
- Practise positive self-talk
- Avoid negative stress
- Join de-stress programmes
- Practise self relaxation
- Stop criticising people
- Do your best and trust in God
- Follow a regular daily routine
- Do daily exercise

Practical steps to combat stress

Potential Risks of Exercise

It may aggravate cardiovascular problems, result in extremely high blood pressure or undue fall in blood pressure and glucose level and cause vitreous haemorrhage. It may also result in traumatic injuries to the feet especially in those with PVD or peripheral neuropathy.

Therefore, a detailed assessment of the health status of the individual patient is mandatory before exercise schedule specific to him is prescribed.

Stretching Exercises (Figs 26.2.1A to H)

- *These exercises are extremely useful in those diabetics who are frail and have osteoarthritis and muscle weakness*
- *These exercises must be done in graduated fashion without tiring the muscles*
- Initially do each stretch 3 times a week. 10 minutes each sessions.
- Hold each stretch for 10 seconds
- Progressively increase to 5 times a week with 20 minutes each sessions. Increase holding time to 20 sec.

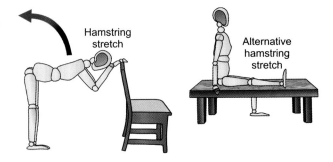

Fig. 26.2.1A: Hamstring stretch exercise

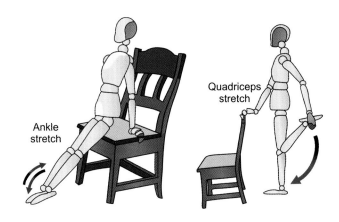

Fig. 26.2.1B: Quadriceps and ankle stretch

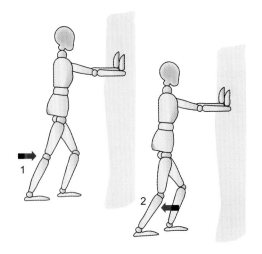

Fig. 26.2.1C: Calf muscle stretch exercise

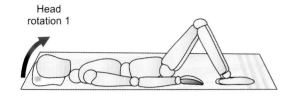

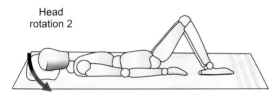

Fig. 26.2.1D: Head rotation

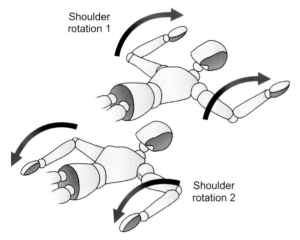

Fig. 26.2.1E: Shoulder rotation

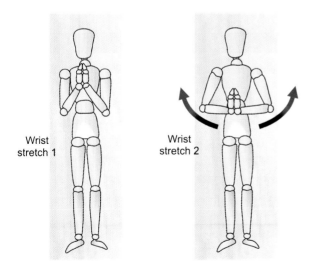

Fig. 26.2.1F: Wrist stretch

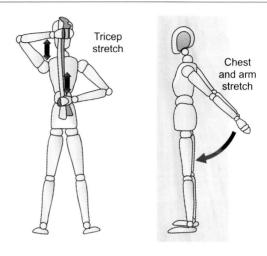

Fig. 26.2.1G: Triceps and chest and arm stretch

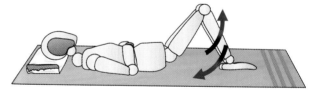

Double hip rotation

Fig. 26.2.1H: Double hip rotation

Muscle Strength Training Exercises (Figs 26.2.2A to E)

- Initially repeat each exercise 5 times, one session a day. After 7 to 8 days, increase to 10 times and thereafter gradually to 20 times one session a day
- Strength training exercises help muscle tone and should precede walking exercises.

Note: Stretch and hold for 10 seconds initially, progressively increase to 30 second.

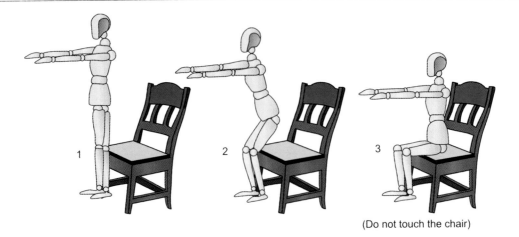

(Do not touch the chair)

Fig. 26.2.2A: Squarts

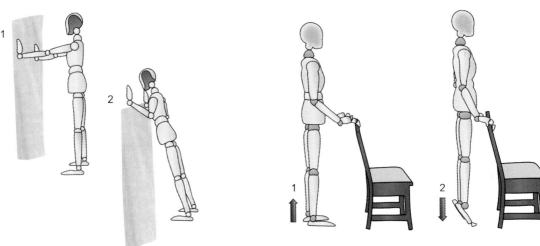

Fig. 26.2.2B: Wall push

Fig. 26.2.2C: Toe standing

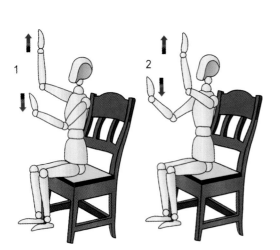

Fig. 26.2D: Finger marching (for small hand muscles)

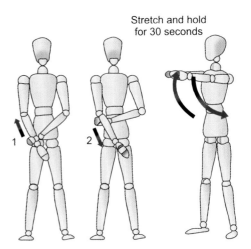

Stretch and hold
for 30 seconds

Fig. 26.2.2E: Wrist, elbow and shoulder muscles
stretching exercises

Advanced Muscle Strength Traning Exercises (Figs 26.2.3A to G)

- Repeat each exercise initially 10 times one session a day
- Gradually increase to 20 times one session a day

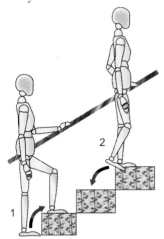

Fig. 26.2.3A: Steps upstairs

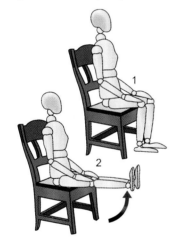

Fig. 26.2.3B: Knee extension

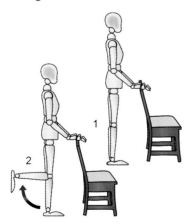

Fig. 26.2.3C: Knee flexions

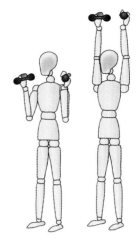

Fig. 26.2.3D: Overhead extension

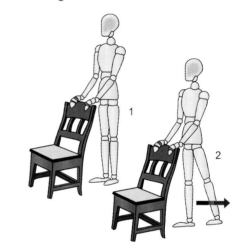

Fig. 26.2.3E: Side hip movement

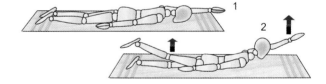

Fig. 26.2.3F: Floor pelvic and back exercise

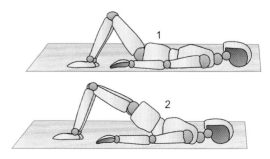

Fig. 26.2.3G: Pevic bridge

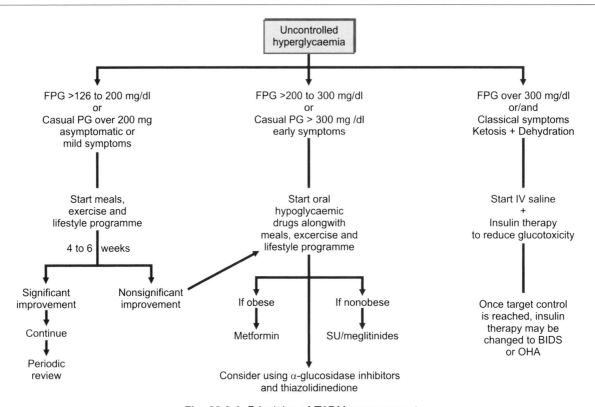

Fig. 26.2.4: Principles of T2DM management.
Note: (a) If monotherapy fails, use one of the combination. If that also fails, try BIDS or insulin therapy
(b) Persist with meal, exercise and lifestyle programme

ORAL HYPOGLYCAEMIC DRUGS

When the blood glucose value is not controlled with diet and exercise, addition of oral hypoglycaemic agents helps control hyperglycaemia in type 2 DM (Fig. 26.2.4).

Sulphonylureas (SU) are secretagogue and stimulate, in a biphasic action, the insulin secretion (but not its synthesis) from the pancreas. The insulinotrophic effect of SU is augmented by glucose and they increase β-cell sensitivity to glucose and other stimuli. Biguanides on the other hand have no pancreatic action. They suppress hepatic gluconeogenesis and glucose production especially in fasting state while in postprandial insulin-stimulated-state they enhance glucose uptake by the muscle. Alpha glucosidase inhibitors interfere with the breakdown of starches, destrins, maltose and sucrose into absorbable monosaccharides, and thus delay the digestion and absorption of carbohydrates in the proximal gut.

Meglitinides stimulate insulin secretion from β-cells by closing ATP-sensitive K^+ channels on cell membrane and are extremely useful in controlling postprandial hyperglycaemia.

Insulin sensitizers (thiazolidinedione, TZD) promote glucose uptake in skeletal muscles, adipose tissue and liver through the specific nuclear receptor, the peroxisome proliferators activator receptor-gamma (PPAR-γ). They exert some effect on intracellular glucose transporters (Fig. 26.2.5). TZD are associated with fluid

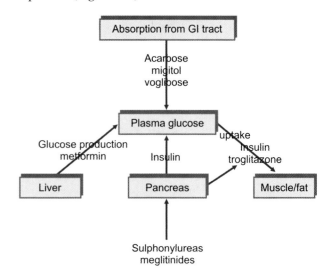

Fig. 26.2.5: Major sites of action

and sodium retention, dependent oedema and congestive cardiac failure as their side effects. Therefore, utmost caution is required when these drugs are used in a patient with clinical oedema or symptomatic heart problem.

Phenobarbitone, an established hepatic microsomal enzyme inducer, has also been recommended (50 to 100 mg per day HS) as an insulin sensitizer to be given along with sulphonylureas in T2DM. Table 26.2.12 presents the expected improvement with various oral antidiabetic therapies.

Incretins

Glucagon like peptide-1 (GLP-1), one of the incretins released from the gut in response to food intake enhances glucose-dependent insulin secretion and has a gluco-regulatory role. It also increases gastric emptying time. Moreover, there is evidence to suggest that GLP-1 not only causes improvement in glucose regulation but it also preserves beta cells and perhaps generates new cells. GLP-1, however, is rapidly degraded in plasma by dipeptidyl peptidase-IV (DPP-IV). This limits its role in improving glycaemic status in T2 DM patient.

Recently "GLP-1 agonist, exenatide, a synthetic exendin-4 compound, has been developed for control of hyperglycaemia in T2 DM. It is degradation resistant and is given 5 to 10 mg × twice a day s/c with meals. From the results available so far, it appears exenatide acts in the presence of hyperglycaemia and helps release insulin from the pancreas. Once normal glucose level is reached, insulin release is stopped. Thus, it is expected to be useful in postprandial hyperglycaemia as a monotherapy and in combination with other oral agents.

DPP IV Inhibitors

Inhibitors of DPP IV lead to the increase in circulating level of GLP-1 allowing it to play its role in increasing insulin secretion with resultant reduction in blood glucose levels. These inhibitors also reduce insulin resistance. In its clinical trials, the drug has proved itself and expected to be available for commercial use in very near future.

The details of oral hypoglycaemic agents are given in the next section.

Role of Antiobesity Drugs in Management of Type 2 Diabetes Mellitus

Antiobesity drugs have so far played only a minor role in the management of obese diabetic patients. These drugs are:
a. *Sibutramine:* It is a centrally acting serotonin and norepinephrine reuptake inhibitor that acts as an

TABLE 26.2.12

		HbA_{1C}	FBG (mg/dl)
Monotherapy	Sulfonylurea	1.5 to 2%	50 to 60
	Metformin	1 to 2%	50 to 60
	Pioglitazone	0.6 to 1.9%	55 to 60
	Rosiglitazone	0.7 to 1.8%	55 to 60
	Troglitazone	0.6 to 1.0%	20 to 40
	Repaglinide	0.8 to 1.7%	30 to 40
	Acarbose	0.5 to 1.0%	20 to 30
Combination therapy	Sulfonylurea + Metformin	1.7%	65
	Sulfonylurea + Pioglitazone	1.2%	50
	Sulfonylurea + Troglitazone	0.9% to 1.8%	40
	Sulfonylurea + Acarbose	1.3%	60 to 40
	Repaglinide + Metformin	1.4%	40
	Pioglitazone + Metformin	0.7%	40
	Rosiglitazone + Metformin	0.8%	50
Insulin therapy	Oral agents + Insulin	Open to target	Open to target

Approximate improvements expected with mono/combination therapy

appetite suppressant. It is not to be used in hypertensive patients and is notorious for drug interactions. It requires careful monitoring when it is used. Its long-term efficiency and safety are debated.

b. *Orlistat:* It acts locally in the gastrointestinal tract where it blocks enzymatic digestion of triglycerides by inhibiting pancreatic lipase. The absorption of up to 30 per cent of ingested fat is thus prevented. Orlistat does induce significant weight loss if consumed over 10 to 12 months but weight is regained subsequently unless due care is taken by the patient to maintain body weight. Gastrointestinal disturbances like flatulance, steatorrhoea and faecal incontinence (especially in elderly) may be seen.

Some patients do not respond to orlistat or lose weight less than 5 per cent in 3 to 4 months time. In such instances it may be advisable to stop the drug and monitor diet control more rigidly. Orlistat is considered by many a useful adjunctive treatment for producing weight loss, improving glycaemic control, lipid and blood pressure levels when used in patients treated with metformin.

Herbal Medicines and Dietary Supplements

The interest in complementary and alternative medicine is increasing all over the world and many diabetics are taking herbal medicines, dietary supplements to control their hyperglycaemia. Guar gum and fenugreek seeds extract taken before the meals slows the absorption of carbohydrates and reduces PP blood glucose values. Fenugreek probably has some insulin sensitizing and insulin secretion effects also. Besides these two herbal products, others which are mentioned to have beneficial effect on insulin sensitivity and blood glucose values are: vanadium, aloe vera, L-carnitine, gymnema sylvestre ('gurnar' of India), American ginseng, momordica charantia (a vegetable indigenous to tropics including India), coccinia indica (ivy gourd) and opuntia streptacantha (Nopal or the prickly pear cactus). Ayurveda, Tibetan, traditional Chinese and native American medicines use these herbs singly or in combination and claim reduction in fasting and postprandial blood glucose levels.

α-lipoic acid, zinc and chromium are the other supplements mentioned in connection with diabetes therapeutics. Enough evidence, however, is not yet available to define definitely their beneficial role and mode of action in management of diabetes mellitus. It is certain, though, that their use does no harm to the users.

MANAGEMENT OF HYPERTENSION IN T2DM

Forty per cent of our T2DM patients have hypertension. ACE-inhibitors (lisinopril, ramipril, captopril, etc.) and angiotensin receptor antagonists (losartan, irbesartan, etc.) are the first choice when lifestyle changes, diet control, salt restriction and other non-pharmacological measures do not bring down the blood pressure. In our clinic we endeavour to bring BP to less than 130/80 mm/ Hg (R3). Other antihypertensive drugs used are calcium channel blockers, vasodilators, diuretic and beta blockers.

Beta blockers inhibit both pancreatic insulin secretion (via B_2 receptors) and peripheral glucose utilization. Weight gain, diminished peripheral blood flow and an unopposed stimulation of α_2 receptor-mediated glycogenolysis are additional potential diabetogenic mechanisms. Therefore, these drugs are not the first choice. However, those β-blockers which have intrinsic sympathomimetic effects and β_1-selective blockers with β_2-agonist properties appear to have minimal detrimental effect on glycaemic control.

Thiazide diuretics worsen glycaemic control in a dose-dependent fashion by impairing insulin secretion and decreasing peripheral insulin sensitivity. Development of hypokalaemia is a precipitating factor and it must be avoided/treated if present. The small doses of thiazide diuretics which are usually used to control hypertension do not affect glycaemic status adversely provided potassium values are not disturbed.

ACE-inhibitors and angiotensin receptor blockers improve glycaemic control by preventing hypokalaemia, promoting adipocyte differentiation and improving insulin sensitivity by enhancing blood flow to skeletal muscle and other tissues. Inhibition of adrenergic activity which impairs insulin secretion (via α_2-receptor) and glucose uptake is another contributory mechanism. Moreover, these drugs do not disturb lipid profile.

Calcium channel blockers cause vasodilatation and improve peripheral blood flow.

α-1 adrenergic blockers like (Terazosin) cause vasodilatation and lower blood pressure without disturbing glycaemic status.

In our experience, combination therapy gives better control than monotherapy in diabetic patients with hypertension and microalbumiuria. A combination of ACE inhibitors, calcium channel blockers has been seen to result in pronounced reduction in systolic and diastolic blood pressure and urinary albumin excretion than single therapy. Some prefer to use a combination of ACE-inhibitors/angiotensin receptor blockers (ARB) with low dose cardioselective beta blockers and diuretics as first line of treatment and add calcium channel blockers later if need arises.

To sum up, it appears that ACE inhibitors/ARB have beneficial effect on glycaemic control, beta blockers worsen the control unless selected agents are used; diuretics in low doses are probably neutral provided potassium balance is maintained. Calcium channel blockers, have minimal good effect (or are neutral) and α-blockers are again beneficial.

SUMMARY

Patient's education about diabetic syndrome and family support are essential for proper management of diabetes. In our clinical practice, we find the glycaemic control can be adequately achieved by diet and lifestyle changes in about 25 to 30 per cent patients while in another approximately 45 to 50 per cent oral drugs along with lifestyle changes ensures near normal glycaemic status. Insulin is required in only 20 to 30 per cent patients out of which many are T1DM type. It is, thus evident that diet and physical activity are the sheet anchor for a good diabetes management. We do not favour use of very low calories diets (VLCD with 400 to 450 calories) or microdiets (Cambridge diets) with 150 to 300 calories and they do not figure in our management strategy. Hypertension in T2DM is better managed by ACE-inhibitors/angiotensin receptor blockers.

FURTHER READING

1. American Diabetes Association. Unproven therapies (position statement). Diabetes Care 2002;25(Suppl 1)S133.
2. Bradley JE, Brown C, Brown RO. Use of intravenous fat emulsions during total parenteral nutrition in glucose-intolerant patients. Nutr Clin Pract 1986;1:136-9.
3. Garg A, Bananome A, Grundt S M, et al. Comparison of a high-carbohydrate diet with a high-monounsaturated fat diet in patients with non-insulin dependent diabetes mellitus. N Engl J Med 1988;319;829-34.
4. Gopalan C, Ramasastri BV, Balasubramanian SC. Nutritive value of Indian foods. NIN Hyderabad 1989;2788.
5. Greenly SM. Dietary Therapy in Diabetes Annual-6. Alberti KGMM, Krall LP (Eds): Elsevier Science Publishers, 1991;169.
6. Kamble SM, Kamalakar PL, Vaidya S, Bambole VD. Influence of coccinia indica on certain enzymes in glycolytic and lipolytic pathways in human diabetes. Indian J Med Sci 1998;52:143-6.
7. Miles M John, Leither Lawrence, Hollander Patel. Effect of orlistat in overweight and obese patients with type 2 diabetes treated with metformin. Diabetes Care 2002;25:1123-5.
8. Nath BS, Murthi MK. Cholesterol in Indian ghee. Lancet 1988;11-39.
9. Nestor W, Bill David, Bonow RO, et al. Thiazobidenedione use, fluid retention and congestive heart failure. A consensus statement from the American Heart Association and American Diabetes Association. Diabetes Care 2004;27:256-63.
10. Payne C. Complementary and integrative medicine emergency therapies for diabetes. Part 1. Diabetes Spectrum 2001;14:129-31.
11. Position of the American Diabetes Association. Health implications of dietary fiber. J Am Diet Assoc 1988;88:216-21.
12. Raheja BS. Ghee, cholesterol and heart disease. Lancet 1987;2:1144.
13. Raheja BS, Murthi MK. Cholesterol and heart disease. Lancet 1987;2:1144.
14. Vinik AI, Jenkins DJA. Dietary fiber in management of diabetes. Diabetes Care 1988;11:160-73.
15. Vinik AI. Report of the American Diabetes Association's Task Force on nutrition introduction. Diabetes Care 1988;11:127-8.
16. WHO. Diet, nutrition and the prevention of chronic diseases. Tech Report Series 1990;797:171.
17. Yeh Gloria, Eisenberg David M, Kaptchuk Ted J, Phillips RS. Systemic review of herbs and dietary supplements for glycaemic control in diabetes. Diabetes Care 2003;26:1277-94.

Management of Hypertension in T2DM

18. Gress TW, Nieto FJ, Shahar E, Wofford MR, Brancati FL. Hypertension and antihypertensive therapy as risk factor for type 2 diabetes mellitus. NEJM. 2000;342 (13):905-12.
19. Hanssan L, Lindholm LH, Niskanen L, et al. Effect of angiotensin-converting-enzyme inhibition compared with conventional therapy on cardiovascular morbidity in hypertension: the captopril prevention project (CAPP). Randomized trial. Lancet 1999;353: 611-6.
20. Komer R, Anderson S. Are angiotensin converting enzyme inhibitors the best treatment for hypertension in type 2 diabetes. Current Opinion in Nephrology and Hypertension 2000;9(2):173-9.
21. Padawal Raj, Laupacis Andreas. Antihypertensive therapy and incidence of type 2 diabetes. Diabetes 2004;27:247-55.
22. Pasanisi F, Imperatore G, Vaccaro O, Iovine C, Ferrara LA. Effects of treatment with terazosin on fasting and postprandial glucose and lipid metabolism in type 2 diabetes mellitus with hypertension. Nutrition, Metabolism and Cardiovascular Disease. 1999; 9(2):73-7.
23. The Allhat Collaborative Research Group. Major outcomes in high-risk hypertensive patients randomized to angiotensin-converting enzyme inhibitor or calcium channel blocker vs diuretic. JAMA 2002;288: 2981-97.

26.3 Oral Antidiabetic Drugs

Surender Kumar

- Introduction
- Classification of Oral Antidiabetic Drugs
- Sulphonyureas (SUs): Mechanism of Action, Clinical Efficacy, Side Effects, Choice of SUs, Cardiovascular Safety, Contraindications for SUs
- Biguanides: Mechanism of Action, Side Effects, Comparison of SUs and Metformin Therapy
- Miglitinides: Mechanism of Action, Pharmacokinetics, Dosage, Side Effects

- Thiazolidinediones: Mechanism of Action, Pharmacokinetics, Indications, Dosage, Combination Therapy, Side Effects, Drug Interaction
- Alpha Glucosidase Inhibitors: Mechanism of Action, Pharmacokinetics, Effect on Carbohydrate Metabolism, Dosage, Combination Therapy, Adverse Effects
- DPP IV Inhibitors
- Miscellaneous: Weight Reducing Agents, Fat Absorption Modulator, Sibutramine, Guar Gum, Fenugreek
- Combination Therapy

INTRODUCTION

In 1926, guanidine derivative, synthalin, was used for the first time to treat diabetes mellitus. Subsequently a chance observation in 1942, revealed that a sulpha derivative has significant hypoglycaemic effect. This led to further research in sulphonylureas and a large number of them were discovered. The biguanide discovery followed sulphonylurea and in recent years, many new compounds for management of diabetes have been found. Recently, weight reducing agents have also been included in the list of agents used in the treatment of type-2 diabetes.

The prevalence of type 2 diabetes mellitus (formerly known as non-insulin-dependent diabetes mellitus) has increased worldwide dramatically over the past two decades and continues to rise. Despite best efforts to improve the management of patients with type 2 diabetes mellitus, attempts at maintaining near normal blood glucose levels in these patients remain unsatisfactory. This continues to pose a real challenge to the physicians as the prevalence of this disease continues to rise.

Type 2 diabetes is defined as a syndrome characterized by relative insulin deficiency, insulin resistance and increased hepatic glucose output. Medications used to treat type 2 diabetes, are designed to correct one or more of these metabolic abnormalities.

Recently, the results of the United Kingdom Prospective Diabetes Study (UKPDS), were released. This study, the largest and longest study of patients with type 2 diabetes, has reinforced the belief that improved control of blood glucose levels can substantially lower the overall morbidity associated with this disease, underscoring the urgency to obtain better glucose control in these patients. Currently, there are five distinct classes of hypoglycaemic agents available, each class displaying unique pharmacologic properties. These classes are the sulphonylureas, meglitinides, biguanides, thiazolidinediones and alpha-glucosidase inhibitors (Table 26.3.1).

Current recommendations include a trial of diet and exercise as first-line therapy for the treatment of patients with type 2 diabetes, if blood glucose is marginally raised. If the desired level of glycaemic control is not achieved with diet and exercise within a three-month period, pharmacologic intervention is required. Once the decision is made to initiate therapy with an oral agent, it is prudent to consider patient-specific (age, weight, level of glycaemic control) and agent-specific characteristics (relative potencies, duration of action, side effect profiles, cost) to make the most appropriate choice.

SULPHONYLUREAS

Sulphonylureas (SUs) have remained the mainstay of antidiabetic therapy since the early 1950s. They lower blood glucose in patients, whose plasma glucose levels cannot be controlled by diet and exercise alone. Following the release of the University Group Diabetes Programme (UGDP) study, which implicated tolbutamide in increased mortality secondary to cardiovascular events, the use of the first generation sulphonylureas (acetohexamide, chlorpropamide, tolbutamide and tolazamide) quickly fell out of favour, recent data supporting the benefits of the sulphonylureas as well as the availability of newer generation sulphonylureas with

TABLE 26.3.1

1. *Hypoglycaemic agents*

   a. Sulphonylureas

      First generation
      - Acetohexamide
      - Chlorpropamide
      - Tolazamide
      - Tolbutamide

      Second generation
      - Glibenclamide
      - Glipizide
      - Gliclazide
      - Glimepiride

   b. Meglitinides
      - Repaglinide
      - Nateglinide

2. *Anti-hyperglycaemic agents*

   a. Biguanides   Metformin

   b. Thiazolidinediones
      - Pioglitazone
      - Rosiglitazone
      - Muraglitazar
      - Tesaglitazar

   c. Alpha-glucosidase inhibitors
      - Acarbose
      - Miglitol
      - Voglibose

   d. DPP IV Inhibitor

3. *Miscellaneous*

   a. Weight reducing agents   Orlistat
                                Sibutramine

   b. Mosapride

   c. Guargum

   d. Fenugreek extract

Classification of antidiabetic drugs

more favourable side effect profiles (glibenclamide, glipizide, gliclazide and glimepiride), have contributed to their renewed popularity.

Sulphonylureas are named for their common core configuration. Substitutions at either end of the sulphonylurea, one at the para position of the benzene ring and the other at a nitrogen residue in the urea moiety, produce pharmacologic and pharmacokinetic differences among sulphonylureas. They are frequently

classified either as 1st generation or 2nd generation agents (Table 26.3.1). First generation sulphonylureas (e.g. tolbutamide, acetohexamide, tolazamide, and chlorpropamide) possess a lower binding affinity for the ATP-sensitive potassium channel and thus require higher doses to achieve efficacy, increasing the potential for adverse events. In addition, the plasma half-life of 1st generation sulphonylureas is extended (e.g. 5 to 36 hr) as compared to the 2nd generation agents. Chlorpropamide was once one of the most commonly used oral agents, but now it is rarely prescribed. Second generation sulphonylureas (e.g. glibenclamide, glipizide, gliclazide) have large nonpolar and more lipid soluble substitutions that more readily penetrate cell membranes, giving them greater potency. Duration of action of these agents can vary; glimepiride and glibenclamide are longer acting agents than glipizide and gliclazide. The 2nd generation sulphonylureas are much more potent compounds (~100-fold), possess a more rapid onset of action, and generally have shorter plasma half-lives and longer duration of action compared to the 1st generation agents. Glimepiride has larger substitutions than other second generation sulfonylureas, but is not yet known whether these differences are sufficient to classify glimepiride as a 3rd generation sulphonylurea.

Mechanism of action

Sulphonylureas are insulin secretagogues, since they control blood glucose levels by directly stimulating insulin secretion in the pancreatic beta cells. The sulphonylureas lead to closure of K-ATP channel. The K-ATP channel is comprised of two subunits, both of which are required for the channel to be functional. One subunit contains the cytoplasmic binding sites for both sulphonylureas and ATP, and is designated as the sulphonylurea receptor (SUR). The SURs are of two types: type 1 and type 2. The SUR type 1 are predominantly found in beta cells of the pancreas, while SUR type 2a, are found in myocardial cells and SUR type 2b are found in vascular smooth muscle cells.

The other sub-unit is the potassium channel (K-ATP), which acts as the pore-forming subunit. An increase in the ATP/ADP ratio or ligand binding (by sulphonylureas, meglitinide) to SUR1 results in the closure of the K-ATP channel. The closure of this channel depolarizes the membrane and triggers the opening of voltage-sensitive calcium channels, leading to the rapid influx of calcium. Increased intracellular calcium causes an alteration in the cytoskeleton, and stimulates translocation of insulin-containing secretary granules to the plasma membrane and the exocytosis leading to release of insulin (Fig. 26.3.1).

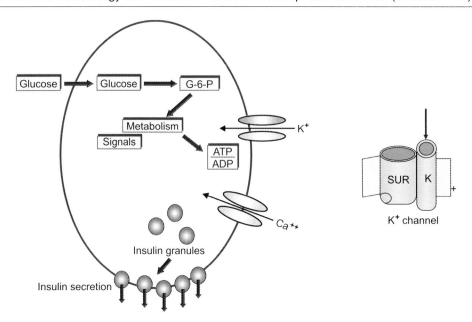

Fig. 26.3.1: Insulin secretion from β-cell

There are several distinct sites on the SUR1 that cause K-ATP channel closure. Some sites exhibit high affinity for glibenclamide and other sulphonylureas, while other sites exhibit high affinity for the non-sulphonylurea secretagogues. Both 1st and 2nd generation sulphonylureas bind at the site labelled as 140 kDa protein on the SUR1, while glimepiride, a novel sulphonylurea binds at the 65 kDa protein at the SUR1. The non-SU secretagogues (meglinitides: repaglinide, nateglinide) bind at a site near 140 kDa protein on the SUR1. The SUs are said to have other effects also, including a decrease in glucagon and hepatic gluconeogenesis, and an insulin binding to target receptors. Sulphonylurea therapy may slightly improve insulin resistance in peripheral target tissues (muscle, fat) and alter lipid metabolism through improvement in glycaemic control. Effectiveness of SU declines as the failure of beta cell function progresses. This results in a 3 to 10 per cent annual secondary failure rate of patients receiving sulphonylureas.

Clinical Efficacy

The clinical efficacy of sulphonylureas in patients with type 2 diabetes is related to the pre-treatment levels of fasting plasma glucose and HbA1c. The higher the fasting glucose level, the greater the effect will be. In patients with a pre-treatment glucose level of approximately 200 mg/dl, sulphonylureas will reduce glucose by 60 to 70 mg/dl and HbA1c by 1.5 to 2%. The most responsive patients are those who exhibit mild-to-moderate fasting hyperglycaemia (<200 to 240 mg/dl), along with adequate residual beta-cell function (evidenced by proportionally elevated fasting C-peptide). When used at maximally effective dose, results from well controlled clinical trials have not indicated a superiority of one generation sulphonylurea over another (Table 26.3.2). Similarly, 2nd generation sulphonylureas exhibit similar clinical efficacy compared to the 1st generation agents. The principal advantage of glimepiride and glibenclamide compared to other agents is the once daily dose regimen.

Approximately 10 to 20% of patients will exhibit a poor initial response to sulphonylureas (primary failures). While these patients are typically those who have severe fasting hyperglycaemia (> 280 mg/dl) and reduced fasting C-peptide levels, tests are not specific enough, to help decide on the usefulness of a sulphonylurea for an individual patient. In addition, treatment with sulphonylureas results in the eventual loss of therapeutic effectiveness (secondary failure) in the range 3 to 10% per year.

Side Effects

The major side effect from sulphonylurea treatment is hypoglycaemia. This side effect is just an extension of the therapeutic objective. Mild hypoglycaemic events occur in approximately 2 to 4% of patients and severe hypoglycaemic reactions that require hospitalization occur at a frequency of 0.2 to 0.4 cases per 1000 patients-years of treatment. In light of this, initiation of treatment with sulphonylureas should be at the lowest recom-

TABLE 26.3.2

Agents	Daily dose	Number of doses per day
First Generation Agents		
• Tolbutamide	500 to 3,000 mg	2 to 3
• Chlorpropamide	100 to 500 mg	1
• Tolazamide	100 to 1,000 mg	1 to 2
• Acetohexamide	250 to 1,500 mg	1 to 2
Second Generation Agents		
• Glibenclamide	1.25 to 20 mg	1 to 2
• Glibenclamide, micronized	0.75 to 12 mg	1 to 2
• Gliclazide	80 to 320 mg	1 to 2
• Gliclazide—MR	30 to 120 mg	1
• Glipizide	2.5 to 40 mg	1 to 2
• Glipizide GITS	5 to 20 mg	1
• Glimepiride	1 to 8 mg	1 to 2

Sulphonylureas for type 2 diabetes

mended dose. An additional undesirable effect of sulphonylurea therapy (as is also the case with insulin therapy) is weight gain. In the UKPDS, sulphonylurea treatment (chlorpropamide, glibenclamide, glipizide) caused a net weight gain of 3 kg, which occurred during the first 3 to 4 years of treatment and then stabilized. In subsequent studies, glimepiride appears to cause less weight gain than all the others, which is most likely due to its insulin-sparing effect. Chlorpropamide is associated with hyponatraemia (SIADH) and an alcohol flushing reaction (disulfram-antabuse reaction). All agents can cause intrahepatic cholestasis. Rarely, maculopapular or urticarial rashes occur. Very rarely, bone marrow depression may be caused by SUs.

In renal failure, the dose of the sulphonylurea agent will require adjustment based on glucose monitoring. The half-life of insulin is extended in renal failure and thus there is an increased risk for hypoglycaemia, especially fasting or pre-meal hypoglycaemia. Secondary failure results when the patient responds well to treatment initially (a decrease in FPG of greater than 30 mg%), but eventually the treatment fails to maintain adequate control. This phenomenon is reported to occur in approximately 3 to 10 per cent of patients per year. Despite these drawbacks, sulphonylureas have been shown to be potent and cost-effective glucose lowering agents.

Choice of SUs

Several sulphonylureas are currently available and selection is determined by side effects, the duration of

action, as well as the patient's age and kidney function. All sulphonylureas may cause hypoglycaemia. They can encourage weight gain and should be prescribed only if poor control and symptoms persist. Generally, sulphonylureas with longer duration of action (e.g. glibenclamide) are not recommended in the elderly or where patients suffer from mild to moderate liver or kidney problems. Other side effects are usually mild and infrequent and include gastrointestinal disturbances. The first generation sulphonylureas, chlorpropamide and tolazamide have been largely superceded by the second generation. Chlorpropamide has also been reported to have the highest number of side effects and this is not or very rarely used these days.

Frequency of Dosing

One of the important parameters in choosing a SU is the frequency of therapy. There are clinical trials that have shown that initiation with once a day pharmacotherapy results in better adherence and persistence compared with a BID regimen, these data suggest that lesser dosing frequency exerts a better impact on patient compliance than number of tablets per dose.

Metabolism and Excretion

Although each agent in this class is metabolized in a slightly different way, sulphonylureas are generally metabolized by the liver in varying degrees and are eliminated by renal excretion (Table 26.3.3). The parent compound may also be excreted by the kidneys. The pharmacokinetics of each agent affects the risk for hypoglycaemia in certain patients. For example, because of a decrease in the renal excretion, glibenclamide can lead to the accumulation of either the parent drug or active metabolites, glibeclamide has generally been associated with a higher incidence of hypoglycaemia,

TABLE 26.3.3

Drugs	Metabolites	Excretion
Tolbutamide	Inactive	Kidney
Chlorpropamide	Active or unchanged	Kidney
Glipizide	Inactive	Kidney 80% Bile 20%
Glibenclamide	Inactive or weakly active	Kidney 50% Bile 50%
Gliclazide	Probably inactive	Kidney 70% Bile 30%
Glimepiride	Probably inactive	Kidney 10% Bile 90%

Metabolites and excretion of SUs

especially in the presence of renal insufficiency. Its use is therefore not recommended in people with compromised renal function and older adults. Glipizide appears less likely to cause hypoglycaemia in this scenario, as its metabolites are either inactive or have minimal hypoglycaemic potency. Glimepiride is completely metabolized by the liver, so it may be more appropriate for patients with renal insufficiency.

Risk of Hypoglycaemia

Glimepiride, glipizide, and the meglitinides have a lower risk for hypoglycaemia than glibenclamide. The duration of action of SUs and the rapidity with which it dissociates from the SU-receptor in the event of development of hypoglycaemia decides about the choice of SUs. The glimepiride associates with SUR, 2 to 3 times faster than glibenclamide but in the event of hypoglycemia, the glimepiride dissociates 8 to 9 times faster than glibenclamide. Thus, the longer acting SU of choice is glimepiride, which has much lower incidence of hypoglycaemia.

Cardiovascular Safety

Sulphonylureas such as tolbutamide and glibenclamide may have adverse effects on the cardiovascular system, mainly because they also close myocardial mitochondrial K-ATP channels, thought to play a central role in ischaemic preconditioning (IPC) protection. Glimepiride has fewer cardiac actions than other sulphonylureas. This would have important implications for its preferred use in the treatment of patients with type 2 diabetes with concurrent coronary artery disease.

Contraindications for Sulphonylureas

1. Type-1 diabetes
2. Pancreatic diabetes (if significant damage of pancreas has occurred)
3. Pregnancy, lactation
4. Major surgery or trauma
5. Severe infection
6. History of sensitivity to sulpha drugs
7. Severe impairment of hepatic and renal function.

BIGUANIDES

The biguanides (phenformin and metformin) are derivatives of guanidine and were introduced in 1957 but phenformin was withdrawn from clinical use in 1970s due to high incidence of lactic acidosis. Metformin

is currently the only agent of this antidiabetic class, in use.

Mechanisms of Action

Metformin works by reducing hepatic glucose output and, to a lesser extent, enhancing insulin sensitivity in hepatic and peripheral tissues. Metformin is absorbed from small intestine and has an oral bioavailability of 50 to 60%. It has mean plasma ½ life of 4 to 6 hours. It is given 2 to 3 times a day, but extended release formulations can be given once a day. It is excreted unchanged in kidneys. The exact mechanism of action of metformin is not fully understood. Metformin decreases basal hepatic glucose output, providing an important mechanism through which the drug lowers fasting plasma glucose concentration. Therapeutic concentration of metformin enhances the suppression of gluconeogenesis by insulin and reduces glucagon-stimulated gluconeogenesis. Metformin also increases the uptake and oxidation of glucose by adipose tissue (Fig. 26.3.2). However, the actions of metformin on peripheral tissues require high concentrations and are slow in onset. Metformin increases the binding of insulin to its receptors, phosphorylation, and tyrosine kinase activity of insulin receptors. Metformin also increases translocation of the GLUT-1 and GLUT-4 isoforms of glucose transporters in different types of cells, and it prevents the development of insulin resistance.

Metformin improves oral glucose tolerance, whereas the plasma insulin response to glucose is unchanged or may be decreased in patients with hyperinsulinaemia. Metformin decreases fatty acid oxidation by 10 to 20 per cent, which, in turn, reduces plasma glucose concentrations by means of the glucose-fatty acid cycle.

Long-term therapy with metformin, particularly in patients with marked hyperglycaemia, results in a moderate (10 to 20%) reduction in plasma triglyceride concentrations due to decreased hepatic synthesis of very-low density lipoprotein. Small decreases (5 to 10%) in plasma total cholesterol and small increases in plasma high density lipoprotein cholesterol have been noted in some studies.

Initiating and Monitoring Therapy with Metformin

Metformin has the potential advantage of targeting insulin resistance, which is an early feature of the disease, and reducing rather than increasing plasma insulin concentrations. Metformin does not cause weight gain and may reduce adipose-tissue mass. Thus, metformin

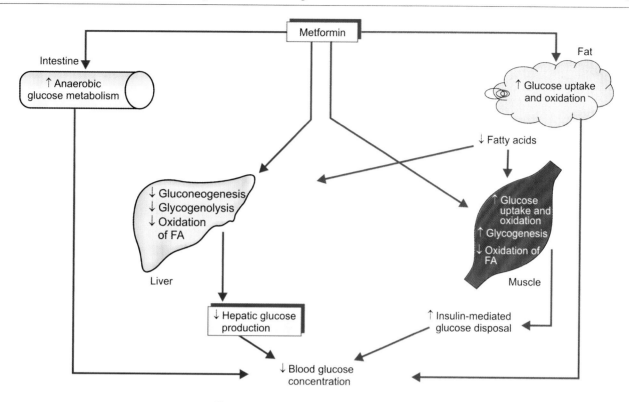

Fig. 26.3.2: Mode of action of metformin

may be preferred in obese. It is also equally useful in non-obese (metabolically obese) patients. The risk of hypoglycaemia is much less with metformin than with sulphonylurea therapy.

Metformin should be taken with meals, starting either with 500 mg or 850 mg dose, at breakfast or with 500 mg dose given with the morning and evening meals. The dose should be increased slowly, 250 mg or 500 mg at a time, at intervals of one to two weeks. A total dose of three to four 500 mg or two to three 850 mg dose is often required, with the maximal dose being 2.5 to 3.0 gm per day. The extended release formulations can be used once a day or twice a day if more than 1 gm dose is required.

To have optimal benefit, combination therapy should probably be instituted before the onset of symptomatic hyperglycaemia. When treatment with a sulphonylurea fails, the addition of metformin to the regimen reduces symptoms but has only a limited effect on glycaemia and in practice, only temporarily defers the need for insulin therapy. Patients in whom metformin therapy is effective, are also prone to subsequent deterioration of glycaemic control, usually because of progressive beta-cell failure rather than loss of effectiveness of the drug.

Metformin should not be used in patients with elevated serum creatinine levels, 1.4 mg per dl or more in women and 1.5 mg per dl or more in men. In patients undergoing contrast studies, metformin therapy should be withheld for approximately 48 hours following the procedure or until it has been determined that renal function has returned to baseline. Other situations in which metformin therapy should be avoided include cardiogenic or septic shock, congestive heart failure that requires pharmacologic therapy, severe liver disease, and pulmonary insufficiency with hypoxaemia or severe tissue hypoperfusion.

Side Effects

Patients on metformin therapy should be advised that they may have minor gastrointestinal side effects. These include diarrhoea, abdominal discomfort, anorexia, nausea, and a metallic taste in the mouth. The symptoms are dose-related and remit if the dose is reduced; sometimes, an increase in the dose can be tolerated later on. More than half of patients can tolerate the maximal dose, but about 5 per cent cannot tolerate any dose of metformin.

Lactic acidosis is a rare but serious adverse effect in metformin treated patients, with an estimated incidence of less than 0.01 to 0.08 case per 1000 patient year. In most patients it occurs because one or more contraindications were overlooked, predominantly renal insufficiency, leading to high plasma metformin concentrations. Additional factors that increase blood lactate concentrations are often present, for example, a major illness causing hypotension with low tissue perfusion, other causes of hypoxia, liver disease, or alcohol abuse. In these situations, the plasma metformin concentration is not necessarily abnormally high. It is important to realize that blood lactate concentrations become elevated in any patient in whom cardiogenic shock or other illnesses that decrease tissue perfusion, and in some reported cases, the metformin was probably an incidental factor and not responsible for the lactic acidosis. The mortality in reported cases is about 50 per cent. The risk of death from lactic acidosis in metformin-treatment patients is similar to that of hypoglycaemia in sulphonylurea-treated patients. Should a patient have lactic acidosis attributable to metformin, the drug can be removed by haemodialysis.

In practice, lactic acidosis is not regarded as a major problem, probably because of adherence to the exclusion criteria. This situation is quite different from the earlier experience with phenformin, which is estimated to have 10 to 20 times greater risk of lactic acidosis than that for metformin. After phenformin was withdrawn from clinical use, it was found that some people (e.g. about 10% of whites) have an inherited defect in the hydroxylation of this drug. Because they are unable to metabolize phenformin adequately, these patients have an increased risk of drug accumulation, which probably accounts for the higher incidence of lactic acidosis with phenformin. This condition does not occur with metformin, which is not metabolized. In addition, metformin does not inhibit peripheral glucose oxidation and does not enhance peripheral lactate production, as occurs with phenformin.

Comparison of Sulphonylurea and Metformin Therapy

Metformin and sulphonylureas cause similar reductions in fasting plasma glucose concentrations in patients. The reductions are greater in patients with marked hyperglyacaemia than in those with moderate hyperglycaemia. Nevertheless, if the fasting plasma glucose concentration is considerably above 200 mg%, neither drug is likely to reduce it to nearly normal level.

Both sulphonylurea and insulin therapy can cause weight gain, but this does not occur with metformin therapy. Sulphonylureas can induce hypoglycaemia, whereas this is rare with metformin therapy alone. Therefore, metformin has an antihyperglycaemic action, whereas sulphonylureas and insulin have hypoglycaemic actions. Sulphonylureas increase fasting plasma insulin concentrations, whereas metformin may decrease them. In theory, the reduced plasma concentrations of insulin and plasminogen-activator inhibitor type 1, thus, could decrease the risk of macrovscular disease.

MEGLITINIDES

Meglitinide analogues are a new non-sulphonylurea insulin secretagogues agents. They are derived from benzamido-non-sulphonylurea portion of glibenclamide. The mechanism of action of the meglitinides closely resembles that of the sulphonylureas. The meglitinides stimulate the release of insulin from the pancreatic beta cells. However, this action is mediated through a different binding site on the "sulphonylurea receptor" of the beta cell. They have somewhat different characteristics when compared with the sulphonylureas. Unlike the commonly used sulphonylureas, the meglitinides have a very short onset of action and a short half-life, thus are useful for postprandial blood glucose control.

Repaglinide

Repaglinide is an oral hypoglycaemic agent for the treatment of type 2 diabetes, and represents a new class of insulin secretagogues.

Mechanism of Action

Repaglinide lowers blood glucose levels by stimulating the release of insulin from the pancreas. This action is dependent upon functioning beta cells in the pancreatic islets. Insulin release is glucose-dependent and diminishes at low glucose concentrations. Repaglinide closes ATP-dependent potassium channels in the beta cell membrane by binding at specific sites (see Fig 26.3.1). Thus, potassium channel blockade depolarizes the beta cell, which leads to an opening of calcium channels. The resulting increased calcium influx induces insulin secretion. The ion channel mechanism is highly tissue selective with low affinity for heart and skeletal muscles.

Pharmacokinetics

After oral administration, repaglinide is rapidly and completely absorbed from the gastrointestinal tract. After a single and multiple oral doses in healthy subjects or in patients, peak plasma drug levels (C-max) occur within 1 hour (T-max). Repaglinide is rapidly eliminated from the blood stream with a half-life of approximately 1 hour. The mean absolute bioavailability is 56%. When repaglinide is given with food, the mean T max is not changed, but the mean C-max and AUC (area under the time/plasma concentration curve) are decreased 20% and 12.4%, respectively.

Repaglinide is completely metabolized by oxidative biotransformation and direct conjugation with glucuronic acid. The major metabolites are an oxidized dicarboxylic acid (M2), the aromatic amine (M1), and the acyl glucuronide (M7). The cytochrome P-450 enzyme system, specifically 3A4, has been shown to be involved in the N-dealkylation of repaglinide to M2 and the further oxidation to M1. Metabolites do not contribute to the glucose-lowering effect of rapaglinide.

Dosage and Administration

Repaglinide is usually taken within 15 minutes of the meal but time may vary from immediately preceding the meal to as long as 30 minutes before the meal. The recommended dose range is 0.5 to 4 mg taken with meals. Repaglinide may be given preprandially 2,3, or 4 times a day in response to changes in the patient's meal pattern. The maximum recommended daily dose is 16 mg. For patients not previously treated or whose HbA1c is < 8%, the starting dose should be 0.5 mg with each meal. For patients previously treated with blood glucose-lowering drugs and whose HbA1c is >8%, the initial dose is 1 or 2 mg with each meal preprandially.

Dose adjustments should be determined by blood glucose response, usually fasting blood glucose. Postprandial glucose levels testing may be clinically helpful in patients whose pre-meal glucose levels are satisfactory but whose overall glycaemic control (HbA1c) is inadequate. The preprandial dose should be doubled up to 4 mg with each meal until satisfactory blood glucose response is achieved. At least one week should elapse to assess response after each dose adjustment.

Nateglinide

Nateglinide is structurally unrelated to the oral sulphonylurea insulin secretagogues. Mechanism of action is similar to repaglinide.

Pharmacokinetics

Following oral administration, immediately prior to a meal, nateglinide is rapidly absorbed with mean peak plasma drug concentrations (C-max) generally occurring within 1 hour (T-max) after dosing. Absolute bioavailability is estimated to be approximately 73%. Nateglinide is metabolized by the mixed function oxidase system prior to elimination. The major routes of metabolism are hydroxylation followed by glucuronide conjugation. The major metabolites are less potent antidiabetic agents than

nateglinide. *In vitro* data demonstrate that nateglinide is predominantly metabolized by cytochrome P450 isoenzymes, CYP2C9 (70%) and CYP3A4 (30%). Nateglinide and its metabolites are rapidly and completely eliminated following oral administration. Within 6 hours after dosing, approximately 75% of the administered C-nateglinide is recovered in the urine.

Dosage and Combination

Nateglinide is indicated as monotherapy to lower blood glucose in patients with type 2 diabetes whose hyperglycaemia cannot be adequately controlled by diet and physical exercise.

Usual dose: 60 mg, 1 to 10 min before each meal. The dose may be increased to 120 mg three times a day before each meal.

Nateglinide is also indicated for use in combination with metformin. In patients whose hyperglycaemia is inadequately controlled with metformin, nateglinide may be added to, but not substituted for, metformin. Patients whose hyperglycaemia is not adequately controlled with other insulin secretagogues, should not be switched to nateglinide, nor should nateglinide be added to their treatment regimen.

Side Effects of Meglitinides

Hypoglycaemia is more likely to occur when caloric intake is deficient, after severe or prolonged exercise, when alcohol is ingested, or when more than one glucose-lowering drug is used. Repaglinide/nateglinide should be administered with meals to lessen the risk of hypoglycaemia. Other precautions are like that of sulphonylureas.

Patients receiving other oral hypoglycaemic agents: When nateglinide/repaglinide is used to replace therapy with other oral hypoglycaemic agents, nateglinide/repaglinide may be started on the day after the final dose is given. Patients should then be observed carefully for hypoglycaemia due to potential overlapping of drug effects. When transferred from longer half-life sulphonylurea agents (e.g. chlorpropamide) to repaglinide/nateglinide, close monitoring may be indicated for up to one week or longer.

THIAZOLIDINEDIONES (GLITAZONES)

The thiazolidinedione (TZD) class of oral hypoglycaemic drugs (popularly known as glitazones) were developed in 1997 and offer a new mechanism for treatment of type 2 diabetes. The agents in this class approved by the US Food and Drug Administration (FDA) and drug controller of India, are rosiglitazone and pioglitazone. In March 2000, the FDA asked the manufacturer of troglitazone, the first agent in this class to receive approval, to remove the product from the market. This occurred following more than 60 reports of severe liver toxicity in patients taking this agents.

The primary effect of TZDs is peripheral; to increase insulin sensitivity and increase glucose uptake. The TZDs have some effect on hepatic glucose uptake and sensitivity but to a lesser degree. They do not stimulate the pancreas to produce more insulin. TZDs are metabolized in liver and thus can be used safely in patients with renal dysfunction. They can be used once daily, although rosiglitazone works better with twice daily dosing. Reports have suggested that rosiglitazone works better in women, but the reason for this is not known.

Mechanism of Action

The antihyperglycaemic effect of thiazolidinedione agent is dependent on the presence of insulin. Glitazone decreases insulin resistance in the periphery and in the liver resulting in increased insulin-dependent glucose disposal and decreased hepatic glucose output.

Glitazone is a potent and highly selective agonist for peroxisome proliferator-activated receptor-gamma. PPAR gamma receptors are found in tissues important for insulin action such as adipose tissue, skeletal muscle, and liver. Activation of PPAR gamma nuclear receptors modulates the transcription of a number of insulin responsive genes involved in the control of glucose and lipid metabolism (Fig. 26.3.3). Clinical studies demonstrate that glitazone improves insulin sensitivity in insulin-resistant patient. Glitazone enhances cellular responsiveness to insulin, increases insulin-dependent glucose disposal, improves hepatic sensitivity to insulin and improves dysfunctional glucose homeostasis. In patients with type 2 diabetes, the decreased insulin resistance produced by glitazone results in lower blood glucose concentration, lower plasma insulin levels and lower HbA1c values.

Pharmacokinetics

Following oral administration, in the fasting state, glitazones are first measurable in serum, within 30 minutes, with peak concentrations observed within 2 hours. Food slightly delays the time to peak serum concentration to 3 to 4 hours, but does not alter the extent of absorption. Glitazones are extensively protein bound in human serum, principally to serum albumin, they are extensively metabolized, the metabolites M-II, M-III and M-IV are pharmacologically active in animal models of type 2 diabetes. The major cytochrome P450 isoform

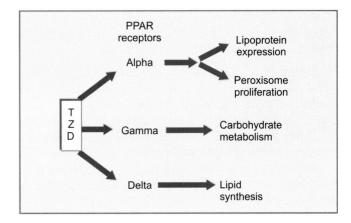

Fig. 26.3.3: Mechanism of action of thiazolidinedione (TZD)

involved in the hepatic metabolism of glitazone are CYP3A4 with contributions from a variety of other isoforms including the mainly extrahepatic CYP1A1.

Serum concentration of total glitazone remains elevated 24 hours after once daily dosing. Steady-state serum concentrations of both free glitazone and total glitazone are achieved within 7 days. At steady-state, two of the pharmacologically active metabolites, metabolites III and IV, reach serum concentrations equal to or greater than that of glitazone.

Following oral administration, approximately 15 to 30% of the glitazone dose is recovered in the urine. Renal elimination of glitazone is 15 to 30% and the drug is excreted primarily as metabolites and their conjugates. It is presumed that most of the oral dose is excreted into the bile either unchanged or as metabolites and eliminated in the faeces. The mean serum half-life of glitazone ranges from 3 to 7 hours.

Indications

Glitazones are indicated as an adjunct to diet and exercise to improve glycaemic control in patients with type 2 diabetes. Glitazones may be used as monotherapy. Glitazones are also indicated for use in combination with a sulphonylurea, metformin, or insulin, when diet and exercise plus the single agent does not result in adequate glyacaemic control.

Dosage and administration

Pioglitazone

The management of antidiabetic therapy should be individualized. Ideally, the response to therapy should be evaluated using HbA1c, which is a better indicator of long-term glycaemic control than fasting blood glucose alone. In clinical use, it is recommended that patients be treated with pioglitazone for a reasonable period of time (3 months or more) to evaluate change in HbA1c unless glycaemic control deteriorates.

Monotherapy: Pioglitazone should be taken once daily without regard to meals. Pioglitazone monotherapy in patients inadequately controlled with diet and exercise may be initiated at 15 mg or 30 mg once daily. For patient who responds inadequately to the initial dose of pioglitazone, the dose can be increased in increments up to 45 mg once daily. For patients not responding adequately to monotherapy, combination therapy should be considered. Monotherapy with these agents has been associated with a 0.5 to 1.5 per cent reduction in HbA1c levels and 25 to 50 mg% reduction in FPG levels.

Combination therapy: Pioglitazone in combination with a sulphonylurea may be initiated at 15 mg to 30 mg once daily. The current sulphonylurea dose can be continued upon initiating of pioglitazone therapy. If patients report hypoglycaemia, the dose of the sulphonylurea should be decreased. Pioglitazone in combination with metformin may be initiated at 15 to 30 mg once daily. The current metformin dose can be continued upon initiation of pioglitazone therapy. It is unlikely that the dose of metformin will require adjustment due to hypoglycaemia during combination therapy with pioglitazone.

Pioglitazone in combination with insulin may be initiated at 15 mg or 30 mg once daily. The current insulin dose can be continued upon initiation of pioglitazone therapy. In patients receiving pioglitazone and insulin, the insulin dose can be decreased by 10 to 25% if the patient reports hypoglycaemia or if plasma glucose concentrations decrease to less than 100 mg/dl. Further adjustments should be individualized based on glucose-lowering response. Maximum recommended dose of pioglitazone should not exceed 45 mg once daily since doses higher than 45 mg once daily have not been studied in placebo-controlled clinical studies.

Pioglitazone has been shown to reduce the intima-medial thickness of vessels; thus, it reduces the progression of atherosclerosis (PROactive Study).

Rosiglitazone

Rosiglitazone may be administered either at a starting dose of 4 mg as a single daily dose or divided and administered in the morning and evening. For patients who respond inadequately following 8 to 12 weeks of treatment, as determined by reduction in FPG, the dose may be increased to 8 mg daily. Rosiglitazone may be taken with or without food.

Monotherapy: The usual starting dose of rosiglitazone is 4 mg administered either as a single dose once daily or in divided doses twice daily. In clinical trials, the 4 mg twice daily regimen resulted in the greatest reduction in FPG and HbA1c.

Maximum recommended dose: The dose of rosiglitazone should not exceed 8 mg daily, as a single dose or divided twice daily. The 8 mg daily dose has been shown to be safe and effective in clinical studies as monotherapy and in combination with metformin. Rosiglitazone may be taken with or without food.

Newer Glitazones

Telsaglitazar and muraglitazar are the newer dual PPAR alpha and gamma receptor agonists. They are known to improve both plasma lipids and glucose.

Future use of these drugs will play an important role in improving glycaemic control and, dyslipidaemia and, thus, help in controlling the complications of diabetes.

Side Effects of Glitazones

Glitazone exerts its antihyperglycaemic effect only in the presence of insulin. Therefore, glitazones should not be used in patients with type 1 diabetes or in the treatment of diabetic ketoacidosis. Patients receiving glitazones in combination with insulin or oral hypoglycaemic agents may be at risk for hypoglycaemia, and a reduction in the dose of the concomitant agent may be necessary.

In premenopausal anovulatory patients with insulin resistance, treatment with thiazolidinediones, may result in resumption of ovulation. As a consequence of their improved insulin sensitivity, these patients may be at risk for pregnancy if adequate contraception is not used.

Glitazones may cause decreases in haemoglobin and haematocrit. Across all clinical studies, mean haemoglobin values declined by 2 to 4% in glitazone-treated patients. These changes may be related to increased plasma volume and have not been associated with any significant haematologic clinical effects.

Glitazones should be used with caution in patients with oedema. In double blind clinical trials of patients with type 2 diabetes, mild to moderate oedema has been reported in patients treated with glitazone. In pre-clinical studies, glitazones have been reported to cause plasma volume expansion and pre-load induced cardiac hypertrophy. In clinical trials that excluded patients with New York Heart Association (NYHA) classes III and IV cardiac status, no increased incidence of serious cardiac adverse events potentially related to volume expansion were observed.

Although available clinical data show no evidence of glitazone-induced hepatotoxicity or ALT elevation, pioglitazone and rosiglatazone are structurally related to troglitazone, which has been associated with idiosyncratic hepatotoxcity and rare cases of liver failure, it is recommended that patients treated with glitazone undergo periodic monitoring of liver enzymes. Serum ALT levels should be evaluated prior to the initiation of therapy with glitazone in all patients, every two months for the first year of therapy, and periodically thereafter. Liver function tests should also be obtained for patients if symptoms suggestive of hepatic dysfunction occur, e.g. nausea, vomiting, abdominal pain, fatigue, anorexia, and dark urine. The decision whether to continue the patient on therapy with glitazone should be guided by clinical judgment pending laboratory evaluations. If jaundice is observed, drug therapy should be discontinued.

Drug Interaction

Administration of thiazolidinedione with an oral contraceptive containing ethinyl oestradiol and norethindrone, reduces the plasma concentrations of both hormones by approximately 30%, which could result in loss of contraception. The pharmacokinetics of co-administration of glitazone and oral contraceptives has not been evaluated in patients receiving glitazone and an oral contraceptive. Therefore, additional caution regarding contraception should be exercised in patients receiving glitazone and an oral contraceptive.

The co-adminsitration of glitazone does not alter the steady-state pharmacokinetics of glipizide, digoxin, metformin or warfarin. In addition, glitazone has no clinically significant effect on prothrombin time when administrated to patients receiving chronic warfarin therapy.

Adverse events that have been commonly reported in placebo-controlled clinical studies of glitazone monotherapy are headache, upper respiratory tract infection, myalgia, sinusitis and pharyngitis. In monotherapy studies, oedema has been reported in 4.8% of glitazone-treated patients versus 1.2% in placebo-treated patients. Mild to moderate hypoglycaemia has been reported, although infrequently, in patients receiving glitazone.

Because these agents do not increase insulin secretion, hypoglycaemia does not pose a risk when thiazolidinediones are taken as monotherapy. Significant weight gain has been reported with these agents. The thiazolidiniones are relatively safe in patients with impaired renal function because they are highly metabolized by the liver and excerted in the faeces; however, caution should be used in patients with hepatic dysfunction because troglitazone and its metabolites have been shown to accumulate in this setting. With use of glitazones, patience on part of both doctor and patient is required. Blood sugar levels may show a significant reduction statistically in as little as two to four weeks, but the maximum effects are not seen until two or three months have passed.

ALPHA-GLUCOSIDASE INHIBITORS (AGIs)

Acarbose, miglitol and voglibose are the three agents available in this class. Acarbose is a pseudo-tetra-saccharide, a natural microbial product derived from culture broths of Actinoplanes strain SE-50. The unsaturated cyclitol component of the molecule has been identified as essential for alpha-glucosidase inhibitory activity.

They bind reversibly, competitively and in a dose-dependent manner to the oligosaccharide-binding site of alpha-glucosidase enzymes in the brush border of the small intestinal mucosa. As a consequence, hydrolysis of oligo- and disaccharides is prevented. This effect lasts for 4 to 6 hours provided that they are present at the site of enzymatic action at the same time as the oligosaccharides. Thus, they must be administered with the first bite of a main meal.

They bind to intestinal sucrase with a 10^4 to 10^5-fold greater affinity than sucrose. The drug delays the intestinal hydrolysis of oligo- and disaccharides by alpha-glucosidases, mainly in the upper half of the small intestine. Consequently, the absorption of monosaccharides after a meal is delayed and transport through the mucosal surface into the circulation is interrupted. The suppression of alpha-glucosidase is reversible, although pharmacological activity is reliable and persistent with long-term use. Effects with continued use can be maintained over years and no report of acarbose failure are present in the available literature.

The relative affinity of acarbose for specific enzymes is as follows: glycoamylase > sucrase > maltase > dextranase. Acarbose has little affinity for isomaltase and no affinity for the beta-glucosidases, such as lactase. Recent evidence also suggests that acarbose inhibits pancreatic alpha-amylase. Acarbose has no direct effect on the absorption of glucose.

With long-term acarbose administration, glucosidase activity increases slowly in the lower half of the small bowel. As the distal part of the small intestine is less exposed to complex carbohydrates, alpha-glucosidase activity is relatively low. This is even more pronounced with a 'fast food' diet with high glycaemic index and little dietary fibre. Alpha-glucosidase activity in the small intestine is subject to inter-individual and racial differences. Initial therapy with an alpha-glucosidase inhibitor often results in carbohydrates appearing in the colon, where bacterial fermentation may occur, accounting for the varying frequency and severity of gastrointestinal adverse effects, predominantly flatulence and loose stools. The quantity of undigested carbohydrates reaching the colon can be determined by analysis of breath hydrogen.

There is no need for dosage adjustment in slight renal insufficiency; however, acarbose should be withdrawn in case of severe progressive renal insufficiency. Acarbose should be started at a low dose followed by slow upward dose titration to reduce or avoid gastrointestinal adverse effects.

Pharmacokinetics

They are poorly absorbed and systemic bioavailability is low. After oral administration, <2% of the unchanged drug is absorbed and enters the circulation, with most remaining in the lumen of the gastrointestinal tract. Acarbose is cleaved in the large intestine by bacterial enzymes into several metabolisable and absorbable intermediates (glucose, maltose, acarviosine), approximately 35% of which will be absorbed, depending on the microbial flora in the intestine. The absorbed material appears in the urine as metabolites, mostly glucose, within 14 to 24 hours. Excretion via the kidneys predominates the absorbed component.

Effect on Carbohydrate Metabolism

After a high carbohydrate meal, acarbose lowers the postprandial rise in blood glucose by approximately 20%, depending on the dose, the extent of hyperglycaemia and the type of carbohydrate ingested. There is a greater effect on postprandial hyperglycaemia after ingestion of starch than of sucrose. This effect is additive with that of dietary manipulation and is more pronounced in patients with newly diagnosed diabetes. Acarbose significantly lowers postprandial blood glucose measured 60, 90 and 120 minutes after a meal. The effects can be seen after the first dose and can last for 3 to 5 hours, although an acute effect is apparent within a few minutes.

The reduction in blood glucose concentration following acarbose treatment is accompanied by decreased plasma insulin, both a significant lowering of fasting insulin and a reduction in the postprandial insulin

rise. The decrease in insulin secretion is secondary to reduced postprandial glucose and is most dramatic in individuals with high insulin secretary rates.

Acarbose Dosage

The drug should be administered just before each meal (as first bite). The dose should be gradually increased: 25 mg OD, BD, TDS then increased to 50 mg before each meal and if required then the dose can be increased to 100 mg TDS before each meal. Therapy should be initiated with the lowest effective dose and titrated slowly over intervals of two to four weeks. Patients should be instructed to take this medication with food. For maximum efficacy, the dietary carbohydrate intake should exceed 50 per cent. Although hypoglycaemia is not typically associated with monotherapy with the alpha-glucosidase inhibitors, it can occur in combination with other drugs. It is important, therefore, to inform patients that the traditional treatment for hypoglycemia may be blocked while using this therapy and to treat hypoglycaemia only with glucose.

The studies consistently reported decreases in:

Fasting glucose	20 ± 5 mg%
Postprandial plasma glucose	50 mg $\pm$ 10 mg%
Falls in HbA1c	0.5 to 1.3% (mean reduction $0.9 \pm 0.25\%$).

Miglitol

It is a pseudomonosaccharide, which is not metabolized. Its mode of action is similar to that of acarbose. It has no drug interaction with digoxin and warfarin. It has greater efficacy than acarbose. The usual dose is 25 to 50 mg three times a day as first bite. The side effects are much less as compared to acarbose. Miglitol is much better tolerated than acarbose and is more effective than acarbose.

Combination Therapy

AGIs can be used in combination with sulphonylureas, metformin and insulin because they lower glucose absorption from the gut. They are consistently effective in lowering postprandial blood glucose as an adjunct to all well-established oral antidiabetic drugs and insulin (Fig. 26.3.4). AGIs improve glycaemic control through different mechanisms to metformin and sulphonylureas, and can provide an additive benefit in glycaemic control when co-administered with these agents. Several major clinical trials have investigated the effect of acarbose in patients with type 2 diabetes inadequately controlled by

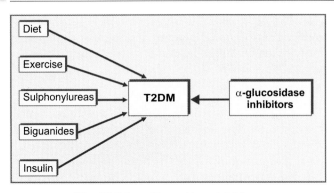

Fig. 26.3.4: α Glucosidase inhibitors
(adjunct to other antidiabetic drugs)

insulin treatment. An analysis of these results revealed an additional average net decrease in the HbA1c of 0.54%. AGIs are equally effective in type 1 diabetes also.

Adverse Effects and Contraindications

The most bothersome side effects observed with these agents are gastrointestinal, including abdominal discomfort, bloating, flatulence and diarrhoea but are reversible with discontinuation. Acarbose causes no hypoglycaemic reaction but induces an additional blood glucose-lowering effect when given in combination with insulin or a sulphonylurea. In the event of hypoglycaemia following acarbose taken in combination with other antidiabetic drug, glucose (but not sucrose) should be administered. Despite an additive effect with glibenclamide in lowering postprandial blood glucose, the risk of hypoglycaemia has been reported to be lower with combined acarbose and glibenclamide treatment (10%) than with glibenclamide monotherapy (29%). Reduced postprandial blood glucose rise and insulin levels are the probably explanation for this.

Few toxic effects have been reported with acarbose. Rare cases (6/100,000) of reversible increases in liver enzymes (ALT and AST) have been reported in Japan and the USA at the maximum recommended dosage; however, hepatotoxicity has not occurred. Two cases of acute, idiosyncratic and severe hepatotoxic reactions in diabetic patients receiving acarbose treatment have been reported (both patients recovered fully). Addition of acarbose resulted in subtherapeutic digoxin plasma concentrations. Decreased absorption of digoxin due to increased gastrointestinal motility and/or hydrolysis of digoxin may have been responsible.

Voglibose

This is the latest addition to previously existing AGIs. It has similar mode of action and is thought to have lesser GI side effects. The dose is 0.2 mg just before each main meal.

DPP IV INHIBITORS

GLP-1, an incretin is quickly degraded by enzyme dipeptidyl peptidase IV (DPP IV). Inhibitors of this enzyme lead to rise in the level of GLP -I; thus, GLP-I, is able to play its important role in increasing insulin secretion and reducing insulin resistance, in addition to many of its actions. Drug trial up to 12 months have been successful. Future of this drug appears very promising especially because it is an oral drug.

Comparison of various oral antidiabetic drugs is shown in Table 26.3.4

MISCELLANEOUS

Weight Reducing Agents

Obesity leads to increase in insulin resistance and weight loss leads to improvement in insulin resistance. Even 5% decrease in body weight leads to significant improvement in insulin resistance. Therefore, drugs which help in weight reduction, indirectly help in improving blood glucose levels.

Fat Absorption Modulator: Orlistat

Orlistat was introduced in 1999. It inhibits the action of pancreatic lipase, thus, preventing the hydrolysis of non-absorbable triglycerides into absorbable components; thus, it decreases fat absorption. It is primarily directed at weight reduction. It is taken before or with food in a maximum dose of 120 mg TDS. It leads to around 6.2% weight reduction by one year.

Sibutramine

It is a centrally acting agent and inhibits re-uptake of both serotonin and nor-epinephrine in CNS. It produces early satiety on eating food. In a dose of 5 to 10 mg/day, sibutramine results in average weight loss of 5 to 10 kg in 6 months.

Guar Gum

Guar gum, is a gum extracted from plant sources. It may be used as a supplement to soluble fibre in diet. It reduces postprandial glycaemia by slowing intestinal glucose absorption. The recommended dose is 5 gm, either sprinkled on food or stirred into 200 ml of water and taken before each major meal.

TABLE 26.3.4

Features	SUs	Metformin	AGIs	Glitazones	Miglitinide
• *Glycosylated Hb*					
Lowers HbA1c	1.5-2.0%	1.5.2.0%	0.5.1.0%	0.5-1.5%	0.6-1.0%
• *Failure rate*					
Primary	10-15%	Similar to SUs	Similar to SUs	Not known	Not reported
Secondary (per year)	3-10%	Similar to SUs	Similar to SUs	Not known	Not reported
• *Effects on lipids*					
TG	Lowers	Lowers	Lowers	Lowers	Lowers
TC	Minimal	Lowers	Minimal	Minimal	Minimal
HDL	Minimal	Minimal	Minimal	Raises	Minimal
• *Hypoglycaemia*	Mild hypoglycemia common but can be severe	None	None	None	Mild hypoglycaemia may occur
• *Weight gain*	Yes	No	No	Yes	Yes

Comparison of oral antidiabetic agents

Fenugreek

Fenugreek seed extract is also used as a supplement to soluble fibre. It may be taken before, with or after each meal. It helps in slowing the absorption of carbohydrates. It is claimed that it may be having some insulin sensitizing and insulin secreting properties, but it has not been proved.

COMBINATION DRUG THERAPY

Diabetes is a multi-factorial disease. Therefore, to tackle it in totality, there is good justification in using combination of those drugs which tackle different pathogenic factors of diabetes. The combination therapy can be very helpful in achieving target blood glucose level. The combination of these drugs could be either in a single formulation in the form of one or two tablets or separately as a tablet for each drug. The sulphonylureas can be combined with metformin or glitazones. The glitazones can also be combined with metformin and such combinations are available in the pharmacopoeia. Double or triple drug therapy trials have shown improvement in glycaemic control. Four drugs (SUs, biguanide, glitazone and AGI) therapy may also be used with greater success. The advantages of combination drug therapy are better compliance (because of lesser number of tablets), lesser side effects due to lesser dosage of drugs used and lesser cost.

The algorithm for management of type 2 diabetes is shown in Figure 26.3.5.

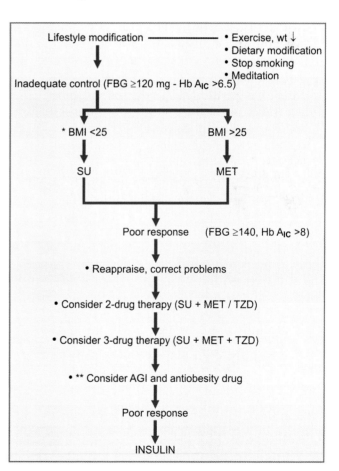

Fig. 26.3.5: Algorithm for management of type-2 diabetes
* *Even if BMI is less than 25, metformin can still be used on individual merits*
** *These drugs can be added at any stage in the above algorithm*

SUMMARY

The purpose of treatment in type 2 diabetes is to ameliorate the symptoms and prevent acute and chronic complications. Drug treatment should not be started without initial management by diet and exercise. Currently, there are five distinct classes of hypoglycaemic agents available, each class displaying unique pharmacologic properties. These classes are the sulphonylureas, meglitinides, biguanides, thiazolidinediones and alpha-glucosidase inhibitors:

1. Sulphonylureas (SUs) stimulate insulin secretion by binding to sulphonylurea receptors on the β-cell membrane and bring down blood glucose levels. The most serious side effect is hypoglycaemia.

2. Metformin is a biguanide that lowers blood glucose by several mechanisms related to insulin sensitivity but mainly by decreasing hepatic glucose output.

3. Meglitinides are short acting agents. They stimulate insulin secretion by binding near the sulphonylurea receptor. These drugs are ideal for postprandial hyperglycaemia.

4. Thiazolidinediones are insulin sensitizers, they bind to nuclear PPAR gamma receptor and enhance the expression of certain insulin sensitive genes, thereby increasing insulin sensitivity. Their use may be associated with weight gain and fluid retention.

5. Alpha-glucosidase-inhibitors (AGI), they inhibit alpha-glucosidase enzymes in the gut, thereby delaying carbohydrate absorption and reducing postprandial blood glucose peaks. The drugs having different modes of action can be used in combination (double, triple or even four drugs) to achieve target blood glucose level.

FURTHER READING

1. Bailey CJ. Potential new treatment for type 2 diabetes. Trends Pharma Sci 2000;21:259-65.
2. Fuhlendorff J, Rorsman P, Kofod H, et al. Stimulation of insulin release by repaglinide and glibenclamide involves both common and distinct processes. Diabetes 1998; 47: 345-51.
3. Garber AJ. Efficacy of metformin in type 2 diabetes: results of a double-blind, placebo controlled, dose response trial. Am J Med 1997;103:491-7.
4. Samraj GPN, Quillen DM, Kuritzky L. Improving management of type 2 diabetes mellitus: thiazolidinediones. Hosp Pract November 2000;123-32.
5. Granberry MC, Fonseca VA. Insulin resistance syndrome: options for treatment. South Med J 1999;92:2-15.
6. Damsbo P, Clauson P, Marbury TC, Windfeld K. A double-blind randomized comparison of meal-related glycemic control by repaglinide and glyburide in well-controlled type 2 diabetic patients. Diabetes Care 1999;22:789-94.
7. Wolffenbuttel BH, Landgraf R, for the Dutch and German Repaglinide Study Group. A 1-year multicenter randomized double-blind comparison of repaglinide and glyburide for the treatment of type 2 diabetes. Diabetes Care 1999;22:463-7.
8. Moses R, Slobodniuk R, Boyages S, et al. Effect of rapaglinide addition to metformin monotherapy on glycemic control in patients with type 2 diabetes. Diabetes Care 1999;22:119-24.
9. Lebovitz He. Alpha-glucosidase inhibitors. Endocrinal Metab Clin North Am 1997;26:539-51.

26.4 Basic Considerations of Insulin Therapy in Diabetes Mellitus

Y Sachdev

- Insulin Preparations
  - Human, Bovine, Porcine
  - Semisynthetic Human Insulin
  - Recombinant DNA (Biosynthetic) Human Insulin
- Insulin Purity
- Types of Insulin
  - Short Acting Regular
  - Intermediate Acting
  - Long Acting

- Premixed
- Technique of Injections
- Insulin Analogues
- Injection Sites
- Storage of Insulin
- Insulin Syringe and Needles
- Noninvasive Insulin Delivery Systems
- Summary

INSULIN PREPARATIONS

Insulin is in therapeutic use since early 1920s and is still the mainstay of treatment of diabetes. Insulin manufactured from the animal source—bovine or pork—is no longer in use in most of the countries. Human insulin differs from bovine insulin by three amino acids and from porcine insulin by one amino acid (Fig. 26.4.1 and Table 26.4.1). Human insulin is manufactured by two processes:

- Semisynthetic human insulin (enzyme modified-porcine insulin), and

- Recombinant DNA techniques (biosynthetic human insulin).

Currently insulin preparations in use are generated by recombinant DNA technology using laboratory strains of *E. coli* bacteria or yeast that have been genetically altered by the addition of the gene for human insulin production. There are two methods of making insulin by the recombinant DNA technique:

a. HI crb-chain recombinant bacterial. Here, the *E. coli* bacteria containing the gene for chain A of insulin make chain A, and the bacteria containing the gene

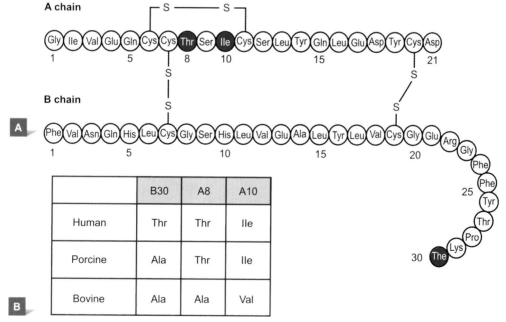

	B30	A8	A10
Human	Thr	Thr	Ile
Porcine	Ala	Thr	Ile
Bovine	Ala	Ala	Val

Figs 26.4.1A and B: (A) The amino acid sequence of human insulin. (B) Amino acid variations in human, porcine and bovine insulin

TABLE 26.4.1

Positions	Chain A			Chain B
	A 8	A9	A10	B 30
Human	THR	SER	ILEU	THR
Porcine	THR	SER	ILEU	ALA
Bovine	ALA	SER	VAL	ALA

Amino acid differences in human, bovine and porcine insulin

for chain B make chain B. The separate chains are isolated from the two ferments and are chemically combined.

b. HI prb-proinsulin recombinant bacterial. In this method the bacteria contain the gene for intact proinsulin. The proinsulin obtained is enzymatically cleaved to obtain intact insulin.

All preparations of insulin have similar physiological effects. They differ only in the rapidity of onset of action, time taken to reach peak and duration of action depending upon their chemical nature. Human insulin is absorbed rapidly and has a shorter duration of action (Table 26.4.2).

INSULIN PURITY

Insulin purity determines the antigenicity of insulin preparations. The quantitative presence of proinsulin contamination is taken as the criterion of purity. Earlier standard insulin preparations contained proinsulin and other impurities in concentration of 10,000 to 30,000 parts per million (ppm). Subsequently insulin preparations were routinely purified by gel-filtration and more recently by ion-exchange chromatography and other molecular sieving techniques. With progressive improvement in the purity standards, presently, the standard insulin preparations have only 10 to 20 ppm of proinsulin while purified monocomponent insulin have less than 1 ppm (Table 26.4.3). These advancements have

TABLE 26.4.2

Preparation	Onset of action	Peak of action	Duration of action
Short acting/soluble/Rapid/regular			
Bovine/porcine	30 minutes	2 to 4 hr	4 to 8 hr
Human	20 minutes	2 to 4 hr	4 to 8 hr
Intermediate acting			
NPH	1 to 3 hr	6 to 8 hr	12 to 16 hr
Lente	1 to 4 hr	6 to 10 hr	12 to 18 hr
Long acting			
Ultra lente	2 to 4 hr	8 to 10 hr	16 to 24 hr
Analogues			
Short acting			
Lispro	15 minutes	1 hr	3 to 4 hr
Aspart	15 minutes	1 hr	3 to 4 hr
Long acting			
Glargine	6 hr	Broad peak lasting for 24 hr	
Detemir	4 to 5 hr	Broad peak lasting for 12 hr	

Pharmacokinetics of commercially available insulin preparations

TABLE 26.4.3

Insulin types	Proinsulin (ppm)
• Conventional insulin (Porcine, bovine)	10,000 to 30,000
• Gel filtration purified insulin	3,000 to 10,000
• Chromatographically purified single peak insulin	300 to 3,000
• Improved single peak purified insulin	<50
• Highly purified	<10
• Mono-component	<1

Proinsulin impurity in commercially available insulin preparations

led to lesser insulin immunogenicity-related problems like insulin allergy, insulin resistance and localized insulin reactions including lipoatrophy. Recombinant human insulin is the best available insulin. However, it is costly and several patients can ill afford it. In such cases, highly purified bovine insulin (with proinsulin < 2 ppm) and monocomponent (proinsulin < 1 ppm) porcine insulin offer a cost effective alternative and may be used.

TYPES OF INSULIN

There are various types of insulin available in the market. They are usually classified as per their therapeutic effectiveness and action profile as:
• Regular/rapid/short acting
• Intermediate acting
• Long acting
• Insulin analogues.

Table 26.4.2 gives the pharmacokinetics of commercially available insulin preparations.

Regular (actrapid) insulin is a short acting soluble clear, crystalline zinc insulin. It is the only insulin which can be given intravenously and is used as low dose insulin infusion in diabetic ketoacidosis. Lente insulin is a mixture of 30% semi-lente and 70% ultralente insulin. Lente insulins are insoluble insulin suspensions made by adding excess zinc ions to insulin. Ultralente is a very slow acting insulin with a prolonged duration of action. NPH is an intermediate acting insoluble suspension of insulin with the highly basic trout or salmon protein, protamine together with zinc ions at neutral (pH 7.1 to 7.4) pH. This is also called isophane as it contains equivalent amount of insulin and protamine. It is called NPH (neutral protamine Hagedoen) after the Hagedoen laboratories in Copenhagen where it was developed in 1940s. Both isophane and lente have action duration of about 8 to 12 hours. A variation of lente called ultralente, with larger, more insoluble crystals, has a duration of over 24 hours when made from beef insulin. Its human formulation has similar duration as isophane and lente.

Stable premixed or biphasic insulin preparations containing regular and NPH in various proportions are also available (Fig. 26.4.2). Frequently used pre-mixed insulin are 30:70 (30% regular + 70% NPH); 25/75, 20/80, 50/50 and so on. These premixed insulin have been made available for convenience of the patient and to cater for their different eating habits.

It has been experienced that to achieve an ideal control, it is necessary to mix short-acting and intermediate acting insulin. For this purpose NPH and

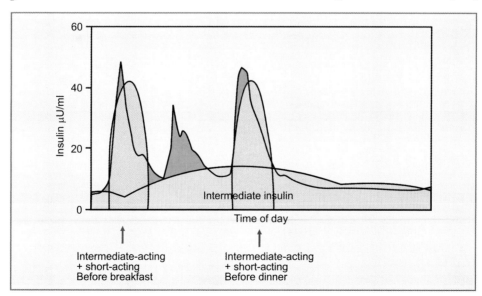

Fig. 26.4.2: Pre-mix insulin injections twice daily

crystalline insulin combination is considered ideal as 'isophane' nature of NPH insulin does not delay absorption of admixed regular insulin.

The excess zinc in lente insulin is liable to bind the soluble insulin and transform it into long acting type and partially blunt its action. If lente and regular insulin are to be mixed then, the mixture must be injected immediately within 3 to 5 minutes of mixing. It is to be remembered that only neutral (and not acidic) insulin preparations are mixed.

In India, insulin is available in two strengths: 40 units and 100 units of insulin per ml. Similarly, two types of disposable plastic insulin syringes with microfine needles are available. It must be ensured that the number of units per ml on insulin vial match with the number of units/ml on insulin syringe. This means, insulin syringe marked 40 units per ml must be used to inject 40 units per ml insulin only. Similarly, 100 units per ml insulin syringe is used for 100 units per ml insulin vial only. Recently, disposable/non-disposable insulin pen devices have been brought out in the market by various pharmaceutical companies. These pens are user-friendly, easy to carry and extremely useful for multiple daily injections.

Insulin syringes are for one time use only. Some patients, however, go on re-using them till the needle becomes blunt. In such cases, needle must be recapped after each use. Most insulin preparations have bacteriostatic additives (such as metacresol and phenol or methylparaben) to inhibit growth of commonly found skin bacteria. Therefore, if due care is taken about needles/pens, the chances of infection by injection are remote.

TECHNIQUE OF INJECTION

Insulin is given subcutaneously for better absorption (Fig. 26.4.3). It is imperative to use a short hypodermic needle with the syringe held perpendicular to the skin (Fig. 26.4.4). If the patient is thin and emaciated, the skin could be lifted up and injection given in raised skin fold with the syringe held at 45° angle (Fig. 26.4.5). It must be ensured that the needle should not penetrate more than 3 to 5 mm. After the injection is completed, pressure with a sterile swab and finger must be kept for about one minute to prevent outward leakage of the injected insulin. No local rubbing should be done. The absorption and response is dependent on the depth of injection (absorption is rapid and erratic if injection is given IM), quantity of injection, type of insulin, exercise of the injected limb/bodypart, antibodies to insulin, insulin receptor problems, local blood flow, ambient temperature and alterations in hepatic and renal functions (Table 24.4.4). Besides these factors, the site of injection is also important. IM injection is given only in shock when subcutaneous absorption is doubtful. Usual sites used (Fig. 26.4.6) are:

- Front of the thigh and abdominal wall where absorption is quickest

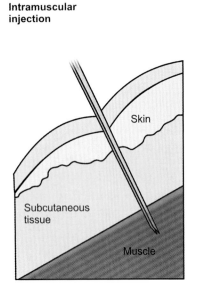
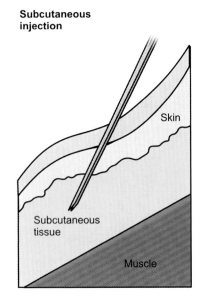

Intramuscular injection

Skin

Subcutaneous tissue

Muscle

Subcutaneous injection

Skin

Subcutaneous tissue

Muscle

Fig. 26.4.3: Modes of insulin injections
(Subcutaneous injection has better and steady absorption. Intramuscular injection has rapid and erratic absorption)

Derby Hospitals NHS Foundation
Trust
Library and Knowledge Service,

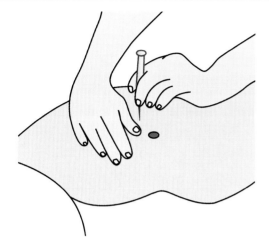

Fig. 26.4.4: Syringe is held perpendicular to the skin

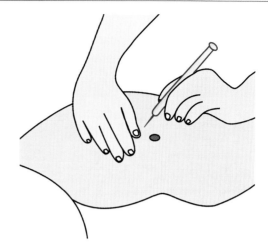

Fig. 26.4.5: Syringe held at 45° to the skin in thin and emaciated patient (correct way to inject)

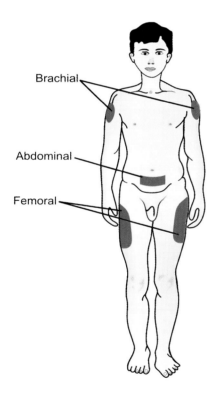

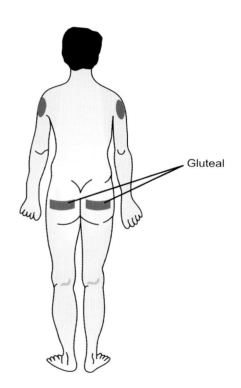

Fig. 26.4.6: Various commonly used sites for insulin injections

- Gluteal region where absorption is slowest, and
- Detoid and outer aspect of the thighs where absorption is intermediate.

The injected site must be changed every time and the distance between two injections sites must be minimum 2.5 to 3 cm. It is always better to use one area of the body (anterior abdominal wall or deltoid/thigh region) for injections so as to standardize insulin absorption. Some prefer to give short acting insulin in abdomen for quick action and long acting insulin in the buttock for slow absorption. When two types of insulin are to be mixed, the following procedure is recommended to be followed:

- The vial having hazy insulin should be gently rolled in the palms to resuspend insulin (Fig. 26.4.7). It should never be shaken
- Inject air equal to the dose of insulin required into the vial to avoid creating a vacuum

Derby Hospitals NHS Foundation Trust

Library and Knowledge Service

TABLE 26.4.4

- Site of injection
- Absorption is quickest from front of the thigh/abdomen while it is slowest deltoid and gluteal region
- Depth of insulin injection
- Quantity of insulin injected
- Type of insulin injected
- Exercise to the injected site
- Local rubbing after injection
- Antibodies to insulin
- Insulin receptors abnormalities
- Blood supply to the injected site
- Ambient temperature
- Hepatic status
- Renal status

Factors which influence insulin absorption and response

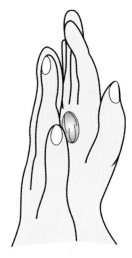

Fig. 26.4.7: Gently roll in the palms. Hazy insulin before injection. Don't shake it

- Draw into the syringe the rapid or short acting insulin first
- Insulin of the same species only should be used for mixing.

INSULIN ANALOGUES

Monomeric insulin analogues have been introduced to speed up the absorption of insulin injection. They have the same biological activity as human insulin. The pharmacokinetics, however, are different. In these analogues certain amino acids of insulin polypeptide chain which are involved in insulin activity or stability

are substituted or interchanged (Fig. 26.4.8). This makes them more effective in certain aspects.

The main disadvantage of exogenous insulin administration is the non-physiological high insulin levels in the peripheral circulation compared to the high portal insulinaemia seen physiologically in the post-prandial state.

In the nondiabetic state, the ingestion of a meal is accompanied by a rapid rise in insulin value which reaches a peak at above ½ to 1 hour time and returns to the baseline after about 4 hours (Fig. 26.4.9).

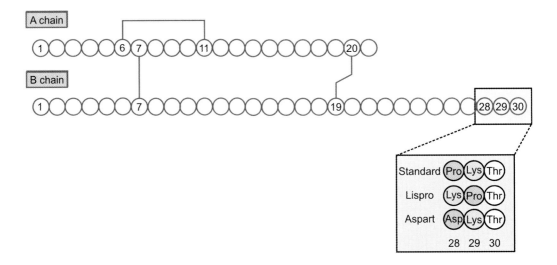

Fig. 26.4.8: Amino acid differences between standard insulin and its rapid acting analogues (lispro and aspart)

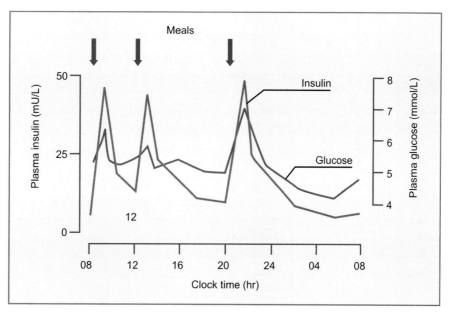

Fig. 26.4.9: Profiles of plasma glucose and insulin concentration in nondiabetic individuals

The absorption pattern of the exogenously administered unmodified insulin preparations is such that it cannot mimic the physiological meal-related events. The absorption of subcutaneously administered insulin in the peripheral circulation is initially too slow and is followed by supraphysiological levels between meals with the consequent risk of hypoglycaemia. The use of the best available human actrapid insulin for multiple daily injections results in too little insulin available immediately after meals and too much insulin between the meals. The delay in absorption of human insulin from the injection site is due to the rate of dissociation from the hexameric units to lower association dimers and monomers states (Fig. 26.4.10).

Genetic engineering technology and increased physiochemical knowledge of the insulin molecule has made it possible for us to create insulin analogues in monomeric state retaining the same biological activity. The interactions between monomers in insulin, dimers and hexamers were analyzed and the tendency for insulin molecule to self-associate was modified by specifically altering the amino acids whose side chains were involved in dimer/hexamer formation. The targets chosen for mutations were those amino acids residues involved in dimer formation but located on the periphery of the putative site for insulin receptor binding, thus retaining the biological activity. The main strategy was to insert more negatively charged amino acids which would decrease the tendency of the molecule to form dimers (see Fig. 26.4.8).

Lispro

It is the first analogue to be marketed (Homalog; Elililly).

In this analogue amino acid lysine which is at position 28 of the β chain and proline which is at position 29 are reversed. This results in an analogue which has more rapid absorption and faster excretion (Peak 99 ± 39 minutes, compared to actrapid 178 ± 93 minutes). These two qualities make lispro a more suitable insulin to control postprandial glucose peaks than the regular insulin (Fig. 26.4.11).

Aspart (Novo Rapid, Novo Nordisk)

It differs from human insulin by substitution of aspartic acid for proline in position 28 on the β chain. This results in a more rapid onset of action and shorter duration (peak action 94±46 minutes, compared to actrapid 173±62 minutes). Like Lispro, it is more suitable for hyperglycaemia and there is a lower risk of postprandial hypoglycaemia. Both these analogues are injected immediately before or after meals. Premix 30:70/25:75 short and intermediate acting analogues are also available in the 'pen' form and are becoming popular. (Novomix 30; Humalog Mix 25).

Insulin Glulisine

It is another rapidly acting analogue which is undergoing clinical trials. Here lysine replaces aspartate at β_3 and glutamate is at β_{29} instead of lysine.

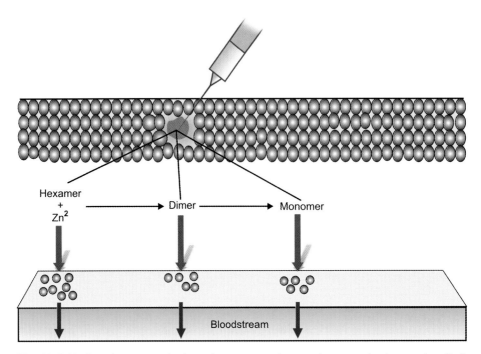

Fig. 26.4.10: Putative events in the subcutaneous tissue where regular human insulin is broken to dimer and monomer insulin

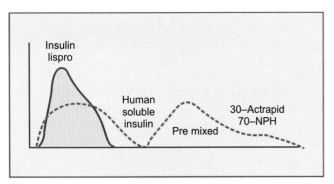

Fig. 26.4.11: Comparison of lispro and human actrapid insulins

Glargine (Lantus; Aventis)

Glargine is a human insulin analogue. It differs from the human insulin by the:
- addition of two arginines to the C terminus of β chain, and
- substitution of the glycine for asparagine at position A 21.

Glargine is produced by recombinant DNA technology from nonpathogenic *E. coli* bacteria. It is soluble at pH 4 but has slow solubility when injected into neutral pH environment. After glargine is injected, micro-precipitates form and the insulin has to be desolubilized. This results in slow insulin absorption and provides a relatively constant level of insulin with practically no peaks over 24-hour time period. This analogue is as potent as human insulin, has a long half-life and requires only one dose in 24 hours (Fig. 26.4.12). Unlike isophane, it causes less nocturnal hypoglycaemia and less variation in fasting blood glucose values. Presently, it is available as clear lavender coloured aquous solution of 100 units/ml.

Detemir (NN 304; Nordisk)

Detemir (NN 304; Nordisk) is another long acting analogue. It is acylated with a fatty acid at the C terminus of β chain (β_{29} and β_{30}). The fatty acid binds to the albumin slowing insulin absorption and prolonging circulation time. It has a shorter action time compared to glargine and twice daily injections are needed.

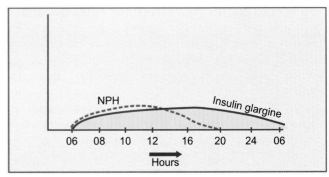

Fig. 26.4.12: Comparison of duration of action of NPH and glargine insulin

The weight gain with insulin analogues is less compared to standard human insulin.

STORAGE OF INSULIN

- Insulin vials should be kept in refrigerator at 2 to 8°C/icebox/in closed cabinets and under clothes. However, they should not be frozen
- Insulin should not be exposed to direct sunlight
- Avoid excessive shaking/agitation of insulin as it results in loss of potency, clumping, frosting, formation of larger particles and precipitation
- Insulin vial in use may be kept at room temperature for 4 to 6 weeks
- Once the vial is opened, discard it after 28 days as its potency gets reduced. Insulin in cartridges and pens probably loses its priority early as compared to vials due to environmental differences
- If regular insulin becomes hazy or changes colour, do not use it as it indicates bacterial growth and contamination.

These instructions are for strict compliance. Patients are advised to read the literature enclosed with insulin vial.

INSULIN SYRINGES AND NEEDLES

The newer insulin needles cause less discomfort compared to previously available needles. They are of a finer gauge, shorter length, sharper point and smooth surface. Insulin pen technology has made insulin administration much easier, convenient and accurate in dosage.

NON-INVASIVE INSULIN DELIVERY SYSTEMS

There are many potential alternative routes for insulin delivery where injections are not required. Some of the routes being tried are: (i) transdermal, (ii) nasal, (iii) oral, (iv) buccal and (v) pulmonary.

Out of all these alternatives, the pulmonary route appears to be the most feasible. Table 26.11.5 describes some of the main features of these routes and their present status. Several pharmaceutical companies are involved in the development of pulmonary insulin delivery systems. The Exubera system (Nektar therapeutics, Cipla and Aventis) delivers a fine dry powder (<5 µm in diameter) of regular short acting human insulin to the deep lung. The powder is packed in a blister containing 1 or 3 mg of insulin (1 mg = 3 Units) and is delivered to the lungs by a inhalation device (nebulizer). The results are quite encouraging. It is expected that this route will enable us to use it as a monotherapy or in combination with oral drugs.

TABLE 26.4.5

High pressure jet injectors
- No injections
- Insulin is delivered in a stream under high pressure across the skin into subcutaneous tissue
- Useful in those who develop reactions with injections like severe lipoatrophy
- Not as comfortable as claimed

Transdermal: Insulin is delivered across the skin barrier by the help of:
a. Iontophoresis: Electrical current is used to enhance transdermal delivery.
b. Low-frequency ultrasound.
c. Transfersomes: Composite phosphotidyl choline-based vesicles with similar permeability to water.

Transdermal administration over 40 cm² skin area may supply significant basal insulin in a classical T1DM patient.

Intranasal
Permeability enhancers (like lecithin, bile salts, laureth-9) are required to increase insulin bioavailability. Nasal irritation and poor absorption are well known limitations. Better results are expected with gelified nasal insulin.

Oral
a. Enteric: Oral enteric insulin delivery has limited bioavailability.
b. Buccal: Liquid aerosol insulin baccal spray with enhancers, stabilizers is being tried.

Pulmonary
Large surface area of the lungs and high permeability are favourable for insulin delivery.
Insulin is rapidly absorbed after inhalation
Comparable to subcutaneous actrapid insulin injection

Various non-invasive insulin delivery routes

SUMMARY

The subsection deals with basic issues of insulin therapy in diabetes mellitus. It describes the various types of insulin preparations available in the market and their differences in pharmacokinetics.

It also deals with the correct technique and various sites for insulin injection, storage of insulin and insulin analogues. The latest situation regarding various noninvasive insulin delivery systems has also been referred to in brief.

FURTHER READING

1. Bethel MA, Feinglos MN. Insulin analogues. New therapies for type 2 diabetes mellitus (review). Cure Diab Reg 2002; 2(5) : 17-30.
2. Cefalu WT. Concept, strategies and faceability of non-invasive insulin therapy. Diabetes Care 2004; 27: 239-46.

26.5 Strategy of Insulin Therapy in T1DM and T2DM

Y Sachdev

INTRODUCTION

For the ideal control of hyperglycaemia with insulin, it is obligatory that:

- Every institution works out its policy/strategy for the control of diabetes laying down in clear terms when insulin therapy is to be initiated and how to overcome resistance/barriers posed by the patient/family.
- Despite institute policy, each patient requires an individualized approach.
- Attending physician must determine how much calories are required to be given and in how many portions it is to be split.
- Insulin: Carbohydrate ratio must be determined, that is, determine how many units of insulin will neutralize 15 or 20 gm of carbohydrate snack in your patient.
- Similarly, determine insulin/snack/exercise relationship.
- Start with a small dose of insulin (unless it is an emergency) and work it up.
- Lay down the targets of glycaemic control in each patient.
- Achieve these targets with once a day insulin/insulin OHA/multiple insulin injection/insulin pump.

INSULIN THERAPY IN TYPE 1 DIABETES MELLITUS

Children with type 1 DM need a careful handling. They are best managed by a combination of:

- Individual and group education
- Intensive self care training, and
- Self insulin injection.

The training is best conducted under medical supervision over at least one week.

This could be provided after admission in a health facility centre (or better still as an outpatient) where patient is permitted to follow the normal daily routine. Mother should be intimately involved in the training and education (see guidelines at the end of the subsection).

The insulin therapy is better started as 0.2 to 0.3 Units per kg/day. Out of this 25 to 30% are given in the form of NPH or Lente at bed time and remaining 75 to 70% is given as regular insulin with three main meals which could be 25% with breakfast and 22.5% with lunch and 22.5% with dinner depending upon the quantum of food intake. In this four-injection (basal-bolus) regimen, intermediate acting insulin provides the background or basal concentration. Its dose is adjusted as per fasting blood glucose value while the regular (bolus) insulin dose is adjusted as per postprandial blood glucose value of the previous day.

Some diabetologists initially start with actrapid (regular) insulin given with three or more main meals and then once the blood sugar is under reasonable control (F 90 to 95 mg/dl; pre-meal 100 to 120 mg/dl, post-meal 130 to 140 mg/dl) they use combination of insulin (regular + NPH/lente) in 2 or 4 doses as indicated above (Figs 26.5.1A to C). In this regimen, the postprandial glycaemia is controlled by regular insulin which encourages the peripheral glucose uptake, while the low and steady concentration of basal insulin is sufficient to restrain the hepatic glucose output during overnight fast and between meals and thus helps maintain normoglycaemia.

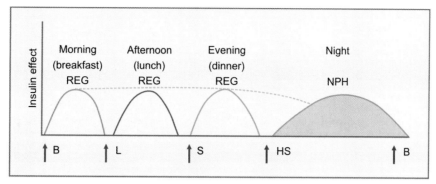

Fig. 26.5.1A: Regular insulin injection with three main meals and NPH at night

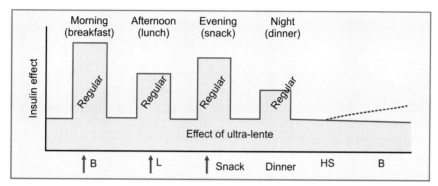

Fig. 26.5.1B: Four injections of regular insulin + one ultra-lente injection at night in 24 hours
(ultra-lente effect is variable and does not lasts for 24 hours in many patients)

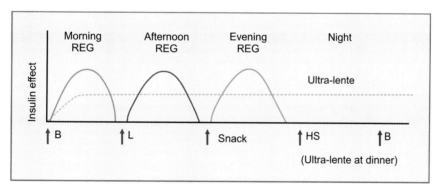

Fig. 26.5.1C: Three injections of regular insulin + one-ultralente at night

Sometimes the insulin requirements are very high and three injections with main meals do not suffice or produce hypoglycaemia, in those patients it is advisable to give multiple injections of short acting regular insulin with each meal—main meal as well as snacks (Figs 26.5.2A to C).

In this 'intensive' or 'optimized' diabetic therapy, the aim of insulin replacement is to mimic physiological insulin delivery and avoid wide fluctuations of hyper or hypoglycaemia. To ensure this, besides the monitoring of premeal and post-meal blood glucose values, it is

advisable to test 3 AM blood glucose value once a week and keep it above 60 mg/dl.

Caution: In most type 1 DM patients, control of symptoms and hyperglycaemia is achieved with relative ease utilizing above mentioned therapeutic approach. In those where hypoglycaemia is frequent, combination of NPH/lente with regular insulin may work better. In some patients, the insulin dose adjustment may be a never-ending exercise with frequent dose changes accompanied by frequent hyperglycaemia/hypo-

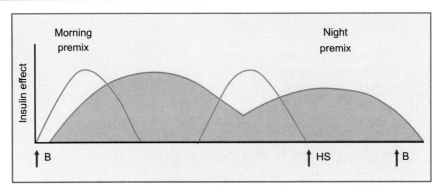

Fig. 26.5.2A: Two injections of premix insulin (regular + NPH) before breakfast and dinner

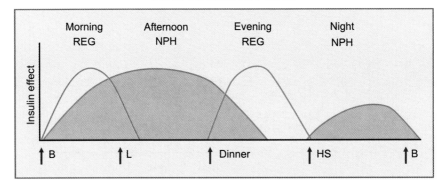

Fig. 26.5.2B: Morning injection (regular + NPH). Regular with dinner and NPH on retiring at night

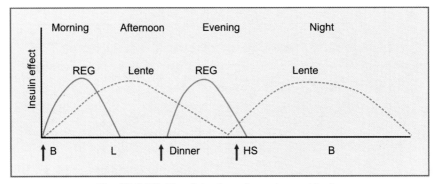

Fig. 26.5.2C: Two injection of regular and lente

Figs 26.5.1 and 26.5.2: Various options for basal-bolus insulin regimens

glycaemic episodes. The reason for this brittleness could be dietary inconsistency, stress, variations in insulin absorption, fluctuating levels of insulin antibodies, alterations in gastric emptying and many other unidentified factors. Brittle control of diabetes demands careful attention to minor details (like technique and site of injection, time interval between meal and injection, check on insulin dose measurement, expiry/in use date of the vial, calorie intake and standards of laboratory testing the blood samples) and more energetic glycaemic management. At the same time, it must be borne in mind

that this insulin replacement regimen is not entirely 'physiological' as the injected insulin is absorbed into the peripheral blood rather than portal bloodstream. Thus effective 'insulinization' of the liver is achieved only at the expense of systemic hyperinsulinaemia. Moreover, short acting insulins are absorbed too slowly to mimic precisely the normal prandial peak and must be given 20 to 30 minutes before meal to optimize the postprandial glucose peak. The slow absorption is due to the fact that injected insulin is in hexameric form (20 to 30% of injected insulin forms aggregates which slows absorption and reduces biologic activity and is required to be converted into dimers and monomers that can be readily absorbed (see Fig. 26.4.10).

Once a reasonable glycaemic pattern is obtained, a sliding scale may be prescribed to the patient to guide daily dose adjustments. Thus, night NPH/morning soluble insulin dose adjustment guidelines could be as under:

- If fasting blood glucose is > 90 mg/dl, add 1 to 2 units of NPH at night
- If it is < 60 mg/dl minus 1 to 2 units of NPH at night
- If PP blood sugar is > 140 mg/dl add 2 units of soluble insulin
- If it is < 120 mg/dl minus 1 to 2 units of soluble insulin.

When multiple daily injections of rapid insulin, insulin analogues are used then the sliding scale could be as given in Table 26.5.1.

If fasting or premeal blood sugar is widely off the target value, insulin dose is to be modified as indicated.

The above mentioned management of type 1 DM with insulin is to be taken only as a guideline as each patient needs a detailed evaluation and individualized management approach.

A common and useful guiding approach to insulin therapy in type 1 diabetes mellitus is:

- Short acting insulin/rapid-acting insulin analogues with each of the three main meals (breakfast, lunch, dinner) or only breakfast and evening meal if lunch is small
- Dose of insulin is adjusted as per carbohydrate content of each meal and postprandial blood glucose value
- Isophane or lente is given either once or twice a day. If the evening dose of isophane/lente is given with the evening meal, it may cause nocturnal hypoglycaemia at about 0100 to 0300 hours. Thereafter, as the insulin sensitivity decreases in the early morning hours because of GH surge during sleep, there is fasting hyperglycaemia (the 'dawn phenomenon'). The problem can be controlled by giving the isophane/lente insulin injection at bed time
- In some patients, duration of glargine insulin effectiveness is substantially shorter than 24 hours. These cases may require twice daily administration of this insulin to be effective.
- The diabetic patients are advised not to observe religious fasts in case their control is brittle and ketosis prone. Those who are on insulin should adjust the insulin timing so as to have a small dose with

TABLE 26.5.1

Blood glucose value (mg/dl)	Insulin dose	Comment
<60	Minus 1 to 2 units insulin	Give insulin during meal. At least 10 gm of simple carbohydrate must be consumed in the meal
60-90	No change	
90-120	Add 1 unit	
120-150	Add 2 units	
150-200	Add 3 units	Inject insulin 10 to 15 minutes before meals
200-250	Add 4 units	Inject insulin 20 to 30 minutes before meals
>250	Add 6 units	

Sliding scale indicating modification in insulin dose in T1DM

morning snack before starting the fast and a larger evening dose with the evening meal when they break the fast.

Insulin Administration by an External Insulin Pump (Figs 26.5.3 and 26.5.4)

External mechanical pump is an alternative method of delivering insulin. These artificial insulin delivery systems can be either, 'open-loop' in which insulin infusion rate is preselected by the doctor/patient or 'closed-loop' in which there is continuous glucose sensing and computer controlled insulin delivery (the so called artificial pancreas). Rapidly acting insulin preparation is delivered by continuous subcutaneous infusion (CS II) through a catheter usually inserted into the subcutaneous tissue of the anterior abdominal wall. The pump is programmed to administer basal infusion as well as patient-directed boluses given before meals and snacks or in response to blood glucose values outside the desired range. The pump is usually worn around the waist and the infusion cannula sited in the abdomen. Currently available pumps infuse insulin basally at the rate of approximately 1 U/hour: they are programmed at predetermined times to increase the rate so that the blood glucose excursions are prevented. Protocols for insulin administration by the pump usually require approximately half the insulin to be administered as a basal infusion and the rest as premeal boluses.

Pumps are costly, tubings require a change every 24 to 72 hours and there is significant risk of infection. Monomeric insulin (Lispro/Aspart) is the pump insulin of choice. Blood glucose must be monitored by the patient

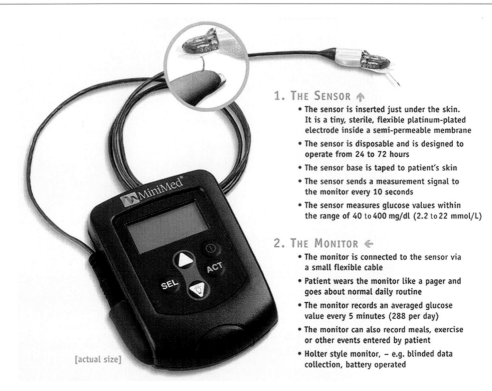

1. THE SENSOR ↑
  • The sensor is inserted just under the skin. It is a tiny, sterile, flexible platinum-plated electrode inside a semi-permeable membrane
  • The sensor is disposable and is designed to operate from 24 to 72 hours
  • The sensor base is taped to patient's skin
  • The sensor sends a measurement signal to the monitor every 10 seconds
  • The sensor measures glucose values within the range of 40 to 400 mg/dl (2.2 to 22 mmol/L)

2. THE MONITOR ←
  • The monitor is connected to the sensor via a small flexible cable
  • Patient wears the monitor like a pager and goes about normal daily routine
  • The monitor records an averaged glucose value every 5 minutes (288 per day)
  • The monitor can also record meals, exercise or other events entered by patient
  • Holter style monitor, – e.g. blinded data collection, battery operated

[actual size]

Fig. 26.5.3: Glucose in the interstitial fluid reacts with glucose oxidase within the sensor generating a tiny electrical signal

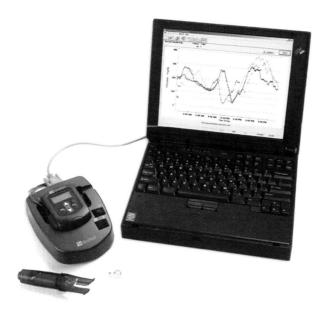

Fig. 26.5.4: The collected data being down loaded on PC with CGMS system software

frequently and he/she should always be alert to the possibility of the failure of the infusion system. In the present Indian scenario, their use appears to be limited.

A typical strategy for starting pump therapy is to calculate the infusion rates by reducing the patients' usual daily dose by 20%; allocating ½ to basal rate (about 0.9 U/hour in adults and 1.3 mU/kg/hour in children) and the other half divided between the three main meals. Basal insulin rate is adjusted as per fasting and 0300 hours blood glucose value while prandial insulin rate is adjusted by postprandial blood glucose value (Fig. 26.5.5). Carbohydrate content of a meal will help in adjustment of prandial insulin dose. The usual guidelines are:
• One unit insulin per 15 gm carbohydrate
• One unit insulin per 10 gm carbohydrate (in insulin resistant cases)
• One unit insulin per 20 gm of carbohydrate (in insulin sensitive cases, e.g. children).

For the success of insulin pump (continuous subcutaneous insulin infusion, CS II) prerequisites are: a willing and motivated patient, who is able to look after and regulate the insulin flow, and can monitor blood glucose, and a health care team (Specialist nurse and health visitor) with special interest in insulin pump therapy. The best established clinical indication for CS II trial is T1DM patients who do not achieve ideal glycaemic control by repeated insulin injections and/or having frequent, unpredictable hypoglycaemic episodes and difficult to control GDM.

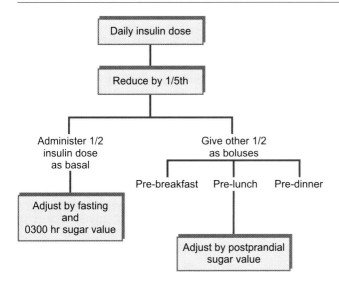

Fig. 26.5.5: Suggested strategy for continuous subcutaneous insulin infusion (CS II)

Inhaled Insulin

Clinical trials are underway with insulin which can be inhaled as an aerosolized dry powder or a liquid formulation using mechanically or electrically controlled inhaler devices. Inhaled insulin is absorbed more quickly than the regular subcutaneous insulin injections and may prove to be useful for meal time control as its bioavailability is only 10 to 20% and peak activity only 30 minutes. Newer modes have been developed for pulmonary administration of human insulin with similar bioavailability and activity as subcutaneous route.

Intranasal and oral insulin are the other alternative routes.

INSULIN THERAPY IN TYPE 2 DIABETES MELLITUS

The management objectives of T2DM are the same as T1DM:
- To achieve ideal glycaemic control,
- Maintain body weight 5 to 6% below standard ideal weight,
- Prevent acute/chronic diabetic complications and
- Ensure that diabetic individual lives a healthy and useful life.

Insulin therapy is not mandatory in T2DM. Insulin therapy is recommended only if diet control, lifestyle changes and oral hypoglycaemic drugs used in combination fail to achieve an ideal glycaemic state. Some diabetologists however, advise insulin therapy as first line treatment along with lifestyle and dietary changes for freshly diagnosed T2DM.

It is recommended that in T2DM cases initially one injection of NPH may be introduced at bed time. Initial dose of NPH or intermediate acting insulin may be calculated as per body weight. In our centre, we usually start with 0.2 to 0.4 U/kg body weight given s/c before dinner. This is the initial dose and is modified on subsequent days as per fasting blood glucose value. The NPH insulin dose can also be calculated as per fasting blood glucose value by the formulae given below:

(a) For normal weight diabetic patient:
Approximate initial insulin dose

$$= \frac{\text{Fasting Blood Glucose (FBG)} - 50}{10}$$

(b) For overweight patients:
Approximate initial insulin dose

$$= \frac{\text{FBG} - 50}{10} \times 2.5 \times \left(\frac{\text{Actual weight (kg)}}{\text{Ideal weight (kg)}} - 1.5 \right)$$

In our experience one injection suffices only if daily insulin requirements are less than 40 units.

This regimen will control fasting hyperglycaemia. If one NPH injection does not control hyperglycaemia throughout the day, oral antihyperglycaemic/hypoglycaemic agents like metformin, glitazone and sulphonylureas may be continued during the daytime. This approach (bedtime insulin, daytime sulphonylureas-BIDS) works quite satisfactory in a number of T2DM patients. The insulin therapy can also be started before breakfast and oral agents in the afternoon/evening with meals.

If single injection does not succeed then two or more injections have to be administered. In such cases either three injections of regular insulin with each main meal may be added to bedtime NPH or two injections of regular insulin mixed with NPH/lente may be given before breakfast and dinner. In majority of type 2 DM patients, this regimen suffices; premixed insulin preparations like 25:75, 30:70 or 50:50 and so on are very handy in such patients. Once a satisfactory control is achieved, glitazones or other oral agents may be re-introduced to insulin therapy. Close glucose monitoring for 7 to 8 days must be done in such situations as many a time insulin dose requirements are markedly reduced on addition of glitazones (Fig. 26.5.6).

There are certain situations where management of T2DM with insulin becomes mandatory. These situations are enumerated in Table 26.5.2. It is to be stressed that it is not true if a type 2 DM is initiated on to insulin treatment, it will become a life long fixture as after variable period, some such patients can be reverted back to oral hypoglycaemic agents.

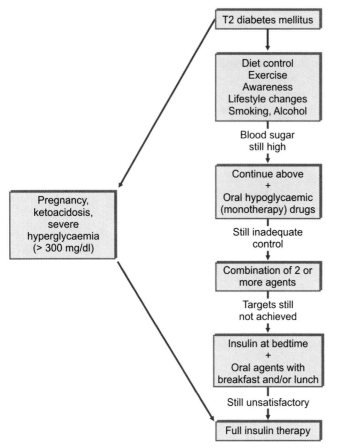

Fig. 26.5.6: Algorithm for treatment of T2DM

TABLE 26.5.2

- Diabetic kitoacidosis
- Hyperglycaemia over 280 mg/dl (fasting)
- Renal decompensation
- Hepatic decompensation
- Pregnancy
- Stessful conditions like
  - Acute myocardial infarction
  - Cerebrovascular accident
  - Fulminating infections
- Before and after major surgery
- Primary and secondary OHA failure
- Adverse reactions to oral drugs

Main indications of insulin therapy in type 2 DM

ADVERSE EFFECTS OF INSULIN THERAPY

- Local reactions:
  - Allergy
  - Lipoatrophy
  - Lipohypertrophy
- Hypoglycaemia
- Body weight gain. It is generally related to the daily injection dose.

Table 26.5.3 presents comparison of various monotherapies in the treatment of T2DM.

MONITORING OF GLYCAEMIC CONTROL

Persistent hyperglycaemia is associated with chronic diabetic complications which, if unchecked and undetected, lead to disastrous consequences. Therefore, it is imperative that regular glycaemic control monitoring is conducted and periodic medical consultations are sought to maintain proper progress. For this purpose, urine analysis for sugar, ketone and protein (proteinuria, microalbuminuria) and blood for Hb, glycosylated Hb and plasma glucose (F, prelunch, predinner) and (if convenient) PP—2 hr after main three meals) is carried out on periodic but well defined basis. Table 26.5.4 enumerates treatment targets followed at our diabetic centre.

Urine analysis for glucose by strips (uro-stripes) is an accepted alternative to blood glucose monitoring. It is definitely inferior to blood glucose monitoring but is cheaper and is still widely practised all over the country. It is recommended that urine glucose testing should be done on second voided urine in a postprandial state and if it is negative it does indicate an adequate control. It also demands a careful supervision of the patient to avoid any possibility of hypoglycaemia. Care must be taken that strips used are not expiry dated and correct procedure is adopted. Otherwise false-positive results may be observed. It must also be recommended that long standing diabetes patients may have higher than normal renal threshold whereas children and pregnant women have low or variable renal threshold. Urine tests are also affected by fluid intake and urine concentration. Some drugs may also interfere with the tests. All these limitations must be explained to the patient.

Urine Test for Ketone

One must look for presence of urinary ketones (ketonuria) if the:
- Blood sugar is 250 mg/dl or more
- Patient is dehydrated and complains of nausea, vomiting, abdominal pain
- Patient is a first time young diabetic
- Patient is pregnant and has poor glycaemic control
- Patient is having acute illness, infection, food deprivation, starvation and compliance of medication has been poor.

TABLE 26.5.3

Clinical profile	Lifestyle	Insulin	Sulphonylureas	Metformin	Glucosidase inhibitors	Glitazones (Piogli/Rosi)	Glinides (Repaglinide/nateglinide)
• Tissue/ system for action for action	• Hypothalamus • Muscle and fat ↓↓	Peripheral tissues Pancreatic insulin supplement	Beta cells	Liver	• Gut • Delays carbohydrates absorption	Muscle	Beta cells
• Fasting sugar	↓	↓↓↓↓	↓↓	↓↓	Hardly any effect	↓↓	–
• PP sugar	↓	↓↓↓↓	↓↓	↓↓	Excellent	↓↓	↓↓↓ (nateglinide is better than repaglinide)
• Glycated Hb	Variable change usually slight	1 to >2%	1 to 2%	1 to 2%	0.5 to 1%	0.5 to 2% 0.5 to 1%	1 to 2% with nateglinide with repaglinide
• Severe hypo-glycaemia	Nil	Yes	Yes	No	No	No	Yes with repaglinide, No with nateglinide
• Body weight	Reduction (especially in obese)	Gain	Gain	Marginal decrease	Marginal decrease	Decrease	Gain
• Lipid profile	Marginal reduction	Marginal decrease	Hardly any effect	Improves	Marginal decrease	Decrease with pioglitazone	No effect

Comparison of monotherapies in T2DM (effects and side effects)

TABLE 26.5.4

Patients profile		DCCT	Treatment	Targets	Our centre targets
a.	Fasting blood sugar mmol/L	Low risk <5.5	Arterial risk >6.5	Microvascular risk >6.0	Fasting <5.5 Premeal <6.6
	PP	<7.5	>7.5	>9.0	Postmeal <7.7
	Hb A$_1$C%	<6.5	>6.5	>7.5	<6.5
b.	Total cholesterol mmol/L	<4.8	4.8 to 6.0	>6.0	<4.65
	HDL	>1.2	1.0 to 1.2	>1.0	>1.03
	LDL	<3.0	3.0 to 4.0	>4.0	<2.5
	Triglyceride	<1.7	1.7 to 2.2	>2.2	<1.12
c.	Blood pressure	Low risk	—	Unacceptable	< 130/80
	General	<130/80	—	>140/90	—
	Patient with microalbuminuria	<125/75	—	—	<120/75
d.	Body mass index (kg/m^2)	Low risk	Acceptable	Increased risk	—
	Men	<25	25-27	>27	—
	Women	<24	24-26	>26	—

Treatment targets for diabetic patients

The ketone bodies are breakdown products of fatty acids. They are β-hydroxybutyric acid, acetoacetic acid and acetone. Urine ketone level is proportional to blood level and is affected by urine volume and concentration. Ketones are present in undetected amount in normal healthy individuals. Positive ketone readings are seen during fasting in some normal individuals and in 30% of pregnant women in their morning urine sample. Many drugs including some of the antihypertensive drugs (captopril) give false-positive results. Urinary strips are used and are reliable. In case of doubt, blood for serum ketones may be checked. This test, however, is time consuming.

Urine for Albumin

Morning sample for urinary proteins should be done in every suspected case of diabetes. If it is positive, 24 hours urine for proteinuria should be carried out. If it is negative, then 24 hours urine for albuminuria may be done and repeated every year. The test provides a fairly correct indication of renal status and is considered a reliable marker for cardiovascular function.

Blood Glucose Test

It is most reliable test for monitoring of glycaemic state and adequacy of therapy. The frequency of this test will depend upon the type of diabetes, therapy used and control achieved. It is always better to test blood glucose before each dose of treatment and in postprandial period. Depending upon the therapeutic management, the test could be twice/four times or even 6 times a day. The basic principle of monitoring is that it should be done with usual activity, diet and medicine intake. Once a person is stabilized then weekly, fortnightly or monthly testing of pre-meal and post-meal (F and PP) blood sugar is sufficient. As a rule, T1DM requires more frequent monitoring than T2DM.

Presently, with the easy availability of gluco-strips and glucometers, self monitoring of blood sugar is an easy, affordable, and cost effective method. It is, however, important to check periodically the measurement techniques and calibrate the glucometer with a standardized laboratory. Once the bottle is opened, the strips should be used within 60 days.

Glycosylated Hb Testing

Glycated proteins (including Hb and serum proteins) provide information regarding glycaemic state over an extended period of time depending upon their half-life in circulation. Usually, glycosylated HbA$_1$C is tested. HbA$_1$C is a specific glycosylated Hb that is an adduct of glucose attached to the β-chain terminal valine residue. The percentage of Hb glycation is proportional to the ambient glucose concentration and is a measure of average glycaemia over the preceding 10 to 12 weeks. As it is expressed in percentage of the total Hb, it is

TABLE 26.5.5

Hb A$_1$C%	Mean plasma glucose value (mg/dl)
6	130
7	165
8	200
9	230
10	265
11	300
12	340

Correlation between HbA$_1$C and mean plasma glucose

necessary that Hb is checked at the same time. Glycosylated Hb, obviously, will be less if total Hb is less. False high values are observed in haemoglobinopathies and haemolytic anaemia.

A change in HbA$_1$C of 1% indicates a blood glucose alteration of about 30 to 35 mg/dl. It is recommended that this test is done initially at diagnosis and repeated every three to six months. Table 26.5.5 gives the correlation between HbA$_1$C% and mean plasma glucose value as seen at our centre.

GUIDELINES AND SOME USEFUL INSTRUCTIONS FOR PARENTS/HEALTH CARE PERSONNEL

General Principles

- Keep diabetes regimen flexible especially in school going children
- Keep plasma glucose levels and HbA$_1$C value relatively at a higher level in infants to avoid hypoglycaemia and its effects on developing brain
- Infants and small children cannot communicate effectively. Therefore attendant should be alert to an 'altered' attitude and 'unusual' behaviour.

Parents Education

Infants

Parents must learn and be taught the:
- Basic of diabetes mellitus
- Skill of daily management of the diabetic infant
- Recognition of hypoglycaemic, altered and unusual behaviour
- Avoidance of wide fluctuations in glucose values
- To cope with extracaring-load of the diabetic infant (medicosocial worker/health visitor must share the burden)
- Appropriate blood glucose values must be defined.

Early Childhood

- With increasing activity and caloric requirements of the child, a workable daily schedule must be initiated and
- Targets of blood glucose levels be revised
- Parents must remember a temper tantrum may be a manifestation of hypoglycaemia
- Parents must monitor blood sugar values more frequently, and
- Share their anxiety, if any, with the care providing team.

Early School Going Child

Train the child to:
a. Take more responsibility of his/her needs (like urine/ blood glucose monitoring, insulin injections (Fig. 26.5.7), extrasnacks ingestion in case of strenuous exercise/games.
b. Recognise early symptoms of hypo-/hyperglycaemia
c. Use of glucometer.
d. Initiate appropriate remedial steps.

Mid School Going Child

By this time, the child understands the problem and is able to manage most of his daily requirements.
- Some children need moral support and encouragement
- Certain families initiate 'pump therapy' at this stage
- In such cases, care of the pump must be understood by the child.

Adolescents

The treatment standards at this age are the same as in adults.

Plasma Glucose Values Targets

These must be individualized. The following values are mentioned as a guidelines.

Infancy	–	90-130 mg/dl before feeds
Early childhood	–	90-130 mg/dl before meals
		120-160 mg/dl after meals
		Glycosylated Hb 7 to 7.5%

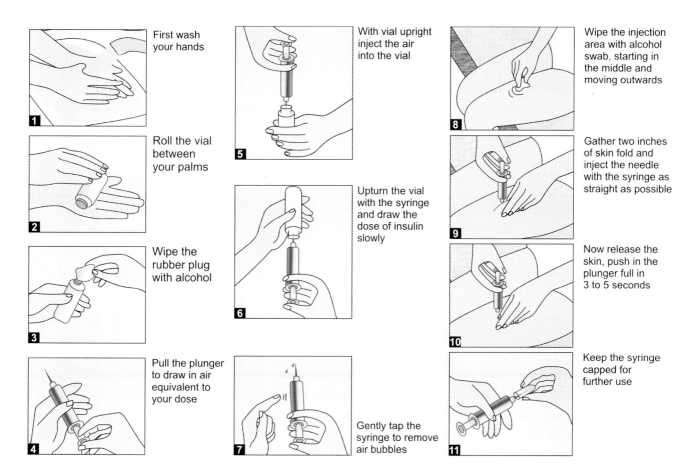

Fig. 26.5.7: Various precautions and steps to be followed for self injection of Insulin by syringe

School going child	–	90-130 mg/dl before meals
		120-160 mg/dl after meals
		Glycosylated Hb 7.0 to 7.5%
Adolescents	–	90-130 mg before meals
		120-150 mg after meals
		Glycosylated Hb 7.0 to 7.5%

Insulin Dose

Newly diagnosed T1DM children usually require 0.2 to 0.3 units/kg body weight initially. The dose is adjusted as per glucose values and growth pattern. At puberty the insulin requirements may go as high as 1.5 to 2 units/kg/day due to growth spurt and hormonal imbalance/upheavel. If a child consumes multiple snacks throughout the day, the insulin injections may be as many as 6 to 7 otherwise 2 to 4 injections per day (with actrapid/actrapid and NPH) will suffice.

Nutrition

Enough nutrition is necessary to gain weight and maintain proper growth (as per growth charts). Therefore, frequent periodic reviews are necessary. If the food intake and timings are consistent insulin dose variations are not necessary.

Physical Activity and Exercise

It must be graduated and last for 30 to 60 minutes every day. Blood glucose monitoring must be done before exercise is recommended, if glycaemic control is not satisfactory. If necessary 10 to 15 gm carbohydrate snack may be taken before strenuous exercise. Blood glucose may be monitored during (if prolonged and strenuous) or after exercise.

Special Occasions

Children camps, interactive discussions, periodic growth and development checks, participation by the parents and teachers are obligatory to ensure appropriate physical and mental growth of the child. Such events also help the care providing personnel to detect any deviation from the normal and seek specialized advice.

SUMMARY

There is enough evidence based on clinical experience and numerous well planned and executed studies that optimized glycaemic control of a patient reduces mortality and morbidity. This involves lifestyle changes, correct activity-rest balance, maintenance of ideal body weight, diet intake and judicious use of oral antidiabetic agents and/or insulin. The secret of success is in individualized approach to each patient, inculcating self monitoring of urine/blood sugar, correcting the abnormal biochemistry and ensuring a proper follow up for periodic regular evaluation of the disease process. For effective management of diabetes, a great deal of time, effort and patience is required besides the cooperation of the patient and family.

FURTHER READING

1. American Diabetes Association. Standards of medical care in diabetes (Position Statement). Diabetes Care 2004; 27 (Suppl): 515-35.
2. American Diabetes Association. Urine glucose and ketone determination (Position statement). Diablutes Care 1992;15 (Supple 2): 38.
3. Bergenstal RM. Optimization of insulin therapy in patients with type 2 diabetes. Endocr Pract 2000; 6: 93-7.
4. Hill RP, Hindle EG, Howey JEA, et al. Recommendations for adopting standard conditions and analytical procedures in the measurement of serum fructosamine concentration. Am Clin Biochem 1990; 27: 413-24.
5. Home P. The challenge of poorly controlled diabetes mellitus. Diabetes Metab 2003; 29:101-9.
6. Kazlausksite R, Fogelfeld L. Insulin therapy in type 2 diabetes (review). Dis Mon 2003; 49(6):377-420.
7. Lepore M, Pampanelli S, Fanelli C, et al. Pharmacokinetics and pharmacodynamics of subcutaneous injection of long-acting human-insulin analog, glargine, NPH insulin, and ultra lente human insulin and continuous subcutaneous infusion of insulin lispro. Diabetes 2000; 49:2142-8.
8. NCCLS: Harmonization of glycohaemoglobin measurements: approved guideline. Wayne PA. NCCLS (document C44-A) 2002.
9. Sacks DB, Bruns DE, Goldstein DE, et al. Guidelines and recommendations for laboratory analysis in the diagnosis and management of diabetes mellitus. Diabetes Care 2003; 25: 750-86.

SECTION

27

HYPERGLYCAEMIC EFFECTS ON OTHER BODY SYSTEMS

Y Sachdev

Hyperglycaemic Effects on Other Body Systems

Y Sachdev

- Vascular Tree: Diabetic Vascular Disease
- Haemopoietic System; Diabetic Vasculopathy; Aetiopathogenesis: Polyol Hypothesis, Non-enzymatic Glycosylation, Activation of Protein Kinase C, Increased Hexosamine Pathway Flux
- Pancreas
- Liver
- Digestive System

- Kidneys, Urinary Tract
- Heart, Blood Pressure
- Lungs
- Nervous System
- Reproductive System
- Thyroid
- Diabetic Retinopathy

VASCULAR TREE

The prevalence of the vascular complications of diabetes has a significant impact on the mortality and morbidity of the diabetic population. T1DM patients have 4 to 5 times more mortality risk than that of the general population. Coronary heart disease (CHD) accounts for approximately 45 to 50 per cent of the deaths and renal failure for 20 to 25 per cent. Blindness due to diabetic retinopathy in at least one eye, occurs in about 30 per cent of T1DM. Amputations of the lower extremities due to peripheral vascular disease and/or peripheral neuropathy is again much high in diabetics above the age of 50 years compared to non-diabetic general population. About 10% of T1DM who survive for more than 40 years escape many of the serious complications. This is attributed to their genetic make-up. In T2DM, macroangiopathic complications appear to account for more of the mortality and morbidity.

Diabetic Vascular Disease

It is usually seen as one of the chronic complications of long standing (15 to 20 years) diabetes mellitus (DM). It has two distinct components:

a. Macrovascular component (atherosclerosis) which is non-specific and is usually independent of diabetic syndrome. It, however, gets accelerated by the diabetic process (Fig. 27.1).

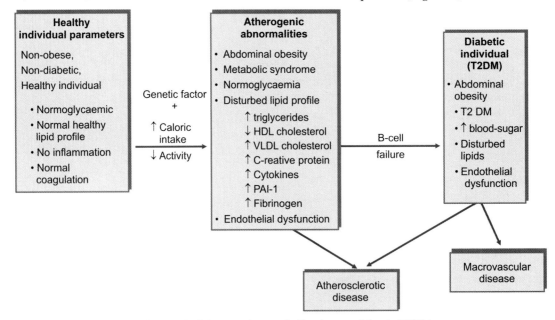

Fig. 27.1: Atherogenic metabolic abnormalities in T2DM

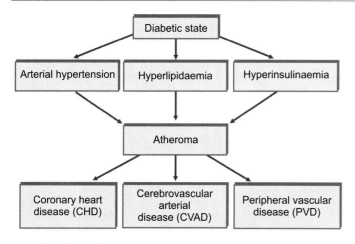

Fig. 27.2: Pathogenesis of diabetic macroangiopathy

Clinically, it manifests as peripheral vascular disease (PVD), coronary artery disease (CAD) and cerebro-vascular arterial disease (CVAD) (Fig. 27.2). The diabetic patients have greater incidence of multivessel disease and larger diseased vessel segments.

b. Microvascular components which is specific to DM is termed as diabetic microangiopathy. The term includes arteriosclerosis, thickening of the capillary walls, involvement of venular walls, impaired perfusion and basement membrane thickening (BMT).

The arteriosclerosis of diabetes is characterized by the concentric hyaline thickening of arteriolar walls which is segmental in nature and involves afferent and efferent glomerular arterioles, pancreatic arterioles resulting in patchy ischaemic acinar degeneration, retinal vessels and arterioles in other organs like adrenals, etc.

The diabetic process affects the arterioles throughout the body and results in thickening of their basement membrane. Hyperglycaemia results in increased dis-accharide synthesis and secretion of peptide portion of basement membrane. These changes in basement memb-rane (due to altered glycoproteins) leads to increased effective pore size and significant continuous, nonselective albumin leak in the kidneys and altered capillary permeability in other tissues (Fig. 27.3).

It is debated if the BMT is related to the severity or the duration of diabetes. Probably both factors contribute as it has been seen that a tight glycaemic control delays the basement membrane thickening and even results in regression of abnormal thickening. Moreover, Pirart's observational study covering 4,400 type 1 and type 2 diabetics (T1DM, T2DM) and followed up to 25 years proved that prevalence of retinopathy, nephropathy and neuropathy increased with duration of diabetes and was highest when the glycaemic control was poor. The

Winconsin Epidemiologic Study of Diabetic Retinopathy (WESDR) also confirms the relationship of incidence and progression of retinopathy in T1DM and T2DM to glycaemic status.

This was further confirmed by the Diabetes Control and Complication Trial (DCCT 1993) where 1440 patients at 29 centres in North America were allocated randomly to either 'conventional' (1 to 2 daily insulin injections, 3 monthly clinic visit, and no insulin adjustment as per self-monitored glucose level) or to the 'intensive therapy (3 or more daily insulin injections or CSII, monthly clinic visit, weekly telephone call and frequent insulin dose adjustment as per self-monitored blood glucose data, with diet and exercise programme). Throughout the 9-year study period, there was markedly better glycaemic control in intensively treated patients. The United Kingdom Prospective Diabetes Study (UKPDS 1998) where over 5000 type 2 DM patients were studied in 23 centres again confirmed that an intensive therapy was associated with marked (25%) reduction in microvascular complications.

Aetiopathogenesis of Microangiopathy

The exact pathogenesis has always been a matter of debate. It is most probably due to relative tissue hypoxia affecting the endothelium resulting in

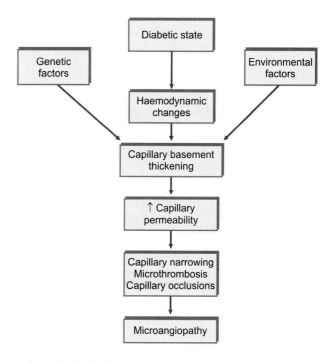

Fig. 27.3: Pathogenesis of diabetic microangiopathy

structural changes and endothelial dysfunction. The endothelial changes induce the secretion of chemokines such as monocyte chemoattractant protein 1 (MCP1), increase the expression of endothelial adhesion molecules for leucocytes and platelets and enhance endothelial permeability to lipoproteins and other plasma constituents. The normal endothelium produces nitric oxide (NO). Stimulation of endothelial cell-nitric oxide (eNO) production is a major anti-atherogenic process as NO is a 'potent inhibitor' of platelets aggregation and adhesion. Moreover, NO controls expression of genes involved in atherogenesis, reduces vascular permeability and rate of oxidation of low density lipoproteins (LDL) to its pro-atherogenic form, and inhibits proliferation of vascular smooth muscle cells.

The hyperglycaemia inhibits arterial endothelial-NO production enhancing atherogenic process. Besides hyperglycaemia, genetic process also plays a part in the aetiopathogenesis. However, the metabolic (hyperglycaemia and dyslipidaemia) hypothesis of microangiopathy is favoured as it has been a common experience that incidence of nephropathy and retinopathy increases with duration and severity of diabetes mellitus.

Genetic basis being different in T1DM and T2DM, the genes appear to play only a secondary role. The genetic role is supported by the presence of familial clustering of diabetic nephropathy. Numerous associations between genetic polymorphism and risk of diabetic complications have been described. All these studies provide no direct indication that polymorphic gene actually plays a definite functional role.

HAEMOPOIETIC SYSTEM

Hyperglycaemia leads to a number of haematological abnormalities which, in turn, lead to decreased tissue oxygenation and hypoxia. These alterations are described in brief as under:

Increased Vascular Protein Accumulation

It is due to:
- Abnormal leakage of plasma proteins which get deposited in the capillary wall stimulating perivascular cells to elaborate growth factors and extracellular matrix.
- Extravasation of growth factors which directly stimulate overproduction of extracellular matrix.
- Hypertension-induced stimulation of pathogenic gene expression by endothelial and supporting cells.

Erythrocytes

Erythrocytes show the following:
- Increased aggregation due to cell surface changes in RBCs and elevated levels of certain plasma proteins.
- Decreased deformity of RBCs leading to reduced homogeneous and rapid perfusion through microcirculation.
- Increased microvascularity
- Reduced oxy-Hb dissociation curve.

Leucocytes

- Polymorphs demonstrate defective granulocytic adherence, reduced chemotaxis, phagocytosis and intracellular bacterial activity.
- Lymphocytes show reduced proliferation response to mitogen stimulation, reduced T- and β-cell surface membrane markers, and cell-mediated immunity.

Platelets

The platelets adhesiveness, aggregation, synthesis of thrombogenic prostaglandin derivatives are increased. The ADP-induced biosynthesis of thromboxone A2, B2 (which is a stimulator of platelets clumping and arterial constriction) is elevated along with increased release of platelets factors 3 and 4 which accelerate coagulation.

Whole Blood

The blood rheology is profoundly altered. There is increased whole blood and plasma viscosity, elevated levels of fibrinogen, haptoglobin, VMF activity, α_2 macroglobulin and α_1 antiprotease. Antithrombin III (AOD) is reduced while CH 50, C_1S, C2, C3 (complement system) are increased. There is increased fibrinogen and α_2 macroglobulin turnover; fibrinolysis is reduced leading to diminished spontaneous fibrinolytic activity, reduced plasminogen activator release and diminished fibrinolytic response to venous occlusion.

Plasma Proteins

They demonstrate elevated levels of blood glycoproteins, fibrinogen, haptoglobin, β-lipoprotein, ceruloplasmin, α_2 macroglobulin leading to increased plasma viscosity. Increased fibrinogen and α_2 globulin result in elevated coagulation factors VIII and V. Fibrinogen survival is reduced and vWF which increases adhesion and aggregation of platelets is elevated. Moreover, due to reduced release of plasminogen activator, there is

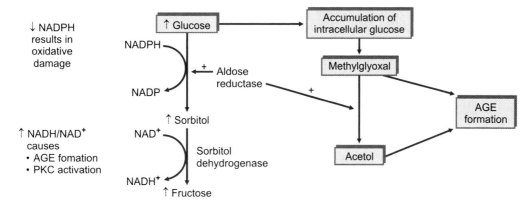

Fig. 27.4: Consequences of increased glucose flux through the polyol pathway
*(AGE = Advanced glycated end-product, PKC = Protein kinase C. Polyol pathway is normally inactive.
It gets activated when intracellular glucose levels rise)*

reduced fibronolytic activity and reduced fibronolytic response to venous occlusion (see above para).

Cell Surface Changes

Insulin deficiency and metabolic disturbances alter synthesis of macromolecules in certain tissues and influence the permeability, and binding properties of mitogen, hormone and lipoprotein receptors.

All these alterations (increased viscocity, coagulability, changes in fibrinolytic systems, RBC, etc.) contribute towards the pathogenesis of diabetic vasculopathy.

Besides these endothelial and blood component changes, there are other important mechanisms as under which play significant role in pathogenesis of diabetic vasculopathy.

The Polyol Hypothesis (Fig. 27.4)

One mechanism by which hyperglycaemia may cause complications is by an increased flux of glucose. In this pathway, the rate-limiting enzyme, aldose reductase, reduces glucose to its sugar alcohol, sorbitol. Sorbitol is then oxidized by sorbitol dehydrogenase into fructose. Aldose reductase is found in tissues such as nerve, retina, glomerulus and the blood vessel wall, where glucose uptake is independent of GLUT-4 and insulin. The pathway is normally inactive because of the high Km of aldose reductase, but hyperglycaemia increases influx through the pathway and leads to accumulation of intra-cellular glucose and glucose-derived substances, such as methyl glyoxal and acetol (which rapidly glycate proteins). Sorbitol does not diffuse easily across cell membranes and damage may occur because of the sorbitol-induced osmotic stress.

Alternative mechanisms may involve decreased NADPH, thereby decreasing reduced glutathione, an important scavenger of reactive oxygen species; or an increased NADH/NAD$^+$ ratio, which inhibits glyceraldehyde 3-phosphate dehydrogenase, increasing intracellular triose phosphate formation of one methylglyoxal and activation of protein kinase C.

Non-enzymatic Glycosylation (Fig. 27.5)

Glycosylation of slow turn-over structural proteins in hyperglycaemic environments results in damage to basement membrane, type IV collagen and collagen in

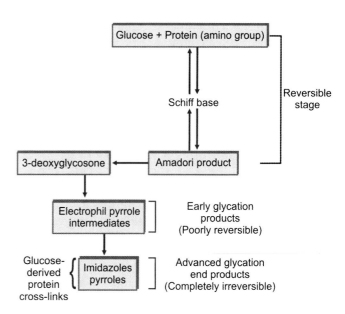

Fig. 27.5: Formation of reversible early and advanced glycation end products

skin and connective tissue. Advanced glycation end-products (AGEs) damage cells by altering cellular protein function and by cross-linking extracellular matrix molecules, such as collagen and laminin, which in the blood vessels increases wall thickness and permeability, and decreases elasticity. AGE-modified circulating proteins bind to a specific receptor (RAGE) on various types of cells including glomerular mesangial cells and endothelial cells. This binding leads to increased vascular permeability. There is also 2-3-fold elevation of minor haemoglobins-HbA_1a, HbA_1b and HbA_1c.

Activation of Protein Kinase C (Fig. 27.6)

The third mechanism by which elevated glucose may induce tissue damage is through excessive activation of protein kinase C (PKC). PKC is an enzyme that phosphorylates several target proteins. It exists in several isoforms and is activated by diacylglycerol. Diacylglycerol is formed *de novo* from glucose via triose phosphates in the glycolytic pathway. Overactivity of PKC has been implicated in increased vascular permeability, blood flow changes and increased basement membrane synthesis. PKC also inhibits nitric oxide (NO) production.

Increased Hexosamine Pathway Flux (Fig. 27.7)

Hyperglycaemia may also cause diabetic complications by shunting glucose into the hexosamine pathway. Here, fructose-6-phosphate is diverted from glycolysis to form UDP-N-acetyl-glucosamine, used in the synthesis of glycoproteins. The rate limiting step in the conversion of glucose to glucosamine is regulated by glutamine: fructose-6-phosphate amidotransferase (GFAT). Possibly, glycation of transcription factors by N-acetylglucosamine increases the transcription factor of key genes such as TGF-B, acetyl CoA carboxylase (the rate-limiting enzyme for fatty acid synthesis), plasminogen activator inhibitor-(PAI-1) and probably many other genes.

Besides, these four known hyperglycaemia-induced abnormalities, hyperglycaemia induced increased mitochondrial superoxide production enhances aldose reductase activity, AGE formation, PKC activity and hexoamine pathway activity. It also induces mutations in mitochondrial DNA. Hyperglycaemia-induced mitochondrial superoxide production probably explains the development of complications during post-hyperglycaemic normoglycaemic phase (hyperglycaemic memory).

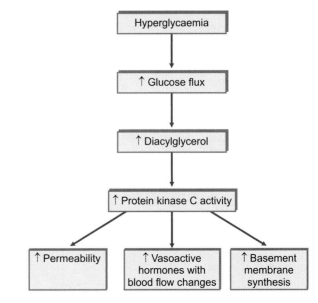

Fig. 27.6: Activation of protein kinase C by *de novo* synthesis of diacylglycerol subsequent to ↑ glucose utilization

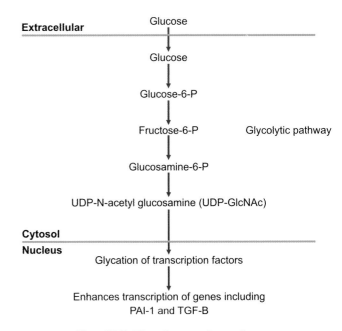

Fig. 27.7: The glucosamine pathway

PANCREAS

The pancreatic changes will obviously depend upon the type of diabetes mellitus as well as endocrine pancreatic status. Thus there will be a variable picture. Essential features in a chronic patient, however, will always be acinar degeneration, fibrosis with or without calcification.

There may be no abnormality in young and mild diabetics.

LIVER

It may be enlarged with variable degree of fatty infiltration. There is decreased lectin binding plasma membrane receptors in liver cells.

DIGESTIVE SYSTEM

Symptoms of gestroparesis like bloating, nausea, early satiety, vomiting, slow food absorption may be present due to involvement of autonomic neuropathy.

KIDNEY

Diabetic nephropathy is a distinct well established entity with various clinical and histopathological grades.

Urinary Tract

Repeated urinary tract infections, neurogenic bladder with residual post-void urine, chronic infections, hydronephrosis and abnormal cystometrics may be seen in diabetics with autonomic problems.

HEART

There is subendothelial thickening and acid mucopolysaccharide deposits in capillaries associated with diabetic process. Besides this, interstitial and perivascular fibrosis, myocardial basement membrane thickening and capillary microaneurysms are also present. A diabetic patient is more prone to develop CAD, unexplained congestive cardiac failure and cardiomegaly.

Blood Pressure

Persistent elevated blood pressure with postural hypotension and syncopial episodes on sudden rising from sitting/lying position are often seen in chronic diabetic patients.

LUNGS

Besides various pulmonary dysfunctions, both bacterial and non-bacterial respiratory infections including pulmonary tuberculosis and fungal infections are more common in diabetes mellitus. Sleep apnoea is common especially in those diabetics who have autonomic neuropathy.

NERVOUS SYSTEM

Cerebrovascular accidents, lacunar infarcts, basal ganglia and mid brain dysfunction due to osmotic disturbances and microvascular complications are commonly seen in chronic diabetics. Various types of neuropathies, sexual dysfunctions, urinary bladder problems may also be present due to autonomic nerves involvement.

REPRODUCTIVE SYSTEM

Infertility/abortions/miscarriages/stillbirths/prematurity/postmaturity, menstrual dysfunction are some of the common features associated with hyperglycaemia. In men erectile dysfunction, retrograde ejaculation is quite a common complaint.

SKIN

Skin changes in diabetes mellitus include 'shin spots', diabetic bullae and necrobiosis lipoidica diabeticorum. Skin infections, eczemas and ischaemic skin lesions may also be seen at the distal limbs especially feet.

THYROID

The chronic effects of diabetes mellitus are due to deficient tissue glucose utilization and are similar to those seen in starvation. The prominent changes are:
- Decreased conversion of T_4 to T_3
- Elevated reverse T_3 value
- Inhibition of TSH response to low T_3 value
- Decreased T_3 receptor capacity (also seen in caloric deprivation).

In diabetic ketoacidoses:
- $FT_3 : T_3$ ratio is increased
- $FT_4 : T_4$ ratio is increased
- TSH secretion is depressed
- TSH response to TRH is reduced.

It appears that the effects of diabetes on receptor capacity is related to local tissue glucose uptake as well as general stress effects.

DIABETIC RETINOPATHY

It is defined as presence of one or more definite microaneurysms or any other more severe lesion of retinopathy formed in any of the 7 stereoscopic fundus photographic fields. It is generally agreed that retinopathy frequently appears after 5 years of untreated diabetes and 50% of patients have some evidence of it in

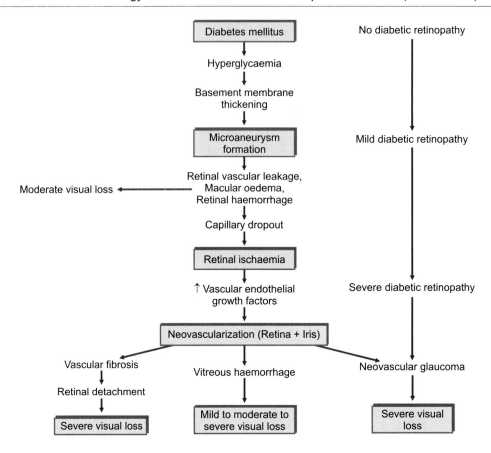

Fig. 27.8: Clinical stages of diabetic retinopathy

less than 10 years. Functional changes in retinal circulation precede structural changes. In uncontrolled type 1 DM it is present in over 60% patients after 6 years and after 10 years in nearly 100%.

Regional retinal ischaemia is the central mechanism for its development. Retinal ischaemia is the result of:
- Capillary vasodilatation and hyperpermeability
- Basement membrane thickening
- Loss of endothelial cells and pericytes
- Focal capillary occlusion
- Formation of AV shunts
- Blood abnormalities, and decreased release of O_2 from Hb due to elevated level of HbA_{1C} and reduced 2,3-diphosphoglycerate.

The retinal ischaemia is reversible in early stage before the capillary occlusion takes place. It becomes irreversible if blood-retinal barrier breaks and if tight endothelial cell junctions open up (Fig. 27.8). The break down of blood retinal barrier is related to duration and severity of diabetes mellitus.

Initially, in uncontrolled diabetes mellitus, there is compensatory increase in retinal blood volume and segmental blood flow along with autoregulatory dilatation of retinal blood vessels. Later on, with development of background retinopathy there is regional hypoperfusion of retina due to 'skimming' where RBCs are shunted through some capillaries and plasma alone through others. Eventually, severity of retinal hypoxia increases microaneurysms, cotton-wool spots, new vessel formation (proliferative retinopathy) and intraretinal oedema and haemorrhage occur. Thus, retinal manifestations of diabetes are:
- Microaneurysms (MA)
- Haemorrhages (H)
- Soft exudates (SE)
- Hard exudates (HE)
- Venous beading (VB)
- Intraretinal microvascular anomalies (IRMA)
- Neovascularisation elsewhere (NVE)
- Neovascularisation of the optic disc (NVD)
- Clinically significant macular oedema (CSME).

Retinopathy before the development of retinal neovascularisation is termed 'nonproliferative diabetic retinopathy' (NPDR). Once proliferation of new retinal vessels occurs, it is referred to as 'proliferative diabetic retinopathy' (PDR).

Role of Growth Hormone (GH) in Diabetic Vasculopathy

In several diabetic patients there is 3-fold increase in GH values. Those who present with proliferative retinopathy have been seen to have higher GH values. Therefore, it has always been postulated that GH has a significant role in causing diabetic retinopathy. This is further supported by the fact that GH deficient dwarfs do not develop retinopathy even when they have glucose intolerance. Despite all this supportive evidence, the role of GH is still not clear as there are many exceptions to this.

SUMMARY

The long-term effects of hyperglycaemia are borne by all body systems—the maximum effects, of course, are on the eyes, nerves, blood vessels, kidneys, heart and skin.

FURTHER READING

1. Nathan DM. Long-term complications of diabetes mellitus. N Engl J Med 1993;328:1676-85.
2. Singh R, Barden A, Mor T, et al. Advanced glycation end-products: a review. Diabetologia 2001;44:129-46.

SECTION

CHRONIC DIABETIC COMPLICATIONS

28.1 Diabetic Retinopathy

DP Vats, VS Gurunadh, M Bhadauria

- Introduction
- Epidemiology
- Aetiopathogenesis
- Retinal Manifestations
- Natural Course of Diabetic Retinopathy

- Cause of Visual loss
- Investigations
- Management
- Summary

INTRODUCTION

Diabetes mellitus has a peculiar affection for the eye. The most important aspect is that all the structures of the eye are susceptible to the deleterious effects of this disease of glucose metabolism. However, among these ophthalmic manifestations of diabetes mellitus, the most vital subject, and the focus of research in the past as well as in the present and that which is the cause of concern and challenge to the internist, the ophthalmologist and the investigative clinician is the affection of the retinal microcirculation.

Diabetic retinopathy is a well-characterized, sight-threatening, chronic ocular disorder that eventually develops, to some degree—in nearly all patients with diabetes. It is characterized by gradually progressive alterations in the retinal microvasculature, leading to areas of retinal nonperfusion, increased vasopermeability, and the pathologic intraocular proliferation of retinal vessels. The complications associated with increased vasopermeability and uncontrolled neovascularization can result in severe and permanent visual loss.

In 1967, in his magnum opus *"The System of Ophthalmology, Sir Stewart Duke-Elder had written,"... diabetic retinopathy is one of the major tragedies of ophthalmology in our present generation; always common and rapidly becoming still more common; affecting the young as well as the aged, predictable but not preventable."* However, extensive data are now available on most aspects of this disease from numerous epidemiological studies and clinical trials that provide a solid basis for developing the evaluation and management guidelines being followed now. With appropriate medical and ophthalmological care, more than 90% of visual loss resulting from diabetic retinopathy, can now be prevented.

With experienced ophthalmic evaluation, diabetic retinopathy can be detected in its early stages. Therapies exist that can be remarkably effective when administered at the appropriate time in the disease process. In addition, improvement of systemic glycaemic control is associated with a delay in the onset and a slowing of the progression of diabetic retinopathy.

EPIDEMIOLOGY

The biggest risk factor for diabetes is diabetes itself. Though there are reports of diabetic retinopathy without diabetes, the DCCT has proved beyond doubt that the complications of diabetes mellitus are direct consequences of long-term hyperglycaemia, perhaps modified by genetic or other features that may vary from one individual to another.

The Indian figures for the prevalence of diabetic retinopathy vary from 4 to 28%. The WHO multinational study of vascular disease in diabetes estimated the prevalence of diabetic retinopathy in males and females in New Delhi as 6.23% and 3.7% respectively.

As far as the duration of diabetes and retinopathy is concerned, in the population study at a South Indian urban setting retinopathy was found in 87.5% of diabetics with duration more than 15 years compared to 18.9% in those with duration of disease less than 15 years.

The incidence of the severity of diabetic retinopathy as seen in the south Indian study among recently detected diabetics revealed non-proliferative diabetic retinopathy at 30.8% including 6.4% with maculopathy and proliferative diabetic retinopathy at 3.4%. In a population based assessment of diabetes and diabetic retinopathy, the age-sex adjusted prevalence of diabetes among people aged 50 years and over was 5.1% and of diabetic retinopathy among diabetics was 26.8% with nonproliferative retinopathy being the most common form (94.1%).

Puberty and pregnancy can accelerate retinopathy progression. The onset of vision - threatening retinopathy is rare in children before puberty regardless of the duration of diabetes. However, if diabetes is diagnosed between the ages of 10 and 30 years, significant retinopathy may arise within 6 years of the disease.

Proliferative retinopathy is present in 25% of patients with type 1 and a duration of 15 years but in 25% of type 2 disease at a duration of 25 years. However, in type 2 disease with less than five years proliferative retinopathy develops in 2% only.

The prevalence of macular oedema is approximately 18 to 19% in patients either with type 1 disease or type 2.

When retinal photographs and fluorescein angiograms were used to detect the onset of the disease, retinopathy was found not to occur before 3 to 5 years of the onset of the systemic disease in either type of diabetes.

AETIOPATHOGENESIS

The key that opens all the mechanisms that lead to the development of diabetic retinopathy (DR) is ischaemia. Though there are many conditions that lead to ischaemia and the end-state of any ischaemic retinopathy appears clinically similar, diabetic retinopathy is different both in the mechanisms and the changes that occur at the microscopic level. The most important initiating and inciting factor has to be the hyperglycaemic state, which sets up a cascade of biochemical reactions. The essential histopathological features that are specific for DR, and which cause the lesions of DR, in particular the microaneurysms (MA) are:
a. Thickening of the basement membrane.
b. Loss of intramural pericytes in the retinal endothelium.

RETINAL MANIFESTATIONS

The retinal manifestations of diabetes are as follows:
• Microaneurysms (MA)
• Haemorrhages (H)
• Soft exudates (SE)
• Hard exudates (HE)
• Venous beading (VB)
• Intraretinal microvascular anomalies (IRMA)
• Neovascularisation elsewhere (NVE)
• Neovascularisation of the optic disc (NVD)
• Clinically significant macular oedema (CSME).

Microaneurysms (MA)

These are small pinheads like, obviously red looking lesions that are usually found in the macular area and around the disc. They are seen ophthalmoscopically as small dots usually varying from 10 to 15 μ in size. But they are clearly delineated after an intravascular injection of fluorescein in an area, which may have appeared as normal on ophthalmoscopy. In numbers, these microaneurysms vary from a few to an astonishing quantity scattered over the retina. They usually, but not invariably, arise from the venous side of the capillary network, as localized distensions of the one side of the vessel wall, generally forming saccular diverticula full of blood; on the other hand, they may arise from the capillary loops, formed perhaps by endothelial proliferation and migration.

Haemorrhages (H)

Haemorrhages in diabetic retinopathy are usually intra-retinal arising from deeper capillaries within the retina located within the compact inner nuclear and outer plexiform layers of the retina and thus assuming the typical dot and blot appearance.

Haemorrhages occurring in the inner retina assume a flame shape due to the trickling of the blood between the nerve-fibre layers of the retina. Though they may be seen with many systemic and other retinal disorders, they are often associated with systemic hypertension and a plethora of these in a case of diabetic retinopathy should lead to a suspicion of uncontrolled hypertension.

Soft Exudates (SE)

Otherwise known as cotton-wool spots, they are seen on ophthalmoscopy as discrete fluffy white like opacification in the inner retina. They represent swelling of nerve-fibre layer and disruption of axoplasmic flow within nerve-fibre layers and thus are signs of focal ischaemia in the retina. However, they are less helpful in predicting progression to proliferative phase.

Hard Exudates (HE)

They have a waxy yellow appearance with sharply defined borders (as compared to the fluffy bordered SE) and represent the residue of oedema that has leaked from abnormal retinal vessels. HE tend to accumulate in the outer plexiform layer (hence deeper to SE), where the tissue is most lax. They usually assume a ringlike or circinate conformation around the site of leakage, such as from a retinal microaneurysm or a diseased capillary leakage.

Venous Beading (VB)

This is the term given to the beaded appearance of the veins that are dilated segments of retinal veins. The veins may also undergo tortuosity and reduplication.

Intraretinal Microvascular Abnormalities (IRMA)

One of the most serious consequences of diabetic retinopathy is the obliteration of retinal capillaries. When patches of acellular capillaries, seen early in the course of the disease, become confluent, the terminal arterioles that supply these capillaries often become occluded. Adjacent to these areas of non-perfused retina, clusters of MA and tortuous, hypercellular vessels often develop. It is difficult to determine whether these vessels are dilated pre-existing vessels or neovascularization in the retina. These vessels have been referred to as intraretinal microvascular abnormalities (IRMA) clinically to include both possibilities (Fig. 28.1.1).

Neovascularisation Elsewhere (NVE)

These are the new vessel proliferations seen in the retina. Their extent, location from the optic disc and their position within the retinal layers or on the surface of the retina represent the extent of ischaemia.

Neovascularisation of the Optic Disc (NVD) (Figs 28.1.2 and 28.1.3)

The development of new vessels on the optic disc or up to 01 disc dioptres of the optic disc is termed as neovascularisation of the optic disc (NVD). The extent of the NVD represents the extent of retinal ischaemia.

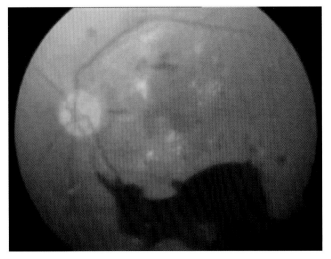

Fig. 28.1.1: Proliferative diabetic retinopathy with preretinal haemorrhage

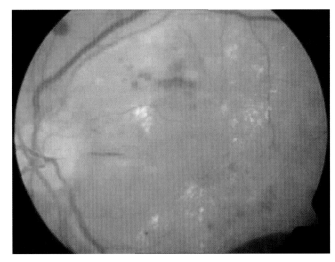

Fig. 28.1.2: Neovascularisation of the optic disc (NVD) and hard exudate (HE)

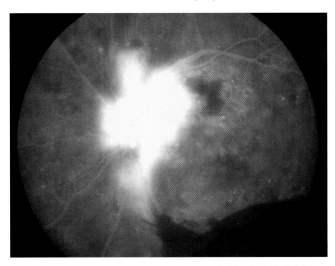

Fig. 28.1.3: Fluorescein angiogram (FA) of NVD (HE)

The appearance of NVD signifies retinal ischaemia of at least five disc dioptres of retinal area and its presence is of critical importance in a case of diabetic retinopathy.

Diabetic Macular Oedema and Clinically Significant Macular Oedema (CSME) (Fig. 28.1.4)

Retinal oedema threatening or involving the macula is an important visual consequence of abnormal retinal vascular permeability in diabetic retinopathy because of the breakdown of the blood-retinal barrier. This is best delineated by fluorescein angiogram.

Diabetic macular oedema may manifest as focal or diffuse retinal thickening with or without exudates. However, simple leakage on the angiogram may not always be associated with retinal thickening in the

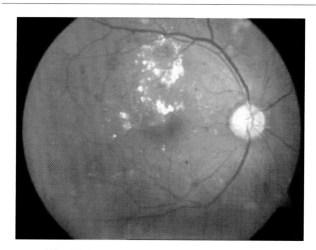

Fig. 28.1.4: NPDR with clinically significant macular oedema (CSME)

macular area. Although an overlap of categories often occurs, two general categories of macular oedema have been described, i.e. focal and diffuse:

Focal Macular Oedema

Areas of focal fluorescein leakage from specific capillary lesions characterise focal macular oedema. It may be associated with rings of hard exudates derived from plasma lipoproteins that appear to emanate from micro-aneurysms. Resorption of fluid components results in precipitation of lipid residues, usually in the outer and inner plexiform layers but occasionally beneath the sensory retina itself (these are the hard exudates).

Diffuse Macular Oedema

Diffuse macular oedema is characterised by widespread retinal capillary abnormalities associated with diffuse leakage from extensive breakdown of the blood-retinal barrier and, often, with cystoid macular oedema.

The diagnosis of macular oedema is best made by slit lamp biomicroscopy of the posterior pole using a non-contact 78 D/90 D or a Goldman contact lens. Important observations include
a. Location of retinal oedema relative to the fovea
b. Presence and location of exudates
c. Presence of cystoid macular oedema.

However, the Early Treatment Diabetic Retinopathy Study (ETDRS) has thrown a pattern of macular oedema, which has been defined by the Study as clinically significant macular oedema (CSME). Its common forms of presentation are as follows:
a. Retinal oedema located at or within 500 µm of the centre of the macula.
b. HE at or within 500 µm of the centre if associated with thickening of the adjacent retina.

c. A zone of retinal thickening larger than 01 disc area if located within the 01 disc diameter of the centre of the macula.

NATURAL COURSE

Some degree of retinopathy occurs in nearly all patients with diabetes of more than 20 years' duration. The natural history of retinopathy has been evaluated in large multicentre clinical trials: the DRS (Diabetic Retinopathy Study), the ETDRS (The Early Treatment Diabetic Retinopathy Study), the DRVS (Diabetic Retinopathy Vitrectomy Study), the DCCT (Diabetes Control and Complication Trial), and the UKPDS (United Kingdom Prospective Diabetes Study).

Background diabetic retinopathy and preproliferative diabetic retinopathy are outdated terms referring to general levels or stages of non-proliferative diabetic retinopathy (NPDR). Since this terminology is not closely associated with disease progression, it should no longer be used and has been replaced by the various levels of NPDR, which correlate closely with disease progression.

Pre-clinical changes in diabetic retinopathy include alternations in retinal blood flow and loss of retinal pericytes. The earliest clinical stages of diabetic retinopathy are characterized by microaneurysms. SE may occur, which represents stasis of axoplasmic flow due to focal ischaemia of the nerve fibre layer. Increased vascular permeability can occur at this or any later stage, resulting in fluid accumulation in the retina. As the disease progresses, gradual loss of the retinal micro-vasculature occurs, resulting in retinal ischaemia. Venous calibre abnormalities, intraretinal microvascular abnormalities (IRMAs), and more severe vascular leakage are common reflections of increasing retinal non-perfusion.

The most advanced stages of diabetic retinopathy are characterised by the onset of ischaemia-induced new vessel proliferation at the optic disc (NVD) or elsewhere in the retina (NVE). The new vessels are fragile and prone to bleed, resulting in vitreous haemorrhage. With time, the neovascularization tends to undergo fibrosis and contraction, resulting in retinal traction and retinal detachment. New vessels can also arise on the iris (NVI) or in the trabecular meshwork of the anterior chamber (ANV), resulting in neovascular glaucoma.

Retinopathy before the development of retinal neovascularization is termed NPDR (Figs 28.1.5A and B).

Once proliferation of new retinal vessels occurs, it is referred to as PDR (Figs 28.1.6 to 28.1.8).

When PDR is associated with defined retinal lesions that increase the likelihood of severe visual loss, it is

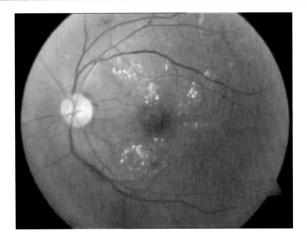

Fig. 28.1.5A: Nonproliferative diabetic retinopathy (NPDR) with CSME

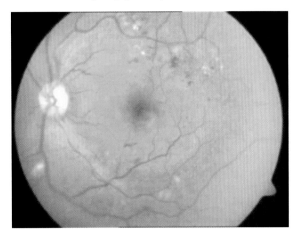

Fig. 28.1.5B: Nonproliferative diabetic retinopathy (NPDR) with regressing CSME (after laser)

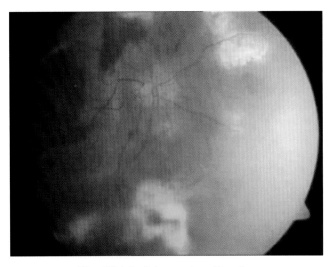

Fig. 28.1.6: Advanced proliferative diabetic retinopathy (PDR)

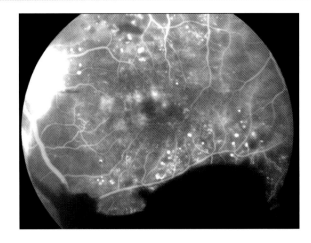

Fig. 28.1.7: Angiogram of advanced PDR

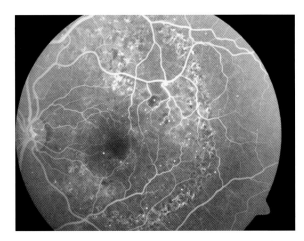

Fig. 28.1.8: Confirmatory fluorescence angiogram of PDR

termed high-risk PDR and prompt treatment is indicated. Treatment modalities are thus primarily directed towards preventing these complications.

CAUSE OF VISUAL LOSS

The predominant cause of visual loss in diabetic retinopathy is CSME or PDR. The latter results in tractional retinal detachment or non-clearing vitreous haemorrhage.

Severe Visual Loss (SVL)

DRS defined this term as the best corrected visual acuity of 5/200 (1/60) or worse at two or more consecutive visits 04 months apart.

Moderate Visual Loss (MVL)

This term was defined by the ETDRS as at least a doubling of the visual angle (e.g. 6/12 to 6/24) (Table 28.1.1).

TABLE 28.1.1

Severity	Lesions present
Non-proliferative	
No retinopathy	No retinal lesions
MA only	No lesions other than MA
Mild NPDR, venous loops or both	MA plus H, HE
Moderate NPDR	Mild NPDR plus SE and/or IRMA
Severe NPDR	Presence of one of the following features as per the "4-2-1" rule : "4" quadrants having H and MA "2" or more quadrants having VB "1" quadrant at least having moderate IRMA
Very severe NPDR	Two or more of the above features described in severe NPDR
Proliferative	
PDR without HRC	New vessels and/or fibrous proliferations; or preretinal and or vitreous haemorrhage
PDR with HRC	NVD < 1/4 of the optic disc with vitreous haemorrhage NVD 1/4 to 1/3 of the optic disc with or without vitreous haemorrhage NVE >1/2 disc area with vitreous haemorrhage
Advanced PDR	Extensive vitreous haemorrhage precluding grading. Retinal detachment involving the macula. Phthisis bulbi. Enucleation secondary to a complication of diabetic retinopathy

Classification of severity of diabetic retinopathy

INVESTIGATIONS

The only ophthalmic investigation required is a fluorescein angiogram (FA). The benefit of the same are enlisted in Table 28.1.2.

Though there are usually no serious side effects of FA, it is not to be done in pregnancy and in the lactating mother as its effects on the foetus and the neonate are not known.

GENERAL PURPOSE AND GOALS OF MANAGEMENT

The primary reason for the evaluation and management of diabetic retinopathy is to prevent, reverse, or delay the visual loss associated with this disease process.

TABLE 28.1.2

Indications	Benefits
• Guiding treatment of CSME	• Identification of" treatable" lesions and methods of photocoagulation
• Determining extent of macular non-perfusion	• Extent and location may alter visual and treatment prognosis
• Evaluating unexplained visual loss	• Additional information
• Searching for subtle neovascularisation	• Rarely helpful as clinical examination is highly sensitive and HRC should usually be clinically identifiable
• Diagnosis of NPDR	• In the absence of other indications
• Diagnosis of PDR before panretinal photocoagulation and before intraocular surgery	• FA is not routinely indicated in these settings since the low likelihood of significant additional information does not usually justify the additional risk, discomfort and cost to the patient
• Post-laser	• A must to determine the efficacy of the laser and the requirement for further sittings

Indications and benefits of fluorescein angiogram (FA)

Appropriate management involves seven primary goals:
a. Identify individuals at risk of developing diabetic retinopathy.
b. Assure appropriate systemic glycaemic control.
c. Provide appropriate life-long evaluation of retinopathy progression.
d. Provide therapy to individuals at risk of visual loss.
e. Minimize the associated visual and functional side effects of this therapy.
f. Provide rehabilitation for those with visual loss from the disease.
g. Educate and involve the patients in the management of their disease.

The actual numbers of persons suffering from various vision affecting entities of DR like CSME and/or PDR is not available in our country. It is known that blindness has been estimated to be 25 times more common in people with diabetes than in those without the disease. Estimates of the medical and economic impact of retinopathy-associated morbidity have been performed using computer simulations in the US. The effects of applying accepted methods for evaluating and treating diabetic retinopathy have been studied for both type 1 and type 2 diabetes. The models predict that, in the absence of good glycaemic control, over their lifetime, 72% of patients with type 1 diabetes will eventually develop PDR, requiring panretinal photocoagulation, and that 42% will develop macular oedema.

Current estimates are that only about 60% of patients in need of retinopathy treatment are receiving such care in a developed country like US. If all patients with both type 1 and type 2 diabetes were to receive currently suggested care, there would be savings of lakhs of rupees and person-year of sight. The indirect costs, in terms of lost productivity and human suffering are even greater. In one study, 55% of patients with high-risk PDR and CSME had never had laser photocoagulation. In fact, 11% of type 1 and 7% of type 2 patients with high-risk PDR necessitating prompt treatment had not been examined by an ophthalmologist in the past 2 years.

The onset of diabetic retinopathy can be delayed and the progression of diabetic retinopathy greatly slowed with glucose concentrations maintained in the near normal range. However, strict glycaemic control may be difficult, and some individuals may still develop sight-threatening diabetic retinopathy.

Dilated ophthalmic examination is superior to no dilated evaluation because only 50% of eyes are correctly classified for presence and severity of retinopathy through undilated pupils. Appropriate ophthalmic evaluation entails a directed detailed history and comprehensive ocular examination, including pupillary dilation, slit-lamp biomicroscopy, examination of the retinal periphery with indirect ophthalmoscopy or mirrored contact lens, and sometimes gonioscopy as detailed below. Indeed, 27% of retinal abnormalities are found outside the central macular region.

Careful management of the metabolic and pathologic aspects of diabetes has positive impact on the patient's visual prognosis, since such systemic processes as renal function, blood pressure, and glycaemic control affect the onset, progression, and prognosis of diabetic retinopathy.

COMPREHENSIVE EYE EVALUATION

A comprehensive eye examination is recommended for any patient with or without diabetes being seen either for the first time or after an extended duration and is of particular importance for patients with diabetes.

The fundamentals of a comprehensive eye examination of the patient with diabetes are shown in Table 28.1.3. The examination should include the items listed in the table, but is not limited to them.

TABLE 28.1.3

Examinations	Examples of particular relevance to patient with diabetes
Best corrected visual acuity	Quantitates level of high-contrast high-frequency visual function. Decline can indicate onset of visually significant macular oedema, vitreous haemorrhage, cataract, macular traction detachment, etc.
Ocular alignment and motility	Evaluates function of oculomotor cranial nerves. Abnormalities can indicate ocular nerve palsies associated with diabetic nerve damage to cranial nerves III, IV and VI.
Pupil reactivity and function	Evaluates pupil-motor pathway and structural integrity of the iris. Abnormalities can indicate neuropathy, iris neo-vascularization, or afferent pupillary defect
Visual fields	Evaluates possible defects in peripheral vision. Confrontational fields provide a qualitative assessment, and perimetry provides a quantitative assessment. Abnormalities can indicate vitreous/pre-retinal haemorrhage, retinal detachment, vascular occlusion.
Intraocular pressure	Measurement of intraocular pressure. Applanation tonometry is preferred. Abnormalities can indicate possible neovascular or open-angle glaucoma.
Slit lamp examination	
i. Cornea	Assessment of ocular surface. Abnormalities can indicate epithelial abnormalities, defects, or infection.
ii. Iris	Assess iris and when indicated gonioscopy for possible angle-closure or angle neo-vascularisation. Abnormalities can indicate neovascular glaucoma.
iii. Lens	Assess lens nucleus, cortex, and posterior capsule. Abnormalities can indicate cataract.
iv. Vitreous	Assess clarity and character of vitreous gel. Abnormalities can indicate vitreous haemorrhage (red cells), retinal tear or detachment (pigment cells), or possible vitreoretinal traction.
Dilated fundus examination Slit lamp biomicroscopy and binocular indirect ophthalmoscopy	Assess, presence, location, and extent of retinovitreal disease. Abnormalities include retinal thickening, HE, H and MA

Elements of eye examinations with particular relevance to diabetes patient

Additional procedures and further evaluation should be tailored to the abnormalities and findings identified during the examination.

MANAGEMENT

In general laser photocoagulation surgery is advised for patients with high risk PDR and for patients with CSME, since both groups have better visual prognosis when treated.

Photocoagulation

The cornerstone of the management of diabetic retinopathy is photocoagulation. Photocoagulation is a therapeutic technique employing a strong light source to coagulate tissue. Light energy is absorbed by the target tissue and converted into thermal energy. When tissue temperature rises above 65°C, denaturation of tissue proteins and coagulative necrosis occur. Most surgeons perform photocoagulation with lasers spanning the visible light spectrum of 400 to 780 nm. The presently favoured laser in this spectrum is the frequency-doubled Nd-Yag system apart from the time-honoured argon blue-green. Diode laser with 810 nm is also in vogue.

Delivery systems may employ a transpupillary approach with slit lamp delivery, indirect ophthalmoscopic application, endophotocoagulation during vitrectomy surgery, and trans-scleral application with a contact probe. Selection of laser setting parameters depends on the intent of treatment, the clarity of ocular media, and the fundus pigmentation. As a general rule, smaller spot sizes require lesser energy than larger spot sizes, and longer duration exposures require less energy than short duration exposures to achieve the same intensity effect.

Laser is applied in the form of spots. When it is applied in a localised area, it is known as focal laser, as would happen when laser is applied to a leaking area in the macular area clinically seen as a circinate ring of HE.

When laser spots are applied over the entire retinal area visualised, it is termed as panretinal photocoagulation (PRP) or scatter laser photocoagulation.

The basic rationale of photocoagulation is to destroy neovascular complexes, to obliterate areas of microinfarction or capillary closure, to destroy leaking vessels in the macular or paramacular area and ultimately produce a chorioretinal adhesion that will resist the later ravages of increasing vitreoretinal traction. The prolife-ration of new vessels is probably a result of localized hypoxia in the region of retinal vessels near the internal limiting membrane. It would seem obvious that these blood vessels are proliferating in response to some biochemical stimulus, and neovascularization appears to be an appropriate defence for the reparative mechanism of the body. However, the in-growth of the neovascularization with support of the glial tissue, as well as the attendant leakage of damaged vessels into the surrounding retinal spaces, the transport of high molecular weight lipoproteinaceous material through the neovascular walls into the retina, the resulting haemorrhages, and the dynamic changes occurring from interposition of fibrovascular membranes can irreversibly damage the macular retina.

Panretinal photocoagulation (PRP) appears to successfully obliterate or cause the regression of neovascularization by one of the four mechanisms:

a. The reduction or destruction of hypoxic retina that is producing the vasoformative factor (could be vascular endothelial growth factor) that is calling forth neovascularization from more healthy areas of the retina.

b. The creation of closer apposition of the inner layers of the retina to the choriocapillaris by multiple scattered photocoagulation scarring around the entire posterior polar region, thereby allowing greater oxygen perfusion from the choroidal layers to the inner retinal layers that have undergone a relatively high degree of microinfarction.

c. The destruction of unhealthy microinfarcted areas of retina and sluggishly perfused capillaries, thereby allowing the blood to increase the nourishment of the remaining retina.

d. The destruction of leaking blood vessels and other abnormal vascular complexes that are creating abnormal haemodynamic situation in the diabetic retina, thereby more nearly normalising the vascular supply of the macular region of the eye.

The entire concept of the vasoformative factor being elaborated by the hypoxic retina, secondary to microinfarction and capillary closure, is a most inviting explanation for the beneficial effects of PRP. If, the vasoformative factor emanating from the hypoxic areas of the retina can be reduced in the posterior vitreous, the neovascular stimulus is thereby decreased, and the new vessels tend to regress or become obliterated. Certainly the better nutrition of the inner portions of the retina by closer apposition of the inner layers to the choriocapillaris and the choroidal blood supply would also appear to be a beneficial result of the PRP technique.

Focal laser in the macular area is termed as a grid laser. Usually this grid is applied in the form of a 'reverse-C' with the arms of the 'C' staring at the origin of the arcades beyond the papillomacular bundle. Upon angiographic evaluation, selective grid laser can be done around a leaking site in the macular area.

PRP of one eye is usually applied in two-three sittings. If focal macular laser is to be done along with PRP, it is usually done with the first sitting of PRP.

PDR is treated with PRP and CSME with focal laser photocoagulation. Some patients with high risk PDR or with severe or very severe NPDR may also benefit from PRP depending upon such factors as:

i. Diabetes type
ii. Medical status
iii. Access to care
iv. Compliance with follow-up
v. Status and progression of fellow eye, and
vi. Family history.

Neovascularization of the angle and iris is also an indication for PRP.

Typical Management Recommendations

It should be noted that the appropriate management for a particular patient depends not only on the level of retinopathy and extent of macular oedema but also on a wide array of additional factors as discussed above.

1. CSME can occur with any level of NPDR/PDR.
2. CSME should be treated. Only consideration for deferral of treatment would be an excellent visual acuity and ability for close follow-up.
3. Treatment of CSME precedes PRP.
4. Treatment of CSME should be performed as part of first treatment session along with initial PRP.
5. Any PRP should include macular grid even if CSME is not present.
6. CSME treatment is recommended to be done after angiographic evaluation as only it can pick-up a case of ischaemic maculopathy wherein laser is contraindicated.

Follow-up

1. Minimal NPDR without CSME can be followed up at 01 year.
2. Mild to moderate NPDR without CSME can be followed up at 6 to 12 months.
3. All the remaining levels of retinopathy with or without CSME should be followed up at 02 to 04 months interval.

High risk PDR *not* amenable to photocoagulation can arise because of:

i. Advanced disease.
ii. Poor retinal visualization (i.e. severe vitreous haemorrhage or cataract).
iii. Active neovascularisation despite complete laser treatment.
iv. Tractional macular detachment.
v. Combined traction-rhegmatogenous retinal detachment.

Therapeutic considerations include vitrectomy or, possibly, cryotherapy.

Vitreous surgery has the potential for serious complications, profound visual loss and permanent pain and blindness, and should be undertaken only after careful consideration of the potential risk and benefits.

Exercise

In general, exercise and physical activity have not been shown to accelerate diabetic retinopathy. On the contrary, physical exercise has a positive effect on reducing the risk of diabetic complications. Strenuous activity in patients with active PDR may precipitate vitreous hemorrhage or tractional retinal detachment. It has been suggested that patients with advanced stages of DR limit strenuous activities that involve extensive Valsalva manoeuvres, pounding or jarring of the head.

Aspirin Therapy

The effect of 650 mg of aspirin was studied in 3,711 patients with all levels of NPDR and with patients with less than high risk PDR during the ETDRS study.

Aspirin:

i. Did not alter the course of DR
ii. Did not affect the development of high-risk PDR
iii. Did not reduce the risk of visual loss
iv. Did not increase the risk of vitreous haemorrhage.

These findings indicate that there are no ocular contraindications to aspirin therapy in patients with DR when required for cardiovascular disease or other medical indications.

Calcium Dobesilate

Calcium dobesilate (Calcium 2, 5 dihydroxy benzene sulphonate). Its recommended dose is initially 1500 mg daily for 2 to 3 months, thereafter 1000 mg daily. Its early

TABLE 28.1.4

Indications	Treatments	Efficacies
CSME	Focal laser photocoagulation	50% reduction in MVL after 03 years
High risk PDR (all levels)	PRP	60% reduction in SVL after 03 years
Development of high risk PDR	PRP	87% reduction in SVL after 03 years
		97% reduction in bilateral SVL after 03 years
		90% reduction in legal blindness after 05 years
Severe PDR and severe vitreous haemorrhage	Vitrectomy	60% increased chance of 6/12 or better after 02 years
Severe PDR and vision 3/60 or better	Vitrectomy	34% increased chance of 6/12 or better after 02 years
No diabetic retinopathy	Intensive glycaemic control	76% reduction in the onset of retinopathy
NPDR	Intensive glycaemic control	63% reduction in retinopathy levels
		47% reduction in the development of severe NPDR and PDR
		26% reduction in the development of macular oedema
		51% reduction in need of laser treatment

Treatment efficacies

administration slows down the disease progression, delays laser treatment and prolongs the sight in diabetic patients. It takes nearly 2 to 3 months before its optimum effects are seen. Once signs of improvement are evident, the dose may be reduced to 1000 mg daily. It is well tolerated though minor side effects like nausea, vomiting, skin reactions and fever may be seen in few patients (3 to 4%). Occasionally bone marrow depression with agranulocytosis, anaemia and liver dysfunction may be seen. All these findings disappear when the drug is withdrawn.

The efficacies of the various treatment protocols are summarised in Table 28.1.4.

SUMMARY

Diabetes is a panophthalmic entity with every layer being affected. Yet, the most important and vision threatening involvement is that of the retina. The essence of management at the present is periodic check-up and prompt intervention under a setting, of course, of a strict glycaemic control. The future might give us a definitive management in the form of antagonists to the various biochemical mediators. From being an entity wherein the exercise of examination was for prognostication, it has now come to stay as an entity requiring immediate therapeutic intervention. Best results are obtained if an ophthalmologist is involved early as a therapeutic team member.

FURTHER READING

1. Aiello LP, Gardner TW, King GL, Blankenship G, Cavallerano JD, Ferris FL, Klein R. Diabetic retinopathy (Technical review). Diabetes Care (Indian edition), Apr-June 1998;1:48-61.
2. Francis AL Esperance Jr. Ophthalmic Lasers. Mosby: Missouri, 1989;347-24.
3. Retina and vitreous (Section 12). The foundation of the American Academy of Ophthalmology 2000;88-111.
4. Ryan SJ. Retina. Mosby: Missouri, 2001;(2):1259-349.

28.2 Diabetic Nephropathy

Y Sachdev

- Introduction
- Natural Course of Diabetic Nephropathy (DN)
- Metabolic and Haemodynamic Changes in DN
- Other Renal Conditions Associated with DM

- Management
- Microalbuminuria
- Summary

INTRODUCTION

Diabetic nephropathy is, probably the main cause of end-stage renal disease (ESRD). The clinical hallmark of diabetic nephropathy is persistent proteinuria greater than 500 mg/24 hours. This is equivalent to urinary albumin excretion rate (UAER) of 300 mg/day (or over 200 µg/min) in a person with diabetes, and without any other renal disease. Microalbuminuria is defined as urinary albumin excretion greater than 30 mg/24 hours (or 20 µg/min) and less than or equal to 300 mg/24 hours (200 µg/min) irrespective of how the urine is collected (Table 28.2.1).

Although proteinuria was observed in diabetic patients as early as 18th century, it was Bright in 1836 who postulated that albuminuria could reflect a serious renal disease specific to diabetes mellitus. It was one hundred years later when Kimmelstiel described the nodular glomerular intercapillary lesion in long-standing diabetics.

Diabetic nephropathy is closely related to the duration and severity of hyperglycaemia. Genetic and environmental factors, delayed diagnosis and less than adequate diabetes care are the contributory causes. The main potentially modifiable diabetic nephropathy initiation and progression factors in susceptible individuals are sustained hyperglycaemia and hypertension. Other putative risk factors are glomerular hyperfiltration, smoking, dyslipidaemia, proteinuria levels, and amount and source of protein intake and fat in the diet.

Glomerulosclerosis is present in nearly all type 1 patients, 2 to 3 decades after the diagnosis. Probably 25 to 27% of these patients, result in renal failure. Nephropathy is relatively less frequent in type 2 patients as the disease develops later in life and many of them have high mortality due to macrovascular disease. Even then, type 2 patients make more than 90% of those who come for renal replacement with the diagnosis of diabetes.

TABLE 28.2.1

Status	24 hr urinary protein (mg/day)	Albumin (mg/day)	UAER (µg/min)	Spot sample (mg/L)
Normal	–	< 30	< 20	< 20
Borderline	–	–	–	20 to 50
Incipient nephropathy		30 to 300	>20 to <200	50 to 300
Clinical nephropathy	> 500	>300	>200	>300

Levels of proteinuria/albuminuria in nephropathy

Natural Course of Diabetic Nephropathy

Glomerular basement membrane (GBM) thickening constitutes the ultimate structural and functional abnormality underlying diabetic nephropathy. Continual thickening of GBM over years causes progressive occlusion of glomerular capillaries leading to continuous proteinuria, decreased glomerular filtration rate (GFR) and ultimately chronic renal failure (Figs 28.2.1A to C). The natural history of diabetic nephropathy can be divided in five distinct stages (Table 28.2.2).

Progressive renal function changes in early stages of diabetic nephropathy comprise of:
- Increased GFR
- Increased filtration function
- Elevated urinary proteins and albumin (4400 to 15000 daltons)
- Increased renal clearance of neutral dextran polymer, and
- Increased glomerular permeability which is due to increased viscosity, microvascular stress, high content of sialic acid, IgG, albumin and fibrin in basement membrane.

TABLE 28.2.2

Approx years after diabetes	Clinical course of diabetic nephropathy
Onset (0 year)	↑GFR, ↑renal size, ↑plasma flow, super normal function, normal microalbuminuria (reversible with treatment)
2 to 5 years	Thickening of GBM, ↑mesangial matrix, normo/microalbuminuria (reversible)
6 to 10 years	Microalbuminuria (20 to 300 μg/min) or (30 to 300 mg/day) especially after exercise (progression preventable)
11 to 15 years	Proteinuria (first intermittent, later persistent) (progression preventable)
16 to 20 years	Azotaemic/uraemic stage, ESRD (? progress can be slowed)

Natural clinical course of diabetic nephropathy

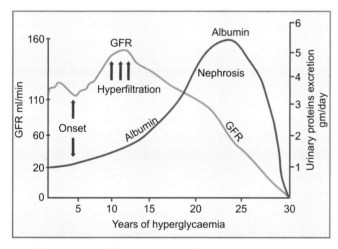

Fig. 28.2.1A: Clinical course of diabetic nephropathy

A few weeks or months later, there is:
- Significant increase in kidney size
- Increased glomerular tuft volume
- Increased capillary luminal volume, and
- Increased capillary filtration surface area.

In later stages, renal changes are:
- Accumulation of serum proteins/degradation products in glomeruli
- Glomerulosclerosis and tubulointerstitial fibrosis
- Excess fibrin due to decreased fibrinolysis
- Capillary occlusion
- Nonenzymatic glycosylation of plasma proteins, leading to capillary occlusion.

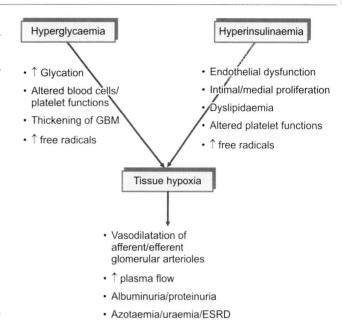

Fig. 28.2.1B: Pathophysiology of diabetic nephropathy

Years	0	3	5	10	15	20	25
GFR ml/min		100	150	150	120	60	<10
Serum creatinine			0.8	0.8	1.9	>2	>3

Incipient stage | Overt stage

Fig. 28.2.1C: Progression of diabetic nephropathy

Overt proteinuria supervenes followed by the development of renal impairment and renal failure.

The histological hallmark of diabetic nephropathy is the classical Kimmel-Steil-Wilson syndrome which consists of a typical nodular glomerulosclerosis. Histologically, a typical nodular lesion is a well demarcated, PAS positive globular structure that occurs at the periphery of the glomeruli. Diffuse glomerulosclerosis, although not specific, is more common. Additionally, hyaline deposits (exudative or insudative lesion), consisting of plasma proteins and lipids may be present in arterioles (hyaline arteriosclerosis), capillary walls (fibrin caps) and Bowman's capsule (capsular drops). Hyaline arteriosclerosis affects both afferent and efferent arterioles. Gradually the entire wall structure of arterioles and capillaries is replaced and complete sclerosis occurs. Besides this, tubular basement membrane also gets thickened and interstitial space expands.

METABOLIC AND HAEMODYNAMIC CHANGES

There are two major functional changes in diabetic nephropathy. They are:

1. Metabolic changes
2. Haemodynamic changes.

Metabolic Changes

Four metabolic changes appear to play a significant role in causation of diabetic nephropathy. These are as under:

Glycosylation

It represents a complex series of reactions which occur when glucose and other reducing sugar react with proteins, lipids and nucleic acids. In diabetes mellitus, there is an acceleration of Maillard or Browning reaction. This results in the formation of a range of advanced glycation end-products (AGEs). AGEs bind to specific receptors in macrophages, endothelial cells and cultured mesangial cells. Interaction of AGEs with their receptors in mesangial cells leads to increased transforming growth factor-B (TGF-B) expression and extracellular matrix synthesis.

Increased Polyol Pathway Flux

In kidney where glucose uptake is independent of insulin, hyperglycaemia results in increased levels of tissue glucose. The excess glucose is subsequently reduced to sorbitol by the NADPH-dependent enzyme, aldose reductase, the first enzyme in the polyol pathway. The increased sorbitol is accompanied by a depletion of free myoinositol, loss of Na^+- K^+- ATPase activity and increased consumption of the enzyme cofactors NADPH and NAD, leading to changes in cellular redox potential. These metabolic derangements result in cellular dysfunction and morphological lesions.

Activation of Protein Kinase C

The adverse effects of hyperglycaemia are attributed to activation of protein kinase C (PKC) which regulates diverse vascular functions including contractility, blood flow, cellular proliferation and vascular permeability

Increased Hexosamine Pathway Influx

This leads to increased TGF-B expression and extra cellular matrix synthesis.

Haemodynamic Changes

Increased intraglomerular pressure in association with vasodilatation of the afferent glomerular arterioles and constriction of the efferent arterioles is a classical feature of early diabetic nephropathy. Intrarenal-renin angiotensin system (RAS) appears to get activated in diabetes and modulates the changes seen in nephropathy. Angiotensin II stimulates TGF-B and matrix protein in renal interstitial fibroblasts and in proximal tubular epithelial cells. ACE inhibitors and angiotensin receptor antagonists normalize the intraglomerular pressure, suppress renal cytokines production and prevent extracellular matrix formation Figure 28.2.2 gives the metabolic and haemodynamic abnormalities of diabetic nephropathy.

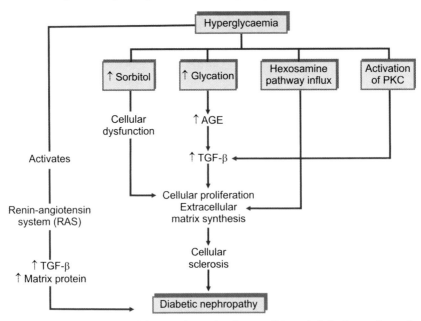

Fig. 28.2.2: Metabolic and haemodynamic abnormalities of diabetic nephropathy

Besides classical diabetic nephropathy as described above, there are other renal conditions which are associated with diabetes mellitus. They are as follows.

Urinary Tract Infection (UTI)

Recurrent UTI is very common in long-standing diabetic patients (F > M). UTI may get aggravated by atony of the urinary bladder which is present in some of the long-standing diabetics. Diabetics are also at risk to develop emphysematous polynephropathy which is characterized by gas in renal parenchyma or perirenal space. Energetic antibiotic therapy and strict glycaemic control are mandatory. Nephrectomy/drainage is often necessary to preserve life.

Renal Papillary Necrosis

It represents severe destruction of renal parenchyma which is due to impaired blood flow to the inner medulla and papilla of the kidney. Renal abscess or carbuncle of the kidney may also occur. Clinically, it manifests as flank pain, haematuria, chills, fever and septicaemia. Papilla fragments may cause ureteric obstruction which requires prompt treatment. Besides diabetes, papillary necrosis is also seen in urinary infections, over use of analgesics and Sickle cell disease.

Diabetes with renal insufficiency may result in radio-contrast-induced renal failure. Hydration before and after contrast injection may reduce this risk. Pretreatment with acetylcysteine may also protect the patient.

MANAGEMENT OF DIABETIC NEPHROPATHY

Persistent microalbuminuria is a clear confirmation of diabetic renal involvement. Such patients require frequent regular clinical assessment and advice to ensure proper dietary intake, tight glycaemic control, and adequate control of systemic blood pressure. The aim is to reduce the dietary protein intake to 0.6 to 0.8 gm/kg body weight depending upon the severity of renal involvement. This helps reduce albumin excretion and hyperfiltration.

- It has been seen that decline in glomerular filtration rate (GFR) is directly related to diastolic blood pressure. Therefore, it is recommended that blood pressure should be kept below 130/80 mmHg (preferably 120 to 125/70 to 75 mmHg) by salt restriction, lifestyle changes (graduated daily exercise, no smoking and no alcohol) and single or combination drug therapy. We recommend antihypertensive therapy in normotensive diabetic patients who have microalbuminuria.

- ACE-inhibitors (Lisinopril, ramipril, captopril, etc.) are the first choice as they are known to be 'reno-protective.' They not only reduce blood pressure, but also reduce albumin excretion rate. They, however, are not to be used in pregnancy and bilateral renal artery stenosis. These drugs are to be used with care if serum creatinine and potassium are high (>3 mg and >5 mEq respectively) and should be stopped if a rising trend is seen. Angiotensin receptor antagonists (Losartan, ibesartan, etc.), calcium channel blockers, vasodilators, selective beta and alpha adrenoceptor blockers, diuretics, and octreotide are the other drugs which can be used singly or in combination. A combination of octreotide and captopril results in significant reduction in renal growth and UAE. There is sufficient evidence to demonstrate that both ACE inhibitors and ARBs have a similar renoprotective effect. In resistant cases, a combination of a loop diuretic like frusemide 80 mg × twice daily and quinazole diuretic like metolazone (Zaroxolyn) 10 mg twice daily is very useful therapy. In isolated systolic hypertension with systolic pressure over 180 mmHg, the initial objective should be to reduce it gradually to 160 mmHg. If this is well tolerated then it can be reduced further gradually. If after 4 to 6 weeks treatment, ideal BP is not reached additional medication may have to be added depending upon cardiac status and fluid overload.

- Lipid abnormality may require statin administration to keep LDL cholesterol below 100 mg/dl.

Glycaemic Control

We endeavour to keep fasting plasma glucose level below 100 mg/dl and pre-meal blood glucose below 130 mg/dl with HbA1C less than 6.5%. This is mandatory to reduce the disease progression and help lesions to regress. In 1980s, the initial studies demonstrated that nearly 80% microabuminuria patients of T1DM progressed to proteinuria over 6 to 14 years. In more recent studies only 30 to 45% patients have been reported to progress to proteinuria over 10-year period. This is the result of intensive glycaemic and blood pressure control. Insulin is the ideal treatment if serum creatinine is 1.5 mg/dl or above. Insulin degradation is compromised in renal failure. Therefore, reduction in oral hypoglycaemics and insulin must be ensured to avoid hypoglycaemia. Metformin is contraindicated if serum creatinine is over 2 mg/dl because of risk of lactic acidosis.

Anaemia

Anaemia may occur even before the onset of advanced renal failure and is related to erythropoietin deficiency.

It is advisable to start erythropoietin therapy if Hb falls less than 10 gm/dl. Aim should be to keep it above 12 gm. Diabetic end stage renal disease (ESRD) patients are now accepted for treatment in ESRD programme where earlier they were refused.

It is advisable to have renal physician and transplant surgeon consultation if serum creatinine is 2.26 mg/dl (200 mol/L) or above.

Best results are achieved by early recognition and energetic treatment of diabetic nephropathy. A suggested algorithm for the management of a patient suspected to have raised urinary albumin excretion is given in Figure 28.2.3.

Use of Aspirin

It should be given in doses of 100 to 150 mg/day as some patients show aspirin resistance. Clopidogrel probably will be better than aspirin.

Newer Drugs on Clinical Trails

Aldose Reductase Inhibitors

Aldose reductase inhibitors have been observed to improve nerve conduction in diabetic neuropathy and are under trial for nephropathy.

Advanced Glycation End Products Inhibitors (AGE Inhibitors)

Hydrazine compound, aminoguanidine is useful in retinopathy. It has proved beneficial in reducing proteinuria and is undergoing multicentric trails.

Protein Kinase C Inhibitors

B-isoform-specific PKC inhibitor-Ly333531 reduces PKC activity in retina and renal glomeruli. Its benefits have been demonstrated in animals and is undergoing clinical trails at present.

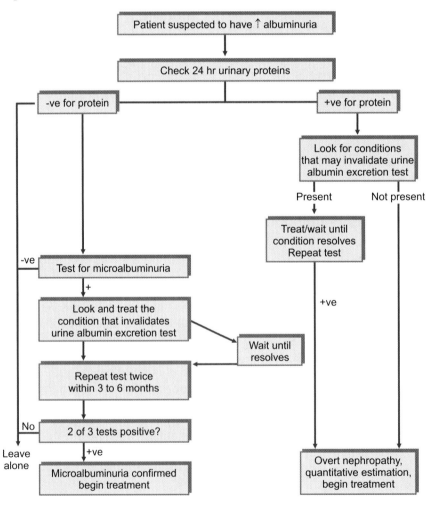

Fig. 28.2.3: Algorithmic approach to annual screening for urine albumin excretion

Anti-thromboxane Agent

Anti-thromboxane agent, picotamide, is another drug which is undergoing clinical trails. It has been observed to reduce microalbuminuria in normotensive T2DM patients.

SUMMARY

Diabetic nephropathy is the most common cause of ESRD in India. Its best treatment is its prevention which can be ensured by aggressive control of hyperglycaemia and elevated blood pressure, diet control, normal lipid profile and lifestyle changes. Male Indians and other Asians are a high risk ethnic group. Microalbuminunia phase lasts for 5 to 10 years and an energetic management of diabetic syndrome during this phase helps delay or avoid full-fledged diabetic nephropathy requiring haemodialysis and renal transplant. ACE inhibitors/ARBs lower blood pressure as well as reduce microalbuminuria. Many new drugs are undergoing clinical trails and may prove useful in time to come.

MICROALBUMINURIA

Microalbuminuria predicts the onset of clinical proteinuria and renal involvement in diabetes (both type 1 and type 2). It is also an independent risk factor for cardiovascular disease in non-diabetic populations. It may also be associated with a number of acute inflammatory conditions. In view of its importance, it is being described in details.

The term 'pathological albuminuria' or mere 'albuminuria' is used to describe the presence of albumin in the urine in the range of 30 to 300 mg/24 hours or 20 to 200 μg/minute or an albumin-to-creatinine ratio greater than 2 mg/mmol in the first morning urine sample. It is undetectable by qualitative chemical dipsticks. It is generally expressed as the albumin excretion rate in μg per minute or as the albumin (mg) creatinine (mg/mmol) ratio to correct for variations in urine flow. Calculation of the albumin excretion rate requires a timed urine collection (6, 12 or 24 hour collection) while the albumin: creatinine ratio can be calculated from a 'spot' urine test. The latter assumes that the subject's urinary creatinine excretion remains constant.

Albumin excretion rate varies with posture. Its over-night excretion rate is significantly lower. It rises three fold during and immediately after strenuous short-term exercise. In a normotensive individual there is no or very little relationship between blood pressure and albumin excretion; but there is a strong positive correlation if the BP is above 150/90 mmHg. It is nearly 30% higher in smokers than non-smokers.

Microalbumin is also seen in chronic obstructive pulmonary disease (COPD), congestive cardiac failure (CCF), hypertension and malignancy. In diabetics and essential hypertension patients, the degree of micro-albuminuria correlates positively with blood pressure reading and falls in response to antihypertensive treatment. Both hypertensive and diabetes patients with microalbuminuria show an increased transcapillary escape rate of radio labelled albumin denoting increased vascular permeability (Figs 28.2.4A and B). Increased vascular endothelial permeability allows the infiltration of low-density lipoproteins into the vessel wall. This

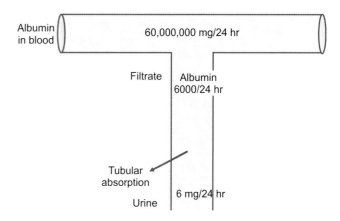

Figs 28.2.4A: Sixty kg of albumin pass through the kidneys every 24 hours. Less than 0.01% reaches the glomerular filtrate. More than 99% of filtered albumin is reabsorbed in the tubules which are near saturation

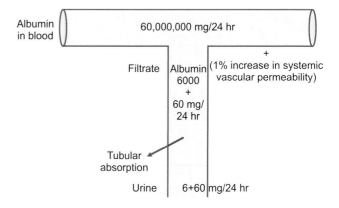

Fig. 28.2.4B: 1% increase in systemic vascular permeability results in 60 mg of additional albumin entering the filtrate which cannot be absorbed and leaks out

forms an important step in the process of atherogenesis and explains the rationale of calling microalbuminuria as an independent predictor for cardiovascular disease in both diabetic and hypertensive patients.

The non-diabetics with a urinary albumin excretion rate of >20 μg/min. have a 4-fold increased risk of peripheral vascular disease and 2-fold increased risk of coronary artery disease. Subjects with urinary albumin concentration of > 30 mg/litre have significantly higher BP, circulating triglycerides, hyperglycaemia and insulin resistance. Those with autonomic neuropathy are in risk for sudden heart failure and death. It is also a predictor of mortality from cardiovascular disease especially in middle aged and elderly population. The predictive power of microalbuminuria for cardiovascular complications and mortality appears to be as strong if not stronger than that of hyperlipidaemia and hypertension.

Microalbuminuria is also associated with many acute and chronic inflammatory conditions indicating increased vascular permeability. In acute conditions like surgery, acute myocardial infarction, severe pancreatitis, bacterial meningitis, etc. the microalbuminuria is an early feather of increased vascular permeability. This response to acute inflammatory process occurs much earlier than a rise in serum C-reactive protein (CRP) concentration which takes 2 to 3 days to reach its maximum. Usually it has a rapid onset and lasts for 1 to 24 hours unless there are complications when it may be prolonged. The degree of microalbuminuria is proportional to the severity of the acute condition. It is believed that glomerular leakage of albumin reflects systemic vascular status making detection of microalbuminuria an independent marker of endothelial dysfunction and predictor of the severity of the disease process.

Therefore, it is mandatory to have at least two elevated albumin to creatinine ratios separated by 3 to 6 months to make the diagnosis of diabetic micro-albuminuria, provided there is no other evidence of renal involvement by diabetes.

SUMMARY

Microalbuminuria reflects increased vascular permeability. It is a predictor of diabetic complications; a powerful cardiovascular risk factor in non-diabetics and a marker for organ failure in a acute inflammatory conditions.

FURTHER READING

Diabetic Nephropathy

1. Alberti K GMM, et al. International Textbook of Diabetes Mellitus (2nd edn). Wiley, Chichister, 1997.
2. American Diabetes Association Clinical Practice Recommendation. Diabetes Care 2001;24 (Suppl.1) S1-S133.
3. American Diabetes Association. Diabetic nephropathy. Diabetes Care 2003;26 (Suppl 1): 1-5.
4. American Diabetes Association. Treatment of hypertension in adults with diabetes. Diabetes Care 2003;26 (Suppl 1): 80-2.
5. American Diabetes Association: Standards of medical care for patients with diabetes mellitus. Diabetes Care 2003;26(Suppl. 1):33-50.
6. Gross JL, De Azevedo MJ, Silveiro SP, et al. Diabetic nephropathy: diagnosis, prevention, and treatment. Diabetes Care 2005;28:176-88.
7. Indian College Physician: Guidelines on management of diabetic nephropathy 2003.
8. Mogensen CE, Christensen CK. Predicting diabetic nephropathy in insulin-dependent patients. N Engl J Med 1984;311:89-93.
9. Perkins BA, Ficociello LH, Silva KH, et al. Regression of microalbuminuria in type 1 diabetes. N Egl J Med 2003;348: 2285-93.

Microalbuminuria

10. Gerstein HC, Mann JF, Pogue J, et al. Prevalence and determinants of microalbuminuria in high risk diabetic and non-diabetic patients in heart outcomes prevention study (The HOPE Study) Diabetes Care. 2000;23:835-9.
11. Gosling P. Microalbuminuria a marker of systemic disease. Jr Applied Medicine 1996;53-62.
12. Keane WF, Eknoyan G. Proteinuria, albuminuria, risk, assessment, detection, elimination (PARADE): a position paper of the National Kidney Foundation. Am J Kidney Dis 1999;33: 1004-10.

28.3 Diabetic Neuropathy

Y Sachdev

INTRODUCTION

Diabetic neuropathy (DN) is one of the most common and most distressing late complications of diabetes mellitus. It affects nearly 50% of diabetic patients. It has varied presentations and treatment is not very helpful in many of the cases. Neglected cases are liable to develop foot ulcers and gangrene which may need foot/leg amputation in certain instances.

The epidemiology and natural history of DN is poorly defined.

DEFINITION

It is best defined as the presence of symptoms and/or signs of peripheral nerve dysfunction in diabetes after the exclusion of other causes (malignancy, chronic alcoholism, nutritional deficiency, infections, iatrogenic, etc.)

PATHOGENESIS (Fig. 28.3.1A)

The affected nerve has diminished nerve conduction indicative of distal axonopathy of dying-back variety. The metabolic initiators are: non-enzymatic glycosylation with production of advanced glycated end-products (AGEs), auto-oxidation of glucose, increased aldose reductase activity leading to elevated sorbitol and fructose, and activation of protein kinase C (PKC).

The physiological mediators for neuropathy are interruption of nerve blood flow leading to micro-vascular inefficiency, impaired neurotrophic support by neurotrophins, cytokines like growth factors and induction of neuronal and Schwann cell apoptosis by autoimmunity and oxidative stress.

Presently, it is felt that both metabolic initiators and physiological mediators are operative and result in various types of neuropathies.

CLASSIFICATION

There are several classifications, the best and most commonly used is one based on clinical patterns of neuropathy (Table 28.3.1) while Figure 28.3.1B classifies diabetic neuropathy as peripheral and autonomic based on pattern of the nervous system involved.

TABLE 28.3.1

1. Length-dependent diabetic neuropathy
   - Distal symmetrical sensorimotor polyneuropathy
   - Small fibre painful neuropathy
     - Acute painful neuropathy
     - Chronic painful neuropathy
   - Long fibre neuropathy
   - Autonomic neuropathies
2. Focal and multifocal neuropathies
   - Cranial neuropathies
   - Limb neuropathies
   - Proximal neuropathy of the lower limb
   - Truncal neuropathies
3. Others
   - Pressure or entrapment palsies
   - Acquired inflammatory demyelinating polyneuropathy

**Classification of diabetic neuropathies
(as per clinical pattern)**

CLINICAL PRESENTATION

It is bizarre and may be in the form of:

Distal Symmetrical Sensorimotor Polyneuropathy (Fig. 28.3.2)

It is the most common form of diabetic neuropathy. It manifests as sensory loss in the toes and feet which is the result of dysfunction in both large and small myelinated and unmyelinated nerve fibres. All sensory modalities are usually affected including vibration and

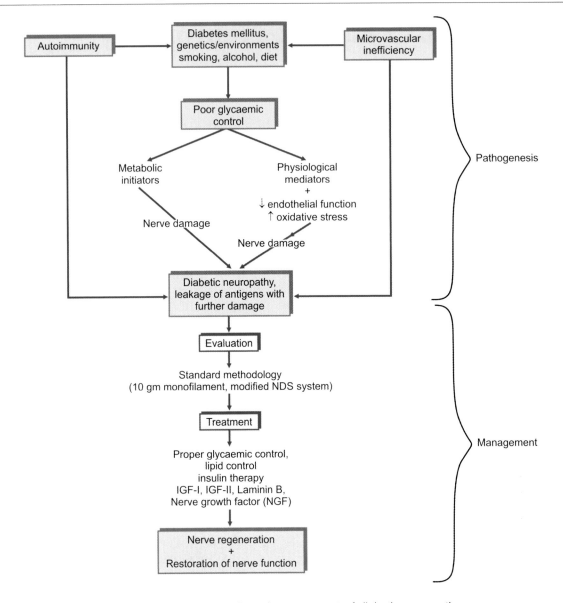

Fig. 28.3.1A: Pathogenesis and management of diabetic neuropathy

joint position sense. It is length-dependent process and sensory loss begins from the toes and ascends upwards in the legs. Ultimately it produces a classical picture of 'glove and stocking' sensory loss. Mild or disabling pain with paraesthesias/dysaesthesias may be experienced by some patients. Ankle jerk may be absent and weakness of intrinsic muscles results in claw toe and foot deformities. Chronic foot ulceration may also be seen if there is associated vascular insufficiency as well.

In 1988, American Academy of Neurology at San Antonio conference on distal symmetrical peripheral neuropathy (DSPN) decided that at least one parameter

from each of the following 5 categories must be present to reach its diagnosis:

i. Symptoms profile
ii. Neurological examination
iii. Quantitative sensitivity test (QST)
iv. Nerve conduction velocity (NCV)
v. Quantitative autonomic function test (QAFT).

Small Fibre Neuropathy

It may manifest as acute or chronic neuropathy.

Acute painful neuropathy (Fig. 28.3.3) It is characterized by acute pain, paraesthesias in patients with diabetes

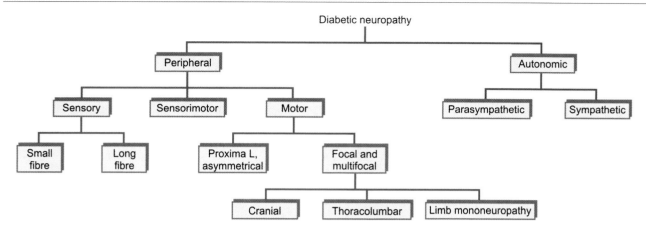

Fig. 28.3.1B: Classification of diabetic neuropathy (as per pattern of nervous system involvement)

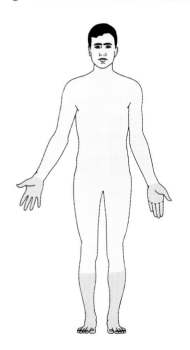

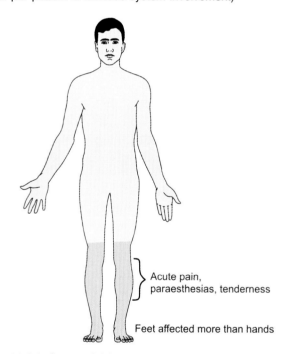

Fig. 28.3.2: Symmetrical diffuse sensorimotor neuropathy (Sensory loss—nil to moderate, pain—mild to moderate, tendon reflexes—normal to decreased, motor deficit—nil to mild)

Fig. 28.3.3: Acute painful neuropathy (Sensory loss—nil to mild, pain—mild to moderate, tendon reflexes—normal to decreased, motor deficit—absent)

mellitus of less than 6 months duration. Pain is more at night, has variable severity and character—may be lancelating, stabbing or sharp. Feet are affected more than hands. Lower limbs are extremely tender to touch.

The patient suffers severe depression and profound weight loss. Some of them recover spontaneously while others need analgesics and antidepressants.

Chronic painful neuropathy It occurs years after onset of diabetes mellitus. It starts slowly and gradually becomes debilitating.

Long-term sequelae of small fibre neuropathy could be foot ulceration and gangrene.

Long Fibre Neuropathy (Fig. 28.3.4)

It may be sensory/motor or both. The early signs may be impaired sense of vibration and position. Tendon reflexes are depressed. Pain could be dull, deep or crushing and accompanied by cramps. In some cases there is sensory ataxia. Small muscles of hand and feet are weak and wasted and may lead to foot deformities and Charcot's neuroarthrosis. Feet may be warm due to increased blood flow.

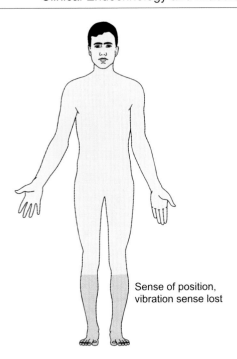

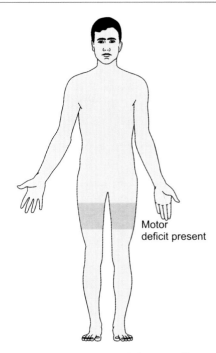

Fig. 28.3.4: Long fibre neuropathy (Vibration sense loss present, sense of position loss present, local pain variable nature, depressed tendon reflexes, hand and feet muscles wasted, foot deformities)

Fig. 28.3.5: Diabetic amyotrophy of Garland (Sensory loss—nil to mild, pain—mild to moderate, tendon reflexes decreased to normal, motor deficit—mild to moderate)

Proximal Motor Neuropathies (Diabetic Amyotrophy of Garland) (Fig. 28.3.5)

Primarily it is seen among the elderly male diabetics. It may have a gradual or an abrupt onset and presents with pain in thighs, hips, or buttocks followed by proximal muscle weakness of the lower limbs. The patient finds it difficult to get up from the sitting/sqatting position (positive Gower's test). Usually the muscle weakness begins as a unilateral event and becomes bilateral later on. It may coexist with distal symmetrical sensorimotor polyneuropathy. The affected muscles may show spontaneous or induced fasciculations. Body weight loss may be another prominent feature.

Mononeuropathies (Fig. 28.3.6)

Isolated peripheral nerve lesions are recognized as more common in older diabetic patients. Many a time it may even be a presenting feature of type 2 DM.

Cranial Mononeuropathies

The III and IV cranial nerves are involved manifesting with ptosis and ophthalmoplegia. The onset is usually rapid and is often accompanied by pain. The pupils are usually spared in 3rd nerve palsy. Diplopia is the common complaint. Less common involvement is that of IVth and VIIth nerves. VIIth nerve involvement leads

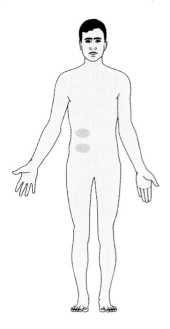

Fig. 28.3.6: Mononeuropathies (Sensory loss—nil to mild, pain—mild to moderate, tendon reflexes—normal, motor deficit—mild to moderate)

to Bell's palsy with unilateral weakness of facial muscles and widening of the palpebral fissure. Some workers have reported increased incidence of trigeminal neuralgia in diabetics.

Truncal Mononeuropathy

It is characterized by pain occurring in a band-like distribution around the lower chest or abdomen in a dermatomal pattern. Usually, it occurs in isolation but may be associated with other long-term complications of diabetes. The pain may be aching or burning in quality; may get superimposed with lancinating character. It shows nocturnal exacerbations with cutaneous hyperaesthesias. Rarely, it may result in muscle weakness with local abdominal bulge.

Isolated and Multiple Mononeuropathies

Any peripheral nerve may be involved; though mostly we see the involvement of the median/ulnar/peroneal nerve (entrapment syndromes) (Fig. 28.3.7) or lateral femoral cutaneous nerve of the thigh (meralgia paraesthetica).

Median nerve entrapment or carpal tunnel syndrome It is the most common entrapment entity in diabetes mellitus. It is due to nerve compression under the transverse carpal ligament. Idiopathic carpal tunnel syndrome is also seen in rheumatoid arthritis, hypothyroidism and obesity. There is painful paraesthesias of the fingers which may progress to a deep-seated ache radiating up the forearm and rarely to the arm. Usually, it occurs at night, but may be initiated during the day by repeated flexion and extension at the wrist. Thenar muscles may waste especially in the elderly patients.

Ulnar neuropathy It is the second most common entrapment neuropathy and is due to ulnar nerve compression immediately distal to the ulnar groove beneath the edge of the flexor carpi ulnaris aponeurosis in the cubital tunnel. Classical symptoms are painful paraesthesias in the fourth and fifth digits with hypothenar and interosseous muscle wasting.

Radial neuropathy It is due to radial nerve compression in the spiral groove and is accompanied by wrist drop. Occasionally sensory symptoms in the dermatomes supplied by radial nerve may be observed.

Peroneal neuropathy It is the most common lower limb mononeuropathy and manifests as weakness of dorsiflexors resulting in foot drop. Sensory deficit is also present but there is usually no pain or paraesthesias. Diabetes is a relatively uncommon cause of this neuropathy. Usual causes are external compression and traumatic bone fractures.

Lateral femoral cutaneous neuropathy It is uncommon and results in pain, paraesthesias and sensory loss in the lateral aspect of the thigh (meralgia paraesthetica). Obesity is the most common cause of this.

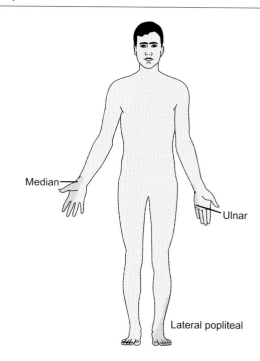

Fig. 28.3.7: Entrapment syndromes (Sensory loss—mild to severe, pain—mild to severe, tendon reflexes—normal, motor deficit—mild to moderate)

OBJECTIVE CLINICAL ASSESSMENT OF DIABETIC PERIPHERAL NEUROPATHY (DPN)

Pain and paraesthesias are the two chief complaints of DPN. Both these complaints are subjective and it has been seen that there could be marked differences between the description of the symptoms given by two different patients having similar pathological findings. This is not surprising as the former depends primarily on the vocabulary and the descriptive quality of the patients. An objective and standardized assessment methodology, therefore, is considered necessary so as to rationalize the clinical assessment.

As such many screening questionnaires with scoring system to conduct an objective assessment of DPN have been prepared and made available. A few of them are as under: Michigan Neuropathy Scoring Instrument (MNSI), Neuropathy Deficit Score (NDS) and Neuropathy Impairment Score (NIS). Table 28.3.2 gives the scoring details of one of these systems which is widely used and has stood the test of the time.

Similarly, standardized hand-held or mechanically operated devices are available to evaluate the patient's response to stimuli like superficial and deep touch, pressure, pain, hot, cold and vibration sensations. One of the hand-held devices is Semmes Weinstein monofilament. The filament assesses pressure perception when gentle pressure is applied to the handle sufficient

TABLE 28.3.2

	Parameter checked	Rt	Lt	Stimulus applied	Site checked	Response	Score
1.	Vibration sense	√	√	Tuning fork 128 Hz	Apex of big toe	• Normal • Abnormal	0 1
2.	Temp perception	√	√	Tuning fork with beaker of ice/warm water	Foot dorsum	• Normal • Abnormal	0 1
3.	Pin prick	√	√	Pin	Proximal to big toe nail (to deform the skin)	• Minimal • Can differentiate sharp and blunt	0 1
4.	Achilles reflex	√	√	Percussion hammer	Achilles tendon	• Absent • Present with reinforcement • Present	2 1 0

Modified NDS for screening DN patient (Total score 10)
(A score over 6 has 6-fold increased risk of foot ulcer)

to buckle the nylon filament. Several filaments of different sizes are available. The most commonly used is the one that exerts 10-gauge of pressure and is known as 5.07 monofilament. The graduated Rydel-Seiffer tuning fork is another hand-held device that is useful for evaluation of sense of vibration. This fork uses a visual optical illusion to allow the accesser to determine the intensity of residual vibrations on a 0 to 8 scale at the point of threshold (disappearance of sensation). Recently introduced 'neuropen' is a device with a neurotip at one end of the pen to assess pain and a 10 gm monofilament at the other end to assess pressure.

In contrast to these simple hand-held devices, more sophisticated Quantitative Screening Test (QST) instruments which are more accurate but expensive are also available though not everywhere.

Other Assessment Procedures

Electrophysiological studies (nerve conduction velocity), endoneural oxygen tension, epineural vessel photography, fluorescein angiography to study the neural microvasculature:
• Skin biopsy
• Nerve biopsy
• MRI spinal cord.

Most of these procedures are highly specialized and available only in specialist research centres.

MANAGEMENT OF DIABETIC NEUROPATHY

Whatever may be the type of neuropathy, it is essential to ensure a tight glycaemic control (to stop the relentless progression of neuropathy) and provide symptomatic relief. Tight glycaemic control also reduces the risk of developing diabetic neuropathy which once established progresses slowly and may become irreversible. Tight glycaemic control improves vibration sense and nerve conduction.

In motor neuropathy, neurovitamines like B_1, B_6, B_{12} supplementation has proved useful along with anabolic steroids which help regain some of the muscle mass and muscle power.

For severe pain, analgesics like aspirin, NSAIDs, opioid analgesics may be of some help. Antidepressants like phenothiazines (e.g. Fluphenezine 2.5 to 5 mg), tricyclic drugs like amitriptyline 25 mg (elderly 10 mg) at bed time, or imipramine (10 mg daily, increase it weekly to a maximum of 150 mg) are of help in some patients. Phenothiazines enhance analgesic effects of tricyclic drugs but aggravate postural hypotension. For this, appropriate instructions to guard against postural hypotension may be stressed.

In other patients, drugs like tramadol (central analgesic up to 400 mg daily), dextromethorphan, carbamazepine (100 mg OD → BD till 800 mg daily in divided doses) and gabapentin (900 to 3600 mg daily in divided doses) may be useful. Gabapentin is an effective anticonvulsant. It has been used as a useful analgesic in treatment of pain and sleep problems and diabetic peripheral neuropathy. Some cases are benefited by transcutaneous electrical nerve stimulation (TENS). In certain circumstances pethidine or morphine may have to be used.

For A-delta fibre pain, clonidine, mexilitine (40 mg/day in divided doses), lidocaine, carbamazepine, calcitonin and intravenous insulin infusion (without lowering blood sugar) is helpful (and results are evident within 48 hours when it can be discontinued) whereas in severe 'C' fibre pain, lidocaine, mexilitine and local application of clonidine/capsaicin is useful. Clonidine can be applied topically. The dose titration, however, is difficult. Capsaicin causes hot chilli sensation and depletes pain transmitting 'C' fibres of substance P. Capsaicin is derived from chilli pepper 1 to 3 TSF of Cayenna pepper added to a jar of cold cream applied locally relieves the pain. After the application cover the affected area with a plastic wrap. It acts on vanilloid receptor (VR1) and produces desensitizing effect. Care must be taken to protect eyes and genitals. It is better to use gloves when applying the cream. Capsaicin cream (0.075%) is available commercially and is applied 3 to 4 times daily for 6 to 8 weeks (maximum).

For restless legs syndrome, clonazepam 0.5 to 3 mg is recommended. For allodynia (contact pain) a leg cradle or opsite adhesive plaster film to the skin may prove useful. Besides above mentioned measures, proper foot care, shoe and socks size need attention so that there is no pressure on any part of the feet.

In the management of distal motor/sensorimotor peripheral neuropathy, the following new therapeutic agents are useful:
a. Aldose reductase inhibitors (ARIs) like tolrestat and zenarestat are beneficial as they reduce the flux of glucose through polyol pathways. However, they have been withdrawn because of the toxicity. Presently, only epalrestat and fidarestat are marketed and some degrees of benefits have been attributed to them.
b. α-lipoic acid which is derivative of octanoic acid is useful in both somatic and autonomic neuropathies. Lipoic acid is a natural co-factor in pyruvate dehydrogenase complex where it binds acyl groups and transfers them from one part to another α-lipoic acid. Lipoic acid is present in food and is also synthesized in the liver. Its intravenous preparation is available in certain European countries.
c. Gamma-linolenic acid supplementation is demonstrated to be of great utility. Linoleic acid is an essential fatty acid. In diabetes, linoleic acid conversion to γ-linolenic acid (GLA) is impaired. GLA is important for preservation of nerves' integrity and its blood flow. Its supplementation helps in management of peripheral neuropathy.
d. Aminoguanidine, an inhibitor of AGEs and a free radicals scavenger, is another drug which has proved its usefulness.
e. Human intravenous immunoglobulin (IVIg). Whenever immune process is suspected to be involved, the human I V immunoglobulins, especially for chronic inflammatory demyelinating polyneuropathy, circulating GMI antibodies, antibodies to necrotizing vasculitis and monoclonal gamma may

be used. Their value, however, is limited. In some cases, it may be necessary to combine it with prednisone and/or azathioprine. Repeated courses may be required in relapses. Anaphylactic reaction is a known side effect. However, its incidence is very low.
f. Selective serotonin reuptake inhibitors (SSRIs) like citalopram, duloxetine hydrochloride or paroxite and other anticonvulsants like iamotrigine and topiramate have also been used with limited success.
g. Transcutaneous electrical nerve stimulation (TENS): It may be occasionally helpful and represents a very benign therapy for painful neuropathy. Care must be taken to move the electrodes around to recognize the most sensitive areas and obtain maximum relief.

SUMMARY

Neuropathy is one of the most common long-term complications of uncontrolled diabetes mellitus. The clinical presentation of diabetic neuropathy shows a very wide spectrum and variable course. This is due to a progressive loss of nerve fibres affecting various peripheral nerves singly or in multiples. The chapter discusses clinical presentation, objective assessment and management of neuropathies. Prolonged hyperglycaemia and accompanying impaired vascular and neurotrophic support are the main factors responsible for the neurones damage.

FURTHER READING

1. American Diabetes Association, American Academy of Neurology. Report and Recommendations of the San Antonio Conference on diabetes neuropathy (Consensus Statemnet). Diabetes Care 1988;11:592-7.
2. Boulton AJM, Gries FA, Jervell JA. Guidelines for the diagnosis and management of diabetic peripheral neuropathy. Diabet Med 1998;15:508-14.
3. Chopra JS, Hurwitz LG, Montgomery DA. The pathogenesis of sural nerve changes in diabetes mellitus. Brain 1969;29: 391-9.
4. Dyck PJ, Thomas PK (Eds). Diabetic Polyneuropathy. Philadelphia: WB Saundes 1999.
5. Dyck PJ, Windebank AJ. Diabetic and nondiabetic lumbosacral radiculoplexus neuropathies: new insights into pathophysiology and treatment. Muscle Nerve 2002;25:477.
6. Feldman EL. Oxidative stress and diabetic neuropathy: a new understanding of an old problem. J Clin Invest 2003;111:431-3.
7. Garland H. Diabetic amyotrophy. Br Med J 1955;2-1287-9.
8. Mendell JR, Sahenk Z. Painful sensory neuropathy. N Engl J Med 2003;43:957-73.
9. Simmonos Z, Feldman EL. Update on diabetic neuropathy. Cura Opin Neurol 2000;15:595.
10. Spence MC, Potter J, Coppini DV. The pathogenesis and management of painful diabetic neuropathy. A Review Diabetic Med 2003;20:88-98.
11. Stewart JD. Diabetic truncal neuropathy. Topography of the sensory deficit. Ann Neurol 1989;25:233.

28.4 Diabetic Autonomic Neuropathy

Y Sachdev

- Introduction
- Pathogenesis
- Clinical presentation: Sudomotor, Postural Hypotension, Neurological Deficits, Resting Tachycardia and Palpitation, Urogenital, Gastrointestinal, Ewing's Tests in Asymptomatic Diabetics

- Clinical Manifestation: Urinary, Cardiovascular, Sexual, Gastrointestinal, Sudomotor, Pupillary, Respiratory
- Management
- Prevention
- Glycaemic and Lipid Control, Symptomatic Management
- Summary

INTRODUCTION

Clinical manifestations of autonomic neuropathy are relatively uncommon. However, if special tests are conducted to study the autonomic functions, widespread abnormalities can be elicited (Fig. 28.4.1). Involvement of the autonomic nervous system (ANS) may occur as early as the very first year of the diagnosis or may be a delayed feature. It can involve any system in the body though the main clinical manifestations are due to cardio-vascular, gastrointestinal, genitourinary and metabolic dysfunctions/disorders. One of the earliest manifes-tations of diabetic autonomic neuropathy is denervation of the cardiovascular system. Loss of heart rate variability may be as high as 22% and decline may be three times faster per year compared to normal individuals.

PATHOGENESIS

Multiple aetiological factors involved are metabolic insult to the nerve fibres, neurovascular insufficiency, auto-immune damage and neurohormonal growth factors.

CLINICAL PRESENTATION

The patient may be completely asymptomatic or present with variable symptoms as under.

In diabetic autonomic neuropathy (DAN), abnor-malities in sweating (sudomotor), postural hypotension, motility disorders affecting oesophagus, GI tract, urinary bladder, erectile dysfunction, painless myocardial infarctions and unexplained sudden cardiorespiratory arrest particularly during anaesthesia and surgery are some of the main problems faced by those diabetics whose autonomic nervous system is involved.

Involvement of autonomic nervous system is more common among those patients who have obvious peripheral neuropathy though it is not mandatory.

Loss of sweating in parts of lower extremities—leg and feet, due to degeneration of the sympathetic fibres is a common feature in diabetics. This may be accom-panied by compensatory hyperhidrosis involving typically the face, neck and upper limbs. Gustatory sweating—sweating over face and neck on food intake is one of the common features.

Microvascular skin flow is under the control of autonomic nervous system and is regulated by the central and peripheral components. In diabetes, the rhythmic contraction of arterioles and small arteries is disordered resulting in microvascular insufficiency to the skin and peripheral nerves. Dry skin and development of skin cracks are common clinical features due to this. Microvascular blood flow is easily measured by laser Doppler flowmetry.

Postural hypotension manifesting as dizziness, unsteadiness and other neurological deficits on sudden standing up are other common symptoms. The involve-ment needs detailed evaluation in all cases of DAN in view of the risk of sudden death. Resting tachycardia, palpitation, painless ischaemia are indicative of auto-matic involvement and are risk factors for silent myo-cardial infarction, respiratory failure and sudden death.

It is advisable to carry out specific bedside tests detailed by Ewing to determine the integrity of autonomic regulation of heart beat and vasomotor tone. In these tests, parasympathetic cardiac regulation is tested by Valsalva manoeuvre (patient steadily blows into a mouth piece for 15 sec. This increases heart rate and is followed by rebound bradycardia), deep breathing R-R variation (patient breaths deeply at 6 breaths a minute), and heart beat response to immediate standing. Valsalva manoeuvre transiently increases intrathoracic, intraocular and intracranial pressures. Therefore, there could be a theoretical risk of intraocular haemorrhage and lens dislocation. Standing causes an immediate rapid

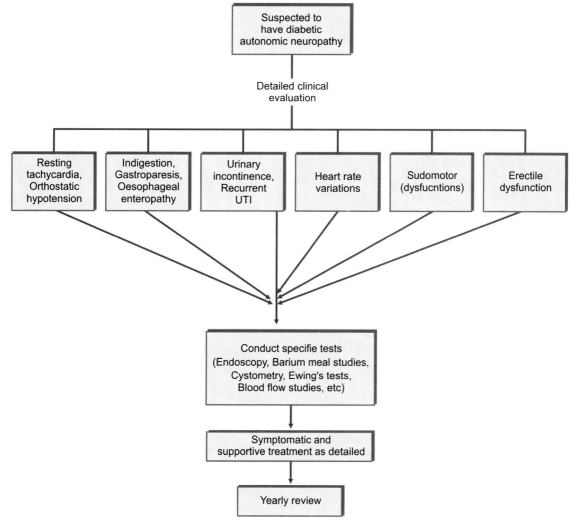

Fig. 28.4.1: Evaluation and management of diabetic autonomic neuropathy (DAN)
*(Note: T1DM patients must be checked 5 years after the diagnosis and then reviewed every 1 to 2 years.
T2DM patients must be evaluated at the time of diagnosis and reviewed every year)*

increase in heart rate with the maximum rate generally found at around the 15th beat after standing. The heart rate slows at or around the 30th beat. The heart rate tracing is used to calculate the ratio of the longest R-R interval (about beat 30th) and shortest R-R interval (about beat 15th) after standing. This measure (30:15 ratio) reflects the overall condition of the parasympathetic fibres.

The sympathetic integrity is tested by systolic blood pressure response to immediate standing and diastolic blood pressure response to sustained hand grip (maintained for 5 minutes). An internationally accepted score system is used to determine normal response, borderline and distinct involvement (Table 28.4.1).

Usually parasympathetic fibres are affected first and later on sympathetic fibres involvement supervenes; this sequence, however, is not always present. Proceedings from a consensus conference (1992) recommended three tests (R-R variation, Valsalva and postural BP check) for longitudinal checking of the cardiovascular autonomic system. As patients' cooperation is necessary to carry out these tests, it may become difficult to conduct these in children.

CLINICAL MANIFESTATIONS (TABLE 28.4.2)

Gastrointestinal System

There may be no symptoms at all in some diabetics or the symptoms may relate to gastrointestinal system like

TABLE 28.4.1

Tests	Scores		
	0	1	2
Valsalva manoeuvre			
Valsalva ratio	>1.20	1.11 to 1.20	<1.10
R-R variations on deep breathing	>15 beats /min	11 to 15 beats/min	<10 beats/min
R-R internal and immediate standing (30:15 ratio)	>1.03	1.01 to 1.03	<1.00
Sustained hand grip and diastolic BP	>15	11 to 15	<10
Systolic BP and immediate standing	<20	20 to 30	>30

Ewing's tests score for autonomic neuropathy
Key: Score 0—Free of neuropathy, < 5—Borderline neuropathy, >5—Distinct neuropathy

anorexia, nausea, epigastric discomfort, indigestion, dysphagia, constipation, abdominal distension, etc. These symptoms are indicative of gastric atony, oesophageal enteropathy, sluggish intestinal movements and decreased gastric acid secretion. Sometimes, intermittent diarrhoea is more prominent a complaint than constipation. Food stasis and decreased intestinal mobility may lead to bacterial colonization in the upper gut with more severe symptoms. Internal anal sphincter may also get affected (neuropathic sphincter) leading to frequent uncontrollable loose motions particularly at night. Nuclear medicine scintigraphy after ingestion of a radiolabelled meal is the best study to document gastric emptying. Presently noninvasive breath tests after ingestion of radiolabelled meal are being developed. It is to be remembered that hyperglycaemia itself can induce delayed gastric emptying. Parasympathetic dysfunction, however, aggravates the problem. Gallbladder may be atonic and enlarged.

Urinary Symptoms

Neuropathic urinary bladder is not an uncommon clinical experience (seen in 37 to 50% diabetics). The earliest bladder dysfunction is sensory abnormality resulting in impaired bladder sensation, elevated threshold for initiating micturition reflex and asymptomatic increase in bladder capacity and retention. Initially increase in residual urine does remain asymptomatic until infection supervenes or retention occurs. Suprapubic fullness is usually noticeable during clinical examination though it could also be easily missed. Hesitancy in micturition is another common feature. Ultrasonography, cystometry and urodynamic studies are essential investigations for assessment of bladder functions.

TABLE 28.4.2

Gastrointestinal symptoms

- Anorexia, nausea, dysphagia, epigastric discomfort, gastroparesis diabeticorum, diarrhoea, constipation, faecal incontinence

Cardiovascular symptoms

- Resting tachycardia, postural hypotension, exercise intolerance, painless angina, silent MI, respiratory failure, sudden death

Urogenital symptoms

- Neurogenic bladder (diabetic cytopathy)
- Other urinary bladder dysfunctions
- Erectile dysfunction
- Retrograde ejaculations
- Loss of vaginal lubrication

Peripheral symptoms

- Anhidrosis, heat intolerance
- Hyperhidrosis/hypohidrosis
- Gustatory sweating
- Pupillary abnormalities (pupillomotor impairmrnt, Argyll-Robertson pupil)
- Impaired peripheral blood circulation
- Dependent oedema

Metabolic symptoms

- Wide fluctuation in blood glucose levels
- Unawareness of hypoglycaemia
- No/hyporesponse to hypoglycaemia

Clinical manifestations of autonomic neuropathy

Cardiovascular System

Cardiovascular autonomic neuropathy (CAN) is due to damage to the autonomic nerve fibres that innervate the heart and blood vessels. Abnormalities in the heart rate control and vascular dynamics are the consequence of this. Reduced heart rate variations is earliest indicator of CAN.

Autonomic dysfunction can impair exercise tolerance. Individuals with CAN show a reduced response in heart rate and blood pressure during exercise. Decreased cardiac output, ejection fraction, systolic dysfunction and impaired diastolic filling restrict the quantum of exercise in CAN. Orthostatic hypotension is another feature of CAN and is considered to be due to damage to the efferent sympathetic fibres particularly in the splanchnic vasculature.

The cause of silent myocardial ischaemia seen in diabetic patients is controversial. Perhaps reduced appreciation of myocardial ischaemia impairs the timely recognition and delays the initiation of the appropriate therapy.

There are several studies which provide consistent evidence for an increased mortality and risk among diabetics with CAN compared with diabetics without it. Ewing et al reported a 2- to 5-year mortality rate of 27.5% that increased to 53% after 5 years in diabetic patients with DAN, compared with a mortality rate of only 15% over the 5-year period among diabetics with normal autonomic function. Half of the deaths in DAN were from renal failure while 29% were sudden deaths.

An autonomic imbalance resulting in QT prolongation may predispose an individual to life-threatening cardiac arrhythmia and sudden death. Inspite of all these, the association of CAN with sudden deaths in the absence of coronary disease and cardiomegaly needs further study to delineate the exact underlying aetiological factor.

There appears to be an association between CAN and diabetic nephropathy that contributes to its high mortality.

Sexual Dysfunction

In females, loss or impaired vaginal lubrication, reduced sexual desire, dyspareunia and reduced orgasm is a common complaint; while in males the common complaint (60 to 75 %) specially in those who are over 50 years is erectile dysfunction. Neurogenic impotence is usually the result of nervi erigentes (parasympathetic outflow S_2-S_4) involvement. The nerve is found to be thickened, beaded and vacuolated. Sympathetic involvement leads to failure of ejection of semen in the urethra and affection of pudendal nerve (somatic reflex) results in failure of ejaculation or retrograde ejaculation.

Sudomotor Dysfunction

This is a common dysfunction of DAN and like peripheral sensorimotor neuropathy, the sudomotor dysfunction occurs as a length-dependent fashion loss of thermoregulatory sweating in a glove and stocking distribution. The first symptom is usually hypohidrosis, as a result of decrease in the number of active sweat glands and a low rate of sweat per unit area of skin and later progresses to anhidrosis. Typically, the symptom starts in the feet, ascends up leg, involves thigh, hands, and anterior abdominal wall. The process then may become global. There may be focal areas of anhidrosis especially over trunk, or in cases of mononeuropathies.

Sometimes, there may be areas of excessive sweating (hyperhidrosis) especially over trunk and head, which may be as a result of compensation for distal anhidrosis. Occasionally, distal hyperhydrosis may occur early in the course of DAN as a result of spontaneous firing of injured neurones.

The third type of sweating disturbance may be gustatory sweating, characterized by abnormal production of sweat that appears over the face, head, neck, shoulders and chest after eating even nonspicy foods. This symptom is often socially embarrassing.

Evaluation

There are a number of tests available for assessing the sudomotor function and help in assessing and localizing the sympathetic nervous system dysfunction.

Thermoregulatory sweat test: This test evaluates the integrity of the central and peripheral aspects of efferent sympathetic nervous system from the hypothalamus to the sweat glands. The body temperature is raised by external heating of the body, and the distribution of sweating is evaluated by the change of colour of an indicator such as iodine with starch, quiniazarin or alizarin red. An increase in oral body temperature by 1°C is sufficient to induce generalized sweating. This test is well standardized, but is unable to differentiate between pre- and postganglionic causes of anhidrosis.

Quantitative sudomotor axon reflex test (QASRT): This test quantifies postganglionic sudomotor function and is mediated by an "axon reflex." It is elicited by iontophoresis of a cholinergic agonist.

Sympathetic skin response: Sweating results in change in the electrodermal activity, which can be recorded by an active electrode placed over the palm or sole, and the indifferent electrode over the volar surface. Various stimuli can be used to evoke sweating, viz. stimulation of a peripheral nerve (e.g. median at the wrist)—the most common method used, and also internal stimuli, viz. deep breathing, startle, mental stress, cough, etc. The method habituates with repeated stimuli, and has inter-subject variability.

Sweat imprint test: A sweat imprint test is formed by secretion of active sweat glands into plastic or silicon mould in response to iontophoresis of a cholinergic agonist. The test helps determine sweat gland density, sweat-droplet size, and sweat volume per area.

Pupillary and Lacrimal Gland Dysfunction

Miosis (reduced pupillary size), impaired light reflexes, and decreased hippus are the pupillary manifestations of autonomic neuropathy in diabetics. The parasympathetic dysfunction is more common than sympathetic. The former is assessed by measuring the latency and constriction velocity of light reflex. The oscillations of the pupil (hippus), measured by focussing a narrow beam of light from a slit lamp on the pupillary margin, may provide a good index of parasympathetic pupillomotor function.

Abnormalities of pupils may be observed within 2 years of diagnosis of both T1DM and T2DM. The indices of pupillary function correlate with disease duration, cardiovascular autonomic dysfunction, small fibre function, and somotic peripheral neuropathy.

In diabetics with autonomic failure, there may be failure of lacrimal gland secretion, resulting in dry eyes.

Disturbances of respiratory control: There have been varied reports of disturbed respiratory control in diabetic patients with autonomic neuropathy. Impaired responses to hypoxia (possibly due to denervation of carotid body chemoreceptor), to hypercapnia, and impaired bronchomotor responses to cold have been reported, while sleep apnoea does not appear to be a significant risk.

Diabetic Foot and DPN

It has been suggested that autonomic neuropathy is a principal cause of foot ulceration. Absence of sweating predisposing to the brittleness of callouses in feet and loss of vasomotor tone with the defective tissue oxygenation due to autonomic neuropathy result in initiation and propagation of diabetic foot ulcer.

MANAGEMENT

Prevention of Autonomic Neuropathy

This is achieved by a tight glycaemic, lipid profile and hypertension control. The use of antioxidants (α-lipoic acid, vitamin E, etc.) and ACE inhibitors substantially reduce the possibility of autonomic neuropathy. Some, however, doubt the 'DAN prevention' properties of ACE inhibitors.

Gastrointestinal System

- Give small frequent meals and reduce fat content (as it delays gastric emptying). Maintain a good glycaemic control
- In severe symptoms, metoclopramide given IV/as a suppository/or in liquid form (10 mg × TDS before meals), domperidone (10 to 20 mg TDS), and erythromycin (IV 100 to 200 mg every 4 to 6 hours, liquid form or suppository) are helpful. Tachyphylaxis is common in metoclopramide therapy. Therefore, its periodic withdrawal is essential to restore effectiveness. Erythromycin acts on motilin receptors and shortens gastric emptying time (Motilin has been called sweeper of the gut).
- If medications are unsuccessful, jejunostomy placement into normally functioning bowel may be needed
- Constipation and explosive diabetic diarrhoea need appropriate treatment including gluten-free diet and antibiotics (metronidazole is probably the best and is recommended for 15 to 20 days).

Retention of bile is often very irritating to the gut and many require bile salt chelation with cholestyramine 4 gm thrice daily mixed with fluids. Diarrhoea control may need diphenoxylate with atropine. In refractory cases, octreotide in small doses may help. With diphenoxylate, toxic mega colon can occur. Therefore, extreme caution is to be exercised. High incidence of cholesterol gallstones has been reported in diabetes due to defective contractility of gallbladder.

Postural Hypotension

Stepwise and deliberate change from supine to erect position, use of supportive stockings and garments is extremely helpful. Total body stockings are more effective than leg stockings alone. α-fluorohydrocortisone, metoclopramide and selective use of α_2-antagonist yohimbine, β-antagonist propranolol, α_2-agonist clonidine, midodrine, dihydroergotamine and octreotide may help in some cases, though one has to be very careful about side effects. Drugs like atenolol, propranolol, metoprolol oppose sympathetic stimulation and may restore parasympathetic-sympathetic balance.

Cystopathy

If initiation of micturition, even when bladder is full, causes problem, it is advised to use Crede's manoeuvre. Use of doxazosin and bethenecol is sometimes helpful. Self catheterization is another useful tool in refractory cases.

Sudomoter Dyfunction

For gustatory sweating, topical application of glycopyrrolate while eating food, an antimuscarinic compound, is found to be effective in reducing severity and frequency of the sweating. Anticholinergic agents such as trihexiphenidyl may be used to treat hyperhidrosis, including gustatory sweating. However, these agents have systemic side effects, such as dry mouth, urinary retention, and constipation. Recently, intradermal injection of botulinum toxin-A in the areas of hyperhidrosis, have shown encouraging results.

Sexual Dysfunctions

In males, erectile dysfunction (ED) is the common diabetic sexual disorder. The cause of this problem is multifactorial like nutritional, neuropathy, vascular involvement, hyperglycaemia, endocrine dysfunction, drugs side effects and psychogenic factor. An objective assessment is essential before treatment. Sildenafil 50 to 100 mg is useful. It, however, should not be started before detailed evaluation of cardiac status.

SUMMARY

Diabetic autonomic neuropathy is an uncommon manifestation of diabetic syndrome. It affects all body systems causing multiple problems. A proper evaluation helps the health care provider an opportunity to offer definitive therapy.

FURTHER READING

1. Abrahamsson H. Gastrointestinal motility disorders in patients with diabetes mellitus. J Intern Med 1995;237(4):403-9.
2. Desautels SG, Hutson WR, Christian PE, Moore JG, Datz FL. Gastric emptying response to variable oral erythromycin dosing in diabetic gastroparesis. Dig Dis Sci 1995;40(1):141-6.
3. Ewing DJ, Campbell IW, Clarke BF. Assessment of cardiovascular effects in diabetic autonomic neuropathy and cardiovascular effects in diabetic autonomic neuropathy and prognostic implications. Ann Intern Med 1980;92:308-11.
4. Ewing DJ, Campbell IW, Clarke BF. The natural history of diabetic autonomic neuropathy. Q J Med 1980;49:95-108.
5. Schiller LR, Santa Ano CA, Schmulen AC, Hendler RS, et al. Pathogenesis of fecal incontinence in diabetes mellitus. Evidence of internal anal splincter dysfunction. N Eng J Med 1982;307:1666-71.
6. Vinik AI, Erban T. Recognizing and treating diabetic autonomic neuropathy. Cleve Clin J Med 2001;68:928-44.
7. Ziegler D, Gries FA, Spuler M, Lassmann F. Diabetic cardiovascular autonomic neuropathy. Multicentric Study Group. The epidemiology of diabetes neuropathy. J Diabetes Complications 1992;6:49-57.

28.5 Sexual Dysfunctions in Diabetes Mellitus

Y Sachdev

INTRODUCTION

Sexual dysfunctions in diabetes mellitus are seen in both male and female patients, though they are much more dramatic and extensive in males. In man, diabetes mellitus is probably the most common organic disease leading to sexual dysfunctions. Many diabetic men dread it more than blindness or loss of a limb to gangrene. Sexuality of women, on the other hand, is less affected by diabetes and they are, therefore, less likely to report with sexual problems.

PHYSIOLOGY OF HUMAN SEXUALITY

The human sexuality or sexual behaviour revolves around sexual appetite or sexual desire, sexual arousal, fantasies, day dreaming, genital response in the form of vaginal lubrication or penile erection, sexual intercourse and orgasm. Sex hormones (testosterone, oestrogen, progesterone, gonadotrophin, prolactin), opioids and other endocrine hormones are involved in this activity besides various neurotransmitters, intact autonomic nerves and microvasculature. Human psyche and cultural background are other two factors which play a major role in this aspect of human behaviour.

In eugonadal male, there is no direct relationship between testosterone and frequency of sexual intercourse, intensity of sexual fantasies, day dreaming and sexual interest. However, an anticipation of sexual activity does result in increased testosterone secretion.

A wide variety of external stimuli including sights, sound or smell as well as internal imagery or fantasy arouse sexual interest or appetite. One of the most powerful sexual stimuli is touch especially on the erotic areas of the body like lips, tongue, nipples, inner thigh and external genitalia. The sexual stimulus may arise from the psyche or it may act via spinal reflex arc. It is obvious, both routes are interlinked.

When the sexual arousal is intense, and prolonged, body responds by undergoing various stages of sexual responses. The blood supply to the external genitalia of both male and female increases resulting in vaso-congestion in about 10 to 30 seconds leading to penile erection in males. The erection is totally dependent on the engorgement of corpora cavernosa and is due to decreased arterial and venous resistance. Blood flow increases by 2 to 3 folds.

A sufficient pressure builds up to ensure stiffness of the erect penis. The corpora cavernosa are surrounded by a strong fibrous coat which allows further penile stiffness and it becomes hard and elongated. Tumescence of corpus spongiosum and glans also occurs. The testes are pulled in due to the retraction of the spermatic cord and contraction of the cremaster muscle, scrotal wall becomes thicker and tighter due to local vasocongestion and contraction of scrotal muscles. In intensified stimulation, testes may reach the perineal floor and increase in size. Neurologically, erection is caused by the parasympathetic fibres reaching the penis via nervi erigentes. Arterial dilatation takes place, increased blood inflow occurs resulting in fullness of erectile penile tissue and engorgement of cavernous venous sinusoids.

In female, the venous plexus surrounding the lower part of vagina and the erectile bulbs of the vestibule become engorged. A 'turgid cuff' is, thus, formed which narrows and elongates the outer third of the coital canal. If the arousal is intense or prolonged, the congestive swelling of the vulva causes redness and pouting of the labia minora. The erect clitoris retracts slightly into a less prominent position against the symphysis pubis. The uterus becomes engorged and increases in size and rises in the pelvis. This results in elongation and ballooning of the upper 2/3rd of the vagina. Some slow irregular contractions of the vaginal vault may also occur if sexual stimulus continues. Simultaneously and at much earlier stage, due to increased blood supply, a fluid appears on the vaginal epithelium quickly forming a lubricating coat (vaginal sweat). It must be appreciated that vaginal lining is of squamous epithelium and it has no mucous gland. Some secretions, in small amounts, are contributed by endocervix and greater vestibular (Bartholin's) glands.

The ultimate outcome of all these responses is orgasm which in male culminates in ejaculation and in female in series of muscular spasms culminating in abrupt release of all tenseness of muscles and body.

From this description, it is clear that for a successful sexual act, the essentials are (Figs 28.5.1 and 28.5.2):
• Functional limbic system, intact neuronal connections, and
• Elevated arterial inflow with venous valvular integrity to block venous run-off.

The arterial blood supply to the cavernous bodies is from the external iliac artery and hypogastric, internal pudendal, penile, bulbourethral, dorsal and deep penile arteries of the internal iliac artery (Fig. 28.5.3).

• <u>Central control</u>

  • Limbic system ⟶ Lateral columns

      Facilitatory   Inhibitory
      effect   effect

• <u>Autonomic nervous system
  (Redistributes blood)</u>

    • Afferent path pudendal nerve
    • Sacral erection centre S_2, S_3, S_4
    • Efferent (parasym) nervi erigentes

Fig. 28.5.1: Neurology of erection

TWO COMPONENTS

• **Arterial impotence**
  • **It is the result of failure of mechanism of erection due to organic insufficiency of the arterial bed supplying the cavernous bodies**

• **Phlebogenic impotence**
  • **It is the result of excessive venous drainage due to inadequate blockage of venous run-off**

Fig. 28.5.2: Vasculogenic impotence

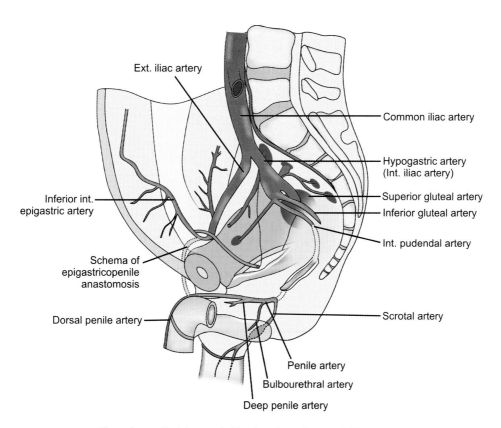

Fig. 28.5.3: Pelvic arterial bed and penile arterial blood supply

SEXUAL DYSFUNCTION IN MALES

Diabetic sexual problems are seen, not only, in those patients who have gross metabolic disturbances; but are also observed in those patients who have only mild metabolic abnormality and lead an unrestricted life. Therefore, these dysfunctions appear to be the result of interplay between various physical and psychological factors.

Aetiopathogenesis

The sexual function of a human being is a complicated psychosomatic phenomenon which is dependent on ill-understood and complex psychophysiological mechanisms where many physical and psychological processes interact. The processes involved are as under.

Physical Factors

Endocrine Hormonal Abnormalities

The relevance of hormonal abnormalities to the disturbed sexual functions in a diabetic is uncertain. Inspite of various animal and clinical studies where reduction in the Leydig cell mass, impaired androgen production and decreased circulating free testosterone levels have been reported, it is not clear whether these changes are responsible for the sexual disturbances or are secondary to the metabolic imbalances or the result of therapy. Many workers have failed to observe any difference in plasma testosterone values between impotent diabetics, potent diabetics and normal individuals; thus further adding to the prevailing confusion. The present ineffectiveness of androgen replacement therapy also points to the impression that androgen deficiency is of little relevance to the sexual problems of male diabetics.

Similarly, there is conflicting opinion regarding hypothalamic pituitary functions in diabetics. Majority of the studies have demonstrated that there is no abnormality in gonadotrophin (Gn) levels and Gn response to dynamic tests. Some investigators, however, found impaired luteinizing hormone (LH) response to gonadotrophin releasing hormone (GnRH) despite normal basal Gn levels, whereas others found high basal LH level with a prolonged response to GnRH stimulation.

In 1983, five hundred diabetic male patients of different age groups were studied by the author who found normal values of Gn (LH, FSH) and total T_e with normal response to GnRH and hCG stimulation tests. The sex hormone binding globulin (SHBG), however, was significantly increased with decreased free T_e levels. These changes were more marked in patients above the age of 50 years. The significance of these changes is uncertain as similar changes were seen by the worker in age-related normal healthy non-diabetic individuals leading a normal life and were attributed to 'ageing process.' In female diabetics also, the endocrine hormonal axes remain unaffected as compared to age-related non-diabetics.

Vascular Factors

An adequate blood supply is essential for the development and maintenance of full erection. Penile blood pressure and angiographic studies in a number of diabetics have demonstrated impaired blood supply to corpora cavernosa. This is frequently due to autonomic nerve damage leading to disruption of both arterial inflow and venous drainage. Thus, structural vascular lesions may not be visible in a number of impotent diabetic males.

Neurological Factors

There is enough evidence to show a close relationship between disturbed erectile function and autonomic neuropathy. Thus, impotent diabetic males may have abnormal cystometrograms, bulbocavernous reflexes and histochemistry of pelvic autonomic nerves. A number of diabetics report with only erectile dysfunction as an isolated feature and without any other evidence of autonomic neuropathy. This is due to an early involvement of the long parasympathetic fibres to the pelvic organs. Majority of these patients develop, in years to come, widespread autonomic dysfunctions and neuropathy.

Other Physical Factors

Many other diseases like alcohol abuse, drug therapy, ischaemic heart disease, hypertension, cerebrovascular accident, etc. may also contribute to the sexual dysfunctions.

Psychological Factors

Depression, poor self esteem and self image, negative attitude towards sex, anxiety over sexual performances, marital disharmony and other psychological factors add to the organically based sexual problems of diabetics especially those who are more vulnerable psychologically. Some patients, however, remain unperturbed by the altered sexual activity while others are able to adjust themselves rather quickly with no significant effect on their daily life.

Clinical Examination

For a proper assessment of the patient's problems, it is necessary to obtain a detailed history of the sexual handicap and contributory factors (drugs, alcohol abuse etc.) responsible. The history is better elicited from the patient and sexual partner separately as well as jointly. A widely accepted erectile function questionnaires are given in Table 28.5.1.

The clinical examination should include detailed physical and endocrine examination, sexual development and neurological examination including bladder and vascular symptoms, if any. The investigations should include the tests for cardiovascular reflexes, cystometrograms, urodynamic studies, penile BP measurement (by digital cuff or ultrasound Doppler system) and determination of blood flow to the penile arteries. Metabolic parameters of diabetes mellitus (blood glucose, lipid profile, ketoacidosis) and endocrine hormones (LH, FSH, T_e, PRL, E_2, etc.) should also be estimated. Dynamic hormonal tests where applicable, should be carried out to define the border line abnormalities. Urine should be tested for retrograde ejaculations.

TABLE 28.5.1

Question	Response options
1. How often were you able to get an erection during sexual activity?	0 = No sexual activity 1 = Almost never/never
2. When you had erections with sexual stimulation, how often were your erections hard enough for penetration?	2 = A few times (much less than half the time) 3 = Sometimes (about the half time) 4 = Most times (much more than half the time) 5 = Almost always/always
3. When you attempted sexual intercourse, how often were you able to penetrate (enter) your partner?	0 = Did not attempt intercourse 1 = Almost never/never
4. During sexual intercourse, how often were you able to maintain you erections after you had penetrated (entered) your partner?	2 = A few times (much less than half the time) 3 = Sometimes (about the half time) 4 = Most times (much more than half the time) 5 = Almost always/always
5. During sexual intercourse, how difficult was it to maintain your erection to completion of intercourse?	0 = Did not attempt intercourse 1 = Extremely difficult 2 = Very difficult 3 = Difficult 4 = Slightly difficult 5 = Not difficult
6. How many times have you attempted sexual intercourse?	0 = No attempts 1 = One to two attempts 2 = Three to four attempts 3 = Five to six attempts 4 = Seven to ten attempts 5 = Eleven plus attempts
7. When you attempted sexual intercourse, how often was it satisfactory to you?	0 = No attempts 1 = Almost never/never 2 = A few times (much less than half the time) 3 = Sometimes (about the half time) 4 = Most times (much more than half the time) 5 = Almost always/always
8. How much have you enjoyed sexual intercourse?	0 = No sexual stimulation/intercourse 1 = Almost never/never 2 = A few times (much less than half the time) 3 = Sometimes (about the half time) 4 = Most times (much more than half the time) 5 = Almost always/always

Contd...

Contd...

Question	Response options
9. When you had sexual stimulation or intercourse, how often did you ejaculate?	0 = No sexual stimulation/intercourse 1 = Almost never/never
10. When you had sexual stimulation or intercourse, how often did you have the feeling of orgasm or climax?	2 = A few times (much less than half the time) 3 = Sometimes (about the half time) 4 = Most times (much more than half the time) 5 = Almost always/always
11. How often have you felt sexual desire?	1 = Almost never/never 2 = A few times (much less than half the time) 3 = Sometimes (about the half time) 4 = Most times (much more than half the time) 5 = Almost always/always
12. How would you rate your level of sexual desire?	1 = Very low/none at all 2 = Low 3 = Moderate 4 = High 5 = Very high
13. How satisfied have you been with your overall sex life?	1 = Very dissatisfied
14. How satisfied have you been with your sexual relationship with your partner?	2 = Moderately dissatisfied 3 = About equally satisfied and dissatisfied 4 = Moderately satisfied 5 = Very satisfied
15. How do you rate your confidence that you can get and keep an erection?	1 = Very low 2 = Low 3 = Moderate 4 = High 5 = Very high

Erectile function questionnaires (to assess erectile dysfunctional status)

Nocturnal penile tumescence (NPT) and psycho-physiological responses to erotic stimuli should also be carried out. NPT occurs during REM phase of sleep. Total tumescence time, erection time, number of maximum tumescence and penile circumference decrease in diabetic mellitus. They also diminish with age.

Sacral outflow (S_2, S_3, S_4) assessment must be carried out to confirm intact nervation that enables the erection to occur by testing anal sphincter tone, perianal sensation, anal wink and bulbocavernous reflex.

Clinical Manifestations

In male diabetics, the sexual disorders may be in the form of nonspecific or specific dysfunctions. Nonspecific sexual problems in the form of decreased sex appetite and erectile failure are attributed to general lethargy, tiredness, malaise and weakness. These problems usually appear at the onset of diabetes mellitus or whenever there is poor control of hyperglycaemia. Therefore, the functions are restored with better metabolic control. The specific diabetic impotence, on the other hand, is organically determined and is characterized by progressive, irreversible decline in an apparently well controlled patient with no mental stress. Erectile function, ejaculation, spermatogenesis and sexual appetite are usually affected to variable degrees.

Erectile Impotence

Erectile dysfunction (ED) is defined as the consistent inability to attain and maintain an erection adequate for sexual intercourse and occurring at least for 25% of the time (some say 50%). The organic erectile impotence develops gradually and all types of erections (during sleep, on waking, masturbation, spontaneous) are affected (Table 28.5.2). Initially there are day to day variations in erectile functions though with progressive decline, the penis ultimately becomes 'dead.' Libido, orgasm and ejaculations may remain unaffected for a long time further adding to the patient's problems. There is no definite relationship between organic diabetic impotence and duration/control of diabetes mellitus, though it is definitely related to diabetic microangiopathy and/or neuropathy. Psychogenic component may also

TABLE 28.5.2

Clinical parameters	Organic dysfunction	Psychogenic dysfunction
Onset	• Gradual	• Rapid
Nature	• Selective	• Absolute
NPT	• NPT affected	• Not affected
Causes	• Neuropathy	• Depression
	• Vascular	• Guilt
	• Endocrine	• Unhappy marriage
	• Drugs	
	• Surgery	

Differences between organic and psychogenic erectile dysfunction

be superimposed, thus further complicating the issue. The frequency of the erectile impotence has been mentioned as 35 to 59% of male diabetics. The author's series comprising 500 Indian male diabetics aged 18 to 67 years had 43% incidence of erectile impotence; age wise incidence being 18 to 30 years 19%, 31 to 40 years 31%, 41 to 50 years 39%, 50 to 60 years 58% and above 60 years 68%.

Ejaculatory Defects

There is a wide and varied spectrum of ejaculatory defects. Ejaculations may be unaffected, reduced or completely absent. There may be even retrograde ejaculations where the patient 'shoots dry' and semen finds its way into the urinary bladder. Some patients may complain of absence of 'pumping sensation' when the semen just seeps out from the erect, semierect or a flaccid penis at the height of orgasm or before it. Retrograde ejaculations are the result of incompetence of internal sphincter of urinary bladder resulting in failure to close during ejaculation. This defect may be the result of autonomic neuropathy, bladder neck surgery, lumbar sympathectomy and adrenergic blocking drugs like guanathidine, etc. Urine examination immediately after coitus confirms the diagnosis of retrograde ejaculation which usually results in male infertility (Table 28.5.3).

Spermatogenesis (Table 28.5.4)

In uncontrolled diabetics, testicular atrophy, and infertility is a frequent complication. However, in the presence of proper diabetic control, the fertility and sperm density are unaffected though the sperm motility is somewhat decreased. The author did not observe any significant decrease in spermatogenesis when diabetic process was mild and well controlled. In uncontrollable diabetics, however, the motility of spermatozoa was never over 15% even when the sperm density showed only marginal variations.

TABLE 28.5.3

Competence of internal sphincter of bladder compromised physically/pharmacologically resulting in failure to close during ejaculation
- Autonomic neuropathy
- Bladder neck surgery
- Lumbar sympathectomy
- Adrenergic blocking drugs
  - Guanethidine
  - Phenoxybenzamine
- RE results in infertility
- It is confirmed by post-coital urine examination

Chief causes of retrograde ejaculation (RE)

TABLE 28.5.4

- In uncontrolled diabetes
  - Grossly affected
  - Testicular atrophy
  - Infertility
- In controlled diabetes
  - Fertility unaffected
  - Sperm density unaffected
  - Sperm motility substandard

Effects of diabetes mellitus on spermatogenesis

Sexual Appetite

Libido and sexual appetite remain unimpaired for a much longer time as compared to erectile and ejaculatory dysfunctions. With period of time, the sex hunger also gets affected and initial sexual problems do not occupy patient's attention any more and the complaints 'disappear' or abate.

Therapeutic Approach

The primary aim of therapeutic management is to ensure that both patient and partner are able to enjoy their sexual life within limits prescribed by irreversible diabetic changes. The reversible physical factors like general health, nutrition, metabolic control should be treated energetically. Inflammatory genital disease, if any, should be attended to. Drug therapy, effect of alcohol and residual effects of urogenital surgery should be evaluated. Drug therapy may be modified/omitted if necessary. Sildenafil is the drug of choice. It is a phosphodiesterane type 5 inhibitor. Recommended dose is 50 to 100 mg an hour before sexual act. It is marginally less effective in diabetic population than in non-diabetic population. A detailed cardiac assessment is necessary before it is used. It is not to be combined with nitrites/nitrates because of profound hypotension which may occur. Todalafil (long acting) and vardenafil are other two available products from the same group. Intracavernosal injections of vasoactive substances like papaverine, phentolamine and prostaglandin E1 (alprostadil—a synthetic analogue is the best in this group) increase blood flow to the corpora cavernosum and help in natural erectile process. Side effects like pain, prolonged erection, priapism, haematomas and fibrosis, however, make this treatment less acceptable. Alprostadil can also be introduced as a pellet by transurethral route (MUSE).

Contributory psychological factors should also be tackled. If necessary, a psychiatrist may be consulted. It may be worthwhile to prescribe non-coital sexual exercises which reduce performance anxiety. It may also be beneficial to suggest alternative sex positions, orogenital contact and other stimulatory techniques. Hormonal replacement therapy is of not much benefit unless there is evidence of hypogonadism.

Surgery

If arterial insufficiency is confirmed by angiography, cavernogram and penile BP studies, corporal revascularization by small arterial grafts may be considered (Table 28.5.5). Vacuum assisted erection devices/surgical penile implants (silicon rod implant or inflatable prostheses) are expected to be useful provided penile sensation is present and the erectile failure is due to diabetic autonomic neuropathy or atherosclerosis and nocturnal penile tumescence is absent or markedly reduced. Tables 28.5.6 to 28.5.9 give brief characteristics of various available implants.

Penile implantation is very helpful provided the patient has stable marital relationship, intact sex appetite, genital sensation and orgasmic capacity. Unfortunately,

TABLE 28.5.5

Revascularization procedures
- Anastomosis of epigastric artery to corpus cavernosum
- Interposition of saphenous vein graft between iliac artery and corpus

Surgery
- Vascular surgery if arterial insufficiency
- Corporal revascularization by small artery grafting
- Assess by cavernosogram the integrity of corpora cavernosa and exclude Peyronie's disease before surgery is undertaken
- Experience limited
- Results poor

Surgical management of erectile dysfunction

TABLE 28.6.6

Types
- Semi-solid Small carrion silicone implant (Small 1978)
- Scott-Bradley inflatable prosthesis (Furlow 1978, Scott, et al 1979)
- Solid penile implant with a silver wire core
- Solid penile implant with a hinged base
- Newer types of solid implant, less conspicuous erection when clothed

Risks of implants
- Penile ischaemia
- Penile gangrene
- Usually within 3 to 4 weeks
- Especially, if diabetic vascular complications present

Types and risks of penile implants

TABLE 28.6.7

Advantages
- Technically simple
- Surgery simple
- Inexpensive
- Hospital stay 2 to 3 days
- Complications few

Disadvantages
- Constant erection, difficult to conceal, embarrassment
- Rod may migrate
- May cause penile fracture
- Glans may slip over
- Penile dimensions less than inflatable device

Advantages and disadvantages of silicone rod prosthesis

TABLE 28.6.8

Advantages
- Mimics normal erection
- Inflated as desired
- Deflated otherwise
- Urinary functions not affected
- Penile girth-length more than rod device

Disadvantages
- More complicated surgery
- Malfunction—mechanical failure
- May require re-operation
- More expensive surgery
- Hospital stay 7 to 10 days
- Complications—infection, inflammation, foreskin tightness, adhesions

Advantages and disadvantages of inflatable prosthesis

TABLE 28.6.9

- **Flexi-rod prosthesis (Finney)**
  - Hinged section along the shaft allows penis to flex in the pubic region without compromising penile regidity
- **Jonas prosthesis**
  - Silicone rubber with core of twisted siliver wire. Malleability allows manual positioning for intercourse

Types and characteristics of semi-rigid prosthesis

implants did not live up to the expectations and many diabetics remain unsatisfied. Arterial grafts again, have not been a great success.

Retrograde Ejaculations

The aim of treatment of retrograde ejaculations is to recover the spermatozoa from the urinary bladder with minimum contamination so that they could be used for fertilization by artificial insemination. Attempts have also been made to encourage anterograde ejaculations by using α-adrenergic stimulants. Results, however, are poor.

SEXUAL DYSFUNCTIONS IN FEMALES

The sexuality in female diabetics is less affected and their main problems are decreased libido (seen in 25% diabetics), dyspareunia (25%), decreased vaginal lubrication (25%), clitoral tumescence and poor orgasm (12%). These problems can be tackled with understanding tender love making and use of local hormonal vaginal lubricant creams. At present, there is enough evidence to suggest that female diabetic with good metabolic control is relatively free from sexual impairment even when there is severe autonomic neuropathy. This has been explained on the presumption that perhaps autonomic nervous system plays a different role in the female and male sexuality.

Our experience is that a diabetic woman feels more tender to her caring husband because he is supportive while a diabetic man may find his dependence on his caring wife as undermining his sense of masculinity and may exert a negative effect on his sexuality.

SUMMARY

Sexual impotence seen in diabetic patient occurs in both types of diabetes mellitus. Its effects are more dramatic and extensive in male than in female diabetics. In males, autonomic neuropathy and vascular pathology are mainly responsible for erectile dysfunction. Psychological overlay is also present in some cases. Endocrine hormonal abnormalities are usually not a contributory factor. With judicious use of diagnostic investigations, a rational therapy is possible to ensure adequate sexual activity. Vascular surgery and penile implants are beneficial in some of the properly selected patients. They however, have not lived up to the expectations and many patients stay unsatisfied.

In females, management is comparatively easy and symptomatic.

FURTHER READING

1. Benecroft J. Sexuality of diabetic women. Clinics Endocrinology and Metabolism 1982;11:785.
2. Boulton AJ, Selam JL, Sweeney M, Ziegler D. Sildenafil citrate for the treatment of erectile dysfunction in man with type II diabetes mellitus. Diabetologia 2001;44:1296-301.
3. Daubresser JC, Nauenier JC, Wilmotta J, Luuyckx AS. Pituitary testicular axis in diabetic men with and without sexual impotence. Diabetes and Metabolism (Paris) 1978;4: 223.
4. Ellenberg M. Impotence in diabetes: the neurologic factor. Annals of Internal Medicine 1971;75:213.
5. Faerman I, Vilar D, Riverola MA, Rosnsr JM, Jadzinsky MN, Fox D, Perez Loret A, Sernatein Hahn L, Saraceni B. Impotence and diabetes—studies of androgenic function in diabetic impotent males. Diabetes 1972;21:23-30.
6. Geisthovel W, Niedergerke U, Norgner KD, Willms B, Nitzket NJ. Androguststus BEI mannlichen Diabetikern, Medizinishe Klinik 1975;70:1417.
7. Janson SB, Nagen C, Froland A, Patterson PB. Sexual function and pituitary axis in insulin treated diabetic men. Acta Medica Scandinavics Supplementum 1979;624:65-8.
8. Kent JR. Gonadal function in potent diabetic males. Diabetes 1966;15:557.
9. Kolodny RC, Kahn CB, Goldstein NH, Bernett DM. Sexual dysfunction in men. Diabetes 1974;23:306-9.
10. Linet OL, Ogrine FG. Efficacy and safety of intraconvernosal alprostadil in men with erectile dysfunction. The Alprostadil Study Group. N Eng J Med 1996;334:873-7.
11. Podolsky. Sexual dysfunction in diabetic men. Pract Diabetol 1982;1(1),1.
12. Podolsky. Diagnosis and treatment of sexual dysfunctions in the male diabetic. Med Clin North America 1982;66:1389.
13. Sachdev Y. Sexual dysfunction in T2DM. Proceedings of workshop on diabetes mellitus. Postgraduate Institute of Medical Research and Education, Chandigarh 1985.
14. Sachev Y. Sex and sexuality in diabetes mellitus. Proceedings Geriatric Society of India, Annual Conference, Varanasi 1989.
15. Schoffing K, Federlin K, Ditchunheit H. Disorders of sexual function in male diabetics. Diabetes 1963;12:519.
16. Vinik AL, Richardson D. Erectile dysfunction in diabetes: pills for pentile function. Clin Diabetes 1998;16:108.
17. Vinik AL, Richardson D. Erectile dysfunction in diabetes. Diabetes Review 1998;6:16.
18. Weight AD, London DR, Holds G, Williams JW, Rudd ST. Luteinizing release hormone tests in impotent diabetic males. Diabetes 1976;25:975.

28.6 Diabetic Foot Syndrome

Y Sachdev

- Introduction
- Pathogenesis: Vascular, Neuropathic, Infections, Role of Proteases
- Symptomatology
- Clinical Examination

- Investigations
- Management
- Prevention
- Summary

INTRODUCTION

The feet of diabetic patients (both T1DM and T2DM) are vulnerable to be affected as are the eyes, kidneys and heart. Estimated 6 to 12% of diabetics give present or past history of foot ulceration and nearly 1% undergo amputation. The foot/leg amputation is 15 times more common in diabetics than in non-diabetics. The male : female ratio of amputees is 30:1 among non-diabetics. It is 2:1 in diabetics. The proper care of a diabetic foot involves a team approach and is an expensive proposition. The diabetic foot is beset with prolonged suffering, crippling disability and high morbidity and mortality. We believe, of all the late complications of diabetes, foot problems are probably the most preventable. Therefore, it is more easy and more cost effective to prevent it than treat it.

PATHOGENESIS

Multiple factors operate; the prominent being vascular, neuropathic, trauma and infection (Fig. 28.6.1).

Vascular Factors

It is the ischaemia of the feet which is partly due to peripheral vascular disease (PVD) and partly due to small vessels involvement resulting in ischaemic ulceration.

Neuropathic Factors

Neuropathy plays a significant role. The skin is dry due to loss of sweating. Sensations are blunt and local injuries (mechanical, chemical, thermal) are common leading to break in the skin and superadded infections. Motor

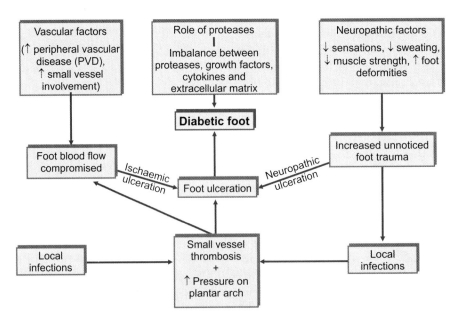

Fig. 28.6.1: Diabetic foot
(Multiple factors, mainly compromised blood supply, peripheral sensations, trauma, infections interplay)

neuropathy causes atrophy of muscles, pareses and foot deformities.

Trauma

It is extremely common among those who walk bare feet. Most of the time the injuries go un-noticed and un-attended providing a fertile soil for infections.

Infections

It is usually a mixed flora (aerobic and anaerobic) which is involved in diabetic foot infections. Deep tissue infections tend to induce thrombosis in small vessels, aggravating local ischaemia. Infection in the interior of the foot also compresses on plantar arch reducing blood supply to the forefeet and toes. Glycosylation of collagen causes rigidity of the joints and increased plantar pressure during walking. All these changes are prone to result in ulceration, gangrene and osteomyelitis. Table 28.6.1 gives some of the major risk factors to develop diabetic foot syndrome.

Role of Proteases

A normal wound healing needs a balanced interaction of growth factors, cytokines, proteases and extracellular matrix. In chronic wounds, the high level of proteases at the wound site leads to a disrupted and uncoordinated wound healing process by degrading matrix proteins and growth factors that are essential for healing. In diabetic foot syndrome, the chronic ulceration is due to low mitogenic activity, high concentration of inflammatory cytokines and proteases.

SYMPTOMATOLOGY

The symptoms of a diabetic foot can be classified as per Wagener's criteria (Table 28.6.2) or as:
a. *Neuropathic foot:* Where neuropathy dominates over reduced blood supply, and
b. *Neuroischaemic foot:* Where occlusive vascular disease is the main feature though neuropathy is also present.

Neuropathic Foot

In neuropathic foot, one must record the history and finding of nocturnal pain, vibration sensation, ankle jerk, motor power, Semmes Weinstein microfilament test and biothesiometry. Neuropathy leads to local fissures, breaks in skin, bullae, neuropathic (Charcot's) joints, neuropathic oedema, digital necrosis and neuropathic ulcers. Ischaemia leads to digital necrosis and gangrene.

TABLE 28.6.1

- Altered foot biomechanics (deformed foot)
- Bare foot walking (inviting unnoticed trauma)
- Impaired peripheral circulation (ischaemic feet)
- Increased pressure-points problems (corns, callosities, erythema)
- Limited joint mobility (intrinsic minus' foot)
- Loss of perspiration (dry skin, cracks, fissures)
- Oedema feet (congestive heart failure, nephropathy)
- Past history of foot ulceration, gangrene, amputation
- Peripheral neuropathy and insensitive foot (loss of protective sensation leading to various types of injury)
- Severe nail pathology (ingrowing nails)

Major risk factors to develop diabetic foot

TABLE 28.6.2

Grade 0:Foot at high risk—no ulceration
Grade 1:Superficial ulceration
Grade 2:Deep ulceration
Grade 3:Deep ulceration with infection and osteomyelitis
Grade 4:Forefoot or localized gangrene
Grade 5:Extensive gangrene requiring amputation

Wagener's classification of diabetic foot lesions

Ischaemic (Neuroischaemic) Foot

In many such cases, history of claudication or rest pain is present. The peripheral pulsations are weak and foot may be cold to touch. Ischaemic foot is the result of macrovascular and microvascular diabetic complications involving infrapopliteal vessels. The lesion is bilateral and blood supply to the feet is compromised. Many of such patients have coronary artery disease as well.

Charcot Foot/Joint (Charcot's Neuroarthropathy)

A Charcot's joint is a relatively painless arthropathy of a single or multiple joints due to underlying neuropathy. The joints, most frequently, involved are tarsometatarsal joints followed by metatarsophalangeal joints. Ankle and subtalar joints may be involved subsequently. In initial stages, the presentation may be in the form of a hot swollen foot which is precipitated by a minor injury.

Charcot's neuroarthropathy is a rare and disabling condition. The actual pathogenesis of this condition is not well understood but patients who have peripheral neuropathy, autonomic dysfunction with increased blood flow to the feet and most vulnerable to unrecognized repeated trauma are the ones who develop this syndrome. There is increased osteoclastic activity and remodelling of the bone. The diagnosis is based on high suspicion and plain radiography. X-ray reveals bone and joint destruction, fragmentation and remodelling. Management is by immobilization usually in a total contact cast, bisphosphonate therapy which reduces osteoclast activity and halts progression.

Other Features

Interdigital fungal infection; nail deformities like ingrowing toe nails (onychocryptosis), thickened nails (onychogryphosis) overgrowth of nails (onychauxis) may lead to subungual ulcers and may even involve adjacent toes. Bones may get infected and osteomyelitis may result if there is chronic fulminating deep seated infection (Table 28.6.3).

CLINICAL EXAMINATION

Besides detailed general clinical examination, ankle/brachial blood pressure and their systolic index (ABI) must be recorded. Ankle/brachial systolic index (ABI) is calculated by dividing ankle systolic pressure by the brachial pressure using a hand-held ultrasound probe. Normally ABI is >1. A ratio less than 0.8 signifies ischaemia. Unusually high ratio may be observed when there is decreased arterial wall compressibility as seen in Monckeberg's sclerosis.

INVESTIGATIONS

Transcutaneous Pressure of Oxygen (TCPO$_2$) Measurement

TCPO$_2$ measurement is of prognostic significance. A heated oxygen sensitive probe is placed on the dorsum of the foot and a reference probe is kept below the clavicle. After an equilibrium period of about 15 minutes, skin oxygen tension (mmHg) is recorded. This reflects the local blood flow. A value below 30 mmHg is a risk factor for ischaemic foot ulcer.

Doppler Studies

With the help of Doppler, blood flow studies and localization of blockage or stenotic lesions in the iliac to the popliteal arteries is determined.

Angiography

Digital substraction angiography is recommended when vascular reconstructive intervention like angiography or

TABLE 28.6.3

- Onychomycosis
- Paronychia
- Infected foot ulcer
- Necrotizing fascitis
- Osteomyelitis
- Charcot's neuroarthropathy
- Gangrene

Progressive diabetic foot lesions

bypass surgery is contemplated. It is also extremely helpful in deciding level of amputation.

MANAGEMENT OF DIABETIC FOOT

The aim is to save the foot/limb and make the patient effectively mobile without any morbidity. A meticulous personalised programme is usually worked out in our centre for each individual patient. The multidisciplinary team involved usually has an educator, physiatrist, physiotherapist, trained nurse, diabetologist and a surgeon. The main principles are off loading (complete avoidance of weight-bearing), debridement, wound dressings, aggressive but appropriate antibiotic therapy, revascularization and limited amputation, if inevitable.

General Measures

It includes a tight glycaemic control, normalization of blood pressure and lipid profile. Patient must stop smoking, tobacco chewing and should avoid exposure to cold, use of tight elastic stockings, prolonged static standing or sitting with cross legs. The physical exercise must be graduated and introduced in a graded manner. CCF, if present, must be controlled. It is advisable not to use drugs like beta-blockers, dopamine and dobutamine.

Foot Wear

An appropriate foot wear and insoles are advised after identifying the high pressure areas on the foot with the help of a computer or using ink pads. It is advisable to wear a pair of shoes or sandals with a heel counter. The foot wear should be a size larger than the actual fit size and it should have a firm cup heel to prevent the heel from spreading. It should have retaining straps or laces and its inside must be smooth. Insoles act as shock absorbers and they are essential in patients with neuropathy. Those patients who have abnormally high pressure under one or two metatarsal heads are at high risk to develop ulceration at these sites. They are advised to use plantar metatarsal pads (PMP) to redistribute the weight from the high pressure areas under metatarsal heads to other metatarsal heads. Necessary alterations/ modifications can also be made by an expert shoemaker. Socks should be a clean pair and changed everyday. The socks with constricting topband should never be worn.

Frequent inspection of feet and foot wear is necessary to ensure no trauma is caused to the foot.

Management of Ulcers

Table 28.6.4 enumerates some of the factors which contribute to development of foot ulcers. The management involves callus removal, eradication and redistribution of the weight-bearing forces. Callus contributes to high plantar pressure and risk of abscess formation while its removal permits proper wound drainage and early healing. If the ulcers are long standing, too large and slow to heal, it is better to immobilize the foot, reduce its weight-bearing activities, treat infection and help it heal by application of contact plaster cast. This gives rest to the wound and ulcers heal over 4 to 6 weeks. Lack of sensations and pain usually results in non-adherence by the patient to the advice not to put pressure on the ulcer. Therefore, it has to be stressed most emphatically that 'off loading' the ulcer area is essential for an early recovery. The local use of recombinant human platelet-derived growth factor (PDGF) gel, becaplermin or dressing the ulcer with human dermal replacement make the ulcer healing faster. In view of its high cost, it is used only in difficult-to-heal neuropathic ulcers.

The human dermal equivalents have been bioengineered and have human fibroblasts and PGDF and other growth factors. Topically applied growth factors (Regranex) are also useful. Regranex is a PDGF. Both these devices are useful only in infection-free ulcer and are recommended for resistant non-healing neuropathic ulcers. Their expensive cost is a limiting factor.

The use of 2% ketanserin ointment has been found to accelerate healing. Oral use has no effect. In one study, an ester of hyaluronic acid has been found to be effective in chronic fibrous ulcers. Protease inhibitor dressings, promogran is also helpful in wound healing.

Management of Infection

Infected foot can be a limb and even life threatening event. Therefore, it requires aggressive treatment. Inappropriate and inadequate treatment of infections

TABLE 28.6.4

- Unnoticed repeated foot trauma
- Loss of sensations
- Compromised blood supply
- Oedema feet
- Ill fitting shoes
- Tight socks
- Development of corns, callosities
- Uncontrolled hyperglycaemia, disturbed lipid profile
- Presence of peripheral vascular disease

Contributory factors for foot ulcerations

delays the healing process. Therefore, aggressive antibiotic treatment is an essential element of ulcer care. Superficial infection requires debridement, daily dressing and oral antibiotics. Deep infections usually involve muscles, tendons and even bones. Such patients need hospitalization, broad spectrum antibiotics (initially empirically but later, on the basis of culture and antibiotics sensitivity report, antibiotics change should be specific (Table 28.6.5). Such patients will require wider debridement and even drainage. In some resistant cases, use of hyperbaric oxygen therapy has provided tremendous relief and success. If surgical intervention is needed it must be done early to prevent permanent damage and prolonged convalescent period.

Management of Decreased Vascular Supply

Exercise of the foot involved and its joints will improve the blood supply. Cessation of smoking, avoidance of exposure to cold will also help in this regard. Regular daily use of pentoxyfylline (400 mg × thrice daily), aspirin

TABLE 28.6.5

Type of lesion	Antimicrobial therapy
Superficial ulcer and non-toxic	Ampicillin+cloxacillin
	Ampicillin + clavulanate Cephalexin + ciprofloxacin + metronidazole
Deep ulcer and toxic	Ampicillin + cloxacillin + metronidazole
	Ampicillin + clindamycin
	Ampicillin + clavulanate
	Amoxycillin + 3rd generation
	cephalosporin + metronidazole

Recommended initial antibiotic cover
(till culture and antibiotic sensitivity report is available)

(100 to 150 mg daily), thrombolytic agents (urokinase, streptokinase, and prostanoids (prostaglandin I_2 (PGI_2), prostaglandin E_1 (PGE_1) or the stable prostacycline analogue is extremely useful, if there is PVD.

Thrombolytic therapy is especially useful in acute onset ischaemia. The locally catheter-delivered thrombolytic agent is better than when used systematically. The prostanoids are used as intra-arterial or intravenous infusion.

Vascular Reconstruction

Critical ischaemia is defined as ulcer/gangrene/rest pains with the blood pressure at or below 30 mmHg and/or ankle BP at or below 50 mmHg. This condition indicates high risk of amputation unless revascularization is done.

The surgical procedures like percutaneous transluminal angioplasty (PTC), surgical construction, intravascular stents, laser therapy for atherosclerotic plaques are some of the available procedures which can be utilized to improve the long-term vascular patency.

Amputation

In some cases, inspite of all efforts, gangrene of the foot sets in and foot or limb has to be sacrificed. Such cases must be referred to a prostheses centre for limb prosthesis.

PREVENTION

It is the earnest desire of every diabetic centre that its patients lead a normal healthy life inspite of diabetes and they do not develop complications like diabetic foot. Table 28.6.6 gives some of the important steps a diabetic should always bear in mind to avoid diabetic foot syndrome. The high risk patients (see Tables 28.6.1) have to be recognised and followed up frequently at short intervals to record their health status and enforce modifications in treatment whenever needed. Table 28.6.7 gives a few guidelines for a health visitor/medicosocial worker while Table 28.6.8 enumerates care of an infected foot. As Joslin wrote that *diabetic gangrene is not heaven sent, it is earthborn,* diabetic foot is the result of how we care about our diabetic patients and how they care for themselves.

SUMMARY

Diabetic foot syndrome is a serious complication which requires energetic and aggressive therapeutic approach.

TABLE 28.6.6

- Wash feet daily, do not soak in hot water
- Dry gently but thoroughly especially between the toes
- Do not walk barefoot indoors/outdoors
- Cut nails straight
- Never indulge in bathroom surgery
- Do not use hawaii slippers and strap slippers
- Sandals are recommended with Velcro
- Shoes with broad front should be used
- Shoes must be roomy and loose fitting
- Never use socks with constricting tops
- Footwear should be ideally purchased in the evening
- For advanced diabetic lesions, to use specially ordered shoes
- Treat cuts, scratches promptly
- Never use hot water bottle

Diabetic foot care advice for diabetic patients

TABLE 28.6.7

- Assess the patient's knowledge and foot care practices
- Advise essential guidelines for preventive foot care
- Advise to consult the doctor if swelling of foot, colour change of toe/nail, pain or throbbing, thick hard skin or corns, breaks in skin, cracks, blisters or sores
- Identification of foot at risk (low and high risk) and take measures to prevent foot ulceration in them
- Assess at each visit for protective sensation (touch, pain and vibration), foot structure, biomechanics, vascular status and skin integrity
- Evaluation for additional risk factors and plan strategies accordingly

Guidelines for a medicosocial/health visitor

TABLE 26.6.8

- Immobilization of the extremity, drainage of pus
- Early surgical intervention (if plantar mid-compartment affected)
- Aggressive debridement of necrotic and infected tissue
- Avoid tight bandage in fulminant infection with soft tissue swelling (it prevents pressure necrosis)
- Suspect osteomyelitis in deep lesions especially if bone felt on probing—confirm by radiography
- Proper local care of wound, removal of slough and dressing
- Consider use of hyperbaric oxygen
- Doppler ultrasound to detect vascular pathology

Care of infected foot injury in a diabetic patient

It involves prolonged treatment, frequent follow-up assessments and a great deal of cooperation from the patient and family. Inspite of all efforts in many instances the disease progresses relentlessly and a foot/limb has to be sacrificed. The strategy in every diabetic centre/hospital, therefore, is to prevent this complication by meticulous control of hyperglycaemia, hyperlipidaemia and other abnormalities and ensuring ideal foot care.

FURTHER READING

1. Boulton AJM, Connor H, Cavanagh PR (Eds). The Foot in Diabetes (3rd edn). Chichester, United Kingdom. John Wiley, 2000.
2. Boulton AJM, Vileikyte L. The diabetic foot: the scope of the problem. J Fam Pract 2000; 49 (suppl):53-8.
3. Bowler J, Pfeifer MA (Eds): Levin and O'Neal's. The Diabetic Foot (6th edn). St. Louis CV Mosby, 2000.
4. Lobmann Ralf, Schultz Gregory, Lehnert Hendrick. Proteases and the diabetic foot syndrome: mechanism and therapeutic implications. Diabetes Care 2005;28:461-71.
5. Smiell J, Wieman TJ, Steel DL, et al. Efficacy and safety of becaplermin in patients with non-healing lower extremity diabetic ulcers: a combined analysis of four randomized; controlled studies. Wound Rep Regen 1999;7:335-46.
6. Veves A, Sheehan P, Pham HT. A randomized, controlled trial of promogran (a collagen/oxidized regenerated cellulose dressing) vs. standard treatment of diabetic foot ulcers. Arch Surg 2002;137:822-7.
7. International concensus on the Diabetic foot by the International Working Group on the Diabetic Foot 1999.
8. Wagener EW. The Dysvascular foot: a system of diagnosis and management. Foot Ankle 1981;2:64-7.

28.7 Peripheral Arterial Disease

Y Sachdev

- Introduction
- Symptomatology
- Clinical examination and investigations
- Treatment
- Summary

INTRODUCTION

Peripheral arterial disease (PAD) is a manifestation of atherosclerosis and is a marker for a atherothrombotic disease in other vascular beds. Diabetes and smoking are the strongest risk factors for its development. Other risk factors are advanced age, uncontrolled hypertension and hyperlipidaemia. Elevated levels of C-reactive proteins (CRP), homocysteine and plasma viscosity are other recognised contributory factors. It appears alcohol in moderate quantities, affords some protection.

Unlike smoking and hypertension which affect mostly the proximal portion of the aorto-iliofemoral vessels, diabetes is most strongly associated with femoral-popliteal and tibial (below the knee) vessels.

SYMPTOMATOLOGY

The most common symptom of PAD is intermittent claudication which patient may describe as pain, cramps or aching in the calves, thighs or buttocks. This appears on walking and is relieved by rest. In severe cases, there may be pain on rest, tissue loss, ulcer or gangrene. In diabetics due to associated peripheral neuropathy, the pain perception of the patient may get blunted and the presence of ischaemic ulcer may be the first indication of PAD.

CLINICAL EXAMINATION AND INVESTIGATIONS

Absence of peripheral arterial pulsations, history of claudication, ankle-bronchial index (ABI) (by hand-held Doppler to record systolic blood pressure and calculating the ratio) are confirmatory of the diagnosis. Normal ABI is 0.91 to 1.30; mild obstruction is 0.7 to 0.8, moderate obstruction 0.4 to 0.69, severe obstruction is <0.40 and poorly compressible and calcified arteries if ABI is > 1.30.

In a diabetic with PAD, the lesions are more diffuse and distal and patient is more prone to sudden ischaemia

TABLE 28.7.1

Clinical features	Non-diabetic	Diabetic
• Male: female ratio	M > F	M > F
• Age	Older age	Younger age
• Clinical course	Slow	Rapid
• Segment involved	Single	Multiple
• Affected arteries	Proximal	Both proximal and distal
• Limbs/extremities	Unilateral (usually)	Bilatreal
• Collateral arteries	Normal (usually)	Involved
• Occlusion	Less severe	Severe

Clinical differences in peripheral arterial disease in non-diabetic and diabetic individuals

of arterial thrombosis ending in neuroischaemic ulcer and infection. Table 28.7.1. presents some of the characteristic features pertaining to the behaviour of PAD in diabetic and non-diabetic persons.

Doppler sonography, MR angiogram (MRA) and contrast angiography help us visualize the site and extent of the lesion.

TREATMENT

Treatment consists of a multiprong approach, viz. strict control of hypertension, hyperlipidaemia, hyperglycaemia, infection, rehabilitative exercises, use of Statins, clopidogrel or aspirin or both (probably clopidogrel is better than aspirin), pentoxyphylline, etc. If these measures fail, surgical revascularisation must be tried.

SUMMARY

Peripheral arterial disease is usually confined to lower limbs and is more common in males. Its chief symptom is intermittent claudication which appears on walking and is relieved by rest. When ischaemia is severe, the pain appears even on rest. Diabetes and smoking are two main factors which contribute to its severity and early onset. The condition is described in brief as it could be a forerunner to diabetic ulcers and diabetic foot.

FURTHER READING

1. American Diabetes Association. Peripheral arterial disease in people with diabetes. Diabetes Care 2003;26:3333-41.
2. Dolan NC, Liu K, Criqui MH, et al. Peripheral artery disease, diabetes and reduced lower extremity functioning. Diabetes Care 2002;25:113-20.
3. Dormandy JA, Rutherford RB. Management of peripheral arterial disease (PAD). TASC Working Group Trans-Atlantic Inter-Society Consensus (TASC). J Vas Surg 2000;31:S1-S296.

SECTION

ACUTE METABOLIC COMPLICATIONS OF DIABETES MELLITUS

29

29.1 Diabetic Ketoacidosis (DKA)

Y Sachdev

- Introduction
- Pathogenesis
- Precipitating Factors

- Clinical Manifestations
- Diagnosis
- Management

INTRODUCTION

Diabetic ketoacidosis (DKA) is one of the most serious acute metabolic complications of diabetes. During pre-insulin era it was an extremely common cause of mortality among diabetics. After the insulin discovery and now with the standardization of the diabetic management strategy, enhanced knowledge of the community and improved communication techniques, the incidence of DKA and its mortality and morbidity have substantially reduced. In young type 1 DM patients below the age 20 years, however, it is still the common cause of death.

PATHOGENESIS

DKA is the result of insulin deficiency with concomitant unopposed action of counter-regulatory hormones. Whenever there is insulin lack, the catabolic effects of counter-regulatory hormones (glucagon, catecholamines, glucocorticoids, GH) dominate the scenario and gluco-neogenesis, glycogenolysis are promoted. The insulin dependent peripheral utilization of glucose by muscles and adipose tissue is also reduced. Simultaneously, there is accelerated lipolysis and protein break down. All these changes result in hyperglycaemia, raised level of free fatty acid (FFA), glycerol, amino acids and lactate. The beta-oxidation of excess FFA in the liver results in increased production of ketone bodies, mostly aceto-acetate, beta-hydroxybutyrate and acetones, leading to acidosis.

The consequence of these biochemical changes are osmotic diuresis, water and electrolytes loss, dehydration and hypotension (Fig. 29.1.1).

PRECIPITATING FACTORS

Missed/inadequate insulin dose, lung/skin/urinary tract infection, gastroenteritis, cerebral/coronary infarction and pregnancy are the common precipitating factors.

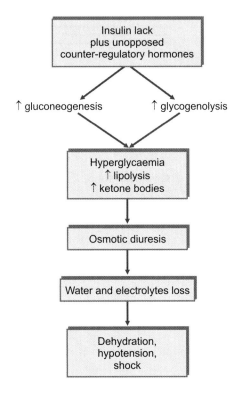

Fig. 29.1.1: Pathogenesis of diabetic ketoacidosis

CLINICAL MANIFESTATIONS

Symptoms

Nausea, vomiting, excessive thirst, polyuria, abdominal pain which is all over the abdomen. It could also be central around the periumbilical area. Usually, it is vague, though sometimes, it is severe and agonizing to be mistaken for 'acute abdomen.' Shortness of breath, dyspnoea on accustomed exertion and altered mental behaviour are the other symptoms.

Clinical Signs

Clinically the patient is obviously dyspnoeic, has dry tongue, reduced skin turgor, soft eyeballs, hypotension,

TABLE 29.1.1

Plasma osmolality	Level of consciousness
324-330 mOsm/kg	Drowsy
340-350 mOsm/kg	Semicoma
360-370 mOsm/kg	Coma

Relationship between plasma osmolality and level of consciousness in DKA

tachycardia, tachypnoea, Kussmaul's breathing, abdominal distension and tenderness, hyporeflexia, lethargy, drowsiness, disorientation and coma. Clinically, the level of consciousness appears to be proportional to plasma osmolality (Table 29.1.1)

DIAGNOSIS

The clinical presentation, presence of dehydration and acidotic breathing suggest the diagnosis. The history of polyuria, polydipsia, fatigue, vomiting (in over 75% patients) and muscle cramps, very strongly support the suspicion. In a large number of patients history of recent infection is present. There may be hypothermia inspite of the infection. The odour of acetone in the breath is a characteristic feature in DKA patients. The biochemical parameters like heavy glycosuria, ketonuria, hyperglycaemia confirm the diagnosis beyond any doubt. Plasma osmolality (by osmometer) will be between

300 and 380 mOsm/L. If osmometer is not available, plasma osmolality can be calculated from the formula given below:

$$2(Na + K) + urea + glucose \text{ (all in nmol/L)} = mOsm/L$$

Two potentially misleading laboratory results are WBC count and plasma sodium. The former is always raised and is not a sign of infection. The plasma sodium is often low and is due to the osmotic effect of glucose draining water from cells and diluting the sodium. Plasma sodium usually falls by 1 mmol/L for every 3 mmol/L that the glucose is raised. The sodium and other analytes will be spuriously low if there is marked hyperlipidaemia. This is referred to as pseudo-hyponatraemia.

MANAGEMENT (Fig. 29.1.2)

The DKA management strategy is based on five objectives:

- Replenish fluid loss by providing appropriate amount of fluids to restore circulation
- Administer rapid acting insulin in adequate and continuous doses to restore normal glycaemic status
- Provide general care and careful monitoring to ensure early and complete recovery
- Search for the underlying precipitating cause to avoid recurrence
- Ensure regular periodic follow-up.

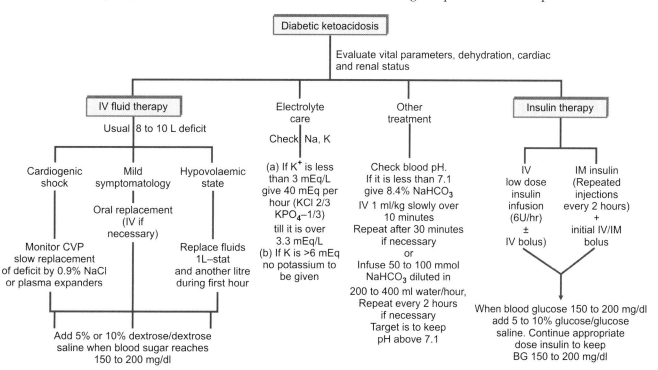

Fig. 29.1.2: Management of diabetic ketoacidosis (Guildelines of fluids and insulin therapy)

The management has to be individualized and modified as per prevailing scenario.

Table 29.1.2 gives the principles and general guidelines for management of DKA.

TABLE 29.1.2

Principles of management
- Maintain airways, vital parameters
- Identify and correct precipitating factors
- Stop further clinical and biochemical deterioration
- Correct metabolic imbalances smoothly and gradually
- Ensure adequate fluid and insulin therapy. Personalised nursing and supportive care

General guidelines
- Confirm diagnosis: History, clinical picture, ↑blood sugar, urinary ketones and metabolic acidosis
- Admit intensive care
- Monitor BP, HR, RR, level of consciousness, intake/output, electrolytes, pH, LFT, lipids, haemogram, BUN, creatinine
- Take ECG
- Replace fluids
- Initiate rapid acting regular insulin therapy
- Monitor and replace potassium and bicarbonate (if needed)
- Continue insulin therapy and saline infusion till plasma glucose is 150 to 200 mg/dl and acetone is controlled
- Switch over to 3 to 4 hours insulin doses and later to intermediate/long acting insulin
- Regulate food intake and insulin doses
- Search for precipitating cause
- Ensure self monitoring of blood glucose (SMBG) values
- Ensure regular periodic check-up
- Educate patient/relative/family members
- Organise health visitor/medicosocial worker

Principles and general guidelines for management of DKA

Fluid Replenishment in DKA (Table 29.1.3)

The first priority is rehydration so that perfusion of insulin sensitive tissues and urine flow are re-established. The body is short of hypotonic fluid, but it is safer to use isotonic saline unless plasma sodium is above 150 mmol/L, when 'half normal' saline should be used. Use of hypotonic replacement fluids throughout is associated with the risk of osmotic disequilibrium with cerebral oedema and adult respiratory distress syndrome. It is appreciated that volume contraction is one of the hallmarks of DKA and it contributes to acidosis through production of lactic acid and decreased renal clearance of organic and inorganic acids. Renal clearance of glucose is decreased contributing to hyperglycaemia. In patients with significant decreased tissue perfusion, the insulin delivery to the sites of insulin-dependent

TABLE 29.1.3

- Define aim
- Fluid therapy is first priority
- Monitor CVP especially in cardiac elderly patients
- Avoid osmotic disequilibrium, adult respiratory distress syndrome (ARDS)
- 0.9% NaCl
  - Ideal, prevents too rapid decline in osmolality
  - Ringer's lactate
- 0.45% NaCl
  - If serum Na >150 mEq/L
  - Give it at a slower rate
- 5 to 10% glucose
  - When BGL 150 to 200 mg/dl
- Calculate total fluids

Principles of fluid therapy

glucose disposal is reduced leading to hyperglycaemia. Catecholamines, glucocorticoids and other stress hormones are increased as a response to stress of reduced tissue perfusion.

Five to eight litres deficit is common in DKA (Table 29.1.4). Therefore, it is advisable to administer 1 litre of normal saline immediately followed by 1 litre during the first hour in case there is clinical evidence of dehydration, otherwise 500 to 600 ml immediately and same quantity during first hour will suffice. This is followed by 200 to 500 ml/hour of fluids in subsequent period. The rehydration status must be assessed at regular intervals to avoid overload and guard against under-therapy. If there is a doubt about cardiovascular status or if the person is old, central venous pressure monitoring is invaluable. When the plasma glucose level reaches 150 to 200 mg/dl, 5 to 10% dextrose/dextrose saline should form a part of all fluids administered. This is recommended to keep the blood glucose level between 150 and 200 mg (9.0 and 11.1 mmol/L) for 18 to 24 hours to allow slow equilibration of osmolatically active substances across cell membrane. We prefer 10% dextrose (at 100 ml/hour, with 20 mmol KCl per 500 ml) to 5%

TABLE 29.1.4

• Water	5 to 8 litres
• Sodium	400 to 600 mmol
• Potassium	300 to 1000 mmol
• Calcium	50 to 100 mmol
• Phosphate	25 to 50 mmol
• Magnesium	25 to 50 mmol
• Alkali	300 to 500 mmol

Average fluid and electrolyte deficit

dextrose as the patient is still catabolic and ketosis clears more rapidly with it. The infusion is continued till oral food intake is established.

Insulin Administration

In the past, there was considerable argument as to how much insulin should be used and 50 units/hour or even more were favoured. These days low dose insulin (0.1 U/kg/hour) is being used as relatively small amounts of insulin are required to inhibit lipolysis and cut off the substrate supply for ketogenesis and acidosis. Two regimens are commonly advocated:

a. The first comprises continuous infusion of insulin at 6 units/hour in normal saline (0.1 U/kg/hour in children) using an infusion pump. Hyperglycaemia is expected to improve at the rate of 75 to 100 mg/dl (4.2 to 5.6 mmol/L) per hour or near about. Alternatively, plasma glucose fall is 10% by 1 hour or 3 to 3.5 mmol/L by 2 hours. If no satisfactory response is found in first 2 hours, it is worth checking on the adequacy of rehydration and if it is adequate, insulin dose should be increased 1½ times or doubled. This is, however, rarely necessary.

b. The second regimen is to give a loading or priming dose of 10 to 20 units IV/IM respectively and then 5 units IM every hour (0.25 U/kg initially and 0.1 U/kg hourly in children). The second regimen is recommended in those health facilities where staffing pattern and expertise are less than ideal. When blood glucose level has fallen to 150 to 200 mg/dl, the IV insulin dose should be reduced to 3 units per hour. In IM insulin regimen, insulin should be reduced to 5 units × 2 to 3 hourly until oral food is re-established.

Treatment of Electrolyte Disturbance

Potassium

Plasma potassium on admission may be normal or high (if the onset is very acute) or low. Despite variable serum potassium values, there is no denying the fact that there is total body potassium deficit (3 to 10 mEq/litre) and with the initiation of therapy, potassium level comes down further. This is due to replacement of intracellular fluid which draws potassium into the cells, specific action of insulin on potassium uptake by cells, loss of K^+ in urine, extracellular volume expansion, and intracellular movement of K^+ as acidaemia is corrected. Therefore, serum potassium is always checked at the time of admission and replenished as per the guidelines given in Table 29.1.5. The patient should be attached to an ECG monitor to look for evidence of hypo/hyperkalaemia. The flat T wave and appearance of U waves indicates

TABLE 29.1.5

Serum potassium (mEq/L)	Suggested replacement of potassium dose (mEq)
Less than 3	40
3 to 4	30
4 to 5	20
5 to 6	10
>6	No potassium

Potassium replacement dose based on serum potassium value

significant hypokalaemia while peaking of T waves indicates hyperkalaemia. Hyperkalaemia may occur during treatment but is less common and is generally associated with Sickle cell syndrome or anaemia.

Bicarbonate

There is argument both for and against the use of alkali in the treatment of ketoacidosis. Over-vigorous alkalinisation causes hypokalaemia while untreated acidaemia is a cause of sustained insulin insensitivity. As such it is recommended to administer 1 ml/kg of 8.4% $NaHCO_3$ slowly over a period of 10 minutes if the blood pH is less than 7.1 or bicarbonate is less than 10 mgEq/L or the patient is having typical acidotic breathing. The $NaHCO_3$ can be repeated after 30 minutes if hyperpnoea persists. Whenever $NaHCO_3$ is given, additional 10 mmol (10 mEq) of K is administered along with it.

Phosphate

Phosphate in the body also gets depleted in DKA and may contribute to muscle weakness and lethargy. Its replacement as a separate entity is hardly needed unless its value is less than 1 mEq/L (Table 29.1.6).

TABLE 29.1.6

- Due to intracellular movement with insulin therapy
- PO_4 deficiency usually silent clinically
- Potential effects
  - Impaired cardiac function, haemolysis, glycolysis
  - Respiration failure, tissue hypoxia
- If initial PO_4 level is low, may give 40 to 60 mmol PO_4
- Intensive PO_4 therapy may result in Ca and Mg decline

PO_4 deficiency in DKA

General Care

There is often pooling of fluid (up to 2 L) in the stomach. Therefore, passage of Ryle's tube and gastric aspiration is done routinely if the vomiting persists or the patient is semicomatose or comatose.

- Oxygen administration is needed if pO_2 is less than 80 mm
- Central venous pressure monitoring is essential especially in elderly patients and those with compromised cardiac status
- Judicious antibiotic cover, both prophylactic and therapeutic, is advocated in frail and serious patients
- DKA, particularly when very hyperosmolar, may be associated with an increased incidence of thromboembolic phenomenon. Increased platelet aggregation and blood viscosity are two major contributory factors. In such cases, prophylactic use of low dose heparin (5000 units S/C 8 hourly) is recommended.
- In severely hypotensive patients where crystalloid infusion is not of much help, support with plasma expanders may be needed
- Sometimes a small dose of IV frusemide may be needed to re-establish urinary flow.

Table 29.1.7 enumerates key points to be observed for effective treatment of DKA. It also gives common therapeutic errors seen by us in handling DKA.

Monitoring of the Progress

- BP, HR, CVP and level of consciousness must be monitored continuously
- Blood glucose must be monitored every hour
- Electrolytes should be done every 4 hours for 12 hours. It is pointless to measure ketones as these may stay positive for 2 to 3 days because of continuous diffusion of acetones and body fat
- It is to be remembered that acidosis takes much longer time to subside than hyperglycaemia.

Complications of Therapy

Besides iatrogenic hypoglycaemia, cerebral oedema especially in children may be encountered and may prove fatal. If blood glucose and other parameters are properly maintained, it should be an extremely rare complication. Acute respiratory distress (ARD) syndrome is seen when plasma osmolality reduces rapidly. Bronchial mucus plugging, especially in elderly, is another complication which must be treated energetically. Fluid overload and arteriovenous thromboembolic events are the other complications of therapy.

Search for Precipitating Factors

Look assiduously for clinical evidence of infection. Rule out myocardial infarction. Enquire about missing of insulin, traumatic injury, indiscrete dietary intake, lack of activity excessive dehydration and excessive use of

TABLE 29.1.7

Key points for effective management
- Correct and complete diagnosis
- Appropriate treatment
- Frequent monitoring of:
  - Clinical status
  - BG, ketones
  - Electrolytes
  - pH, osmolality
  - Precipitating factors
- Proper nursing support

Common therapeutic errors
- Too early or too late 'K' administration
- Too rapid correction of hyperglycaemia
- Insufficient rehydration
- Too much insulin dose
- Insufficient and delayed glucose administration
- Thromboembolic episodes, gastric atony
- Infections—mucormycosis, candidiasis

Key points and errors in management of DKA

alcohol, fried and fast food without appropriate insulin/OHA therapy.

Periodic Regular Check and Follow-up

It is necessary to ensure a meticulous continuous periodic communication/interaction with the patient who should be educated regarding self care, self monitoring of glycaemic control by periodic urine/blood check.

SUMMARY

Diabetic ketoacidosis (DKA) is one of the very serious complications of diabetes. It is still the most common causes of mortality in young T1DM patients. Its early detection and prompt treatment with appropriate fluid and rapidly acting insulin therapy are life saving.

Infection and inadequate medication are the two common precipitating causes.

Patients' education and regular follow-up are necessary to avoid its recurrences.

FURTHER READING

1. American Diabetes Association. Continuous insulin infusion. Diabetes Care 2002;25 (suppl 1):116.
2. Kitabchi AE. Low insulin therapy in diabetic ketoacidosis: fact or fiction? Diabet 1989;5:337-63.
3. Sachdev Y. Clinical and biochemical status in diabetic ketoacidosis treated with low dose insulin infusion. JAPI 1983;31:621-5.
4. Sachdev Y. Kinetics of ketone bodies and shift of electrolytes with low dose infusion in diabetic ketoacidosis. AFMC Project 1150/83 Final Report 1983.

29.2 Hyperglycaemic Hyperosmolar State

Y Sachdev

INTRODUCTION

Hyperglycaemic hyperosmolar state (HHS) is due to relative insulin deficiency and inadequate fluid intake. Insulin deficiency enhances hepatic glucose production by glycogenolysis and gluconeogenesis and impairs peripheral utilization of the glucose.

PATHOGENESIS

Hyperglycaemia induces an osmotic diuresis that leads to intravascular volume depletion which is aggravated by inadequate fluid replacement. The absence or minimal presence of ketosis in this condition is probably due to relative and less severe insulin deficiency (compared to DKA), lower levels of FFA, and counter-regulatory hormones.

CLINICAL MANIFESTATIONS (TABLE 29.2.1)

The condition is usually seen in type 2 DM individuals with a history of persistent polyuria, weight loss and

TABLE 29.2.1

- 20% of diabetic coma
- Elderly, rarely young IDDM
- High renal threshold for glucose
- No or littel acidosis
- High mortality
- Adequate residual insulin secretion
- Severe dehydration, very high BGL (>700 mg/dl)
  - ↑ Blood urea, Na, creatinine, ketones <3 mmol/L
- Hyperviscosity syndrome
- Rapid infusion 0.45/0.9% NaCl
- Plasma expanders, insulin, α-adrenergic agents

Main features of hyperosmolar non-ketolotic state

reduced oral intake. The patient may be confused, lethargic, drowsy or even semicomatose/comatose. There is profuse dehydration, hypotension, tachycardia, altered mental status and profound hyperosmolality. There is very frequently concurrent illness in the form of pneumonia, infection, myocardial infarction or stroke.

BIOCHEMICAL TESTS

Biochemical investigations reveal very high blood glucose level (600 to 1300 mg/dl; 33.3 to 66.6 mmol/L), plasma osmolality of 330 to 380 mOsm/ml and plasma ketone bodies absent or only marginally raised. There is pre-renal azotaemia while serum sodium may be normal or slightly low. Table 29.2.2 enumerates representative biochemical parameters of DKA and HHS.

TREATMENT

Broadly speaking, the treatment of hyperglycaemic hyperosmolar state is similar to that of DKA. Careful monitoring of patient's hydration status, laboratory results and response to insulin infusion is crucial. Fluid replacement of 1 to 3 litres of 0.9% normal saline over a period of 2 to 3 hours will stabilize the haemodynamic status in most of the patients. If the serum sodium is over 500 mEq/L, it might be better to infuse 0.45% saline rather than 0.9% saline. The usual fluid deficit in hyperglycaemic hyperosmolar state is 8 to 10 litres. This deficit should be replaced very gradually over a period of 1 to 2 days to avoid worsening of the neurological status. Potassium deficit may be quite large and its replacement is usually necessary. Therefore, it is advisable to test serum potassium repeatedly. Magnesium and phosphate deficiency may also be observed and needs correction. Besides rehydration, insulin therapy as in DKA must be initiated and precipitating factor(s) sought out and treated energetically. A low dose of heparin may be useful in avoiding vascular thrombosis and intravascular

TABLE 29.2.2

Biochemical parameters	Normal range	Diabetic ketoacidosis	Hyperglycaemic hyperosmolar states
Glucose mg/dl (mmol/L)	80 to 120 (4.4 to 6.0)	300 to 800 mg/dl (16.7 to 33.3)	600 to 1200 (33.3 to 66.6)
Sodium (mEq/L)	136 to 142	125 to 135	135-145
Potassium (mEq/L)	3.8 to 5.0	Normal ↑	Normal
Magnesium (mEq/L) (mg/dl)	1.3 to 2.1 1.8 to 3.0	Normal	Normal
Chloride (mEq/L) (mg/dl)	95 to 103 (95 to 103)	Normal	Normal
Phosphate (mg/dl) (mmol/L)	2.5 to 4.3 (0.8 to 1.4)	↓	Normal
Creatinine (mg/dl) (µmol/L)	0.6 to 1.2 (53 to 106)	↑(slight)	↑(moderate)
Osmolality (mOsm/ml)	280 to 295	300-320	330-380
Plasma ketones	–ve	++++	+/–
Sodium bicarbonate (mEq/L)	21 to 28	<15	Normal or ↓ slight
Arterial pH	7.38 to 7.44	6.8 to 7.3	>7.3
Arterial pO$_2$ (mmHg)	35 to 40	20 to 30	Normal
Anion gap			
Sodium + potassium minus (Chloride + HCO$_3$) mEq/L		↑	Normal or ↑ slight

Representative biochemical parameters of diabetic ketoacidosis (DKA) and hyperglycaemic and hyperosmolar states (HSS)

coagulation. The patient may be discharged on insulin/ OHA once he/she is stabilized. As the patient is usually an elderly person, help of medicosocial worker/health visitor must be incorporated for a strict follow-up in order to avoid recurrence.

SUMMARY

Hyperglycaemic hyperosmolar state (HHS) is comparatively an uncommon acute complication of diabetes mellitus. It is seen mostly in elderly diabetic patients and treated by fluid and insulin therapy as the diabetic ketoacidosis

FURTHER READING

1. Pickup J Williams (Ed). Textbook of Diabetes. London: Blackwell Science, 1997.
2. Rosenbloom AL. Intracerebral crisis during treatment of diabetic ketoacidosis. Diabetes Care 1990;13:22-33.

29.3 Lactic Acidosis

Y Sachdev

- Introduction
- Aetiological Causes
- Clinical Manifestations

- Biochemical Findings
- Treatment
- Summary

Lactic acid (LA) is present physiologically in all body tissues especially in the brain, red cells and skeletal muscle. LA formation is due to glycolysis and it generates energy (ATP) without the consumption of oxygen. The normal serum lactate is between 0.4 and 1.0 mmol/L. It rises to 1.5 mmol/L after feeding. When LA dissociates, the hydrogen ion combines with bicarbonate diminishing its level. However, if the lactate ions are utilized by oxidation or in gluconeogenesis, bicarbonate ion is restored. Liver and kidney are the main sites of lactate utilization. Both these organs play a special role in lactate homeostasis (liver clears 70% and kidneys 30% of lactate).

Lactic acidosis develops when there is over-production or underutilization of lactic acid and it accumulates to reach a level of 5 mmol/L or over. When this happens, there is significant production of hydrogen ions, reduction in pH and serum bicarbonate.

AETIOLOGICAL CAUSES

Mostly lactic acidosis is secondary to conditions where there is poor tissue perfusion as seen in acute myocardial infarction, severe internal bleeding, acute necrotizing pancreatitis, respiratory failure and carbon monoxide poisoning. It is also seen in diabetics who are treated with high doses of biguanides, have compromised hepatic or renal functions and suffer alcohol abuse or tissue hypoxia.

CLINICAL MANIFESTATIONS

The onset is usually sudden. There is marked hyperventilation, air hunger, tachycardia, vomiting, abdominal pain, hypotension and ultimately consciousness is impaired.

BIOCHEMICAL FINDINGS

Biochemically, there is profound metabolic acidosis without significant ketonaemia and ketonuria. The blood sugar is usually normal, low or slightly elevated. Serum potassium is high. The lactate-pyruvate ratio exceeds the normal of 15. Anion gap is above 20 mmol/L. Anion gap is calculated by the formula given blow:

Sodium + potassium − (chlorides + bicarbonate) = 16 ± 2 mEq

A value above this is indicative of a widening of anion gap and is characteristic of lactic acidosis. This finding may also be seen in parenteral nutrition with fructose and sorbitol which are converted to glucose and lactate in the liver, in starvation, alcoholic ketoacidosis and DKA. Table 29.3.1. gives comparative biochemical picture in various acute metabolic emergencies seen in diabetic patients.

TREATMENT

Lactic acidosis is an extremely serious disease having high mortality. Therefore, it is better to take all

TABLE 29.3.1

	Blood pressue	Blood sugar	Plasma ketone	Dehydration	Hyperventilation
Hypoglycaemia	Normal	< 2 mmol	0	0	0
DKA	Normal or ↓	> 13 mmol	+ to +++	+++	+++
Hyperosmolar nonketotic (HONK) coma	N ormal or ↓	>13 mmol	0 to +	++++	0
Lactic acidosis	Low	Variable	0 to +	0 to +	+++
Non-metabolic coma	Variable	N ormal ↑	0 to +	0 to +	0 to +

Comparative biochemical situation in various metabolic emergencies seen in diabetic patients

precautions to prevent this complication. The biguanides should not be used in those diabetics who have renal and hepatic dysfunctions. It should also be used with caution in frail and elderly. Out of biguanides, metformin is safer: even than it is advisable to withhold it in those diabetics who have cardiac, respiratory or circulatory disorders likely to result in tissue hypoxia. It is, again, better avoided in those patients who are addicted to alcohol abuse. Under no circumstances, dose should exceed 2 gm per day.

The therapeutic management of lactic acidosis aims at correcting hypotension, improving oxygenation and tissue perfusion. Isotonic sodium bicarbonate in large amounts (500 to 1500 mmol) should be infused to raise the pH to 7.25. It is essential to raise pH above 7 so that the hepatic production of lactate is reduced, myocardial contractility and tissue perfusion improve. Caution is needed to avoid hypokalaemia and sodium overload. Serum potassium and ECG should be monitored frequently. Small dose of insulin with IV dextrose is useful to control hyperkalaemia. In nonresponding patients, peritoneal dialysis using bicarbonate fluid instead of usual lactate may help remove excess of hydrogen ion, lactate, ethanol and biguanides. In alcohol-associated lactic acidosis, intravenous thiamine is beneficial.

SUMMARY

Lactic acidosis is mostly secondary to those conditions where there is poor tissue perfusion. In diabetes mellitus it is usually seen when high doses of biguanides are used especially in patients with hepatic/renal dysfunctional status. It is a serious complication with high mortality and needs a prompt energetic treatment. Injudicious use of biguanides must be avoided to safe guard against it.

FURTHER READING

1. Fulop M. Alcoholism, ketoacidosis and lactic acidosis. Diabetes Mellitus Rev 1989;5:365-78.
2. Madias NE. Lactic acidosis. Kidney Int 1986;29:752-74.

SECTION

30

SPECIAL TOPICS IN DIABETES MELLITUS

30.1 Drug-induced Hyperglycaemia

GR Sridhar

INTRODUCTION

There are many drugs which impair insulin secretion and may precipitate diabetes in a predisposed individual. Many diabetics take a number of drugs, which may interact and lead to hyperglycaemia.

DRUGS WHICH AFFECT GLUCOSE BALANCE

The commonly used drugs which affect the glucose tolerance adversely are:
- Antihypertensive agents including beta-blockers and diuretics
- Oestrogen-progesterone
- Corticosteroids
- Sympathomimetics
- Immunosuppressive drugs (post-transplant diabetes mellitus)
- Protease inhibitors
- Clozapine
- Recombinant interferon
- Caffeine, cyproheptadine, ascorbate
- Vacor
- Pentamidine
- L-asparaginase
- Diazoxide.

These drugs impair glucose tolerance in various ways:
- Impair insulin secretion
- Reduce insulin efficacy
- Reduce insulin sensitivity and secretion
- Increase nutrition flux.

Antihypertensive Drugs

Conventional antihypertensive drugs may lower blood pressure but they seem to have an unfavourable influence on other cardiovascular risk factors.

Diuretics

Thiazides impair glucose tolerance, elevate LDL cholesterol and triglycerides. Beta-adrenergic blockers increase serum triglycerides and lower HDL cholesterol. Used together, thiazides and beta-blockers further impair glucose tolerance than when used independently. In general, effects on glucose metabolism are greater with thiazide diuretics than with loop diuretics. The likelihood of hyperglycaemia is more when hydrochlorothiazide is used in a dose exceeding 25 mg/day.

The Gothenburg study was a prospective population study of women in Sweden, which showed an increased risk of developing diabetes in women who used diuretics or beta blockers as antihypertensive agents compared to other women. The risk was higher when both were combined.

Hydrochlorothiazide impairs insulin release from beta cell, possibly by decreasing calcium uptake, aside from causing insulin resistance. However, if used in low doses and hypokalaemia is avoided, thiazides are safe, cheap and effective antihypertensive agents.

Beta Blockers

They induce insulin resistance and impair glucose utilization.

Atenolol used in a dose of 100 mg once a day was shown to worsen insulin resistance in individuals who had angina pectoris with angiographically normal coronary arteries. In another study, the drug used in a dose of 50 to 100 mg, impaired insulin sensitivity by 23% at the end of 48 weeks of use. However, glucose tolerance was not adversely affected when used with terbutaline to halt premature labour. They are, however, liable to induce gestational diabetes mellitus.

Clonidine

Clonidine, an antihypertensive agent now less commonly used was shown to cause transient hyperglycemia though there were no long-term diabetogenic effects.

A combination of ACE inhibitor that decreases insulin resistance and calcium channel blocker that lowers heart rate, is useful in insulin resistant type 2 diabetes mellitus

Oestrogen-progesterone

Oral contraceptive agents are reported to be diabetogenic. Gonadal steroids have been shown to worsen insulin resistance in experimental animals. But low dose oestrogens were shown to be free of diabetogenic effects. Ethinyl oestradiol in a dose of 0.03 mg and dinorgestrel in 0.15 mg when given to 19 women with diabetes mellitus and/or high risk of diabetes mellitus, were devoid of diabetogenic effect. Sequential low dose oestrogen-progesterone agents were shown to be non-diabetogenic in experimental animals. In general, the risk of significant hyperglycaemia is greater with the use of oestrogen in a dose larger than 70 μg.

A recent multicentric clinical study using once a month injectable contraceptives showed no clinically relevant changes in carbohydrate tolerance.

However, it is prudent to monitor women using oestrogen-progesterone agents, especially those in high-risk group, such as those with previous history of gestational diabetes mellitus. High dose oestrogen pills must also be avoided.

There may be a lag period of two years before hyperglycaemia manifests in women using oestrogen-progesterone.

Corticosteroids

Corticosteroids are well known to cause or worsen hyperglycaemia, independent of the route administered. Corticosteroid-induced hyperglycaemia may take weeks to months to return to normalcy after steroid use has been stopped. These drugs increase gluconeogenesis, decrease peripheral utilisation of glucose and also have receptor and postreceptor effects on insulin action. Whether alternate day steroid use is less diabetogenic is not adequately studied. However, all persons with diabetes who are on corticosteroids should be closely monitored for hyperglycaemia.

Sympathomimetics

Commonly used sympathomimetics drugs such as ephedrine and pseudoephedrine can mildly raise blood glucose. Albuterol and terbutaline can also cause hyperglycaemia by stimulating glycogenolysis and gluconeogenesis. One must keep in mind that some of these agents may be present in over the counter preparations.

Growth Hormone

With the availability of recombinant DNA derived growth hormone (rGH), and the increasing list of indications for its use, one may expect greater use of rGH and; hence, its possible adverse effects on glucose tolerance.

In experimental animals, growth hormone treatment increased serum glucose and insulin levels, causing insulin resistance through a post-binding site.

If the dose of GH is adjusted to normalise the levels of IGF-1 level, the risk of glucose intolerance can be minimized.

A recent study evaluated the effect of GH in girls with Turner's syndrome (GH dose: up to 8 $IU/m^2/d$). There was no adverse effect on glucose tolerance, although insulin levels were elevated suggesting insulin tolerance. It is not known what the long-term effects of hyper-insulinaemia could be. A large study of more than 20,000 children treated with GH reported that type 2 diabetes developed six times more frequently.

When growth hormone was given to patients who were critically ill, the diabetogenic and lipolytic effects were shown to be mediated via specific GH receptors, in contrast to the effects on protein metabolism, which were mediated via IGF receptors.

Immunosuppressive Drugs

Post-transplant Diabetes Mellitus (PTDM)

With advancing transplant techniques and immunology, a greater proportion of subjects are taken up with other risk factors for glucose intolerance. Post-transplant diabetes has emerged as a significant problem, with attendant complications of infection and vascular disorders. PTDM is believed to be mainly due to the immunosuppressant drug use such as corticosteroids and cyclosporin following transplantation.

Cyclosporin A induces glucose intolerance by impairing insulin production and action. Improved understanding of the effects of immunosuppressants on glucose tolerance, as well as attempts to withdraw corticosteroids and maintain on cyclosporin and azathioprine are likely to reduce the risk of PTDM. One should be aware of the trade-off between the risk of PTDM and immune rejection. In general, lower doses are less diabetogenic.

Protease Inhibitors in HIV

Use of antiretroviral drugs such as protease inhibitors has increased following dramatic increase in HIV infection. Even though they are relatively safe, they can impair insulin sensitivity and lead to hyperglyceridaemia. It is advisable that blood glucose and serum lipids are monitored every three months, and specific therapy for dysglycaemia or dyslipidaemia instituted should either develop.

In a clinical study, 46% (n:18) of patients given the protease inhibitors developed impaired glucose tolerance and 13% (n:5) frank diabetes mellitus. A combination of beta cell dysfunction and peripheral insulin resistance is responsible.

Recombinant Alpha 2 Beta Interferon

This agent is used in patients with chronic hepatitis C, and has been shown to hasten type 1 diabetes mellitus in HLA susceptible individuals. However, the effects on carbohydrate tolerance were shown to be reversible in a later study.

Clozapine and Olanzapine

Clozapine and olanzapine, used in treatment of schizophrenia, cause diabetes mellitus and ketoacidosis, which were reversible on stopping the drugs.

Caffeine

Caffeine, given in a dose of 200 mg by mouth increases blood glucose level, independent of insulin levels.

Cyproheptadine

Cyproheptadine was shown to be diabetogenic in experimental animals when given to pregnant rats.

Ascorbate

Ascorbate was also shown to be cytotoxic to islet cells by free-radical generation

Vacor

Vacor is a rodenticide, which results in rapid death of pancreatic beta cells. It antagonizes the nucleotide niacinamide.

Pentamidine

Pentamidine, an antiparasite agent is cytolytic to beta cells of pancreas. When given in repeated courses, permanent diabetes may result.

L-asparginase

L-asparginase is an antineoplastic agent, which reduces insulin production by lowering asparagine levels, thus impairing insulin production. It is not directly cytotoxic to beta cells of pancreas.

Diphenylhydantoin

Diphenylhydantoin, used as an antiepileptic drug, reduces insulin secretion. In individuals at risk, impaired glucose tolerance may result.

Diazoxide

Diazoxide, which was used in management of malignant hypertension has been shown to reversibly reduce insulin secretion.

Nicotinic Acid

Nicotinic acid is an agent used in hyperlipidaemia. It increases blood glucose levels by increasing glucose output from the liver through increased gluconeogenesis. Clinically, relevant adverse effects include hyperglycaemia, hyperuricaemia and insulin resistance.

TREATMENT OF DRUG-INDUCED HYPERGLYCAEMIA

Ideally, the offending drug should be withdrawn to improve glucose tolerance. When this is not always possible, as with chronic corticosteroid use, other immunosuppressive drugs such as azathioprine may be substituted. Frequent monitoring of plasma glucose and attainment of target glycaemic control must be aimed. Higher levels of glucose may be acceptable, if the offending drugs are used for short-term. However, in long-term use, insulin may be required to attain glycaemic control. In those already controlled with oral antidiabetic drugs, use of corticosteroids may necessitate titration of OHA dose.

SUMMARY

The possibility of drug interaction and hyperglycaemia must always be borne in mind if a patient is taking multiple drugs and is at risk for diabetes mellitus.

FURTHER READING

1. Behrens G, Dejam A, Schmidt H, Balks HJ, Brabant G, Korner T, Stoll M, Schmidt RE. Impaired glucose tolerance, beta cell function and lipid metabolism in HIV patients under treatment with protease inhibitors. AIDS 1999;13:F63-70.
2. Bengtsson C. Incidence of diabetes during antihypertensive treatment. Horm Metab Res (Suppl) 1990;22:38-42.

3. Bulow B, Erfurth EM. A low individualized GH dose in young patients with childhood onset GH deficiency normalized serum IGF-I without significant deterioration in glucose tolerance. Clin Endocrinol (Oxj) 1999;50:45-55.

4. Colli A, Cocciolo M, Francobandiera G, Rogantin F, Cattalini N. Diabetic ketoacidosis associated with clozapine treatment. Diabetes Care 1999;22:176-7.

5. Cutfield WS, Wilton P, Benmarker H, et al. Incidence of diabetes mellitus and impaired glucose tolerance in children and adolescents receiving growth-hormone treatment. Lancet 2000;355:610-3.

6. Fabris P, Betterle C, Greggio NA, Zanchetta R, Bosi E, Biasin MR, de Lalla F. Insulin-dependent diabetes mellitus during alpha-interferon therapy for chronic viral hepatitis. J Hepatol 1998;28:5l4-7.

7. Ferrari P, Rosman J, Weidmann P. Antihypertensive agents, serum lipoproteins and glucose metabolism. Am J Cardiol 1991;67:26B-35B.

8. McMahon CD, Elsasser TH, Gunter DR, Sanders LG, Steele BP, Sartin JL. Estradiol/progesterone implants increase food intake, reduce hyperglycaemia and increase insulin resistance in endotoxic steers. J Endocrinol 1998;159:469-78.

9. Menegazzo LA, Ursich MJ, Fukui RT, Rocha DM, Silva ME, lanhez LE, Sabbage E, Wajchenberg BL. Mechanism of the diabetogenic action of cyclosporin A. Horm Metab Res 1998; 663-7.

10. Pusztay M, Nemesanszky E. Effect of interferon therapy on carbohydrate metabolism in chronic hepatitis C patients. OrvHetil 1999;140:1579-81.

11. Rett K, Jacob S, Wicklmayr M. Possible synergistic effect of ACE inhibition and calcium-channel blockade on insulin sensitivity in insulin-resistant type II diabetic hypertensive patients. J Cardiovasc Pharmacol 1994; 23(Suppl l):S29-33.

12. Sandstrom PE. Inhibition by hydrochlorothiazide of insulin release and calcium influx in mouse pancreatic beta cells. Br J Pharmacol 1993;10:1359-62.

13. Sas TC, de Muinck Keizer-Schrama SM, Stijnen T, Aanstoot HJ, Drop SI. Carbohydrate metabolism during long-term growth hormone (GH) treatment and after discontinuation of GH treatment in girls with Turner syndrome participating in a randomized dose-response study. Dutch Advisory Group on Growth Hormone. J Clin Endocrinol Metab 2000;85:769-75.

14. Teuscher AU, Weidmann PU. Requirements for antihypertensive therapy in diabetic patients: metabolic aspects. J Hypertens Suppl 1997;15:867-75.

15. Weir MR, Fink JC. Risk for posttransplant diabetes mellitus with current immunosuppressive medications. Am J Kidney Dis 1999;34:1-13.

16. White JR, Campbell K. Dangerous and common drug interactions in patients with diabetes mellitus. Endocrinol Metab Clin NA 2000;29:789-802.

30.2 Type 2 Diabetes Mellitus in the Young

AK Das

INTRODUCTION

The projected WHO forecast of 65 million of diabetes by the year 2025 will occur mostly in the young people in our country in contradistinction to above 65 years in the USA. Type 2 diabetes generally occurs a decade earlier in Indians. Further, fibrocalculous pancreatic diabetes (FCPD) and malnutrition modulated diabetes mellitus (MMDM) (did not find a place in 1997 ADA classification) are also diabetes in the young people in our country. The end of 20th century has witnessed a dramatic rise in the incidence of type 2 diabetes in children. It has been recognized that this type 2 diabetes in children is one of the most rapidly growing forms of diabetes in the USA and elsewhere in the world. This increase in type 2 diabetes in children parallels the increase in the obesity in childhood which has assumed epidemic proportion.

Yet another facet of type 2 diabetes in the young is the maturity onset diabetes in the young (MODY). The genetic and morphological characterization of MODY has witnessed rapid strides and today we have about 6 types of MODY characterized. Diabetes in the young comprises in addition to type 1 diabetes (both autoimmune and non-immune forms), LADA, FCPD and MMDM, MODY and type 2 diabetes in children. The focus is on true type 2 diabetes in young people, its heterogeneity, MODY, FCPD and MMDM.

DEFINITION AND TYPES OF DIABETES IN THE YOUNG

By definition the 'diabetes in the young' is defined as diabetes mellitus occurring in people with onset before the age of 30 years. The various types include:

- Type 1 diabetes in young
- True type 2 diabetes in young
- Fibrocalculous pancreatic diabetes
- Malnutrition modulated diabetes
- MODY
  a. Glucokinase MODY
  b. Transcription factors MODY
- Non-autoimmune type 1 diabetes
- Latent autoimmune diabetes in the adult (LADA)
- Type 2 diabetes in children.

The categories of type 1 and type 2 diabetes are usually clinically defined and the classification depending on clinical features alone may be flexible. It is a well known clinical practice that diabetes in the young classification may require a future revision as the clinical course progresses and the treatment options also may change. Sometimes, the obese type 2 diabetes in children may require insulin for initial control of diabetes mellitus and subsequently oral agents may be good enough to control the diabetes. It is useful not to make hasty statements regarding long-term requirement of insulin if one suspects type 2 diabetes in an obese child.

Maturity Onset Diabetes of Young

MODY is a clinically heterogeneous group of disorders characterized by:

i. non-ketotic diabetes mellitus,
ii. an autosomal dominant mode of inheritance,
iii. an onset usually before age of 25 years and frequently in childhood or adolescence and
iv. a primary defect in the function of beta cells of pancreas. It accounts for 1 to 5% of all diabetics in the United States and other industrialized countries.

MODY can result from mutations in any one of at least 6 different genes leading to beta cell dysfunction.

MODY types	Genes
MODY 1	Hepatocyte nuclear factor 4α (HNF4α)
MODY 2	Glucokinase
MODY 3	HNF 1α
MODY 4	Insulin promoter factor 1 (1PF-1)
MODY 5	HNF 1β
MODY 6	Neurogenic differentiation factor 1 (Neuro D1) (or) Beta cell E-box transactivator 2 (BETA 2)

These genes are also expressed in other tissues as liver and kidney. Dysfunction of these organs also may be seen in MODY. One of the associated anomalies is the cystic disease of the kidney. Factors that affect insulin sensitivity as infection, puberty, pregnancy and rarely obesity may trigger the onset of diabetes and worsen hyperglycaemia in patients with MODY. But, otherwise non-genetic factors have no important role in the development of this disorder.

Glucokinase

Glucokinase functions as the glucose sensor in beta cells by controlling the rate of entry of glucose into the glycolytic pathway by phosphorylation. Glucokinase in the liver plays a key role in the ability of that organ to store glucose as glycogen. Heterogeneous mutations in the gene encoding glucokinase leads to a partial deficiency of the enzyme and are associated with MODY 2. Homozygous mutations result in a complete deficiency of this enzyme and lead to a permanent neonatal diabetes mellitus.

HNF-1a, HNF-1b 7, HNF-4a

These constitute part of a network of transcription factors that function together to control gene expression during embryonic development and during adulthood in the liver, pancreatic islets, the kidneys and genital tissues. In pancreatic islets, these factors regulate the expression of insulin gene as well as the expression of genes encoding proteins, glucose transport and metabolism.

IPF-1

This acts as a regulator of the transcription of insulin, somatostatin and other genes in pancreatic islets. It also plays a central part in the development of the pancreas.

Neuro D1

This acts as an activator of transcription of insulin gene and is also required for normal development of pancreatic islets.

Clinical Features

The most common clinical presentation of MODY is mild, asymptomatic hyperglycaemia in nonobese children, adolescents and young adults who have a prominent family history of diabetes, often in generations. In most patients, the onset is in adolescence or childhood. Some patients have mild fasting hyperglycaemia for many years, while others have varying degrees of glucose intolerance for several years before the onset of persistent fasting hyperglycaemia (Table 30.2.1).

TABLE 30.2.1

Characteristic	MODY	Type 2 diabetes
Mode of inheritance	Monogenic, auto-somal dominant	Polygenic
Age at onset	Childhood, adolescence or young adulthood (25 yr)	Adulthood (usually 40 to 60 years; in India a decade earlier)
Pedigree	Usually multigenerational	Rarely multigenerations
Penetrance	80 to 95%	Variable (10 to 40%)
Body habitus	Nonobese	Usually obese
Metabolic syndrome	Absent	Usually present

Difference between MODY and type 2 diabetes

Clinical Features of Subtypes of MODY

MODY 1 and MODY 3

MODY 3 is the most common cause of MODY. The clinical and pathophysiologic features of MODY 1 and 3 are very similar. Most patients present with a mild form of diabetes. The hyperglycaemia in these patients tend to increase over time resulting in the need for treatment with oral hypoglycaemic drugs or insulin (30 to 40% require insulin). These forms of MODY are associated with a progressive decrease in insulin secretion (at the rate of about 1 to 4% per year). Patient with MODY 1 and 3 have the same spectrum of complication of diabetes. Microvascular complications, especially those involving the retina and kidneys are as common as in other diabetics.

It is possible to distinguish persons with HNF-1 alpha mutation from those with HNF-4 alpha mutation according to the ability of glucose to prime the insulin secretion response to a glucose stimulus. In the prediabetic state, the normal priming effect of mild hyperglycaemia on insulin secretion is retained in persons with HNF-1 alpha mutations, but it is lost in those with HNF-4 alpha mutations. A deficiency of HNF-4 alpha activity may affect the function of beta, alpha and pancreatic polypeptide cells of the pancreatic islets.

HNF-1α and 4α affect renal and hepatic function also. Patients with HNF-1α mutation have a low renal threshold for glucose. A deficiency of HNF-4α affects triglyceride and apolipoprotein biosynthesis and is associated with a 50% reduction in serum triglyceride concentration and a 25% decrease in apolipoprotein AII and CIII and LP (a) lipoproteins.

MODY 2

It is a common form of MODY. Heterozygous mutations in glucokinase are associated with a mild form of nonprogressive hyperglycaemia that is usually asymptomatic at diagnosis and is treated with diet alone. About 50% of women who are carriers may have gestational diabetes. Less than 50% of the carriers have overt diabetes. 2% of the carriers require insulin therapy. Diabetes-associated complications are rare in this form of MODY.

Homozygous mutations cause a complete deficiency of glucokinase and are associated with permanent neonatal diabetes mellitus, necessitating insulin treatment within the first few days of life.

The hyperglycaemia in persons with glucokinase related MODY appears to result from a reduction in the sensitivity of beta cells to glucose as well as a defect in postprandial glycogen synthesis in liver. There is an increase in the threshold concentration of glucose necessary to stimulate insulin secretion, from a normal basal concentration of about 90 mg/dl to approximately 108 to 126 mg/dl. In patients with glucokinase mutations, physiologic adaptations within the pancreatic beta cells limit the severity of hyperglycaemia.

MODY 4

IPF 1 gene mutations are rare cause of MODY. It presents with neonatal diabetes and pancreatic exocrine insufficiency resulting from congenital agenesis of the pancreas.

MODY 5

Mutation in gene encoding HNF-1β is characterized by both diabetes mellitus and renal cysts (hypoplastic glomerulocystic kidney disease). Internal genital anomalies as vaginal aplasia, rudimentary uterus and bicornuate uterus are seen in female carriers.

Genetic Screening for MODY

With identification of genes responsible for MODY, it is possible to identify members of pedigrees who have inherited the specific mutation affecting their family, even before carbohydrate intolerance develops. If a child does not carry the mutation, further clinical testing is unnecessary. If a child does carry the mutation, periodic testing for slight abnormalities of carbohydrate metabolism is recommended.

Identification of the specific MODY-related mutation is important. Glucokinase gene mutation needs limited therapy and follow-up. But patients with mutation in gene for HNF-1α and HNF-4α should be monitored frequently so as to achieve normoglycaemia and prevent diabetic complications.

A better understanding of the causes and pathophysiology of MODY is emerging from genetic molecular biologic and physiological studies. This knowledge will lead to new therapeutic approaches and agents that will prevent, correct or at least delay the decline in pancreatic beta cell function that characterizes not only MODY but also type 2 diabetes.

TYPE 2 DIABETES IN CHILDREN AND ADOLESCENTS

Epidemiology

The type 2 diabetes mellitus with the associated obesity, insulin resistance and other co-morbidity are constantly on the rise. It is reported that in school going children type 2 diabetes is seven times more common than type 1 diabetes in Japan. Further, American Indians, Spanics and African Americans and Asians have more prevalence of type 2 diabetes in children and adolescents. In Mexican Americans, the incidence of undiagnosed type 2 diabetes in a middle school population was 1%. The increase in incidence of type 2 diabetes is also evident in Japanese, Canadian, Australian and Libyan children.

Risk Factors for Type 2 Diabetes in Children

Obesity is the singularly most important risk factor for type 2 diabetes in children. Obesity is also familial Table 30.2.2 depicts the risk of obesity in the offspring.

TABLE 30.2.2

Parental obesity	Risk of obesity in offspring
Both parents obese	Risk 66%
One parent obese	Risk 55%
Nil parent obese	Risk 9%

Risk of obesity in offspring

Poor nutritional habits, consumption of fast foods, sedentary lifestyle, increased caloric intake, frequent snacking are the other important determinants of childhood obesity and diabetes.

Clinical Features

The clinicians must always keep in mind to exclude type 2 diabetes in obese children. The other accompaniments may also be prevalent in these children. They include:
1. Hypertension
2. Dyslipidaemia

3. Menstrual irregularities or various spectrum of polycystic ovarian syndromes
4. Orthopaedic problems
5. Depression
6. Obstructive sleep apnoea
7. Acanthosis nigricans.

Out of all these, acanthosis nigricans (AN) is a very useful tool to diagnose type 2 diabetes in children and insulin resistance. This sign needs a special mention as a marker of type 2 diabetes in the absence of immunological antibody studies.

Acanthosis Nigricans (AN)

Acanthosis nigricans is a dark rough thickening of the skin on the areas exposed to repeated flexion or friction. These areas are usually found in the cutaneous folds, nape of the neck and other areas. AN is a recognized cutaneous marker of hyperinsulinaemia in children and serves as a very useful tool in distinguishing true type 2 diabetes in young from LADA, MODY and all others.

Histologically, AN is characterized by papillomatosis and hyperkeratosis with hyperplasia of all dermal layers. In some parts of the world such as in Texas State Legislature Programme, the endemic type 2 diabetes in children is screened by compulsorily examining all school children for acanthosis nigricans by well trained nurse.

Management of Type 2 Diabetes in Children and Adolescents

Once properly diagnosed, type 2 diabetes in children should be treated with the following goals:
1. Weight control and/or weight reduction
2. Maintenance of normal physical growth
3. Near normal fasting blood glucose
4. Near normal glycosylated haemoglobin
5. Effective treatment of co-morbid problems (i.e. hypertension, dyslipidaemia)
6. Prevention of complications
7. Maintenance of emotional well-being.

The principles of managing children with type 2 diabetes include:
1. Diabetes self-management education
2. Medical nutrition therapy
3. Exercise prescription
4. Pharmacological management
5. Psychosocial consideration.

Latent Autoimmune Diabetes in Adults

Slow onset type 1 diabetes is now designated as Latent Autoimmune Diabetes in Adults (LADA). Its onset is usually between 20 and 40 years with obvious polyphagia and weight loss and the BMI is usually less than 25 kg/m^2.

This LADA enters into differential diagnosis of type 2 diabetes in the young and it is very important to distinguish between the two both clinically and laboratory-wise since the management is different.

The important clinical features of LADA are depicted in Table 30.2.3.

TABLE 30.2.3

- Fasting C peptide values are low
- GAD antibodies are positive
- Autoimmune destruction of beta cells of pancreas accounts for the insulin deficiency
- These patients are characteristically non-obese and have low to medium basal insulin levels due to progressive loss of beta cell function
- Early and aggressive insulin treatment appears to be beneficial in a newly diagnosed T1 diabetes patients
- Patients with LADA should take insulin therapy as early as possible to prevent further destruction of residual beta cells and reduce diabetic microvascular complications.

Clinical features of LADA

Criteria for Classifying LADA Patients

1. Age 20 to 48 years
2. Insulin requirement within 5 years of diagnosis
3. BMI less than 27 kg/m^2
4. Fasting hyperglycaemia more than 250
5. GAD antibody positivity.

MALNUTRITION MODULATED DIABETES MELLITUS

In 1985 classification, two distinct types of diabetes were classified both occurring in the young and enter into close differential diagnosis for type 2 diabetes in the young. They include malnutrition modulated diabetes (MMDM) which did not find a place in the 1997 ADA classification, and the fibrocalculous pancreatic diabetes (FCPD) which is now classified as secondary form of diabetes.

The clinical features of MMDM has been described in Table 30.2.4.

The proposed pathogenesis is depicted in Figure 30.2.1.

FIBROCALCULOUS PANCREATIC DIABETES

Fibrocalculous pancreatic diabetes is an important diabetes occurring in the young people in the tropics and

TABLE 30.2.4

1. Onset by 30 years of age (mean 19.8 ±97)
2. Poor socioeconomic status
3. Invariable rural origin (35 years of observation)
4. History of malnutrition in infancy and early childhood and maternal undernutrition during pregnancy
5. Leanness, BMI less than 17.0 kg/M^2
6. Severe diabetes (FPG seldom less than 250 mg/dl)
7. Absence of ketosis and ketonuria at diagnosis and on withdrawal of insulin for long periods
8. Persistent high insulin requirement most often over 60 U/day (2.0-3.0 U/kg)
9. Absence of radiographic or sonographic evidence of pancreatic calculi, ductal dilatation or fibrosis and laboratory evidence of pancreatic exocrine dysfunction.

Clinical features of MMDM (n = 1038)
(Modified from Tripathy BB, Samal KC, et al)

is distinct from the alcohol induced pancreatitis and diabetes found in the continents.

The clinical triad of the diagnosis include abdominal pain in childhood, pancreatic calculi either on X-ray or on ultrasonography and diabetes mellitus.

Old Terminology

- Tropical calcific pancreatitis
- Tropical chronic pancreatitis
- Tropical pancreatic diabetes.

The clinical features and differences from alcoholic chronic pancreatitis are described in Table 30.2.5.

The various aetiopathogenetic mechanisms given below are postulated and considered responsible either singly or in combination.
1. Malnutrition
2. Dietary toxins—cassava hypothesis
3. Antioxidant theory
4. Genetic factors
5. Immunological factors.

SUMMARY

Diabetes mellitus in the young child could be due to many factors. Therefore, to label every diabetic child or adolescent as type 1 diabetes mellitus is not correct. Due to changes in children's lifestyle, eating habits and physical activity, obesity is on massive increase and is

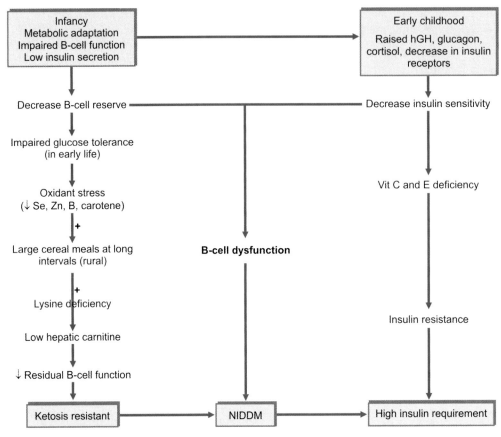

Fig. 30.2.1. Pathogenesis of undernutrition and diabetes (Prolonged protein undernutrition during foetal and early life) (Modified from Tripathy BB, Samal KC, et al)

TABLE 30.2.5

	Chronic tropical pancreatitis	*Chronic alcoholic pancreatitis*
Sex ratio M:F (%)	70 : 30	Almost all male
Age at onset	2nd and 3rd decades	4th and 5th decades
Socioeconomic	Usually poor, may occur in others as well	All strata of society equally affected
Course of disease	More aggressive and accelerated	Slower rate of progression
Diabetes	Occurs in >90%	About 50% of cases
Pancreatic calculi	Occurs in >90%	About 50 to 60% of cases
Appearance of pancreatic calculi defined margins	Large and dense with discrete margins	Usually small and speckled
Location of calculi	Always in large ducts	Usually in small ducts
Ductal dilation	Usually marked	Usually mild
Fibrosis of gland	Marked	Less severe
Alcoholism	Absent by definition	Heavy alcohol abuse
Pancreatic cancer	High	Low

Clinical features of chronic tropical and alcoholic pancreatitis

certainly contributory to diabetes. Similarly, with ever increasing knowledge about genetic abnormalities in MODY, it is obligatory that definite diagnosis is reached before commenting on long-term prognosis. The chapter discusses various types of diabetes seen in young and how to manage them.

FURTHER READING

1. Anand BS. In Balakrishnan V (Ed): Chronic Pancreatitis in India. St. Josephs Press, Trivandrum, 1987.
2. Hoet JJ, Tripathy B, Rao RH, Yajnik CS. Malnutrition and Diabetes in the Tropics. Diabetes Care 1996;19:1428-36.
3. Mohan V, Albert KGMM. Diabetes in the tropics. In Alberti KGMM, Zimmet P, DeFronzo RA, Keen H (Eds): International Textbook of Diabetes Mellitus. John Wiley and Sons Ltd., Chichester 1991;171-96.
4. Mohan V, Premalatha G. Fibrocalculous pancreatic diabetes. Int J Diabetes 1995;3:71-82.
5. Report of the Expert Committee on the diagnosis and classification of diabetes mellitus. Diabetes Care 1997;20:1183-97.
6. Stephen W Ponder, Susan Sullivan, Grete McBath: Type 2 diabetes mellitus in teens. American Diabetes Association - Annual Review of Diabetes 2001; pp 76-89.
7. Tripathy BB, Samal KC. Overview and consensus statement on diabetes in tropical areas. Diabetes/Metabolic Reviews 1997;13:63-76.
8. WHO study group report on diabetes mellitus. WHO Technical Report Series No.727, Geneva: WHO, 1985.
9. Workshop report: Consensus Statement from the International Workshop on Types of Diabetes Peculiar to Tropics, 17-19 Oct. 1995 Cuttack, India. Acta Diabetol 1996;33:62-4.

30.3 Pancreatic Transplant

Y Sachdev

- Introduction
- Pancreatic Transplantation
  - Whole or Part of Pancreas
  - Isolated Pancreatic Islets
- Engineered Pancreatic Beta Cells
- Virtual Pancreas
- Islet Neogenesis

INTRODUCTION

The greatest success in diabetes research has been the advancement of its treatment. The understanding of aetiopathogenesis of T2DM, insulin resistance and beneficial effects of lifestyle changes has resulted in more rational management of the syndrome. Tighter glycaemic control in T1DM has also resulted in delaying the chronic diabetic complications. There has been, however, very little progress in the cure of the disease. It has been envisaged that a successful pancreatic islets transplant in T1DM patients will provide complete correction of the glucose metabolic abnormalities and prevent its microangiopathic complications if the transplant is done at an early stage of the disease and recipient's immune system does not destroy it. Nearly 1500 T1DM patients receive pancreatic/islets transplants every year.

PANCREATIC TRANSPLANTATION

The first human pancreatic transplant was done at university of Minnesota in 1966. The transplant, unfortunately, got rejected after a few weeks. Since then several research workers have been involved in perfecting the technique and presently transplantation of pancreas as a vascularised graft is the most practised procedure.

Transplantation of the Whole or Part of Pancreas as Vascularised Graft

It is not feasible to carry this out at an early age as it is accompanied by high perioperative mortality and requires immunosuppressive drug therapy to prevent its rejection. This, unfortunately, cannot be recommended at an early and tender age. Therefore, this technique is performed only along with renal transplantation in chronic diabetic renal failure patients (Fig. 30.3.1). Obviously at this stage of the disease, diabetic microangiopathic changes are well advanced and irreversible. Pancreatic graft, therefore, is unable to influence these complications. The combined transplant generally offers reduced rates of immune rejection and

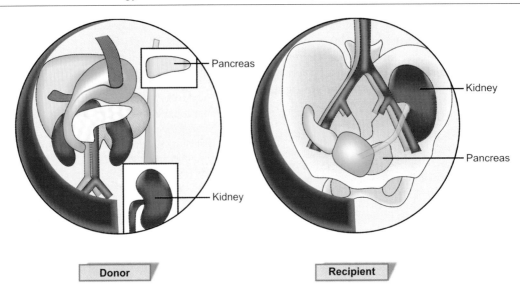

Fig. 30.3.1: Pancreas transplantation as a vascularised graft
(Kidney and pancreas are transplanted from the same donor at the same time)

the graft and the patient survival is better with latest immunosuppressive drugs.

Typically an intact pancreas donated by a person who has died is placed into the pelvis of the recipient and the native pancreas is left untouched. Most grafts receive arterial blood and return venous blood to iliac vessels.

Sometimes, a hemipancreas is donated by a healthy living related donor who has undergone hemi-pancreatectomy.

When a cadaveric organ is used, a small portion of the donor's duodenum containing the exit of the pancreatic duct is included and oversewn onto the urinary bladder. Alternately enteric drainage may be used. Advantages of bladder drainage over enteric drainage are the use of urinary amylase to monitor for rejection. The advantages of enteric drainage over bladder are the avoidance of urinary infection, cystitis, haematuria and reflux pancreatitis.

Complications

Transplanted pancreas can undergo acute and chronic rejection despite immunosuppressive drugs. Other complications seen in clinical practice are intra-abdominal infection and abscess, vascular graft thrombosis, metabolic bone disease and anastomotic and duodenal stamp leak.

Transplantation of Isolated Pancreatic Islets: An Another Option

Paul E Lacy was the first to describe the method for isolation of islets from the rodent pancreas in 1969 and a

few years later succeeded in first successful islet transplantation in rodents. It was a formidable challenge to the researchers to extract hundreds of thousands of islets scattered all over human pancreas. It became relatively much easier only in 1986 when Camillo Ricordiwas was able to introduce an automated method for human islets isolation.

Presently this isolated islet transplant technique makes only 10% of T1DM patients insulin independent in one year. Therefore, currently a great deal of work is being done to make this option a viable cure for a larger number of diabetic patients. Efforts have been made to isolate the islets and place them into semiporous capsules. The goal is to allow the emission of insulin and access of glucose as the primary insulin secretagogue, but prevent infiltration and destruction by the immune system of the recipient. Identification of such a material that allows the passage of glucose and insulin freely but blocks the access of immune effectors is creating technical problems.

The alternative approach is to carry out islets transplants and then use immunosuppression to maintain them. The islets transplant is prepared by chopping two distended cadaveric pancreas into small pieces, followed by digestion with collagenase. Islets are then separated on a ficoll density gradient. This technique provides a pure islets preparation. Islets are then placed via portal vein infusion within portal system of the liver, within spleen or beneath the renal capsule. Islet transplant reduces surgical morbidity. A successful transplant improves quality of life, exerts a beneficial effect on microvascular diabetic complications and ensures a variable insulin independent period. The most serious

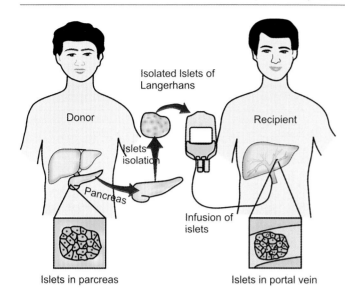

Fig. 30.3.2: Transplantation of isolated islets infusion in portal vein

problem faced at present is that a large number of islets must be harvested to make transplant successful, as islet cells preservation techniques are imperfect and damage to β cells is inevitable. The present efforts, therefore, are directed to develop meticulous islets isolation and preservation techniques and an ideal immuno-suppressive regimen.

The details of the portal route in brief are as under:

Once sufficient amount of pure islets has been prepared, then under local anaesthesia, a 22 mm Hg gauge chelra needle is advanced under fluoroscopic guidance into the portal vein. A guide wire is then inserted into the main portal vein and a catheter is positioned with confirmation by venogram. Purified islets are then infused and portal pressure is checked frequently to ensure it does not go beyond 22 mm Hg. If it does, the infusion is halted till it resolves. If it does not resolve, infusion is discontinued. After the islets have been infused, catheter is removed and patient is sent to her bed (Fig. 30.3.2).

Engineered Pancreatic Beta Cells

There is another approach, that of cell engineering, by which insulin-producing cells are procured for transplantation. This technique involves the development of cells targeted for transplantation with a unique gene complement that will produce insulin in response to glucose. It is one of the procedures which is undergoing research and it is hoped that in time to come, this form of gene therapy may offer cure for T1DM.

Virtual Pancreas

This involves development of an artificial pancreas. Essentials to an artificial pancreas are: (i) ability to recognise the stimulus, say, glucose and (ii) to deliver an appropriate amount of insulin on demand. A number of pilot studies are currently underway.

Islet Neogenesis

In this, biochemicals that initiate and control islets development *in situ* are recognized in an effort to stimulate islet formation from stem cells in the diabetic patient's own islet cells depleted pancreas. The obvious potential advantage of this approach is that the patient's own pancreatic cells are induced to make islets, possibly eliminating or reducing the need for immunotherapy. Recently, Argentine researchers demonstrated that autologous bone marrow stem cells implanted into T2DM patients, in direct form into the pancreas, improved the production of endogenous insulin and C-peptide resulting in decrease in blood glucose and glycated Hb values. It is most likely that the implanted stem cells resulted in regeneration of destroyed β cells in the islets as well as of new β cells formation which produced their own insulin. This appears to be a landmark step towards diabetic cure.

SUMMARY

Presently most commonly performed pancreatic transplantation is one that is combined with renal transplantation and is done in those patients who have end-stage renal disease. The other procedures like transplantation of islets or foetal stem cells or other mentioned alternatives are still to be perfected or to be recommended as a diabetic cure therapy at an early stage of diabetes so as to prevent diabetic complications.

FURTHER READING

1. Morris PJ, Gray DW, Sutton R. Pancreatic islet transplantation. British Medical Bulletin 1989;45:224-41.
2. Caldara R, La Rocca E, Maffi P, Sacchi A. Effects of pancreas transplantation on late complications of diabetes and metabolic effects of pancreas and islet transplantation. Jr Pediatric Endocrinology and Metab 1999;12 (suppl 3):777-87.
3. Sutherland DE. Pancreas and islet cell transplantation. Now and then. Translation Proceedings 1996;28(4):2131-3.
4. Proceedings 45th Annual Meeting of the American Society of Cell Biology held in San Francisco, California. December 2005.
5. Ricordi Camillo. Islet transplantation: A Brave New World. Lilly Lecture 2002. American Diabetes Association. Annual Review of Diabetes 2004;155-63.
6. American Diabetes Association Position Statement. Pancreatic transplantation for patients with type 1 diabetes mellitus. Diabetes Care 2000;23:585.

30.4 Stem Cell Therapy in Diabetes Mellitus

Velu Nair

INTRODUCTION

Diabetes mellitus (DM) both T1DM and T2DM are chronic lifelong diseases which carry a significant burden of mortality and morbidity. All present therapies revolve around either replacement (as in T1DM) or stimulation of insulin release (T2DM) but do not address the basic defect of insufficient beta cells. Stem cell therapy holds promise in this direction for regeneration of beta cells, as is being tried in many other fields (cardiology, neurology) but is purely in the experimental stage today. It will be for a while before it translates from the bench to bedside.

Success in islet transplantation has been proven to restore the physiological secretion of insulin in patients with T1DM and in some patients with severe forms of T2DM. Each year 1300 to 1500 people with T1DM receive whole organ pancreatic/islet cell transplant. However, beta-cell replacement therapy is significantly hampered by an acutely limited source of transplantable human islets from cadaveric donors. Another drawback of this therapy is the prolonged immunosuppressive therapy, which makes the recipient vulnerable to a host of infections. The possibility of using stem cells to treat DM is now gaining credibility as it has been amply demonstrated that these stem cells have a unique property to transdifferentiate across germ layers.

STEM CELLS

Stem cells (SC) are defined by their ability to undergo differentiation and generate specialized mature terminally differentiated cells while possessing the potential for relatively infinite self-renewal.

Stem cells are of two types:
a. Embryonic stem cells (ESCs), which are sourced from the inner cell mass of blastocyst, are totipotent cells, which can give rise to the trophoblast and a complete organism. There are important ethical issues to be addressed when using ESCs for research purpose. Once ESCs are taken out of an embryo, the embryo is sacrificed. This issue is largely circumvented when using embryos, which would be otherwise wasted, from infertility clinic.
b. Adult stem cells are more committed than the totipotent cells. They are pluripotent in character and can give rise to a complete organism but not the trophoblast. These cells reside in various organ systems such as the bone marrow (Haematopoietic stem cells (HSC)) and nervous system (Neural stem cells). However, no stem cells have been identified in the pancreas as yet. Adult stem cells, like totipotent cells have the capability of self-renewal while retaining the capacity to terminally differentiate into specialised cells. When adult stem cells are committed to any organ system they become multipotent.

Stem cells have a unique property to transdifferentiate, which is also referred to as plasticity. This is defined as the capacity to differentiate across the germ layers; for example, HSC, which originates from the mesoderm, can be used to generate cells from the endoderm (liver, lung, GI tract) and ectoderm (neurones, oligodendrocyte cells).

The important differences between ESC and adult stem cells is as given in Table 30.4.1 while Figure 30.4.1 outlines the hierarchy of the stem cells into toti-, pluri-, multi- and unipotent cells. Figure 30.4.2 highlights the possible fate of a HSC.

WHAT IS STEM CELL THERAPY

Stem cell therapy is defined as administration of stem cells that have been selected, multiplied and pharmacologically treated or altered outside the body (*ex vivo*) followed by transplantation of these cells into the patient. These stem cells can be either from the embryo (ESC) or the adult stem cells like HSC or mesenchymal stem cells (MSC). These cells can be either

TABLE 30.4.1

Embryonic stem cells	Adult stem cells
• Totipotent cells	• Pluripotent/multipotent cells
• Ethical objections	• No ethical objections
• Difficult to isolate	• Easily obtainable
• Risk of rejection	• No risk of rejection
• Immune-suppressive therapy required	• Not required in autologous setting
• High risk of teratocarcinomas	• No risk
• Clinical application not feasible for atleast 10 to 20 yr	• Clinical application already realised
• Lack of specific identification markers	• Different expansion ability:
	• Uni-, bi-, multi- or pluripotent
	• Lack of specific identification markers

Embryonic stem cells vs adult stem cells

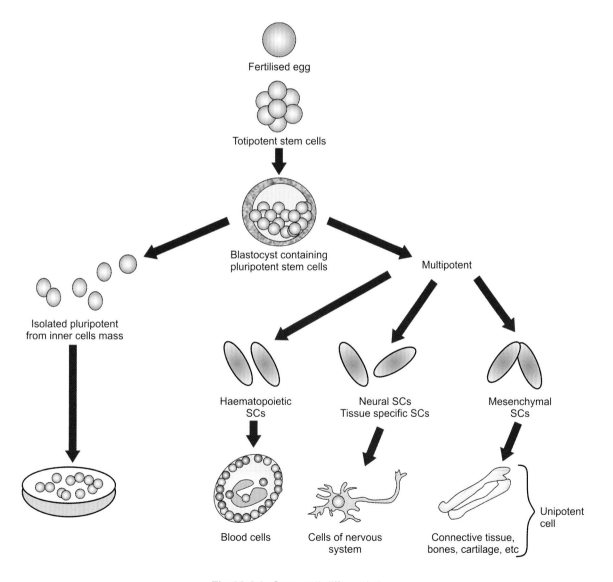

Fig 30.4.1: Stem cell differentiation

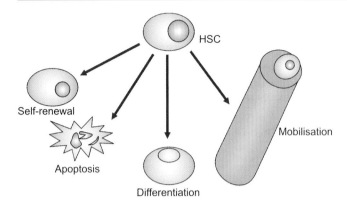

Fig 30.4.2: Fate of a haematopoietic stem cell (HSC)

autologous (stem cells taken from the patient itself) or allogeneic (stem cells sourced from another member of the same species). In the allogeneic setting immunosuppressive treatment will be needed to prevent rejections. Its aim is to replace, repair or enhance the function of damaged tissues or organs. It is related to and overlaps with several other established technologies, such as gene therapy, tissue engineering and regenerative medicine.

To prove that stem cells derived from any source, including HSCs are indeed transformed into solid organ specific cells, several conditions must be met. First, the origin of the exogenous cell integrated into solid organ tissue must be documented by cell marking, preferably at the single cell level. Cells should be processed with a minimum of *ex vivo* manipulation (e.g. culturing), to minimise susceptibility to crossing lineages. Second, the exogenous cell must be shown to have become an integral morphologic part of the new acquired tissue. Third, and most important, the transformed cell must be shown to have acquired the function of the particular organ into which it has been integrated, both by expressing organ-specific proteins and by showing organ-specific functions.

PANCREATIC STEM CELLS

Insulin-secreting cells have been shown to develop from stem/progenitor cells isolated from a variety of tissues, such as in bone marrow, liver and intestinal epithelium. However, no clearly identifiable pancreatic stem cells (PSCs) have been found until now, despite considerable evidence that such cells are present in the islet or ductal cells of the pancreas. An established neuroepithelial protein, nestin, has been reported as a marker for endocrine progenitor cells. These nestin-positive putative PSCs when exposed to different growth factors or microenvironments, give rise to islet-like cell clusters (ICCs), which temporarily express multiple endocrine hormones.

BASIS OF STEM CELL THERAPY IN DIABETES MELLITUS

Animal experiments have shown that mesenchymal stem cells (MSC) could successfully differentiate into pancreatic islet beta-like cells. These cells are morphologically similar to pancreatic islet cells. More importantly, they could also transcript, translate and secrete insulin. High glucose concentration was considered as a potent inducer for pancreatic islet differentiation. A promising therapy in diabetes patients would be using MSCs to generate beta cells by exploiting this transdifferentiation potential. Autologous MSCs can be isolated, expanded *ex vivo* and reinfused. Since these cells are autologous; there is no danger of rejections and hence no need for immunosuppression.

There is no peer reviewed clinical study to suggest a clinical benefit of stem cell based therapy in the treatment of diabetes mellitus. A recent publication of a clinical trial looking at the role of stem cell based therapy in the treatment of peripheral vascular disease, secondary to diabetes mellitus found an improvement in glucose tolerance following stem cell infusion. Whether this improvement was secondary to the correction of the peripheral vascular disease related inflammation and infection as observed in this study or due to β cell generation has not been addressed.

From the available data the possibility of β cell generation from adult HSC cannot be excluded, though the currently available evidence for the same is limited. While data for the role of stem cell based therapy in the management of peripheral vascular disease secondary to diabetes mellitus and other aetiologies are promising and have not been reviewed here, its role in β cell regeneration needs to be further studied, preferably in animal models. There are insufficient data yet to initiate a clinical trial in this area.

ANIMAL STUDIES

Transplantation of ESC derived insulin-producing cells reverses diabetes in rodents, indicating that these cells do synthesise and release insulin. ESC, genetically selected for insulin expression and injected into diabetic rats, improves glucose control in rodents. Haemopoietic organs harbour cells that can also differentiate into functional pancreatic endocrine cells. Similar experiments have been done in overtly diabetic mice whose beta cells have been destroyed by streptozotocin. After bone marrow transplantation, blood glucose and insulin concentrations were normal, and survival was better. In islets, marrow-derived cells had differentiated into both endothelial cells and occasional insulin expressing cells.

Although, stem cell therapy as a therapeutic approach for beta cell replacement is a possibility, the immunological destruction of newly regenerated beta cells in T1DM remains a problem. However, in one mouse model of autoimmune study pancreatic tissue showed increased proliferative activity and regeneration of beta cells. Thus marrow transplantation to induce immunological control plus maintenance of normoglycaemia allowed local beta or progenitor cells to proliferate as an adaptive response. Further, rodent-liver stem cells and human foetal-liver cells have been differentiated *in vitro* into insulin-secreting cells by culture methods and/or introduction of beta cell-specific genes. When transplanted, these cells reverse diabetes mellitus in rodents.

Studies have reported partial correction of murine diabetes with syngeneic hepatocyte transplants. Implantation of autologous insulin-secreting hepatocytes in diabetic pigs as treatment protocol which combines surgery, cell isolation, transfection with a non-viral vector and re-implantation, has shown partial but significant metabolic correction of several indices, i.e. fasting hyperglycaemia, hypertriglyceridaemia and raised levels of serum fructosamine. Preliminary observations suggest that implantation of insulin secreting autologous hepatocytes may also protect diabetic pigs against target organ damage compared to untreated diabetic pigs.

WHERE ARE WE NOW?

As is the case with every emerging field in biology, early reports seem confusing and conflicting. Embryonic and adult stem cells are potential sources for beta cell replacement and merit further scientific investigation. Discrepancies between different results need to be reconciled. Fundamental processes in determining the differentiation pathways of stem cells remain to be elucidated, so that rigorous and reliable differentiation protocols can be established. Encouraging studies in rodent models may ultimately set the stage for large scale animal studies and translational investigation. Regulatory and ethical guidelines applicable to any biological therapies were already in place before the controversy surrounding the embryonic stem cells arose. However, the possibility of autologous stem cell/adult stem cell use will bypass such controversies.

SUMMARY

In less than a decade, the initial zeal of stem cell plasticity and potential cure of any condition inherited or acquired is gradually being replaced by guarded optimism. The stem cell related research findings in the last decade have been revolutionary and the hope remains that at least a few of these findings have the potential to move from the bench to the bedside. The excessive enthusiasm to rapidly move to clinical trials in the absence of substantial preclinical research is of some concern and requires regulation at a national level. More concerning and alarming is the frequent reports of stem cell based therapy being conducted and offered outside the setting of a clinical trial, this needs to be more than just discouraged. The clinical scenarios associated with desperation, with no other alternative therapies, are not sufficient grounds to justify experimental stem cell based therapy. While clinical trials have their time and place, currently, the focus needs to be on painstaking preclinical research to address the relevant issues before moving forward.

PSCs are definitely a potential approach to islet cell replacement therapy; however, much more work is essential for full maturation of the *in vitro* growth of insulin-secreting cells. There is no peer reviewed clinical study to suggest a clinical benefit of stem cell based therapy in the treatment of diabetes mellitus. The identification of a specific marker for the lineage-tracing studies, temporal gene expressions during the development of PSC-derived islets, and appropriate growth factors or microenvironments essential for beta-cell differentiation will represent a major breakthrough for the therapeutic intervention for T1DM in the near future.

In this brief overview, it has not been possible to address every study related to the clinical areas that have been discussed; the aim was to give a flavour of the controversies in this field.

FURTHER READING

1. Blyszczuk P, Czyz J, Kania G, et al. Expression of Pax 4 in embryonic stem cells promotes differentiation of nestin-positive progenitor and insulin-producing cells. Proc Natl Acad Sci USA 2003;100:998-1003.
2. Daley GQ, Goodell MA, Snyder EY. Realistic prospects for stem cell therapeutics. Haematology ASH Education Program. 2003:398-418.
3. Hess D, Li L, Martin M, et al. Bone marrow-derived stem cells initiate pancreatic regeneration. Nat Biotechnol 2003;21:763-70.

4. Hori Y, Rulifson IC, Tsai BC, Heit JJ, Cahoy JD, Kim SK. Growth inhibitors promote differentiation of insulin-producing tissue from embryonic stem cells. Proc Natl Acad Sci USA 2002;99:16105-10.

5. Huang P, Li S, Han M, Xiao Z, Yang R, Han ZC. Autologous transplantation of granulocyte colony stimulating factor mobilised peripheral blood mononuclear cells improve critical limb ischemia in diabetes. Diabetes Care 2005;28:2155-60.

6. Kon Ozlian. Cell based treatment of diabetes mellitus: of mice and pigs. National Cancer Centre, Singapore stem cells and cellular therapies 15 Dec 2005.

7. Li-Bo Chen, Xiao-Bing Jiang, Lian Yang. Differentiation of rat marrow mesenchymal stem cells into pancreatic islet beta-cells. World Journal of Gastroenterology 2004;10(20):3016-20.

8. Lumelsky N, Blondel O, Laeng P, Velasco I, Ravin R, McKay R. Differentiation of embryonic stem cells to insulin-secreting structures similar to pancreatic islets. Science 2001;292:1389-94.

9. Marin Korbling, Zeev Estrov. Adult stem cell for tissue repair—a new therapeutic concept? NEJM 349;6 2003:570-82.

10. Mehboob A Hussain, Neil D Theise Stem-cell therapy for diabetes mellitus. Lancet 2004;364:203-5.

11. Ryan EA, Lakey JRT, Rajotte RV, Korbutt GS, Kin T, Imes S, et al. Clinical outcomes and insulin secretion after islet transplantation with the Edmonton protocol. Diabetes 2001;50:710-9.

12. Seaberg RM, Smukler SR, Kieffer TJ, Enikolopoz G, Asghar Z, Wheeler MB, et al. Clonal identification of multipotent precursors from adult mouse pancreas that generate neural and pancreatic lineages. Nat Biotechnol 2004;22:1115-24.

13. Soria B, Skoudy A, Martin F. From stem cells to beta cells. Diabetologia 2001;44:407-15.

14. Zalzman M, Gupta S, Giri RK, et al. Reversal of hyperglycemia in mice by using human expandable insulin-producing cells differentiated from fetal liver progenitor cells. Proc Natl Acad Sci USA 2003;100:7253-8.

15. Zovina TD, Subbotin VM, Bertera S, et al. Recovery of endogenous cells function in NOD model of autoimmune diabetes. Stem Cells 2003;21:377-88.

16. Zulewski H, Abraham EJ, Gerlach MJ, Daniel PB, Moritz W, Muller B, et al. Multipotential nestin-positive stem cells isolated from adult pancreatic islets differentiate ex vivo into pancreatic endocrine, exocrine, and hepatic phenotypes. Diabetes 2001;50:521-33.

30.5 Diabetes Mellitus in Elderly

Y Sachdev

- Introduction and Review of Literature
- Pathogenesis
- Clinical Presentation
- Management
- Summary

INTRODUCTION AND REVIEW OF LITERATURE

The prevalence of IGT and T2DM is higher above the age of 60 years. Both fasting and 2-hour postprandial plasma glucose values rise with age. Some investigators have observed a rise of 1 to 10% in postprandial blood glucose values per decade above the age of 45 years while others recommend a flat 5% allowance per decade in the blood sugar values after the age of 50 years. The higher blood sugar values in the elderly have been attributed to lack of physical activity and increased food intake and abdominal fat. Some researcher measured plasma glucose response to oral glucose intake in physically active, generally healthy and fit individuals (both men and women) aged 47 to 90 years and did not find any correlation between age and glucose response in men while in women there was only a modest correlation

(p < 01) after due adjustments was made for overweight and obesity. Some other investigators observed a definite but minor contribution (<6%) by age to glucose response in women.

PATHOGENESIS

The author studied glucose and IRI response to OGTT in over 5000 male individuals belonging to 17 to 75 years age group and found increased 2-hour post GTT glucose and IRI values in those above 55 years. Several of them (65%) could be labelled as IGT/DM applying the prevailing diagnostic criteria. However if the PP time interval was shifted from 2 hours to 2½ hours, many values fell within normal range in nearly 55% of them (Tables 30.5.1 and 30.5.2; Fig. 30.5.1). This observation

TABLE 30.5.1

Age (years)	Blood glucose values (mg/dl)		
	F	2 HR PP	2½ HR PP
17 to 25 years	69.72 ± 8.06	83.73 ± 14.40	—
26 to 35 years	77.62 ± 7.82	80.20 ± 11.13	—
36 to 45 years	80.84 ± 9.21	90.75 ± 15.42	—
46 to 55 years	85.77 ± 11.12	95.35 ± 25.15	90.27 ± 7.24
56 to 65 years	88.82 ± 10.24	99.70 ± 24.25	92.71 ± 20.47
66 to 75 years	98.22 ± 16.23	126.71 ± 37.03	120.01 ± 18.60

Mean fasting and PP blood glucose

TABLE 30.5.2

Age (years)	Plasma insulin (IRI) values (mU/L)		
	F	2 HR PP	2½ HR PP
17 to 25 years	2.31 ± 1.49	3.48 ± 2.17	—
26 to 35 years	2.79 ± 1.72	2.30 ± 1.99	—
36 to 45 years	3.57 ± 1.12	5.92 ± 2.70	—
46 to 55 years	3.82 ± 2.01	5.78 ± 1.28	4.44 ± 1.75
56 to 65 years	4.78 ± 2.12	7.27 ± 1.78	5.71 ± 1.27
66 to 75 years	5.21 ± 1.59	8.27 ± 2.12	5.47 ± 1.86

Mean fasting and PP insulin value

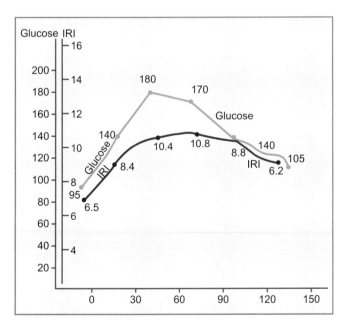

Fig. 30.5.1: Glucose and IRI values in a normal healthy generally fit male of 67 years during OGTT

was explained on an altered pattern of insulin secretion in elderly compared to younger adult population of the study. In the elderly, the second phase of insulin secretion was blunted and prolonged.

Besides ageing factor, lifestyle changes, overweight, obesity, insulin resistance, use of various medicines, lack of physical exercise, reduction in daily activity and increase in sedentary habits are the other contributory factors for this changed pattern of carbohydrate tolerance. Moreover, there is increased deposition of amyloid (which produces amylin) in pancreas with advancing age.

CLINICAL PRESENTATION IN ELDERLY

Besides the usual presentation seen in T2DM, the special features encountered in elderly diabetics are:
a. Recurrent ophthalmic (especially errors of refraction) and neurological problems.
b. Mild diabetic elderly may present with diabetic amyotrophy—asymmetrical progressive muscle

weakness associated with muscle pain and wasting of pelvic and shoulder muscles.

c. Diabetic neuropathic cachexia characterized by weight loss, peripheral neuropathy, generalized muscular pain, severe depression, emotional lability and anorexia. This is seen more frequently in men.

d. Acute abdominal or chest pain due to painful intercostal mononeuropathy. The pain has a dermatome distribution. Electromyography confirms the diagnosis.

e. Painful limitation of the glenohumeral joint (periarthrosis of the shoulder or frozen shoulder). This is due to increased glycosylated aminoglycan deposition in the joint capsular tissue.

f. Diabetic dermopathy is more common in elderly and may be a presenting features in many.

g. Disseminated/pulmonary tuberculosis and other systemic infections especially mucormycosis and other fungal infections are seen more frequently in elderly diabetics than the younger group.

h. 10 to 15% of elderly diabetics may show decreased serum zinc value due to impaired zinc absorption and hyperzincuria.

i. Silent myocardial infarction, peripheral and autonomic neuropathy and peripheral vascular disease are more common in elderly as is the incidence of diabetic foot.

Diagnosis

One could debate if the adult standard of glucose tolerance should be applied to the elderly population or some allowance must be made for the age factor. Perhaps use of a nomogram of the community, if available, may be of some help (see Fig. 26.1.5). We, in our centre, extend the OGTT to 150 minutes in the elderly as a general practice otherwise too we ask for 2 and 2½ hours PP blood glucose values in the elderly.

Management

All elderly diabetics must be treated, as ageing process and diabetes combined together hasten the chronic diabetic complications. The management strategy remains the same. Diet control, lifestyle changes, weight reduction, increased graduated physical activity and use of medication, form the sheet anchor of the diabetic approach. In view of the defective vision, it must be ensured that there is no incorrect administration of insulin dose. A little less tight glycaemic control is aimed at our centre and we are satisfied if fasting plasma glucose is 100 to 105 mg/dl and postprandial 140 to 150 mg/dl (2 hr) and 130 to 135 mg/dl as 2½ hours with glycylated Hb at 7.5%.

SUMMARY

T2DM is a common condition in geriatric practice. It may have a bizarre presentation and requires a holistic treatment approach and not-too-tight a diabetic control.

FURTHER READING

1. Morley John E, Kaiser Fran E. Unique aspect of diabetes mellitus in the elderly. Clinics in Geriatric Medicine 1990;6:693-701.
2. Garland H. Diabetic amyotrophy. Br Med J 1955;2:1287-90.
3. Glucose tolerance test in elderly population. Proceedings of Annual Conference of Geriatric Society of India 1991 at Udaipur.
4. Sachdev Y. Glucose and IRI response in healthy generally fit Indian men (17 to 75 year age group) to oral glucose tolerance test. Research project 1977-1980. Final report of Sachdev Y.

30.6 Prevention of Diabetes Mellitus

Y Sachdev

INTRODUCTION

Diabetes mellitus is a continuum. Its onset or progression can be prevented if it is possible to predict its occurrence. A positive family history, presence of islet cell antibodies, genetic predictors helps us in doing so in a reasonably good number of high risk patients. Moreover, in T1DM, immune system gets involved in the destruction of B cells. Humans have mastered many immunity problems and have managed to manipulate immunity to their advantage by immunosuppressive medication and vaccines. Therefore it is hoped that one day we may succeed to prevent T1DM also.

TYPES OF PREVENTION

The WHO study group (1994) defined prevention of diabetes mellitus into three activities:

Primary prevention: Those activities where the aim is to prevent its occurrence in high risk susceptible individuals.

Secondary prevention: It is aimed at early detection and initiation of prompt and effective strategies to reverse the condition and prevent its progression.

Tertiary prevention: Here the aim is to prevent/delay the complications and associated sequelae and disabilities.

PREDICTION OF DM

Prediction of T1DM or Recognition of High Risk T1DM individuals

T1DM predictors are: strongly positive family history, presence of genetic and immunological markers. HLA DQ2 and DQG are the most susceptible alleles while HLA DQBI 0602 (DQG) confers the strongest protection against T1DM. The presence of circulating autoantibodies like islet cell antibodies (ICA), insulin autoantibodies (IAA), glutamic acid decarboxylase (GAD) and protein tyrosine phosphatase (ICA 512ab) of the islet cell are predominant immunological markers.

Prediction of T2DM or Recognition of High Risk T2DM individuals

The aetiology of T2DM being multifactorial/polygenic, there are only few direct predictive factors like monogenic genetic markers in various forms of MODY and polygenic genetic defects in GLUT system and insulin receptor gene. Recognition of insulin resistance, presence of obesity, sedentary habits, history of low birth weight, consumption of cow's milk (instead of breast milk) are some of the other predictive factors of T2DM which help us recognise high risk individuals.

PREVENTION

Primary Prevention

Nicotinamide therapy, subcutaneous daily insulin injection or annual IV insulin infusion as cytoprotective measures to protect B cells in high risk children have not succeeded. Genetic counselling and engineering are accepted methods of prevention and need to be perfected. Environmental factors like overweight, inactivity, consumption of high caloric-density fried foods, carbonated drinks, smoking, alcohol and no-exercise lifestyle must be changed to active daily routine with healthy food habits and time for self health care, relaxation and yoga to prevent/delay onset of T1DM and T2DM.

Secondary Prevention

This involves an early diagnosis by regular screening of high risk subjects, institution of healthy habits, regulating diet intake, aerobic exercises maintaining body weight and tackling insulin resistance if present. Lifestyle changes are relevant specially in T2DM patients. Tight glycaemic control, correction of lipid abnormalities and maintaining normotensive BP reading with salt restriction and medication, delay the disease process and achieve the objectives of secondary prevention.

Tertiary Prevention

This is primarily the extension of activities carried out in secondary prevention. The objective of tertiary prevention activities are to limit the progress of the diabetic complication and look after the rehabilitation of the patients wherever, needed.

SUMMARY

Community education is the hallmark of primary prevention while lifestyle changes and intensive therapeutic management form the sheet anchor of secondary and tertiary prevention. Genetic engineering, in time to come, may be of great help to eradicate/control T1DM .

FURTHER READING

1. 15th International Diabetes Federation Congress. KOBE. Japan, 1994.
2. ENDIT Group. Preventing before the onset of type 1 diabetes. Baseline data from the European Nicotinamide Diabetes Intervention Trial (ENDIT). Diabetologia 2003;46:339-46.
3. Joslin EP. The prevention of diabetes mellitus. JAMA 1991; 76:79-84.
4. Kolb H, Burkart V. Nicotinamide in type, diabetes. Mechanism of action revisited. Diabetes Care 1999;22(Suppl 21):B16-28.
5. Simone EA, Wegmann DR, Eisenbarth GS. Immunologic 'vaccination' for the prevention of autoimmune diabetes (type 1A). Diabetes Care 1999;22(Suppl 2):137-315.
6. WHO Study Group on Prevention of Diabetes Mellitus. Geneva: World Health Organisation, 1994 (WHO technical report series no 844).

APPENDICES

Appendix 1: Diabetic Dietary Menus

Shaveta Vedehra

INTRODUCTION

Diabetic diet need not be a complete deviation from the normal diet. A diabetic patient should consume wholesome diet with carbohydrates providing 60 to 65%, fat providing 15 to 25% of total calories and rest is derived from proteins. Fibre is good for diabetics as it hampers absorption of lipids and glucose. Dietary fibre is that part of food that is not digested by the gut and is considered as unavailable carbohydrate. It also delays gastric emptying time. Foods rich in fibre are considered beneficial in the treatment of diabetes.

Fibre are of two types: Water soluble and water insoluble. Water soluble-gums, pectins and mucilages are helpful in diabetic diets. Rich sources of water soluble fibre include fruits and vegetables. It has been found that use of soluble fibre contained in barley, oatmeal, fruits and dried beans, helps considerably in reducing blood sugar level. The diabetics should therefore gradually introduce such soluble fibre into their diet. There are certain foods like bitter gourd, garlic, jamun, lettuce, onion, soyabean, fenugreek seeds, etc. that help control diabetes.

GENERAL PRINCIPLES

The following general principles are to be kept in mind for diabetic diet.

Foods to be Avoided

- Sugar, sweets, honey, jams and jellies, ice-cream, cakes, pastries, canned fruit juices, chocolates, etc.
- Deep fried foods.
- Vegetables to be avoided—potato, arbi, zimikand, shakarkandi, kathal.
- Fruits to be avoided—mango, banana, cheeku, lichi, grapes
- Dried fruits and nuts.

Foods to be Used Freely

- Most vegetables contain very little amount of carbohydrates and calories and can be freely used by diabetics. These include leafy vegetables like amaranth, cabbage, celery, coriander leaves, fenugreek leaves, mint, lettuce, spinach and other vegetables like ash gourd, bitter gourd, brinjal, cucumber, cauliflower, drumsticks, French beans, ladies' fingers, unripe green mangoes, onion stalks, pumpkins, radish, ridge gourd, snake gourds, turnips.
- High fibre foods
- Clear soups, lime water, black tea.

For Milk and Milk Products, Use Skimmed Milk

Some of the recommended diabetic menus are given below. An attempt has been made to cater for North Indian, South Indian and Continental tastes.

DIET MENUS

1200 kcal Diabetic Diet (North India)

Bed tea	Tea—1 cup Fibre biscuit/Salto/Marie biscuit—2/2-3/2
Breakfast	Chapatti stuffed with vegetables— 2 (20 gm atta each) or Bread slice—2 (large) or Cornflakes—5 to 6 tablespoons or Porridge (Cooked)—1½ katori (medium size katori) + Milk—240 ml (skimmed milk)
Midmorning	Fruit—1 serving (100 gm)
Lunch	Chapatti—3 (60 gm atta) or Boiled rice—8 to 10 tablespoon Dal—1 katori (25 gm) Green vegetables—1 katori (125 gm) Curd/Buttermilk plain—125 ml/1 glass
Evening	Tea/coffee—1 cup Fibre biscuit/Salto/Plain toast—2-3/3-4/1
Dinner	Chapatti—2 Dal—1 katori Green vegetables—125 gm Paneer—30 gm
Bed time	Milk—½ cup
Cooking oil	2 TSF/day
The above menu provides approximately	
Carbohydrates	190 gm
Proteins	50 gm
Fats	30 gm
For non-vegetarians	

Fish/chicken (75 gm) = 1 katori dal + ½ katori curd.

1200 kcal Diabetic Diet (South India)

Bed tea	Tea—1 cup Fibre biscuit—2 (like diet bik)/salto 2 to 3/ Marie biscuit—2
Breakfast	Idli—2 (medium size) or Dosa Plain—9" diameter or Suji upma—1½ plate (150 gm cooked weight) + Milk—240 ml
Midmorning	Fruit—100 gm
Lunch	Rice (boiled)— 8 to 10 tablespoon Dal/Sambhar—1 katori (25 gm) Rasam—1 katori Green vegetables—125 gm Papad Curd—125 ml
Evening	Tea/coffee—1 cup Poha with vegetables—¾ katori
Dinner	Boiled rice—6 to 8 tablespoons Dal—1 katori (25 gm) Green vegetable curry—1 katori (125 gm) Paneer curry/egg curry—30 gm/1 egg
Bedtime	Milk—½ cup
Cooking oil	2 TSF/day

The above menu provides approximately:

Carbohydrates	190 gm
Proteins	50 gm
Fats	30 gm

1200 kcal Diabetic Diet (Continental)

Bed tea	Lemon tea—1 cup
Breakfast	Vegetable sandwich—2 bread slice (large) or Cornflakes—5 to 6 tablespoons + Milk—240 ml
Midmorning	Fruit—100 mg
Lunch	Noodles or pasta with vegetables—100 gm (cooked weight) or Vegetable pulao—8 to 10 tablespoons Curd—125 ml (1 katori) Sweet 'n' sour vegetables/ Baked vegetables—125 gm Sprout salad—25 gm (without dressing)
Evening	Coffee/tea—1 cup Plain toast—1
Dinner	Clear vegetable soup—1 bowl Vegetable pulao—6 to 7 tablespoon Paneer dish—30 gm Sauted vegetables—125 gm Sprout salad—25 gm Curd—½ katori
Bedtime	Milk—½ cup
Cooking oil	2 TSF/day

The above menu provides approximately

Carbohydrates	190 gm
Proteins	50 gm
Fats	30 gm

1400 kcal Diabetic Diet (North India)

Bed tea	Tea—1 cup Fibre biscuit (like diet bik)—2/salto—2-3/ Marie biscuit—2
Breakfast	Chapatti stuffed with vegetables—2 (20 gm atta each) or Bread slice—2 (large) or Cornflakes—5 to 6 tablespoons or Porridge (cooked)—1½ katori (medium size katori) + Milk—240 ml + Paneer/egg—30 gm/1 egg
Midmorning	Fruit—100 gm
Lunch	Chapatti—3 (60 gm atta) Or boiled rice—8 to 10 tablespoon Dal (25 gm)—1 katori Green vegetables—125 gm Curd/buttermilk—125 ml/1 glass Fruit—100 gm
Evening	Tea/coffee—1 cup Biscuit/salto/plain toast—2-3/3-4/1 number
Dinner	Chapatti—3 Dal—1 katori Green vegetables—125 gm Paneer—30 gm
Bed time	Milk—1 cup
Cooking oil	2-3 TSF/day

The above menu provides approximately

Carbohydrates	230 gm
Proteins	53 gm
Fats	35 gm

1400 kcal Diabetic Diet (South Indian)

Bed tea	Tea—1 cup Fibre biscuit (like diet bik)—2/salto 2-3/ Marie biscuit—2
Breakfast	Idli—2 or Dosa plain—9″ diameter or Suji upma—1½ plate (150 gm cooked weight) + Milk—240 ml + Paneer/egg—30 gm/1
Midmorning	Fruit—100 gm
Lunch	Boiled rice—8 to 10 tablespoons Dal/Sambhar—1 katori (25 gm raw weight) Rasam—1 katori Green vegetables—125 gm Papad Curd—125 ml Fruit—100 gm Oil—1 teaspoon
Evening	Tea/coffee—1 cup Poha with vegetables—¾ katori
Dinner	Boiled rice—8 to 10 tablespoons Dal—1 katori Paneer curry/egg curry—30 gm/1 egg
Bedtime	Milk—1 cup
Cooking oil	2 -3 TSF/day

The above menu provides approximately

Carbohydrates	230 gm
Proteins	53 gm
Fats	35 gm

1400 kcal Diabetic Diet (Continental)

Bed tea	Lemon tea—1 cup
Breakfast	Vegetable sandwich—2 bread slice (large) or Cornflakes—5 to 6 tablespoons + Milk—240 ml + Egg/paneer—1/30 gm
Midmorning	Fruit—100 gm
Lunch	Noodles or pasta with vegetables—100 gm (cooked weight) or Veg. pulao—8 to 10 tablespoons Curd—125 ml Sweet 'n' sour vegetables/ Baked vegetables—125 gm Sprout salad—25 gm (without dressing) Fruit—100 gm
Evening	Tea/coffee—1 cup Plain toast—1
Dinner	Clear vegetable soup (without cream) Vegetable pulao—8 to 10 tablespoons Paneer curry/egg curry—30 gm/1 egg Sauted vegetables—125 gm Sprouted dal salad—25 gm Curd—½ katori
Bed time	Milk—1 cup
Cooking oil	2-3 TSF/day

The above menu provides approximately

Carbohydrates	230 gm
Proteins	53 gm
Fats	35 gm

1600 kcal Diabetic Diet (North India)

Bed tea	Tea—1 cup Fibre biscuit (like diet bik)—2/ Salto 2-3/Marie biscuit—2
Breakfast	Chapatti stuffed with vegetables—2 (20 gm atta each) or Bread slice—2 (large) or Cornflakes—5 to 6 tablespoon or Porridge (cooked)—1½ katori + Milk—240 ml + Paneer/egg—30 gm/1 egg
Mid morning	Fruit—100 gm
Lunch	Chapatti—4 (80 gm atta) or Boiled rice—10 to 12 tablespoon Dal—1 katori (25 gm) Green vegetables—125 gm Curd/buttermilk—125 ml/1 glass Fruit—100 gm Oil—2 teaspoon
Evening	Tea/coffee—1 cup Biscuit/salto/plain toast—2-3/3-4/1 number
Dinner	Chapatti—4/Boiled rice 10 to 12 tablespoon Dal (25 gm)—1 katori Green vegetables—125 gm Paneer—30 gm
Bedtime	Milk—1 cup
Cooking oil	3 TSF/day

The above menu provides approximately

Carbohydrates	255 gm
Proteins	60 gm
Fats	43 gm

1600 kcal Diabetic Diet (South India)

Bed tea	Tea—1 cup Fibre biscuit (like diet bik)—2/salto—2/ Marie biscuit—2
Breakfast	Idli—2 or Dosa plain—9" diameter or Suji upma—1½ plate (150 gm cooked weight) + Milk—240 ml + 1 egg/paneer—30 gm
Midmorning	Fruit—100 gm
Lunch	Boiled rice—10 to 12 tablespoon Dal/sambhar (25 gm raw weight)—1 katori Rasam—1 katori Green vegetables—125 gm Curd—125 ml Papad Fruit—100 gm Oil—2 teaspoon
Evening	Tea/coffee—1 cup Poha with vegetables—¾ katori
Dinner	Boiled rice—10 to 12 tablespoon Dal—1 katori Curry green vegetable—125 gm Curd—125 ml Paneer curry/egg curry—30 gm/1 egg
Bedtime	Milk—1 cup
Cooking oil	3 TSF/day

The above menu provides approximately

Carbohydrates	255 gm
Proteins	60 gm
Fats	43 gm

1600 kcal Diabetic Diet (Continental)

Bed tea	Lemon tea—1 cup
Breakfast	Vegetable sandwich—2 bread slice (large) or Cornflakes—5 to 6 tablespoons + Milk—240 ml + Egg/paneer—1/30 gm
Midmorning	Fruit—100 gm
Lunch	Noodles or pasta with vegetables—100 gm (cooked weight) or Vegetable pulao—10 to 12 tablespoons Curd—125 ml Sweet 'n' sour vegetables/Baked vegetables (with 1 teaspoon butter)—125 gm Sprout salad—25 gm Fruit—100 gm Oil—1 teaspoon
Evening	Tea/coffee—1 cup Plain toast—1
Dinner	Clear vegetable soup (without cream—1 bowl) Vegetable pulao—10 to 12 tablespoon Paneer/egg—30 gm/1 Sauted vegetables—125 gm Sprout dal salad—25 gm Curd—½ katori
Bedtime	Milk—1 cup
Cooking oil	3 TSF/day

The above menu provides approximately

Carbohydrates	255 gm
Proteins	60 gm
Fats	43 gm

1800 kcal Diabetic Diet (North India)

Bed tea	Tea—1 cup Fibre biscuit (like diet bik)/ Salto—2-3/Marie biscuit—2
Breakfast	Chapatti stuffed with vegetables—2 (20 gm atta each) or Bread slice—2 (large) or Cornflakes—5-6 tablespoon or Porridge (cooked)—1½ katori + Milk—240 ml (+ Paneer/egg—30 gm/1 egg) + Oil—1 teaspoon + Fruit—100 gm
Midmorning	Fruit—100 gm
Lunch	Chapatti—4 (80 gm atta) or Boiled rice—10 to 12 tablespoon Dal—1 katori (25 gram) Green vegetables—125 gm Curd—250 ml (big katori)
Evening	Tea/coffee—1 cup Biscuit/salto/plain toast—2-3/3-4/1 number
Dinner	Chapatti—5 Dal—1 katori Green vegetables—125 gm Paneer—30 gm
Bedtime	Milk—1 cup
Cooking oil	3 TSF/day

The above menu provides approximately

Carbohydrates	270 gm
Proteins	65 gm
Fats	50 gm

1800 Kcal Diabetic Diet (South India)

Bed tea	Tea—1 cup Fibre biscuit (like diet bik)—2/ Salto—2-3/Marie biscuit—2
Breakfast	Idli—2 or Dosa plain—9" diameter or Suji (upma)—1½ plate (150 gm cooked weight) + Milk—240 ml Paneer/egg—30 gm/1
Midmorning	Fruit—100 gm
Lunch	Boiled rice—10 to 12 tablespoon Dal/Sambhar (25 gm raw weight)—1 katori Green vegetables—125 gm Curd—250 ml (Big katori)
Evening	Tea/coffee—1 cup Poha with vegetables—¾ katori
Dinner	Boiled rice—12 to 14 tablespoon Dal—1 katori Curry green vegetable—125 gm Curd—1 katori Paneer curry/egg curry—30 gm/1 egg
Bedtime	Milk—1 cup
Cooking oil	3 TSF/day

The above menu provides approximately

Carbohydrates	270 gm
Proteins	65 gm
Fats	50 gm

1800 kcal Diabetic Diet (Continental)

Bed tea	Lemon tea—1 cup
Breakfast	Vegetable sandwich—2 Bread slice (large) or Cornflakes—5 to 6 tablespoons + Milk—240 ml + Egg/paneer—1/30 gm Butter—1 teaspoon Fruit—100 gm
Midmorning	Fruit—100 gm
Lunch	Noodles or Pasta with vegetables—100 gm (cooked weight) or Vegetable Pulao—10 to 12 tablespoons Sweet 'n' sour vegetables/Baked vegetables (with 1 teaspoon butter)—125 gm Sprout salad—25 gm Paneer—30 gm Fruit—100 gm
Evening	Tea/coffee—1 cup Plain Toast—1
Dinner	Vegetable Pulao—12 to 14 tablespoon or Macaroni with vegetables—10 to 12 tablespoon Paneer/egg—30 gm/1 egg Sauted vegetables—125 gm Sprout salad—25 gm Curd—1 katori Butter—1 teaspoon
Bedtime	Milk—1 cup
Cooking oil	3 TSF/day

The above menu provides approximately

Carbohydrates	270 gm
Proteins	65 gm
Fats	50 gm

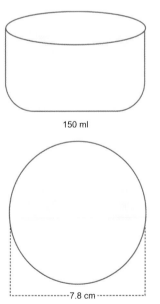

150 ml

7.8 cm

Fig. A.1.1: Actual size of katori

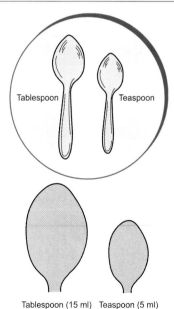

Tablespoon   Teaspoon

Tablespoon (15 ml)   Teaspoon (5 ml)

Fig. A.1.2: Actual sizes of spoons

Appendix 2: Iodine Content of the Common Food Items and Drugs

IODINE CONTENT OF SOME OF THE COMMON FOODS

Food items	Unit (G)	Iodine content per unit (μg)
Iodized salt	100	3000
Bread	100	360 to 390
Milk	250	52 to 56
Fish		
Cod	100	102
Shrimp	100	35 to 40
Tuna	100	17 to 20
Egg (whole)	50	13 to 18
Fruits (in general)	100	4 to 6
Spinach	100	8 to 10
Broccoli	100	5 to 6
Potato (baked) with peel	One medium	63

SOME OF THE COMMON IODINE CONTAINING DRUGS

Drugs	Iodine content
Radiology contrast agents	
Iodized oil	380 mg/ml
Omnipaque	140 mg/ml
Iopanoic acid (telepaque)	333 mg/ml
Urovideo 75%	370 mg/ml
Iothalamate (angio-conray)	480 mg/ml
Ipodate (oragrafin)	308 mg/cap
Metrizamide (amipaque)	483 mg/ml (before dilution)
Oral and local agents	
Amiodarone	75 mg/tablet
Calcium iodide syrup	26 mg/ml
Collosol syrup	1.6 mg/ml
Iodine containing vitamins	0.15 mg/tablet
Proloid	0.15 mg/tablet
Idoxurizine ophthalmic solution	18 μg/drop
KI	245 mg/tab, 24 mg/ml
Lycored (kI) syrup	10 μg/ml
Lugol's solution	6.3 mg/drop
SSKI	38 mg/drop
Recupex	16.5 μg/50 gm
Treptin micromix	2 μg/gm
Nutrocal DM	35 to 85 mg/50 gm
Parenteral	
NaI 10% solution	85 mg/ml
Topical	
Tinc iodine (topical)	40 mg/ml
Povidone-iodine (betadine sol) topical	10 mg/ml

Appendix 3: Unitage Used in the Text and Patients' Identification Bracelet

UNITAGE USED IN THE TEXT

•	1 attogram	=	1 ag	=	10^{-18} G	
•	1 femtogram	=	1 fg	=	10^{-15} G	
•	1 picogram	=	1 pg	=	10^{-12} G	
•	1 nanogram	=	1 ng	=	10^{-9} G	
•	1 microgram	=	1 µg	=	10^{-6} G	
•	1 milligram	=	1 mg	=	10^{-3} G	

PATIENT'S IDENTIFICATION CARD/BRACELET/NECKLACE

Identification card/bracelet/necklace with following particulars must always be carried/worn by an endocrine patient:

1. Name of the patient with other relevant personal particulars

   ....

   ....

2. Name and address and contact telephone number of the treating doctor/hospital

   ....

   ....

3. Medical diagnosis

   ....

   ....

4. Treatment being taken

   ....

   ....

5. Action to be taken in case of an emergency

   ....

   ....

Appendix 4: Hormones Normal Reference Values

THYROID HORMONES

Thyroid hormones	Conventional units	Conversion factors	SI units
Thyroxine (T_4)			
• Total	50 to 120 ng/ml	1.29	60 to 150 nmol/L
Free	8 to 18 pg/ml		10 to 22 pmol/L
Tri-iodo thyronine (T_3)			
• Total	0.65 to 1.7 ng/ml	1.54	1 to 2.6 nmol/L
Free	3.6 to 6.5 pg/ml		5 to 10 pmol/L
Reverse T_3	0.1 to 0.4 ng/ml		0.15 to 0.61 nmol/L
TBG	1 to 2.6 ng/ml	100	100 to 260 µg/L
At birth (5th day)			
• Total T_4	78 to 194 ng/ml	1.29	100 to 250 nmol/L
• Total T_3	0.32 to 2.08 ng/ml	1.54	0.5 to 3.2 nmol/L
Young children			
• Total T_4	50 to 120 ng/ml		60 to 155 nmol/L
• Total T_3	0.65 to 1.7 ng/ml		1 to 2.6 nmol/L
Pregnancy 1st trimester			
• Total T_4	66 to 124 ng/ml		85 to 160 nmol/L
• Total T_3	0.97 to 2.27 ng/ml		1.5 to 3.5 nmol/L
3rd trimester			
• Total T_4	66 to 147 ng/ml		85 to 190 nmol/L
• Total T_3	1.3 to 2.6 ng/ml		2.0 to 4.0 nmol/L
Thyrotrophin (TSH)	0.5 to 6 µU/ml (RIA)	1 (Range is same in men, women,	0.5 to 6.0 mU/L (RIA)
	0.4 to 5 µU/ml (IMRA)	and children)	0.4 to 5 mU/L (IMRA)
Average	1.6 µU/ml (male)	1	1.6 mU/L (male)
	1.4 µU/ml (Female)		1.4 mU/L (Female)
C-cell hormone (calcitonin) (basal value)	< 18 pg/ml	1	<18 ng/L

Contd...

Contd...

Dynamic tests

TSH response (μU/ml)
- TRH test

(200 μg IV)	Male	Female
0 minute	1.6	1.4
20 minutes	9.5	13.5
60 minutes	6.8	9.8

- Twenty minutes technetium (^{99m}Tc) uptake studies

Euthyroid without goitre	1.5% (0.2 to 3.9%)
Euthyroid with goitre	2.1% (0.4 to 4.4%)
Hyperthyroid	10.6% (3.3 to 37.3%)

- Radioactive iodine uptake studies

2 hours	4 to 12%
6 hours	6 to 15%
24 hours	8 to 30%

- TSH stimulation test (Inj TSH 10 IU × 3 days)
  Normal response
  - Doubling of basal hormone values
  - > 15% increase in thyroid uptake values

- Perchlorate test (600 mg potassium perchlorate)
  Normal response
  < 10% fall in thyroid uptake value at 90 or 120 minutes

ANTERIOR PITUITARY HORMONES

Hormones	Conventional units	Conversion factor	SI units
• Adrenocorticotrophic hormone (ACTH)			
0800 to 0900 hr	10 to 80 pg/ml	0.22	2.3 to 18 pmol/L
10 pm to 0200 hr	<10 pg/ml		<2.3 pmol/L
• Follicle stimulating hormone (FSH)		1	
• Female			
Follicular phase	1.4 to 9.6 mU/ml		1.4 to 9.6 IU/L
Midcycle phase	2.3 to 21 mU/ml		2.3 to 21 IU/L
Luteal phase	0.5 to 2.4 mU/ml		0.5 to 2.4 IU/L
Postmenopausal	34 to 96 mU/ml		34 to 96 1 IU/L
• Male	0.9 to 8 mU/ml		0.9 to 8 IU/L
• Prepubertal children	< 5 mU/ml		<5 IU/L
• Luteinizing hormone (LH)		1	
• Female			
Follicular phase	2.8 to 21.4 mU/ml		2.8 to 21.4 IU/L
Midcycle phase	20 to 60 mU/ml (approx 3 times basal value)		20 to 60 IU/L
Luteal phase	< 15 mU/ml		<15 IU/L
Postmenopausal	>35 mU/ml		>35 IU/L
• Male	3 to 15 mU/ml		3 to 15 IU/L
• Prepubertal children	< 5 mU/ml		<5 IU/L
• Prolactin			
• Woman	< 20 ng/ml	20	<400 mU/L
• Men	< 18 ng/ml		<360 mU/L
	(Women have slightly higher normal values than men)		
• TSH (see thyroid hormone section)			

GROWTH HORMONE (GH)

Hormone	Conventional units	Conversion factor	SI units
• Adult (fasting)	<l0 ng/ml (Polyclonal ab assay)	1	<10 μg/L
• Foetal serum (20th week)	100 to 150 ng/ml		100 to 150 μg/L
• Cord blood	30 to 40 ng/ml		30 to 40 μg/L
• Adults range	6.33 ± 5.7 μg/L		
• Preadolescents/adolescents	8.37 ± 5.62 μg/L		
• Elderly	15 to 20% of the adult values (GH declines approx 12 to 14% per decade)		
• Adult (fasting)	< 1 ng/ml (monoclonal ab assay)		<1 μg/L
• 1 GF-1 (varies with age)	180 to 760 ng/ml (young adults)		180 to 760 μg/L

Dynamic tests

• Insulin induced hypoglycaemia (ITT)
  Normal response
    GH rises to over 20 μg/L level or increases at least by 5 μg/L over the basal value

Glucagon test
  Normal response
    GH rises by 5 to 7 μg/L in male and 7 to 10 μg/L in female

Arginine test
  Normal response
    GH rises by 7 μg/L

POSTERIOR PITUITARY HORMONES

Plasma and Urinary Osmolality

Normal subjects	Plasma (mOsmol/kg)	Urine (mOsmol/kg)
Basal values	280 to 288	155 to 800
After 8 hours dehydration	286 to 294	830 to 1160

ADRENAL GLAND

Adrenal Cortex

Hormones	Conventional units	Conversion factor	SI units
• Plasma cortisol			
0700 to 0900 hr	5 to 25 µg/dl	27.59	150 to 690 nmol/L
1600 to 1700 hr	3 to 15 µg/dl		83 to 420 nmol/L
mid night	1.5 to 2 µg/dl		41 to 55 nmol/L
• Dehydroepiandrosterone (DHEA)	2 to 9 µg/dl	3.467	7 to 31 nmol/L
• DHEA-S	10 to 600 µg/dl	10	100 to 6000 µg/L
• 11 Deoxycortisol	< 1 µg/dl	28.96	<30 nmol/L
• 17 Hydroxyprogesterone		3.026	
Female			
Follicular Phase	0.2 to 1 µg/L		0.6 to 3 nmol/L
Luteal Phase	0.5 to 3.5 µg/L		1.5 to 10.6 nmol/L
Male	0.6 to 3 µg/L		1.8 to 9 nmol/L
• Aldosterone			
(Upright-normal diet)	5 to 20 ng/dl	27.74	140 to 560 pmol/L
• Androstenedione			
Female	1 to 2 ng/ml	3.492	3.5 to 7.0 nmol/L
Male	0.8 to 1.3 ng/ml		3.0 to 5.0 nmol/L
• Dihydrotestosterone			
Female	0.05 to 0.3 ng/ml	3.467	0.17 to 1 nmol/L
Male	0.25 to 0.75 ng/ml		0.87 to 2.6 nmol/L

Urine

• Free urinary cortisol			
(Male)	<100 µg (20–100 µg/D)	2.76	55 to 270 nmol/D
(Female)	<145 µg/D		<400 nmol/D
• Aldosterone	5 to 19 µg/D	2.8	14 to 53 nmol/D
• 17 hydroxycorticosteroids	2 to 10 mg/D	2.76	5.4 to 27.6 µmol/D
• 17 ketosteroids			
Male	7 to 20 mg/D	3.47	24 to 70 µmol/D
Female	5 to 15 mg/D		17 to 55 µmol/D

Dynamic tests

- **Single dose dexamethasone suppression test**
  Normal response. Plasma cortisol suppressed to less than 3.0 µg/dl (or <90 nmol/L)
- **Low dose dexamethasone suppression test**
  Normal response. Plasma cortisol suppressed to less than 1.5 µg/dl (or 40 nmol/L)
- **High dose dexamethasone suppression test**
  Normal response in pituitary dependent Cushing's disease at least 50% suppression of basal plasma or urinary cortisol level seen in over 90% cases

Adrenal Medulla

	Conventional units	Conversion factor	SI units
Patient is lying and resting—Blood is taken through a cannula			
Plasma adrenaline (Epinephrine)	0.01 to 0.19 ng/ml	5.46	0.06 to 1.07 nmol/ml
Noradrenaline (Norepinephrine)	0.07 to 0.56 ng/ml	5.99	0.46 to 3.08 nmol/L

Urine

	Conventional units	Conversion factor	SI units
Catecholamines	<100 µg/day	5.911	<590 nmol/day
Epinephrine	<50 µg/day	5.5	<275 nmol/day
Metanephrine	<1.3 mg/day	5.46	<7 µmol/day
Norepinephrine	15 to 89 µg/day	5.911	88.7 to 526 µmol/day
Vanillylmandelic acid (VMA)	1 to 7 mg/day	5	5 to 35 µmol/day
	98 to 106 mEq/L	1	98 to 106 µmol/L
5-Hydroxyindolacectic acid (5-HAIAA)	2 to 9 mg/day	5.24	10 to 45 µmol/day

SEX HORMONES

	Conventional units	Conversion factor	SI units
Oestrogens			
• Male	13.2 to 23.4 pg/ml	3.671	48.45 to 85.9 pmol/L
• Female			
Follicular phase	0.5 to 68 pg/ml		1.83 to 250 pmol/L
Midcycle	68 to 272 pg/ml		246.6 to 998.5 pmol/L
Luteal	22 to 163 pg/ml		80.7 to 598 pmol/L
Postmenopause	< 20 pg/ml		<75 pmol/L
Oral contraceptives	100 to 300 pg/ml		367 to 1100 pmol/L
• Progesterone			
• Male	0.02 to 0.14 ng/ml	3.18	<2 nmol/L
• Female			
Follicular phase	0.01 to 0.44 ng/ml		0.0318 to 1.39 nmol/L
Midcycle	0.44 to 1.27 ng/ml		1.39 to 4.03 nmol/L
Luteal phase	2.35 to 7.27 ng/ml		7.50 to 23.1 nmol/L
• Prepubertal girls	< 2 ng/ml		<6.36 nmol/L
• Testosterone: Free: Female	0.2 to 3.1 pg/ml	3.437	0.69 to 10.7 pmol/L
Male	12 to 40.0 pg/ml		41.2 to 137.4 pmol/L
Total: Female	<1 ng/ml		<3.5 nmol/L
Male	3 to 10 ng/ml		10 to 35 nmol/L
Male: 21-30 years	3 to 8 ng/ml		
31-40 years	3 to 8 ng/ml		
41-50 years	3 to 7.1 ng/ml		
51-60 years	2.5 to 7.1 ng/ml		
61-70 years	2.0 to 6.1 ng/ml		
> 70 years	2.0 to 6.0 ng/ml		

Hormonal values (range) in normal healthy males and normal cycling (age 18 to 30 years) females (n 25)

	LH (mU/ml)	FSH (mU/ml)	Prolactin (PRL) (ng/ml)	Oestradiol (E_2) (pg/ml)	Progesterone (PR) (ng/ml)	Testosterone (Te) (ng/dl)
Females						
Follicular phase	0.8 to 18	0.5 to 5.0	3 to 18	0.5 to 68	0.01 to 0.44	20 to 60
Midcycle	up to 50	up to 20	5 to 22	68 to 272	0.44 to 1.27	
Luteal phase	0.8 to 18	0.4 to 5.0	5 to 20	22 to 163	2.35 to 7.27	
Males	0.5 to 4.3	0.2 to 3.1	3 to 18	13.2 to 23.4	0.02 to 0.14	260 to 800

BIOCHEMISTRY

	Conventional units	Conversion factor	SI units
Blood glucose (Whole blood)	• Umbilical cord 50 to 70 mg/dl (10 to 15% higher if serum/plasma is used)	0.05551	2.7 to 4.0 mmol/L
	• Young Children 50 to 70 mg/dl		2.7 to 4.0 mmol/L
	• Adults <90 mg/dl		5 mmol/L
	• Maternal blood (plasma) First trimester F 70.2 ± 9.8 mg/dl pp 110.3 ± 18.7 mg/dl		
• Insulin Plasma			
Fasting	4 to 24 µU/ml	7.175	29 to 172 pmol/L
During hypoglycaemia (BG <50 mg/dl)	<5 µU/ml		<35 pmol/L
• C-Peptide	0.5 to 2 pg/ml	1	0.5 to 2 ug/L
• Glucagon	50 to 100 pg/ml	1	50 to 100 ng/L
• Microalbuminuria	Urinary albumin excretion > 30 mg/24 hours (or 20 µg/min)		
• *Semen analysis*			
Volume	3 to 5 ml per ejaculate		
appearance			
pH	Alkaline		
Fructose Citrate Alkaline phosphatase Prostaglandins	Present		
Sperm count	> 40 millions per ml or Total of 125 million per ejaculate		
Motility	50 to 60% actively motile (grade 3) 2 to 3 hours after ejaculation		
• Plasma calcium			
Total	7.0 to 10.4 mg/dl or 3.5 to 5.2 mEq/L Ionized 30-55% of the total value	0.2500 0.5000	1.75 to 2.6 mmol/L
• Plasma phosphate (inorganic)	2.5 to 4.4 mg/dl	0.3229	0.8 to 1.4 mmol/L
• PTH (Intact PTH)	10 to 65 pg/ml	1	10 to 65 ng/L
• Plasma renin activity			
Supine	3.2 ± 1 ng/ml/hr		3.2 ± 1 µg/L/hr
Standing	9.3 ± 4.3 ng/ml/hr		9.3 ± 4.3 µg/L/hr
Serum lipids			
Desirable values			
Cholesterol			
Total	<200 mg/dl	0.02586	<5.17 mmol/L
HDL	>60 mg/dl		>1.50 mmol/L
LDL	<100 mg/dl		<2.56 mmol/L
Triglycerides	10-90 mg/dl	0.1129	0.11 to 1.02 mmol/L

Urinary values

Urinary calcium excretion	100 to 300 mg/day	0.02495	2.5 to 7.5 mmol/D
Urinary phosphate	90 to 130 mg/day	0.3229	29 to 42 mmol/D

Index

Note: Letters in the parentheses indicate 't' for table and 'f' for figure.

WITHDRAWN

Derby Hospitals NHS Foundation
Trust
Library and Knowledge Service